Anatomy of

Orofacial
Structures

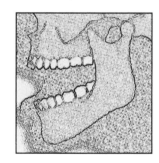

Anatomy of
Orofacial Structures

Richard W. Brand
B.S., D.D.S., F.A.C.D., F.I.C.D.
Assistant Dean for Admissions and Student Affairs
Professor of Biomedical Sciences
Washington University School of Medicine
St. Louis, Missouri

Donald E. Isselhard
B.S., D.D.S., F.A.G.D., M.A.G.D., M.B.A.
Private Practice
St. Louis, Missouri

Sixth Edition

with 547 illustratons

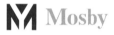 Mosby

St. Louis   Baltimore   Boston   Carlsbad   Chicago   Minneapolis   New York   Philadelphia   Portland
London   Milan   Sydney   Tokyo   Toronto

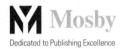

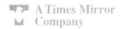

Publisher: John Schrefer
Acquisitions Editor: Penny Rudolph
Associate Developmental Editor: Angela Reiner
Project Manager: Mark Spann
Production Editor: Holly Roseman
Book Design Manager: Judi Lang
Manufacturing Manager: Betty Mueller

SIXTH EDITION

Copyright © 1998 by Mosby, Inc.

Previous editions copyrighted 1977, 1982, 1986, 1990, 1994

Printed in the United States of America
Composition by The Clarinda Company
Printing/binding by R.R. Donnelley & Sons

Mosby, Inc.
11830 Westline Industrial Drive
St. Louis, Missouri 63146

ISBN 0-8151-1000-6

97 98 00 01 / 9 8 7 6 5 4 3 2 1

We dedicate this 6th edition to our families

*To the memory of my father, **Dr. Charles Brand,**
and my uncle, **Dr. Thurlow Brand.**
To my wife **Marie,** our **children,**
and to my extended family for
all their love and support.*

Richard W. Brand

*To my wife **Annette** and
Kerstin, Nissa, Michele, and Tara*

Donald E. Isselhard

PREFACE

With the completion of the sixth edition we celebrate the twentieth year of *Anatomy of Orofacial Structures*. We feel it is only appropriate to thank the many instructors who have helped guide us with their changes in each edition through their continuing input to Mosby, Inc. and their representatives. Of course, much of this input originated through their students, and we also wish to thank those students who have used our book and who continue to help in the development of each new edition. We have tried to follow a number of the suggestions we have received and we hope that you realize that we are unable to incorporate everyone's suggestions into this new edition. There are times when we are faced with conflicting suggestions and we have tried to sort them out and do what we feel might be best. One should never be satisfied. We hope we, as the authors, will never be satisfied, and we hope the time will never come when the instructors and the students cease to give us input, for without them we would truly be lost.

As we have said from the first edition, this book is written for students beginning their study of the anatomic sciences relating to dentistry. We have always attempted to begin at a very basic level and carry forward from there. However, with the various dental educational programs using this book we know that we will never be able to meet one group's needs without the possibility of creating a problem with another program. There are some areas of the book that will always have too much detail for one group and not enough for another. Some topics will be discussed and others will not, but it is our feeling that combining the three subjects of oral histology, head and neck anatomy, and dental anatomy in one edition outweighs the perceived shortcomings.

We are excited about this sixth edition! A second color has been used in this editon, and the addition of the second color really sets off the various subject areas as well as numerous illustrations. We have maintained the general format of objectives at the beginning of the chapters and review questions at the end of the chapters. We have increased the review questions in almost every chapter and have placed the answers at the back of the book along with the answers to the large unit exams. The use of bolding important terms, which are then defined in the glossary, has also been continued in this new edition. Some chapters have been expanded to include new material, and portions of other chapters have been rewritten. Chapters 3, 11, and 18 have entirely new illustrations, and there are also new illustrations in Chapters 2, 4, 13, and 19. The removable flash cards at the back of the book were well received in the last edition, and we have continued them in this edition with full dental arches of both deciduous and permanent dentition.

We would like to recognize and thank the various people who have made this book possible. We have thoroughly enjoyed working on this editon with the following people from Mosby, Inc.: Penny Rudolph, acquisitions editor for dentistry;

Angie Reiner, associate developmental editor for dentistry; and Holly Roseman, senior production editor. These are the people that really make the book, and without them we would not have gotten this far. We are also very fortunate to have back with us Marci Hoffman Hartstein and Vicki Moses Friedman who produced the new illustrations for this edition. They have been with us since the second edition, and we are fortunate to have their talents, once again, added to this book. Finally, we would like to thank all of those authors and publishers who have given us permission to use their illustrations in this sixth edition as well as in previous editions.

There is also a student study guide to accompany this sixth edition. The study guide presents the concepts from this book accompanied by different types of review questions and case studies. There are numerous illustrations to be identified, and there are also crossword puzzles and word search puzzles related to each of the subject areas in the book. We hope you will find this book useful and enjoyable. We also hope that you will be willing to give us input on this new venture so that we can continue to provide the best possible learning situations for each and every one of you. We wish all of you a long and happy future in the profession of dentistry.

Richard W. Brand
Donald E. Isselhard

Contents

UNIT IV

DENTAL ANATOMY

Unit I

Introduction

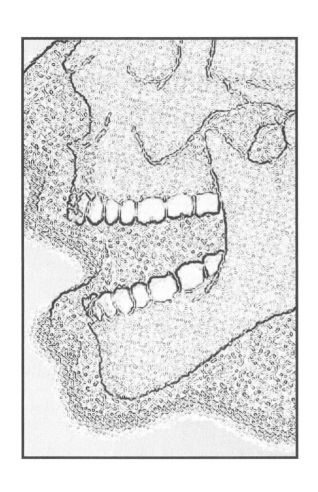

Chapter 1

Oral Cavity

As students of the dental profession you will be concentrating your studies on the head and neck, and more specifically on the structures that make up the oral cavity. It is imperative that you are extremely familiar with the normal makeup and the structures of this area. Therefore this chapter has been set forth to serve as an introduction to your studies of the head and neck region.

The oral cavity is the upper end and the beginning of the digestive system and at its posterior end forms a common pathway with the respiratory system. The oral cavity begins at the lips and cheeks and extends posteriorly to the area of the **palatine tonsils,** which are usually referred to as the *tonsils.* These lie on the sides of the throat between two folds of tissues, one in front and one in back, called the **tonsillar pillars.** Posterior to the tonsillar pillars the oral cavity ends and the **oral pharynx,** a shared pathway of the digestive and respiratory systems, begins. The area from the oral pharynx to the **laryngeal pharynx** is shared with the respiratory system and then goes on to the esophagus and the rest of the digestive system. The respiratory system starts at the nasal cavity and includes the **nasal pharynx,** oral pharynx, laryngeal pharynx, larynx, trachea, bronchi, and lungs. The oral cavity

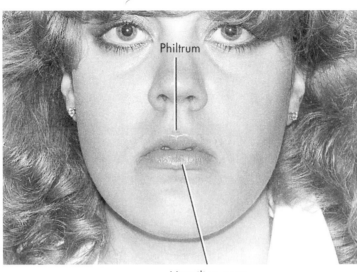

Philtrum

Vermilion zone

FIG. 1-1.   Vermilion zone of lips and philtrum of upper lip.

can be logically divided into two parts: (1) the **vestibule,** which is the potential space that exists between the lips or cheeks and the teeth (in an edentulous person—one without teeth—it would extend between the lips or cheeks and the alveolar ridges where the teeth were at one time); and (2) the **oral cavity proper,** which is the area from the teeth or alveolar ridges back to the area of the palatine tonsils.

VESTIBULE

In considering the vestibular area you should begin by examining the lips. The lips are the junction between the skin of the face, which is a dry epithelium, and the mucosa of the oral cavity, which is a moist epithelium. Between these two areas lies a transitional zone of reddish tissue known as the **vermilion zone** of the lip. It is along the border between the skin and the vermilion zone that one commonly encounters cold sores, which are generally caused by a herpesvirus. The skin of the upper lip has an indentation

at the midline known as the **philtrum,** which is derived from the embryonic medial nasal processes (Fig. 1-1). It is at the lateral junction of this philtrum that a cleft lip would be seen.

Anterior and Posterior Borders

By elevating the mandible so that the teeth are in contact and then retracting the lips and cheeks, you can see the vestibule. Anteriorly it is bounded by the lips (**labia**) and laterally by the cheek (**bucca**). A finger placed in the posterior portion of the vestibule will be impeded by two obstacles—the bony anterior border of the ramus of the mandible and the soft tissue. The cheek is formed to a great extent by the buccinator muscle, covered with skin on the outside and moist mucous membrane on the inside. This muscle extends back from the corners of the mouth to join with the muscles of the upper throat wall. As it passes backward, it crosses in front of the mandibular ramus from a lateral position to a medial position, limiting the posterior extent of the vestibule. As you run your finger in the upper posterior vestibular space, you can feel the ridge of bone that is the beginning of the anterior part of the zygomatic arch (cheekbone). This is frequently referred to as the **zygomaticoalveolar crest.** Run your finger along the cheek area of the vestibule and note the landmarks and structures just mentioned.

Superior and Inferior Borders

The point at which the mucosa of the lips or cheeks turns to go toward the gingival or gum tissue is known as the mucobuccal or mucolabial fold. The mucosa lying against the alveolar bone is loosely attached and movable and known as *alveolar mucosa.* This mucosa is generally reddish because of the presence of blood vessels underneath the relatively thin mucosa. The point at

which it becomes tightly attached to the bone is the beginning of the gingiva. This is known as the mucogingival junction (Fig. 1-2). The normal color of the gingiva is pink because the mucosal layer is thicker and therefore the blood vessels do not impart as much color. In patients with darker skin color, there generally is some pigmentation to the gingiva.

Pull outward on the lips or corners of the mouth and you will see that there are several areas where the tissue is attached in folds to the alveolar mucosa. At the midline in both the upper and lower lips there is a fold of connective tissue known as the **labial frenum.** The frenum contains no muscle tissue, only connective tissue. The upper frenum is usually more pronounced than the lower, but problems may occur with ei-

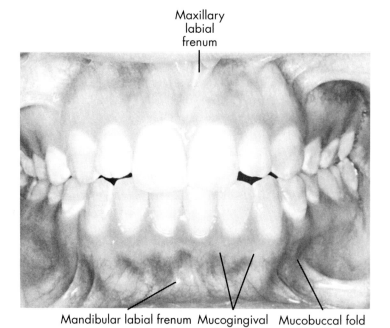

Maxillary
labial
frenum

Mandibular labial frenum   Mucogingival   Mucobuccal fold
junction

FIG. 1-2.   View of vestibule. There is a change in color at the mucogingival junction. The maxillary labial frenum is more evident than the mandibular labial frenum. Mucobuccal folds are quite evident.

ther one. The attachment of the upper (maxillary) frenum may extend to the crest of the alveolar ridge and even over the ridge. This band of tissue is so firm that the erupting central incisors might not penetrate it but be pushed slightly aside so that a space exists between them. This space is known as a **diastema** (Fig. 1-3, *A*). Correction of a diastema usually involves the surgical removal or cutting of the frenum tissue between the teeth. After this the teeth will generally move together into normal contact. If they do not come back into normal contact, minor orthodontic treatment may be required. This procedure is best done when a child is 6 to 8 years old.

The mandibular labial frenum seldom extends up between the teeth, but there are times when it extends close enough to the gingiva to contribute to gingival recession in that area by pulling downward on the tissue when the lip is tensed (Fig. 1-3, *B*). In this instance the frenum attachment needs to be incised with possible periodontal follow-up.

There are also less well-defined frena in the maxillary and mandibular canine areas. These can be seen in Fig. 1-2 at the area labeled mucobuccal fold and in a similar area above it in the maxillary arch. Although these are not as well developed, they and the midline frena still have to be taken into consideration in the construction of a denture. If a groove is not reproduced in the **flange** or edge of the denture at that point, the appliance will cause irritation and possible ulceration of the frenular tissue.

Other Clinical Manifestations of the Vestibule

The coronoid process

As we continue to consider the structure of the vestibule in relation to clinical dentistry, it is interesting to notice what happens to the vestibule when the mouth is opened wide. Place the teeth together, with the lips and cheeks relaxed. Position your index finger in the superior part of the vestibule, adjacent to the maxillary third molar area, move your finger as far posteriorly as you can, and open the mouth wide. You can feel

your finger being pushed anteriorly out of the area; this is the **coronoid process** of the mandible moving into that vestibular space. The coronoid process is of important consideration for several clinical reasons.

In radiology, for example, you can take two periapical films of the maxillary molar area—one using a **bisecting angle technique** with the mouth open and the patient holding the film, and the other using a **paralleling technique** with the mouth closed on a film-holding device. The coronoid process intrudes into the vestibular space on the film taken with the mouth open, making it difficult to get a clear image on film. However, on the second film, taken with the mouth closed, the coronoid process does not impinge on the space, thereby demonstrating the benefit of a film-holding device.

The coronoid process may also cause some problems when you are trying to take maxillary study models. When the mouth is open wide, the coronoid process may tend to push on the posterior part of the impression tray and cause it to be displaced, making it difficult to obtain a good impression of the third molar and the maxillary tuberosity regions. It may also impinge on the posterior-lateral portion of a patient's maxillary denture and cause possible dislodgement of the denture. It is necessary to remove as much bulk as possible on the denture in that area so this does not happen.

Alveolar bone loss and tooth replacement

Other problems arise in endentulous patients (see Figs. 11-12 and 11-15, where the dotted lines mark the alveolar process, or alveolar bone.) When teeth are lost there is generally some loss of the alveolar bone that formed the sockets for the teeth. It tends to happen to a greater extent in the mandible than in the maxilla. If the bone loss is too great there may be problems constructing a denture that will be stable. For the past 40 years there have been attempts to provide some stabilization and retention of dentures through the use of implants. Some of the first implants looked like the metal

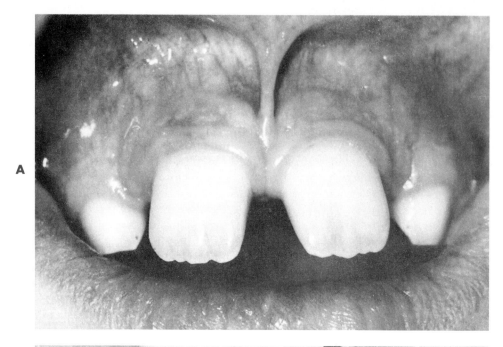

A

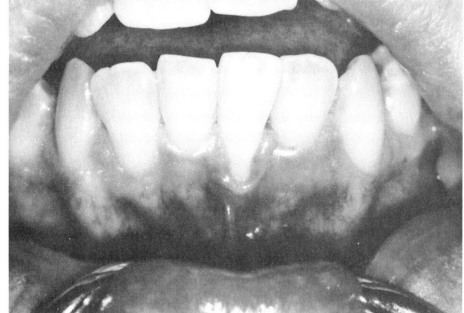

B

FIG. 1-3. **A,** Notice how the labial frenum extends between the maxillary teeth, causing separation or diastema. **B,** Notice how the mandibular labial frenum attaches close to an area of gingival recession and contributes to that condition. (Courtesy Dr. David Vandersall.)

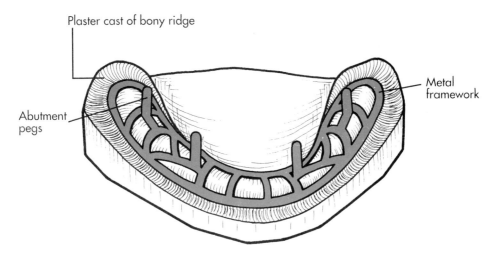

FIG. 1-4.   Subperiosteal implant. The metal framework implant sits on a cast of an edentulous ridge with the mucosa reflected away. It will be attached beneath the covering periosteum of bone and gingiva. The pegs stick up through the gingiva and a denture or bridgework can be constructed on them after the implant has healed as much as possible.

framework of a partial denture with pegs sticking up from it. The gingiva of the ridge was incised, the implant was attached to the bone, and the gingiva was then sutured over the implant. The pegs of the implant fit into sockets constructed in the denture and gave it stability, or the peg(s) may have served as an **abutment** for a fixed bridge. These implants were referred to as **subperiosteal implants** (Fig. 1-4).

Later on a **blade-vent implant** was developed, (Fig. 1-5) which looked like a metal wedge with a peg. The gingiva was incised, a bur cut a trough in the bone in the area of placement, and the blade of the implant was driven into the bone and then sutured over. It too left a peg sticking up through the gingiva. The problems with these implants were many, but the major one was the opportunity for infection or loss of tissue, which could have caused implant failure. There were also problems of the blade entering the mandibular canal or the maxillary sinus.

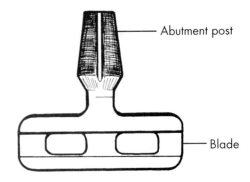

FIG. 1-5.   Blade-vent implant. An incision is made in the gingiva and a trough is cut in the bone. Then the bottom blade of the implant is driven into the bone, and the bone fills in the openings in the blade. A removable or fixed denture can be constructed on several of these.

The most recent type of implant is called an **osseointegrated implant** (Fig. 1-6). There are many varieties to this implant. The one illustrated in Fig. 1-6 has screw threads on the outside, contains some holes, and a small screw fills an opening in the top. For insertion, an incision is made in the gingival tissue, and a precise bone hole is drilled to fit the implant. The implant is firmly secured by screwing it into the socket; the gingiva is sutured over it, and the tissue is allowed to heal. While the tissue is healing, connective tissue and bone are growing into the holes and around the screw threads in the implant, which stabilizes it. After healing and stabilization have taken place, a small incision is made over the screw in the top of the implant. The screw is removed, and one of many types of pegs or attachment apparatuses is screwed into the hole. This implant has had tremendous acceptance because of its success rate. When inserted correctly, success is in the high

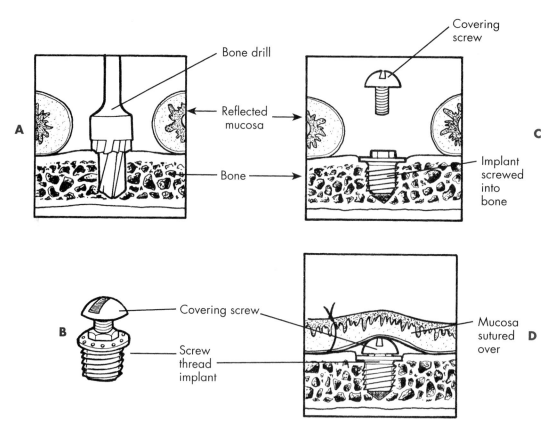

FIG. 1-6.   Osseointegrated implant. **A,** Tissue has been reflected, and a hole is being bored into the bone. **B,** The implant with the covering screw. **C,** The implant will be screwed into the bone, and the covering screw will be inserted in top. **D,** Tissue is sutured over the implant. Time allows the mucosa to heal and bone to fill in. Then a small hole will be made and the covering screw will be removed and replaced by one of many varieties of posts or abutments.

90% rate. The peg may be used to stabilize a removable denture or serve as an **abutment** for a fixed bridge.

Mucosa

Study the texture of the inner surface of the lip. Pull the lower lip down, dry it with a tissue and stretch it. Notice the small drops of fluid on the lip, indicating the openings of small salivary glands. These of course are also found in many other areas of the oral cavity (see Chapter 10).

The mucosa of the lips, cheeks, and **retromolar pad** area, posterior to the mandibular molars, are also the most frequent sites of misplaced **sebaceous glands** frequently referred to as **Fordyce granules.** These glands are normally associated with hair follicles, which are normally only found on skin. In about 60% to 80% of the population some sebaceous glands may be located on mucosa in areas of the oral cavity. They appear as yellowish granular structures embedded in the mucosa. These may be of some concern to patients, but with verification of their true identity, the patients should be reassured that they are harmless and are only a cosmetic situation. Look for these harmless glands in your own mouth.

Buccal Alveolar Bone

Another condition found on the buccal **cortical plate** of the mandible and maxillae in a large portion of the population are small bony growths called **exostoses.** They are generally seen more frequently on the mandible than on the maxilla. They are normally of no consequence unless they become tender from brushing in the area or if dentures are being constructed. Under these circumstances the exostoses may have to be removed, which is a relatively simple surgical procedure. However, be aware that these exostoses may recur over the years and have to be removed again.

ORAL CAVITY PROPER

When the mouth is opened you can see the oral cavity proper. First examine the roof of the mouth and study the hard and soft palates.

Hard Palate

Read Chapter 11 on the osteology of the skull for the extent and makeup of the hard palate. In the anterior portion of the hard palate are transverse ridges of epithelial and connective tissue known as **rugae.** During speech and mastication the tongue contacts these rugae. They are covered with keratinized epithelium and are frequently burned by hot foods, which can cause an ulcerated area of mucosa lingual to the maxillary incisor.

Also within the hard palate is a singular bulge of tissue at the midline immediately posterior to the central incisors known as the **incisive papilla.** Beneath this papilla is the **incisive foramen,** which carries the nasopalatine nerve to the mucous membrane lingual to the maxillary incisor teeth. This is a point of injection for anesthetizing the area. At the posterolateral part of the hard palate, lingual to the second and third maxillary molars, are two openings in the bone, the greater palatine foramina, for the rest of the nerves to the hard palate. This area may also be an injection site (Figs. 1-7 and 1-8).

The tissue beneath the palatal epithelium varies from region to region in the palate. In the midline of the hard palate the connective tissue is rather thin, and the palate feels very hard and bony in that part. In the anterolateral part of the hard palate the connective tissue contains fat cells and is thicker than at the midline. In the posterolateral portion the fat cells are still present, but there are numerous minor salivary glands that secrete mucus. The soft palate also contains these mucus-secreting minor salivary glands, which serve to keep the epithelium moist.

The shape and size of the hard palate vary from individual to individual. It may be wide or narrow, have a high, arching curvature or vault, or be quite flat in its contours. Not infrequently there may be some excess bone growth in the midline of the hard palate. This is referred to as a **torus palatinus** (Fig. 1-9). It may grow to vary-

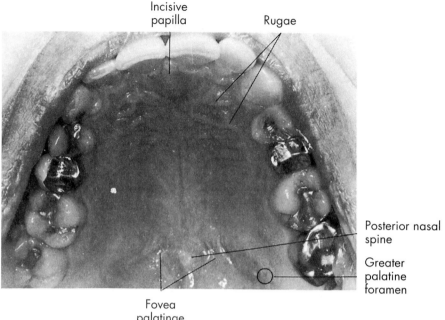

FIG. 1-7.   View of palate. Position of the greater palatine foramen *(circle)*. See the incisive papilla and rugae as well as the area of posterior nasal spine indicating the end of the hard palate.

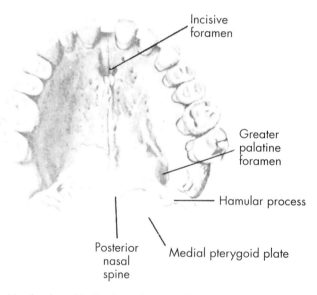

FIG. 1-8.   Hard palate. Notice how the posterior area curves toward the posterior nasal spine. Laterally, notice the hamular process of the medial pterygoid plate. (From DuBrul EL: *Sicher's oral anatomy,* ed 7, St Louis, 1980, Mosby.)

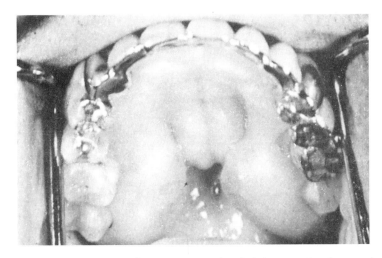

FIG. 1-9.   Typical torus palatinus. Notice the slightly constricted area where it attaches to the hard palate. Modified from Bhaskar SN: *Orban's oral histology and embryology,* ed 8, St Louis, 1976, Mosby.

ing sizes and is generally only a problem when construction of an upper denture is necessary. Under these circumstances the denture cannot be accurately adapted to the palate area, and proper retention cannot be achieved without surgically removing the growth.

The junction of the hard and soft palates forms a double curving line, with the **posterior nasal spine** of the palatine bone being the primary landmark at the midline (see Figs. 1-7 and 1-8). Although you cannot see this posterior nasal spine, you can palpate it. Additionally, there are two small depressions, one on each side of the spine, known as **fovea palatinae,** which mark the spine as a landmark in the construction of an upper denture.

Soft Palate

Most of the posterior portion of the soft palate is actually part of the oral pharynx; however, it seems appropriate to describe it here. The soft palate stretches back from the hard palate and in its most posterior portion at the midline is a downward projection known as the **uvula.** In a relaxed state the soft palate has a slightly arching form from one side to the other. However, in speech and swallowing the soft palate moves into various positions and closes off the oral pharynx from the nasal pharynx. This is accomplished by the **levator veli palatini** muscle, which pulls the soft palate up and back until it contacts the posterior throat (**pharyngeal**) wall.

In Chapter 3 on development of the face and oral cavity, the cleft lip and palate are discussed. Both are drastic medicodental problems and are generally treated by a team of dental and medical professionals. Another variation of cleft palate is the **short palate.** The soft palate may look normal, but does not contact the posterior pharyngeal wall when it is elevated during swallowing or speech, producing a nasal or cleft speech sound. With a dental appliance and/or speech therapy this problem can be corrected with gratifying results.

Lateral Borders

The lateral borders of the oral cavity proper are bounded primarily by the teeth and associated mucosa. In the posterior lateral part of the oral cavity the boundary is the palatine tonsil and its associated **pillars.** The more prominent fold behind the tonsil, extending from the soft palate downward into the lateral pharyngeal wall, is referred to as the **posterior pillar** or **palatopharyngeal arch** or **fold.** Immediately in front of the palatine tonsil is the **anterior pillar** or **palatoglossal arch** or **fold.** These folds are formed by the palatopharyngeal and palatoglossal muscles, respectively (Fig. 1-10).

Posterior Borders

Just posterior to the mandibular third molar is a small elevation of tissue known as the retromolar pad (Fig. 1-11). This structure is a consideration in lower denture construction. The posterior extent of the oral cavity is the space between the left and right tonsils and their pillars known as the **fauces.** Looking into the oral cavity you can see the tongue and soft palate. If you depress the tongue with a tongue depressor blade and ask the patient to say "ahhh," the soft palate will rise, enabling examination beyond

the oral cavity into the oral pharynx. The posterior pharyngeal wall can be an indicator of the health status of the patient.

Tongue and Floor of Mouth

Tongue

Chapter 9 contains descriptions of structures on the tongue such as filiform, fungiform, vallate or circumvallate papillae, and the roughened lateral surface of the tongue opposite the vallate papillae, which represents rudimentary foliate papillae. These foliate papillae should be carefully examined in a routine oral examination because it is a difficult area to see and might hide early signs of oral cancer. There may also be enlargements of lymphoid tissue at the base of the tongue, which are referred to collectively as the **lingual tonsils.**

If you ask the patient to elevate the tongue, you will see that the underside or ventral side of

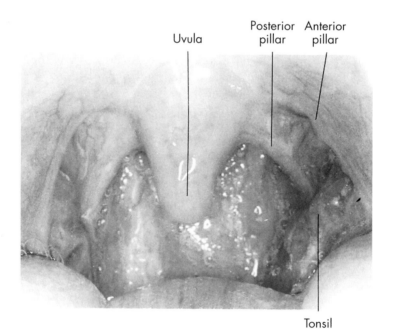

FIG. 1-10.   Various posterior palatal structures.

the tongue has many blood vessels close to the surface. Extending from an area near the tip of the tongue down to the floor of the mouth is a fold of tissue known as the **lingual frenum** or **frenulum.** If this frenum is attached close to the tip of the tongue and is rather short, the tongue will have limited movement. This condition is known as **ankyloglossia** or, as it is commonly called, **tongue-tie.**

Floor of mouth

At the base of the lingual frenum is a small elevation on each side known as the **sublingual caruncle.** This is the opening for the ducts of two of the major salivary glands, the submandibular and sublingual glands. Extending from the sublingual caruncle back along the floor of the mouth on either side is a fold of tissue called the **sublingual fold.** Along the anterior and middle parts of this fold can be found a number of small openings of the multiple ducts

of the sublingual salivary gland. This fold of tissue also marks the paths of a number of structures as they run forward in the floor of the mouth (Fig. 1-12).

There may frequently be some bony swellings on the lingual surface of the mandible at the canine area. These are similar in nature to the palatal tori and are called **mandibular tori** (Fig. 1-13). They may present a problem in radiology because correct film placement may be difficult and sometimes painful for the patient. If the patient requires a lower denture, it is usually necessary to remove these mandibular tori to eliminate undercuts or improper contours that would make denture construction and fit difficult. The same condition can present problems when you are trying to take study models. The flange of the tray may strike the area and cause irritation and may also make it difficult to correctly seat the impression tray.

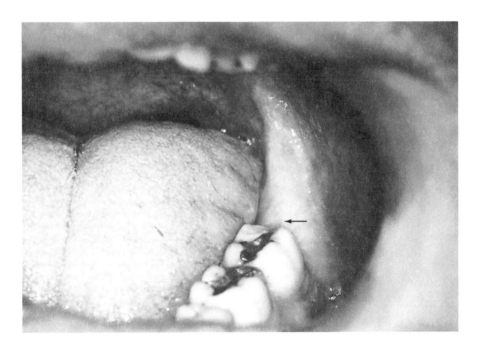

FIG. 1-11.   Arrow indicates retromolar pad behind mandibular third molar.

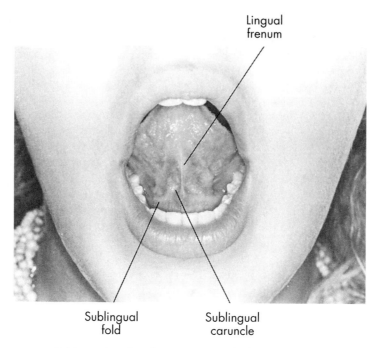

Lingual
frenum

Sublingual   Sublingual
fold   caruncle

FIG. I-I2.   Sublingual region demonstrating the lingual frenum, sublingual caruncles, and sublingual folds.

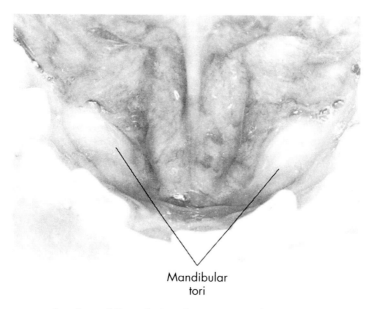

Mandibular
tori

FIG. I-I3.   Another sublingual view demonstrating bony mandibular tori.

The floor of the mouth is supported by the paired mylohyoid muscles, which form a sling from the mylohyoid line on one side of the medial surface of the mandible to the same line on the other side. Contraction of these muscles raises the tongue and floor of the mouth (see Chapters 11 and 13). If you look in a mirror while raising your tongue as high as possible, you will see the movement and get an idea of where the mylohyoid muscle is attached to the mandible. This area of attachment is important in denture construction and determines how far into the floor of the mouth the denture flange should extend on the lingual side. If it extends below the mylohyoid line, the denture may be dislodged during elevation of the tongue or may irritate the lingual mucosa in that area.

The oral tissue beneath the tongue in the floor of the mouth is one of the thinnest in the oral cavity and therefore quite sensitive to trauma. Of course any of the oral tissues may be traumatized, but some are more susceptible than others. Some of the common injuries you will see in the dental office may relate to hot foods and liquids. Potato chips or bony foods may cause cutting injuries to various areas of the oral cavity, especially the gingiva. *Be aware that these tissues may be readily injured.*

OTHER CLINICAL MANIFESTATIONS OF THE ORAL CAVITY

Although many other chapters in this book will refer to the oral cavity, it is important to stress that all who use this book be aware of the need for a solid background in the normal anatomy of the oral cavity. It is the responsibility of all who view the intraoral anatomy of the patient to be aware of what the normal anatomy of the oral cavity looks like, whether they be the dental assistant, laboratory technologist, dental hygienist, or dentist. Legally, the dentist bears the primary responsibility for much of the diagnosis and treatment of the patient, but everyone should look carefully for anything that appears abnormal. Because there are significant differences within the oral cavity, it is beneficial for students to examine as many other students in their class as possible. This will give a good idea of anatomic variation within the general population.

Frequently we think about the effects of oral diseases on other parts of the body and we consider the spread of dental infections, oral cancers, and the like. However, we should never lose sight of the fact that problems in other parts of the body may show up, early or late in the disease state, in the oral cavity. Early stages of measles show up as spots in the oral cavity. Many times acquired immunodeficiency syndrome (AIDS) may be suspected because of oral lesions relating to Kaposi's sarcoma, a disease that may be found in association with AIDS. Many types of cancer from other parts of the body may spread to the oral cavity. A young child may be brought to the office because of bleeding gums. The child may have good oral hygiene, and the tissues may not appear notably abnormal, and yet the gums, or gingiva, bleed readily upon brushing. One should seriously consider having blood tests run because bleeding gingival tissues in a mouth with good oral hygiene are a possible early sign of leukemia. A reddened, painful tongue may be a sign of vitamin deficiencies, and there are oral lesions that may be associated with a number of diseases.

This list is not meant to be comprehensive; rather it is meant to reinforce the fact that all members of the dental team have the responsibility to be observant as they work within the oral cavity. We all owe our patients the very best care and concern we can provide, and a good, solid knowledge of the normal anatomy of the oral cavity will enable any member of the team to spot something that does not appear to be normal and to have the dentist look carefully at the area of concern.

Review Questions

1. What are tori and exostoses, and what may need to be done with them?
2. What is the vestibule?
3. Do the frenum attachments of the lip contain muscles?
4. Why is the alveolar mucosa more red than the gingiva?
5. What are the divisions of the palate, and what are the transverse ridges in the anterior palate called?
6. Where and what is the posterior nasal spine?
7. Which muscle supports the floor of the mouth?
8. What and where is the sublingual caruncle?
9. What makes up the anterior and posterior pillars, and what lies between them?
10. What is the fauces?
11. What are the two parts of the oral cavity, and what are their boundaries?
12. Why is knowledge of normal anatomy of the oral cavity so important?
13. Name three generalized disease states that can be detected by the presence of oral lesions or signs.
14. What are Fordyce's granules? Where are they found, what is their appearance, and are they a clinical problem?

UNIT II

ORAL HISTOLOGY AND EMBRYOLOGY

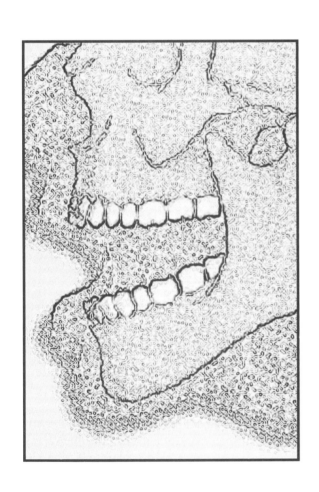

Chapter 2

Basic Tissues

THIS CHAPTER on the basic tissues of the body is in no way meant to be a complete discussion, but rather an introduction to the basic concepts and structure of the body's tissues.

The body is composed of four basic tissues: **epithelium, connective tissue, muscle, and nervous tissue.** A tissue is an accumulation of cells, fibers, crystals, or fluids; any one or all might compose a tissue. The basic description of a **cell** should be the starting point for discussing basic tissues.

CELL STRUCTURE

A cell can be thought of as a bag of fluid, generally varying in size from 0.01 to 0.05 mm in diameter. The wall of this bag is called the **cell membrane,** and its function is to keep the cellular fluid in and unnecessary foreign materials out. The cell membrane does have the potential to allow molecules of different sizes to pass through, and it can incorporate other membranes into it or add to it by itself. In Fig. 2-1, notice that the area inside the cell membrane is a fluid medium known as **cytoplasm.** Within the

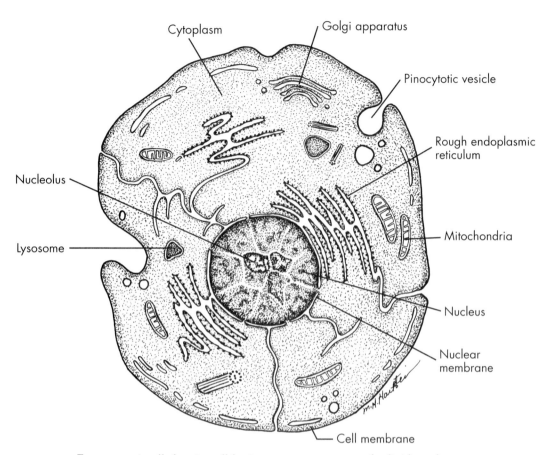

FIG. 2-1.   A cell showing all basic components, except for lipid or glycogen inclusions.

cytoplasm are other components of the cell, but looking through a light microscope you can probably distinguish only one structure—the **nucleus.** The nucleus is the master control of the cell. It contains deoxyribonucleic acid (**DNA**) and ribonucleic acid (**RNA**), which control the operation of the cell. DNA is found in the chromosomes, which during nonmitotic times are found throughout the nucleus. Most of the RNA is found within the **nucleolus.** The nucleolus is a circumscribed dense area within the nucleus. There is generally one nucleolus per cell, but in

some instances there may be more than one. The function of RNA is to carry genetic information or instructions from the DNA to the manufacturing parts of the cell.

Organelles

Looking through an electron microscope, which further enlarges cellular structures, you can see other parts of the cell. Most cell parts are called **organelles,** which are small functioning parts. They allow the cell to remain alive and carry out its particular function.

Small, usually oblong organelles known as **mitochondria** are responsible for energy production and for the rate at which the cell uses energy—commonly called the **metabolism** of the cell. If the mitochondria are injured, the cell will not be able to function and may die. The number and location of the mitochondria are an indication of cellular activity and where the majority of activity is located within the cell. The mitochondria in Fig. 2-1 show the infoldings of the inner membrane of the mitochondria that form leaflike projections called **cristae.** The cristae have **enzymes** on their surface that aid in cell metabolism. Just as an increased number of mitochondria indicates increased cellular activity, an increase in cristae also indicates a more active cell.

Another organelle, called the **endoplasmic reticulum,** is a sort of network within the fluid of the cell. The endoplasmic reticulum is a series of interconnecting tubules in the cell that are responsible for the manufacture of various products to be used inside or outside the cell. This function is controlled by several types of RNA from the nucleus and from the cytoplasm itself. Some endoplasmic reticulum have small granules of RNA known as **ribosomes** on its surface and are referred to as rough endoplasmic reticulum. In other instances the ribosomes are found floating in the cytoplasm. Rough endoplasmic reticulum is responsible for the production of **protein.** The RNA attaches to various amino acids and, by putting them in a certain order, forms different types of proteins. For example, the rough endoplasmic reticulum of salivary glands produces protein components of saliva.

Once the protein material is produced, it is frequently necessary to "package" it, as one would do in the shipping room of a factory. The organelle in the cell that takes care of this packaging is known as the **Golgi apparatus.** The Golgi apparatus produces a thin membrane to surround the material produced by the endoplasmic reticulum so it can be moved around and later out of the cell without mixing with the cell's cytoplasm. To accomplish this type of cell secretion, known as **merocrine** secretion, the Golgi apparatus moves to the inner surface of the cell membrane and fuses to it. At the point of fusion there is a rupture in the cell membrane and in the membrane produced by the Golgi, and the contents of the Golgi are released without any loss of cytoplasm. The Golgi membrane is then incorporated into the cell membrane.

One other small organ found in many cells is called a **lysosome,** a circular structure that acts as a scavenger for the cell. If any other organelles of the cell die, or if the cell takes in some kind of foreign material, the lysosome will digest the substances. The one problem with this organelle is that it contains some very powerful digestive enzymes to perform its job, and if it is injured the enzymes will leak out and consume the cell. The person who discovered these organelles called them "suicide bags."

To some degree cell shape is dictated by the pressure of cells around it if they are in tight contact. However, without that pressure and sometimes in spite of that pressure, most cells maintain their shape because of the presence of organelles known as **microtubules** or **microfilaments.** These structures are ultrastructural, meaning they are so small they can only be seen with an electron microscope. The microtubules are hollow rods formed of ball-like subunits of proteins called **alpha-tubulins** and **beta-tubulins.** They are frequently associated with the motile part of some cells called *cilia* or *flagella.* Microfilaments are solid rods and are found in all cells except mature erythrocytes. They are composed of the protein actin, which is also a component of muscle cells. They run in many directions throughout the cell and often bind to the cell membrane or to other microfilaments.

Cellular Inclusions

Organelles are intermixed in many cells with what are called **cellular inclusions.** This term indicates that the contents of the inclusions are not produced by the cell but rather are stored in the cell to be used at a later time and possibly another place. These inclusions may be little spheres of fat, known as **lipid droplets,** or multiple units of the sugar glucose, known as **glycogen.** Both lipid droplets and glycogen are storage forms of energy. When the body requires energy, they are released from the cell that stores them to travel to other parts of the body to be used as needed (Fig. 2-2). Many of these inclusions enter the cell by a process known as **pinocytosis,** which means "a drinking in." The product pushes into the cell membrane from outside, and the membrane caves inward, finally pinching itself off and surrounding the inclusion without any loss of cytoplasm.

Although this is only a brief discussion of cells and their components, there are a number of different types of cells with different functions. This chapter will further explore the similarities and differences of these cells and their functions within the four basic tissues of the body.

EPITHELIAL TISSUE

Epithelium is a group of cells that makes up the skin and lines the inside of the cavities of the body. Examples of these lining layers include the inside of blood vessels or the digestive tract as well as the lining of the walls of the thoracic (chest) and abdominal cavities. Glands such as salivary glands, sweat glands, pancreas, and liver also originate from epithelium. Shapes of these epithelial cells differ, and they are arranged in a variety of relationships. Because of these differences each type of epithelium has a different classification according to its number of cell layers—single-layered, or simple, epithelium and multiple-layered, or stratified, epithelium.

Simple Epithelium

Simple squamous epithelium

The word *squamous* means "flat" or "plate-like." If you looked at the surface of **simple squamous epithelium,** it would look like a collection of fried eggs side by side in a big pan. If

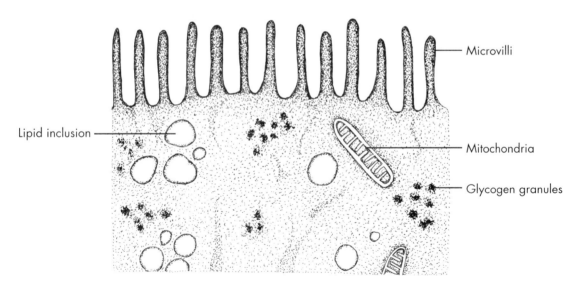

FIG. 2-2. A portion of an absorptive cell showing glycogen and lipid inclusions.

Microvilli

Lipid inclusion

Mitochondria

Glycogen granules

you cut down through this epithelium and looked at a cross section, it would look like an overdone fried egg cut right through the yolk (Fig. 2-3). Looking at it from this side view you can imagine that such a thin layer would not be an extremely protective type of structure but might be thin enough for some materials to pass through between the cells. This type of epithelium is found lining the lungs, blood vessels, abdominal cavity, thoracic cavity, and small fluid-carrying tubes called **lymphatic vessels,** just to name a few. Simple squamous epithelium allows for the exchange of oxygen and carbon dioxide between the lining of the lungs and the capillar-ies of the lungs. It also enables the lungs and the chest wall as well as the heart and the sac that covers the heart, called the **pericardium,** to rub together without any irritation because the layers of the epithelium are lubricated with a fluid substance.

Simple cuboidal or simple columnar epithelium

As the names indicate, **simple cuboidal** and **simple columnar epithelium** are either cuboidal or rectangular. Again, these kinds of epithelial cells are only one layer thick, but that one layer is much thicker than the squamous layer (Fig. 2-4). They are found in a number of areas in the

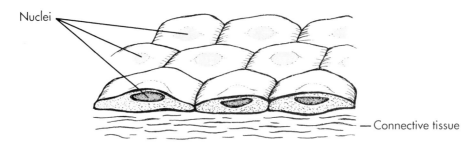

Fig. 2-3.   Simple squamous epithelium. In the cross-sectional picture at the front, you can see that the cells and nuclei are flat. On the upper surface the nuclei are slightly raised, like the yolk of an egg.

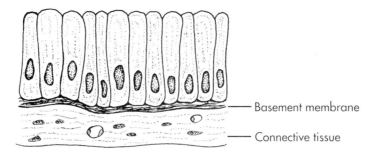

Fig. 2-4.   Simple columnar epithelium. The cells are tall and all the same height. They rest on a basement membrane with connective tissue deep to it. Simple cuboidal epithelium would be similar, but the cells would be short and cuboid in shape.

body. The columnar cells line the digestive tract from the stomach to the anal region. In this location the main function of the epithelium is absorption of the break-down products within the digestive tract. To do a more thorough job in this process, the end of the cell facing toward the lumen has small ultrastructural projections known

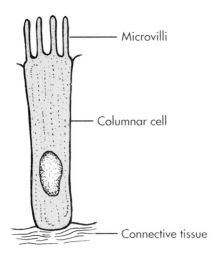

FIG. 2-5.   Simple columnar cell with microvilli. Microvilli are exaggerated in length and width so that you can see how they would increase the surface area of the cell membrane.

as **microvilli.** These microvilli increase the surface area of the cell end by many times its original surface, thereby increasing the amount of nutrients that can be absorbed in the digestive tract (Fig. 2-5). The cuboidal cells are found in the ducts of various glands, such as the kidney, salivary glands, pancreas, and others. When these cuboidal cells are packed together to form small ducts, they tend to form a pyramid shape (Fig. 2-6) and are frequently referred to as **pyramidal cells.** These cells also frequently have microvilli for the same purpose as cuboidal cells.

Looking at the arrangement of these kinds of cells, one can see that the cells adjoin on two sides, and of the other two sides, one rests on underlying connective tissue and the other faces a free border or lumen of a duct. The side facing the underlying tissue is called the **basal end** of the cell. Facing the free surface is the side frequently referred to as the **apical end** of the cell. This terminology makes sense when you look at a pyramidal cell and see that the apical end is the apex of the pyramid and the basal end is the base of the pyramid. Later we will discuss cells that secrete a product from their apical end.

Pseudostratified columnar epithelium

The term **pseudostratified columnar epithelium** means "falsely layered epithelium" or epithelium that looks like more than one layer.

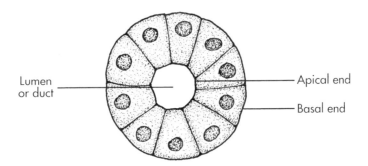

FIG. 2-6.   Columnar cells forming a tube or duct pushed into a pyramidal pattern. Apical ends are narrower than basal ends. Secretions come from the apical ends.

Some texts consider this as a separate classification of epithelium from simple epithelium. Viewed under a microscope it appears that there are several rows of nuclei, which would suggest more than one row of cells. However, on closer examination it is evident that all the cells reach all the way down to the underlying tissue, the **basement membrane.** Some of the cells are very short, but others begin on the basement membrane with a very narrow stem and then expand once they reach the upper part of the cell layer. This type of epithelium is seen in several areas of the body, but the most prominent is the respiratory tract. In the respiratory tract as well as in other places the epithelium has many small single-celled glands called **goblet cells** intermixed with the epithelium (Fig. 2-7). These glands secrete a mucous substance and lubricate the surface of the epithelium for a number of functions. Along with the goblet cells, this epithelium also has small hairlike projections known as **cilia,** which perform a waving, beating motion. These cilia are coated with mucus from the goblet cells and then trap contaminants in the air passing through the respiratory passages. These trapped particles are passed along from cilium to cilium by means of the beating motion until they reach

the nasal opening or the opening of the oral cavity where they are removed from the body. There are cilia on some simple columnar epithelia as well.

Stratified Epithelium

There are three varieties of multiple-layered, or stratified, epithelia, only two of which are commonly found in the body.

Stratified cuboidal or stratified columnar epithelium

A type of epithelium not commonly found is **stratified cuboidal** or **stratified columnar epithelium.** It consists of two or possibly more rows of cuboidal or columnar cells on top of one another and is generally only found forming large ducts of glands.

Transitional epithelium

The term *transitional* indicates change, and that appropriately describes **transitional epithelium.** It changes in thickness and appearance as the need arises. Composed of multiple layers of cells and varying in thickness, it is found in the urinary system, with the primary concentration in the urinary bladder and ureter. When the bladder is empty, the epithelium is relaxed and there are about eight to ten layers of cells, the

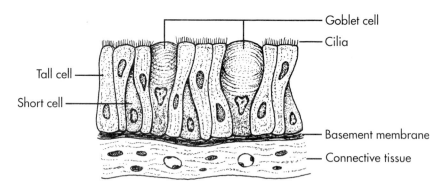

FIG. 2-7. Representation of pseudostratified columnar epithelium from the trachea. Notice goblet cells intermixed. There appears to be more than one row of cells, but there is only one because all cells rest on the basement membrane. Also notice cilia at the cells' surface.

deepest layers composed of cuboidal cells and the surface layers slightly flattened but with rounded bulging nuclei (Fig. 2-8, *A*). When the bladder is full, the epithelium is stretched and may appear to be only three to five layers thick, the deepest cell layers somewhat flattened and the surface layers and the nuclei extremely flattened (Fig. 2-8, *B*). This change in appearance accounts for the name transitional and represents a very functional arrangement of cells.

Stratified squamous epithelium

The most common type of epithelium is **stratified squamous epithelium.** As skin it covers the body and also makes up the mucosa of the oral cavity, pharynx, esophagus, and anal region. In a discussion of this type of epithelium it seems appropriate to consider the changes seen in the cells at different layers of the stratified squamous epithelium.

Stratum basale or stratum germinativum. A single layer of cuboidal cells that rests on the underlying connective tissue of the basement membrane is known as **stratum basale** or **stratum germinativum.** It is in this layer that the cells divide and form more cells to maintain the supply and replace the cells that are lost.

Stratum spinosum. As more cells form in the **basal layer,** they become displaced because of the crowding; thus they are pushed out of the basal layer into the layers above them toward the surface. The **stratum spinosum** varies in its number of cell rows from two or three to ten or more. This layer, like the basal layer, is also sometimes referred to as a *stratum germinativum,* because you can see cell division in this layer as well. In this layer the cells are no longer cuboidal but seem to be star shaped or having many small points; hence the adjective spinosum. The reason for the star-shaped appearance is that the cells are attached at points of intracellular modifications, called **desmosomes,** on the cell walls of adjacent cells. These points almost resemble a series of "spot welds" on the adjacent cell walls. During preparation of tissue for study under a microscope, the cells dehydrate and shrink away from each other, but are held together at the points of desmosomal attachments and thus appear star shaped. The cells continue to be pushed toward the surface by the newly forming basal cells and eventually reach the next layer.

Stratum granulosum. Not clearly seen in many areas of the mucosa of the oral cavity, stra-

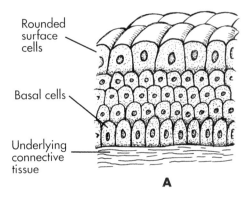

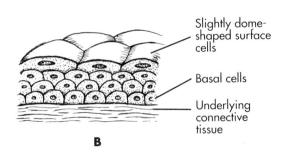

FIG. 2-8.   **A,** Relaxed transitional epithelium of bladder. There are about five rows of cells. **B,** Stretched transitional epithelium. Notice that there are fewer rows, and the surface cells and their nuclei are more flattened.

tum granulosum is particularly evident in thick skin. When seen, it appears as two or three layers of flattened cells that contain granules or spots within their cytoplasm. These granules are made up of a material called **keratohyalin** and eventually cause the cell to die when the amount of **keratin** becomes great enough.

Stratum corneum. The term *corneum* is the same as the term *keratinized;* it means "hornlike," resembling the tissue of the fingernail, only less dense and therefore softer. In many instances **stratum corneum** is misnamed because the top layers of cells are not always cornified or keratinized. Three different situations can be seen in this layer:

1. The cells may be alive and the epithelium referred to as **nonkeratinized** stratified squamous epithelium. In this type there is no stratum granulosum.
2. The cells on the surface, although still showing signs of nuclei, may be in the process of dying and are referred to as partly or **para-**keratinized stratified squamous epithelium. Here the stratum granulosum is very thin.
3. The cells on the surface may be dead and referred to as **keratinized** stratified squamous epithelium. Here the upper layer have no nuclei, and they appear somewhat opaque when they are not stained with dyes for microscopic study (Fig. 2-9; see also Fig. 8-1).

The thickness of this upper dead layer varies, depending on the amount of trauma or rubbing the tissue is subjected to. As you know, working with a shovel or rake will eventually cause a callus to form, a result of a thickening of the stratum corneum as well as a thickening of the stratum spinosum. In thick skin such as the palms of the hands or the soles of the feet a clear layer known as the **stratum lucidum** can be seen between the stratum granulosum and the stratum corneum. The cells are continually produced in the basal layer of the epithelium and move up through the other layers until they reach the surface where they are shed. This process can be

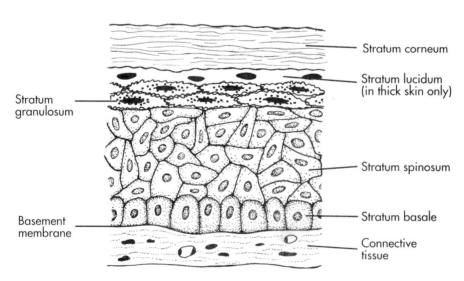

Fig. 2-9. Stratified squamous epithelium. The stratum spinosum and stratum corneum would be thicker. Because this is thick skin, we can see a stratum lucidum.

seen when one sits in a tub of hot water for a while without using soap, a ring begins to develop around the tub. This ring is not readily visible but can be felt. The primary component of this ring is dead epithelial cells, which **slough** off and float to the edge of the tub. Just think of the mechanism that regulates the rate of cells produced with the rate of those lost and that adjusts to meet any changes. Without this control we would either have skin as thick as an elephant or have no skin whatsoever.

Another important mechanism relating to cell replacement in skin has to do with pigment in the skin and changes in that pigment level. Skin normally has a yellowish color because it contains the pigment **carotene.** There is also some pink color imparted to it by the underlying blood vessels. Immediately beneath the basal layer of cells in all persons except albinos are cells called **melanocytes,** which produce a pigment called **melanin.** These cells, when stimulated by **ultraviolet rays,** produce more pigment, which becomes incorporated into the epithelial cells and is carried to the surface. As this happens, the skin darkens. After the person is no longer subjected to these ultraviolet rays, the pigment level is reduced, the cells containing it are eventually lost, and the skin lightens in color. In darker colored races, there are more melanocytes present, and they are constantly producing more melanin, thus maintaining the darker color of their skin. In the absence of melanocytes, or with a limited number of them, the skin imparts a more pinkish color.

Glands

Most of the glands of the body are developed from epithelium. As the epithelium develops, some of the basal cells begin to grow downward into the connective tissue beneath it. As they grow downward, they form a cord of epithelial cells that later hollows out to form a tube. When these tubes have reached a certain depth, they form a number of bulblike or tubelike processes on their ends, which are generally referred to as acini or **tubules,** respectively. Glands can be classified in a number of ways.

Distributive mechanisms

A distributive mechanism is the manner in which the secretory products are carried away from the gland. There are **exocrine** glands, whose products are carried away by ducts leading from the gland, and **endocrine** glands, whose ducts are lost after the gland develops and whose products are carried away from the gland in the bloodstream. Salivary glands are an example of exocrine glands.

Secretory mechanisms

A secretory mechanism is the manner in which the product is secreted from the gland. In **holocrine** glands the entire cell dies, and the secretion is expelled when the cell membrane breaks up. This sort of process is seen in the sebaceous glands of the hair follicles. The oil of the hair is a result of the death of the cells of the gland. The secretory products of **merocrine** glands pass through the cell wall without allowing any cell cytoplasm to escape. This is how the salivary glands secrete, without any loss of cytoplasm. Merocrine secretion was described earlier in the discussion on the Golgi apparatus (see p. 20).

Arrangement of components

Exocrine glands have secretory and excretory portions. The secretory portion is composed of the cells that actually secrete and modify the substance being produced by the gland. The excretory portion is that part of the duct system that carries the product to the surface epithelium without changing the makeup of the secretory substance. The arrangement of these components varies depending on whether the gland is a simple tubular gland, which is just a straight tube, or a **compound tubuloalveolar** gland, of which salivary glands are an example. A compound gland has numerous levels of branching within its duct system, similar in appearance to a bunch of grapes—tubelike secretory parts with a rounded alveolus or acinus at the end of each tube (Fig. 2-10).

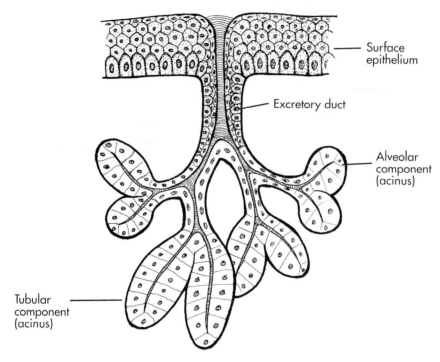

FIG. 2-10. Representation of compound tubuloalveolar glands. There are branchings of ducts with rounded alveolar end pieces as well as elongated tubular endpieces.

Products

Salivary glands produce the following types of secretions:

1. **Serous** secretion–a thin watery substance containing most of the digestive enzymes found in saliva
2. **Mucous** secretion–a thicker, more viscous substance
3. **Seromucous** secretion–produced by many of the glands that have both serous and mucous cells, in varying quantities within the same gland

Embryonic Origin

The next point to consider, which concerns the other basic tissues as well, is embryonic origin. You know that an individual begins development from a single cell, the fertilized ovum. From this one cell the following occurs: The fertilized ovum divides into two cells, the two into four, and so on. This multiplication forms a ball of cells, which becomes hollow with a thickened inner layer on one side. This hollow ball is called a **blastocyst** (Fig. 2-11). The outer layer of cells of this blastocyst is called the **outer cell mass,** and the thickened inner layer is called the **inner cell mass.** The outer cell mass becomes part of the membranes surrounding the developing embryo and the placenta. The inner cell mass forms the actual embryo itself, one of the membrane layers, and a sac called the *amnion*. At first this inner cell mass is an elongated flat structure made up of two layers of epithelial cells. The outer layer of epithelial cells is called the **ecto-**

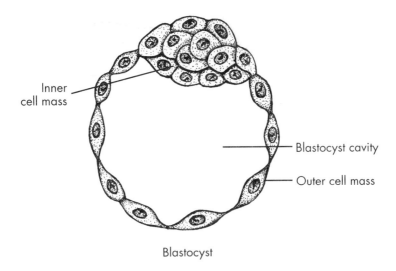

Inner
cell mass

Blastocyst cavity

Outer cell mass

Blastocyst

FIG. 2-11.   Blastocyst. A blastocyst cavity is formed, and the inner cell mass, forming the surrounding membranes, and part of the placenta are developing.

derm layer. The inner layer of epithelial cells will be replaced eventually by cells from the ectoderm layer and become the **entoderm.** Later, more cells of the ectoderm layer work their way in between these two layers and become the **mesoderm** or middle layers. All the other cells of the body develop from these three layers. Different kinds of epithelium may come from any one of these three basic embryonic layers—the skin from the ectoderm, the epithelium of the digestive tract from the entoderm, and the squamous lining of the abdominal and thoracic cavity and the inner lining of blood vessels from the mesoderm (Fig. 2-12). Glands generally arise from either the ectoderm or entoderm.

CONNECTIVE TISSUE

The term *connective tissue* seems self-explanatory in that it implies that tissue connects parts of the body together, and to some extent this description is true. However, because blood is classified as a component of connective tissue, this definition can be confusing. All the various types of connective tissues originate from mesoderm. Connective tissues can be divided into the categories of general connective tissue and more specialized connective tissue, such as cartilage, bone, and blood.

General Connective Tissue

General connective tissue comprises cells, fibers, the fluidlike material referred to as <u>ground substance,</u> and a filtrate of blood plasma called *extracellular fluid.* Connective tissue is subdivided into irregular connective tissue, which is found primarily beneath epithelium, and regular connective tissue, such as **tendons** and **ligaments.**

Irregular connective tissue

If we examine some epithelia, such as the skin on an arm, we can feel that it is quite movable. Epithelium has no blood vessels, and yet its cells are active and therefore must have a nutrient source somewhere. The irregular connective tissue immediately below the skin serves as this source. Besides the cells, fibers, and ground substance, irregular connective tissue also contains

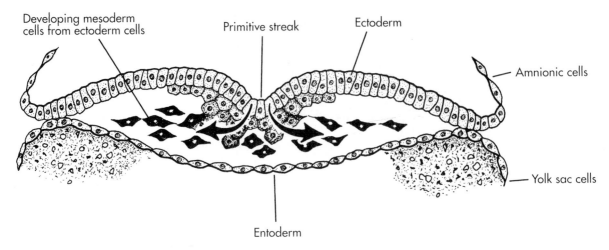

FIG. 2-12. Cross section through a flat plate of cells of a 16-day embryo. There are three germ layers and mesoderm originating from downgrowth of the ectoderm through a central area of primitive streak.

nerves and blood vessels that supply the area (Fig. 2-13). There are many different types of connective tissue cells, but for our purposes one of the most important cells is the **fibroblast.** The suffix *blast* means "sprout." Therefore the word *fibroblast* refers to one of the cells that sprouts or forms fibers. These are known as **collagen** fibers. They are nonelastic and function by holding the epithelium to the underlying muscles or bone, holding bones together, or attaching muscles to bone. The collagen fiber is also the fiber that attaches the tooth to its socket. We will also see later that collagen fibers can be formed by cells that produce bone, cartilage, dentin, and cementum. There are numerous varieties of collagen fibers, each with a Roman numeral designation. The most common one in irregular connective tissue is designated **Type I collagen.**

Another type of cell found in the connective tissue is a primitive cell of mesodermal origin called the **mesenchymal cell.** This is the first cell seen when mesoderm develops in the early embryo. This cell has the potential of changing into a number of other cell types that produce bone,

cartilage, muscle, and fibroblasts. The presence of mesenchymal cells in the tissue allows for the replacement of some components of connective tissue that are lost through injury.

There are cells present in the connective tissue that produce antibodies to fight off or resist certain microorganisms or foreign substances entering the body. The most common of these is the tissue lymphocyte, which is virtually the same as the lymphocyte that travels in circulating blood. These lymphocytes are designated as either **B-lymphocytes** or **T-lymphocytes.** The B-lymphocyte originates from bone marrow and then passes to many lymphoid organs, such as the spleen, lymph nodes, and others, where they multiply. When stimulated antigenically by foreign substances, they duplicate and enlarge to form **plasma cells,** which secrete **antibodies.** T-lymphocytes also originate from bone marrow but then migrate to the **thymus gland** and multiply there to form cells that have numerous functions. The most common of these functions is to combat virus-infected cells, various tumors, and grafted tis-

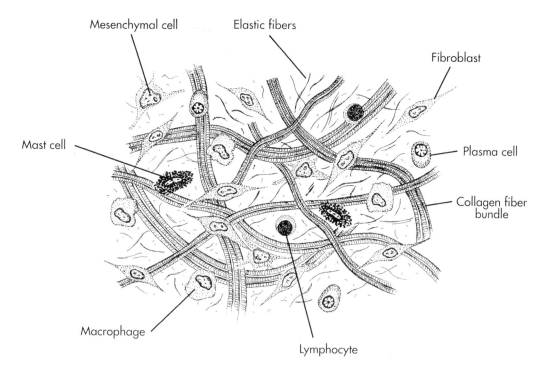

FIG. 2-13. Irregular connective tissue with fibroblasts, collagen fibers, and other cells and fibers of connective tissue. Invisible ground substance holds it all together.

sues and organs. These cells therefore have to be destroyed or have their function suppressed by chemotherapeutic agents before one can transplant tissues or organs. If they are not destroyed, the T-lymphocytes will attack the newly transplanted tissues and cause them to be rejected.

Other cells, called **macrophages,** act as scavengers and devour dying cells and microorganisms. Because of their function macrophages contain lysosomes, the scavenger organelle found in many cells (see p. 20). Macrophages may be fixed in certain areas or may be capable of wandering freely throughout the connective tissue.

Another type of cell that is found in varying quantities within connective tissue is the **fat cell** or **adipocyte.** They can be found in large quantities in the bottom layers of connective tissue. Areas like the abdomen, the gluteal region, and the thighs can accumulate large quantities of fat cells.

In addition to these cells found within connective tissue, there are also other fibers. One, a **reticular fiber,** primarily functions as a framework for a number of organs. This reticular fiber is formed by a cell that looks virtually identical to a fibroblast. Another fiber is an **elastic fiber,** which stretches and then returns to its original length. The elastic fibers found beneath skin are depleted with age, and the results can readily be seen in bags under the eyes and wrinkles in the face because it is most easily visualized in areas of thin skin such as the face.

Irregular connective tissue is so named because its fibers run in all directions. It is further subdivided into loose irregular connective tissue and dense irregular connective tissue. The former primarily contains reticular fibers, elastic fibers, lymphocytes, and plasma cells, as well as the cells already discussed. Dense irregular tissue, however, replaces most other types of fibers with coarse bundles of collagen fibers.

The third major component of connective tissue, the ground substance, is a gluelike substance that holds the cells and fibers together. This is supplemented with varying amounts of gel-like water found as intercellular fluid, which is a filtrate of blood plasma. The gel consistency results from several groups of combinations of proteins and carbohydrates called **proteoglycans** and **glycoproteins.**

Regular connective tissue

The term *regular connective tissue* simply means that the collagen fibers run parallel with one another with fibroblasts squeezed between them. Regular connective tissues are found as tendons, which attach muscle to bone, and ligaments, which attach bone to bone. The collagen fibers are arranged in parallel rows with fibroblasts aligned between the rows. The presence of fibroblasts indicates the ability for tendons or ligaments to repair themselves much of the time. If either is completely torn, then surgery is required.

Special Connective Tissue

Let us now consider the somewhat more specialized components of connective tissue—cartilage, bone, and the blood vascular system.

Cartilage

Cartilage is a noncalcified supporting component of the body, although sometimes cartilage does calcify in areas such as the larynx. It is composed of cells called **chondroblasts** or **chondrocytes,** fibers of either collagen or **elastin,** and a ground substance. There are three types of cartilage—**fibrocartilage, elastic cartilage,** and **hyaline cartilage.**

Fibrocartilage contains a great deal of collagen fibers and functions as a cushioning substance. It is found in areas such as intervertebral discs between vertebrae of the spinal column and, in the adult, the temporomandibular joint of the jaw.

Elastic cartilage contains elastic fibers, and the cartilage is therefore very flexible. It is found in the firm but flexible part of the ear as well as in the epiglottis over the larynx and in the septum of the nose.

The third type, hyaline cartilage, is firmer than the other two and contains smaller amounts of collagen fibers. It can be seen in an adult in such areas as the larynx, trachea, and certain parts of bones. During a person's development from the embryonic stage into adulthood, many of the areas that originate as hyaline cartilage later change into bone. It is also this hyaline cartilage that allows the bones of the arms and legs to lengthen. One significant characteristic about cartilage is that it grows in two ways. First, it grows by adding to its surface, which is known as **apposition** or **appositional growth.** Cartilage is surrounded by a double layer of tissue known as **perichondrium** (meaning "around the cartilage"). The outer layer is composed of collagen fibers, and the inner layer contains cells that become chondroblasts and form cartilage. This layer is what causes appositional growth. Second, the chondrocytes found inside the cartilage undergo cell division and enlargement and cause growth from within. This is known as **interstitial growth.** If it were not for this process of interstitial growth, it would not be possible for long bones of the body to grow in length.

Bone

We know that bone is a hard substance, but what makes it hard? Bone is made up of cells called **osteoblasts** (meaning "bone formers") or **osteocytes** (meaning "bone cells") as well as collagen fibers and ground substance. Bone also has microscopic crystals of a substance called hydroxyapatite. These crystals of calcium and phosphates are found packed into the ground substance and fibers between the cells, giving bone its hardness. If a bone is placed in an acid substance, the crystals will dissolve and only the other three components will be left. Consider the following experiment in which a chicken bone is placed in vinegar. After a few days the bone can be bent into a pretzel shape. Vinegar is acetic acid and dissolves the crystals, leaving the bone flexible.

Intramembranous formation. Similar to cartilage, bone has more than one way to form. One way is by **intramembranous bone formation** or formation within tissue. The bone forms in regular connective tissue by some of the primitive mesenchymal cells becoming osteoblast cells. These osteoblast cells are soon surrounded by a double-layered structure called **periosteum.**

The outer layer is made up of collagen, and the inner layer is made up of osteogenic cells that become osteoblasts and form more bone. This cell secretes ground substance, collagen fibers, and then hydroxyapatite crystals. The crystals grow and pack tightly together, and the forming bone hardens. Osteoblasts that get entrapped within their own matrix quit forming more bone and become known as osteocytes. These cells play a role in nutrition of bone. Most of the bone growth in the head area is of the intramembranous type (Fig. 2-14).

Endochondral formation. The second way in which bone forms is called **endochondral bone formation.** With this type of bone formation, cartilage is first formed, covered by perichondrium (see p. 32); the inner layer of the perichon-

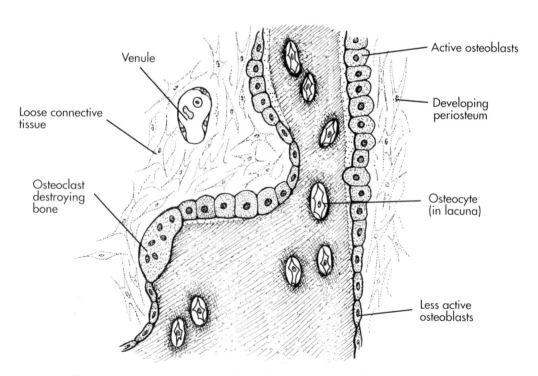

FIG. 2-14. Intramembranous bone formation. Osteoblasts secrete components and become trapped in the mix. They are then referred to as osteocytes. Space occupied by these osteocytes is referred to as *lacuna*. To the left see a multinucleated osteoclast destroying bone.

drium contains cells that become chondroblasts, which produce a cartilage model of the future bone shape. The cartilage is then invaded by bone cells, which replace the cartilage with bone (Fig. 2-15). As the bone replaces the cartilage, it does so in two end sections called the **epiphyses** and a center section, the **diaphysis.** Between each epiphysis and the diaphysis is a block of cartilage known as the **epiphyseal plate.** Within this plate there is interstitial growth of cartilage (see p. 32) that causes the plate to lengthen; then some of either side of the plate is converted to bone, and the bone therefore grows in length. Without that block of cartilage the bone would be unable to

have a directional growth. The perichondrium is eventually replaced by a periosteum. When the pituitary gland stops producing growth hormone, the epiphyseal plate disappears and the bone is no longer in three sections but unites as one. In addition to this type of growth in the long bones and vertebrae, certain important areas of the bones in the bottom of the skull also grow endochondrally, which allows for lengthening of the bones from within as well as at the bone surface.

Bone structure. Once bone has developed, it all tends to appear the same microscopically. Without studying the bone while it was developing you would not be able to determine from the

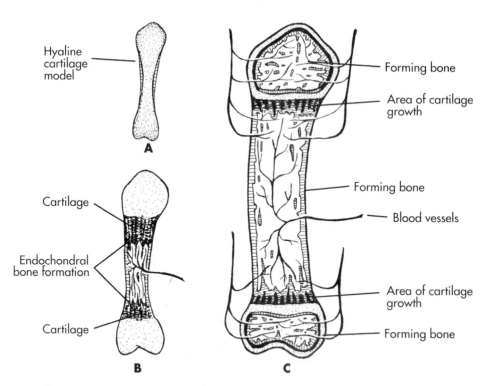

FIG. 2-15. Endochondral growth in a long bone. **A,** A cartilage model of a future long bone. **B,** Center of the model is now converted to a bony shell, and areas toward the ends are where cartilage is changing to bone and elongating. **C,** Here we see bone at either end and in the middle with a cartilage plate between them. This is where elongation of the bone takes place.

final microscopic appearance whether it developed intramembranously or endochondrally. Bone is about 50% hydroxyapatite crystals with the rest collagen, ground substance, and water. It is covered on the outside with a double layer of periosteum. As was indicated earlier, the outer layer of the periosteum is fibrous, and the inner layer is composed of cells that become osteoblasts and can form bone. In the center of bone is a cavity, generally referred to as the **marrow cavity.** This space serves as a site of blood cell production. Later in life the marrow cavity in many bones changes into storehouses for fat. The inner wall of the marrow cavity is lined by an **endosteum,** which forms modified bone on the inside during remodeling of bone-in-bone growth.

The hard structure between the periosteum and the marrow cavity, known as *cortical bone* or *plate,* has numerous blood vessels running through it to keep it vital. Around these blood vessels are gathered many trapped bone cells, referred to in their trapped state as *osteocytes.* This arrangement of blood vessels and osteocytes is called a **Haversian system** (Fig. 2-16), a series of blood vessels running parallel to one another along the length of the bone. As bone grows, these blood vessels lying on the surface of the bone go through a series of changes whereby the bone surrounds the blood vessels, resulting in a hollow tube in the bone with a blood vessel in the middle. The osteoblasts lining this tube begin to secrete bony layers and eventually entrap themselves as osteocytes. These layers continue building and fill in the tube until the blood vessel is completely surrounded. Fig. 2-16 shows the openings of these Haversian systems as circular structures known as **Haversian lamellae.** The longitudinal blood vessels of the Haversian systems are connected with other blood vessels running perpendicular to them and traveling through tubes called **Volkmann's canals** or *nutrient arteries.* These arteries interconnect with one another, bringing blood to the inside of the bone. Within the

Haversian system nutrients are passed on to the entrapped osteocytes closest to the blood vessel, and they in turn pass it on to the cells farther from the blood vessels. Blood is also carried into the marrow spaces where more blood cells are manufactured and passed out of the bone. Before the arteries reach the marrow cavity, they actually go through a capillary bed and enter the marrow cavity as venules. Therefore the endosteal lining of the marrow cavity is similar to an endothelial lining of a vein. There are then veins that carry the blood and new cells produced by the marrow cavity back out of the bone and into the venous circulation of the body and back to the heart.

The area between Haversian systems also has entrapped bone cells and layers known as **interstitial lamellae.** These are parts of older Haversian systems that have been partly destroyed and replaced by newer systems. This bone resorption and apposition is known as *bone remodeling.* Bone is also deposited on its own surface by the periosteum. These layers formed by the periosteum and lying immediately adjacent to it are known as **circumferential lamellae.** On the inside, adjacent to the marrow spaces, are layers produced known as **endosteal lamellae.**

Haversian systems are best seen in a cross section of long bones of the arms or legs (see Fig. 2-16). These same systems do exist in the flat bones and in some irregular-shaped bones of the skull. In flat bones the marrow cavities are very narrow and are known as **diploe.**

It is important that bone be nourished with blood because it is a constantly changing structure. A perfect example is orthodontic treatment. The moving of teeth is only possible because bone is able to change and remodel itself as the tooth moves. Cells called **osteoclasts** are involved in this remodeling process. The suffix *clast* means "something that destroys," and the prefix *osteo* means "bone"; thus osteoclasts are bone-destroying cells. Osteoblasts and osteoclasts work together to change bone constantly as stresses are placed on it.

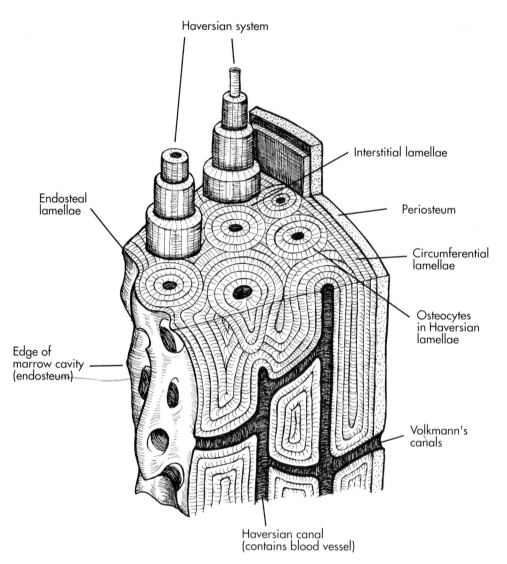

Haversian system

Interstitial lamellae

Periosteum

Endosteal lamellae

Circumferential lamellae

Osteocytes in Haversian lamellae

Edge of marrow cavity (endosteum)

Volkmann's canals

Haversian canal (contains blood vessel)

FIG. 2-16.   Section through a portion of a long bone of an extremity. To the left side would be the inner marrow cavity lined with endosteum. We can see the arteries entering the bone through Volkmann's canals and feeding into the Haversian system. Around the Haversian artery is the Haversian bone containing osteocytes. You can also see the circumferential lamellae around the outside and the interstitial lamellae representing old Haversian systems that are being replaced.

Blood

Blood is another type of special connective tissue. The arteries, veins, and capillaries that carry it, as well as the heart that pumps it, are part of the organ system known as the cardiovascular system. Blood is made up of two components: the fluid part and the cellular part. The fluid part is called plasma and is similar in composition to the fluid found between the cells of the body. The cellular part is divided into **red blood cells, white blood cells, and platelets.**

Red blood cells. Every cubic millimeter of blood contains 4.5 to 5 million red blood cells. Red cells are unusual in that they have no nucleus in their mature state. They are described as **biconcave discs,** in that they are very thin in the middle and thick at the edges. They have an iron-containing element called **hemoglobin.** Hemoglobin has the ability to attach oxygen molecules to its structure and carry them from the lungs to the cells where oxygen is needed. Hemoglobin also has the ability to carry the waste product carbon dioxide from the cell to the lung for elimination. These cells have a life span of about 4 months. They are eliminated by the spleen, located in the upper left abdominal area, when they are worn out.

Any significant decrease in the number of red blood cells, or their ability to carry oxygen, brings on a condition known as anemia. There are several types of anemia—one of them is brought on by a deficiency of vitamin B_{12} and another by a lack of iron in the body. Both of these are **acquired** deficiencies. There is also an **inherited** anemia, found primarily in African Americans, in which the red blood cell is C shaped rather than round and lacks sufficient hemoglobin. This is known as **sickle cell anemia.** Although the cause of sickle cell anemia has been found, there is still a significant death rate; we do not yet have the knowledge to prevent it.

White blood cells. There are far fewer white blood cells than red, numbering only 8000 to 10,000 per cubic millimeter of blood. White blood cells are divided into two groups by the presence or absence of granules in their cytoplasm. Those with granules are referred to as **granulocytes** and those without are **agranulocytes.**

Granulocytes. Granulocytes have three varieties based on the staining properties of their granules.

NEUTROPHILS. Of white blood cells, 50% to 70% have granules that do not stain readily and are therefore referred to as **neutrophils.** They live only about 2 days. During that time they function as **phagocytes,** killing and devouring microorganisms. When microorganisms enter the body where they are not normally found, they trigger an **inflammatory reaction.** The four signs of inflammation are redness, warmth, swelling, and pain. The redness and warmth are attributable to more blood being sent to that region; the swelling and pain are caused by an increase in **extracellular fluid.** This increase in fluid between the cells is caused by blood plasma that leaks from the smallest of blood vessels, the capillaries and venules, of the area. As the fluid leaks out of the blood vessels, so too do neutrophils. They move to the area of the invading microorganisms and begin devouring them.

EOSINOPHILS. Of white blood cells, 1% to 4% stain red with a dye known as eosin. These **eosinophils** function to help combat **allergic reactions** and inflammatory reactions.

BASOPHILS. Of white blood cells, 0.5% stain blue with a basic stain and are known as **basophils.** These cells, along with connective tissue cells known as **mast cells,** contain a substance known as **histamine,** which is released in reaction to an **allergenic** substance. Histamine causes fluid to leak from blood vessels and the local tissues to swell. To decrease this swelling we use a drug that combats this histamine reaction and is therefore known as an **antihistamine.** This combats the action of the histamines, which stops the leakage of the vessels, and the swelling decreases.

Agranulocytes. There are two types of white cells that have no granules and are therefore referred to as agranulocytes. They are the **lymphocytes** and **monocytes.**

LYMPHOCYTES. Of white blood cells, 20% to 40% are lymphocytes. They are found in the circulating blood and in **lymphoid tissues** such as lymph nodes, the spleen, and the tonsils. There are two different types of lymphocytes, both having to do with providing **immunity**. One of these lymphocytes produces a cell known as a plasma cell, also associated with immune responses and seen readily in tissue where there have been long-lasting infections.

MONOCYTES. Of white blood cells, 2% to 8% are monocytes. Monocytes become macrophages in acute inflammation. In such cases, neutrophils, lymphocytes, and monocytic macrophages can all be found within the inflamed tissues. Monocytes fuse together in mitotic multiplication and are believed to form osteoclasts, which are large, multinucleated cells that destroy bone and other hard tissues of the body such as dentin, cementum, and possibly enamel.

During the disease process, the number of white blood cells increases, particularly neutrophils and lymphocytes. **Leukemia** is a disease of white blood cells in which one type of white cell starts multiplying rapidly, choking out the production of red blood cells. Most blood cells are produced in bone marrow, as well as in the spleen, thymus, lymph nodes, and tonsils, where lymphocytes are formed. We frequently read of persons who have bone-marrow transplants. They are first treated with drugs that kill their own defective marrow and then receive new marrow, which should produce a normal blood cell population.

Platelets. There are 250,000 to 350,000 platelets per cubic millimeter of blood. Platelets are a membrane-bound particle of a larger cell called a **megakaryocyte,** which is found in bone marrow. These platelets play an important role in the clotting of blood. When platelets reach a broken blood vessel, they may break and release a substance called **serotonin,** which causes blood vessels to contract, similar to other **vasoconstrictors** such as **epinephrine** that are used in dental anesthetic agents. Other platelets simply stack up in the leakage area and begin forming what

will eventually be a blood clot. Today there is a process known as **pheresis,** in which blood is removed from a donor's arm, run through a centrifuge, which separates out the platelets, and run back into the donor's other arm. This provides the platelets that are necessary for leukemia patients who have clotting problems. Platelets exist for only 8 or 9 days, so they are replaced generally within 72 hours. It is possible to be a pheresis donor more than once a week. Contact your nearest hospital or American Red Cross unit about becoming a pheresis donor. Unlike blood donations, pheresis does not weaken you, and you can go on with fairly regular exercise.

MUSCLE TISSUE

The third basic tissue, muscle, is found throughout the body. There are three types of muscle tissue—skeletal, cardiac, and smooth. All muscle tissue, through its contraction, or shortening in length, accomplishes work.

Skeletal Muscle

The most widely studied muscle is skeletal muscle, also known as striated **voluntary muscle.** The term *striated* refers to the striped appearance of the muscle fibers under a microscope. The word *voluntary* means that the contraction, or shortening, of the muscles is under the willful control of the person or animal. A skeletal muscle, such as the biceps in the upper arm, is made up of thousands of individual muscle fibers, or muscle cells. Each of these skeletal muscle cells has not just one but hundreds of nuclei. This cell is referred to as a **myofiber.** The myofiber runs the full length of the muscle. (To avoid confusion it should be noted that there are various muscle shapes, and some muscles have tendons positioned throughout. Therefore a muscle fiber may run into a tendon and not really run the full length of the apparent muscle; in some instances it may be an inch long, while in other muscles it may be several feet long.) Each fiber is made up of many smaller cell components called **myofibrils.** Between the myofibrils are the usual components of

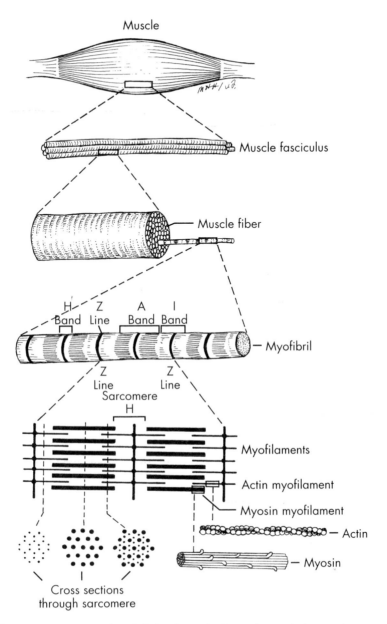

FIG. 2-17.   Entire realm of skeletal muscle tissue, from whole muscle to components of sarcomere. Thin and thick filaments slide over one another in contraction.

cells, such as the mitochondria and endoplasmic reticulum. These myofibrils also have the striated appearance indicative of skeletal muscle. It was originally believed that myofibrils were the smallest component of muscle and that for muscle to contract it was necessary for these myofibrils to shorten. Later it was discovered that myofibrils are made up of two smaller **myofilaments** called **actin** and **myosin.** The thinner actin filaments slightly overlap the thicker myosin filaments, and a chemical reaction causes the two filaments to slide over one another. The overall fiber shortening takes place by this sliding mechanism. This whole process is repeated hundreds of times in a single myofibril. There are hundreds of light and dark staining bands in a fibril. The light band is called the **I band,** and the dark band is called the **A band.** Halfway through the I band is a thin dark line called the **Z line.** The distance between two Z lines is called a **sarcomere,** and within one sarcomere are all the components necessary for this sliding filament mechanism of skeletal muscle. Therefore the sarcomere is the functional unit of skeletal muscle (Fig. 2-17).

Cardiac Muscle

Heart muscle or cardiac muscle is referred to as striated **involuntary muscle,** meaning it has striping similar to the skeletal muscle. The term *involuntary* means that control of the heart is not under willful control of the individual but rather is regulated automatically by the body. Cardiac muscle differs from skeletal muscle in that it has only one or two nuclei per cell and the muscle cells or fibers branch as they meet one another (Fig. 2-18). Similar to skeletal muscle, cardiac muscle has banding, and the sarcomere is the smallest functioning unit. The heart muscle is also unusual in that it has specialized muscle cells, **Purkinje's fibers,** that act like nerves in the heart and conduct messages through the heart to help it contract or beat properly.

Smooth Muscle

Smooth muscle is the third kind of muscle tissue and is nonstriated involuntary muscle. This means that it does not have stripes and cannot be willfully controlled. These muscle fibers are found lining such areas as the digestive tract

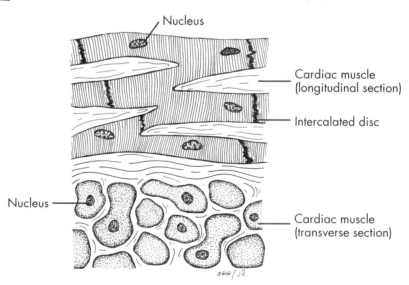

FIG. 2-18.   Cardiac muscle is striated, with branches and only one or two nuclei in each cell. The heavy dark line running across the fiber is the intercalated disc, the point at which two cells join.

(where they move the food through the tract), in blood vessels (where they regulate the flow of blood to different parts of the body), in the lungs (where they contract the air passages and alveolar sac areas), and in many other organs. Smooth muscle has actin and myosin components as is found in the other two kinds of muscle; however, these components are not regularly arranged, and as a consequence the muscle fibers do not appear striped (Fig. 2-19).

NERVOUS TISSUE

Nervous tissue serves as the communicating system of the body. Sensory or **afferent** messages are carried from the outer parts of the body toward the brain. They provide information for the brain, and it reacts accordingly. The messages leaving the brain for distant parts of the body are referred to as motor or **efferent** messages; they usually cause some kind of action to take place.

The cell of the nervous system is called the **neuron.** There are three parts to the neuron: the **cell body,** the **axon,** and the **dendrite.** A neuron functions to carry a message by sodium and potassium ions passing in and out through the cell membrane. This sets up a small electrical charge that passes along the cell wall. These changes in the polarity of the neuronal cell membrane are referred to as depolarization and repolarization. This current does not have a message in it, only a wave of electricity. It is the brain itself that converts the current to information based on the type of neuron carrying the message, where it is from, and at times the relation to a past experience. Neurons carry messages generally in only one direction. The wave of electricity passes

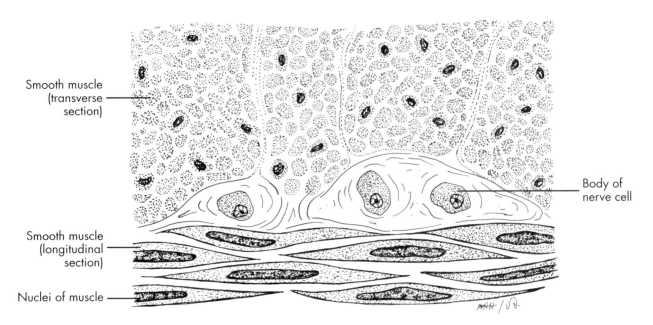

Smooth muscle (transverse section)

Body of nerve cell

Smooth muscle (longitudinal section)

Nuclei of muscle

FIG. 2-19. Smooth muscle cut in transverse (cross) section and longitudinal section. Notice that nuclei are in the center and the fiber is only as wide as the nucleus. Also notice the elongation of smooth muscle fibers.

from the dendrite to the cell body and out along the axon. When it gets to the end of the axon, it contacts the dendrite or cell body of the next neuron and passes the message or impulse to the adjacent neuron via small vesicles or droplets that are made up of **acetylcholine** or **epinephrine.** The wave of depolarization travels along that neuron until it reaches its destination. Thus there are neurons carrying messages to the brain and other neurons carrying messages away from the brain (Fig. 2-20).

Many of these nerve cells, or neurons, have a protective covering around their axons called a **myelin sheath;** therefore some nerves are referred to as **myelinated** nerves. This myelin sheath plays a very important role in some nerves. The

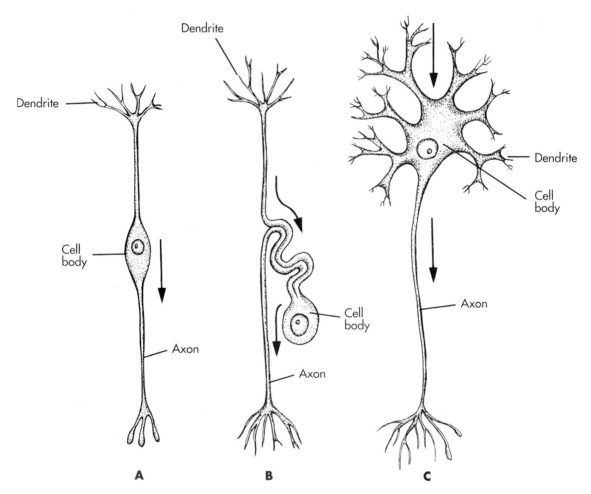

FIG. 2-20.   Some different shapes of neurons. A, Bipolar. B, Pseudo unipolar neuron. C, Multipolar neuron. Multipolar is most commonly found. The impulse passes from dendrites and the cell body down along the axon to meet with another neuron.

size of the axon and degree of myelinization controls the speed at which the message travels along the nerve. Another role it plays is in regeneration of damaged nerves. For example, consider a lower tooth extraction in which the lip and jaw in that area are numb after surgery. In many instances the numbness disappears after a period of time. Following is a simplified explanation of what may occur.

The dendrite is injured and part of it may die. When it dies, it breaks down but may leave portions of the protective myelin sheath cells in place. The nerve, or more accurately the dendrite or axon, regrows down this re-forming tube until it reaches the point where it once supplied sensation; then the numbness disappears. If the myelin sheath is damaged, there is a good possibility that when the dendrite starts to regenerate, it will be unable to locate the old area, which will remain numb.

Neurons are found in the nerves that run out into the body as well as in the spinal cord and brain. Most nerves have neurons carrying messages both ways. Frequently it takes two or three neurons in a chain to relay the message to the brain and another two or three to transfer it from the brain back to the various parts of the body.

See Chapter 19 for additional discussion on the nervous system.

Review Questions

1. Name the organelles of the cell and their general functions.
2. What is pinocytosis?
3. What is the difference between cell organelles and cell inclusions?
4. What is the function of the cell membrane?
5. Define epithelium.
6. Which is the most common type of epithelium?
7. How do the epithelial cells arise in skin, and what happens to them?
8. What are desmosomes?
9. Where do glands come from?
10. How are glands classified?
11. Name the embryonic germ layers. Which layer or layers does epithelium come from?
12. What forms from the outer cell mass and inner cell mass of the blastocyst?
13. Name the components of general irregular connective tissue.
14. How do cartilage and bone differ?
15. What makes bone hard?
16. What is a Haversian system?
17. What are the components of endochondral bone development?
18. What are the divisions of blood cells?
19. What are the functions of each of the white blood cells and platelets?
20. Where do we find hemoglobin, and what is its function?
21. Name the three types of muscle tissue and give examples of their locations.
22. Define or describe the following:
    a. Myofiber
    b. Myofibril
    c. Myofilament
23. What is a sarcomere?
24. How does skeletal muscle contract?
25. What are the parts of a neuron?
26. Define afferent and efferent.
27. What is a myelin sheath?
28. What is the role of the myelin sheath in nerve regrowth?
29. In what direction does a current or message travel in a neuron?

CHAPTER 3

DEVELOPMENT OF OROFACIAL COMPLEX

OBJECTIVES

* To list the developmental stages of the human from fertilization to birth
* To list the embryonic structures that form the face and discuss the approximate age of formation
* To discuss the mechanism involved in the development of the upper lip
* To name the structures involved in the formation of the palate and the timing of its development
* To describe the mechanism involved in the development of the palate
* To describe the other structures arising from the pharyngeal arches
* To discuss the embryonic structures involved in the development of the cleft lip and palate

EMBRYOLOGIC STAGES

From the time of fertilization of the ovum until full-term development is reached, the developing human goes through the following stages:
1. Fertilization through 2 weeks is the period of the ovum.
2. Weeks 3 through 8 is the period of the embryo.
3. Weeks 9 through 36 is the period of the fetus.

During the period of the ovum, the cells are differentiating into the tissues that will form the three germ layers of the body, the ectoderm, mesoderm, and entoderm, as well as the surrounding membranes that protect and nourish the human as it develops.

PREFACIAL EMBRYOLOGY

One can begin to see the early features of the face developing by the embryonic age of 3 weeks. By that time the embryo has gone from a flat, disclike structure consisting of the three germ layers to an elongated structure with a developing spinal cord and brain and a body wall. The body is relatively hollow with the exception of a tube closed at its upper and lower ends and running through the middle of the body cavity whose lining has developed from entoderm. This tube is the developing digestive tract and is divided into three parts. The upper part is the **foregut,** which forms the digestive tube from the throat region to the duodenum. The middle portion is the **midgut,** which forms the rest of the small intestine as well as the cecum, ascending colon, and most of the transverse colon. The lower portion is the **hindgut,** which forms the descending colon, sigmoid colon, and rectum of the large intestine.

By the time the embryo is about 3 weeks old, its length measures approximately 3 to 4 mm from the top of the head to the tail area. Even at that small size, the forerunners of the structures that will become the face can be seen. Fig. 3-1 is a lateral view of the embryo, and several important features can be seen. There is the umbilical cord (shown cut here), which attaches the embryo to the placenta embedded in the wall of the uterus. The heart bulge appears as it does because it develops in an extremely anterior position and pushes out on the upper body wall, which will later become the thorax. As the thorax and ribs develop, the heart will assume a position inside the thoracic cage and will no longer bulge outward. Finally, there are three ridges of tissue visible, the **pharyngeal arches,** which can be seen bulging out laterally. The pharyngeal arches seen in Fig. 3-1 are actually U-shaped bars of tissue. The open end of the U faces posteriorly and surrounds the upper end of the foregut and part of the primitive oral cavity. Eventually six of these arches will develop. The fifth one, however, will degenerate and form nothing of any consequence. The fourth and sixth arches are poorly developed and are not readily seen on the embryonic surface. The ones closest to the head are the largest, and those farther down are smaller in size.

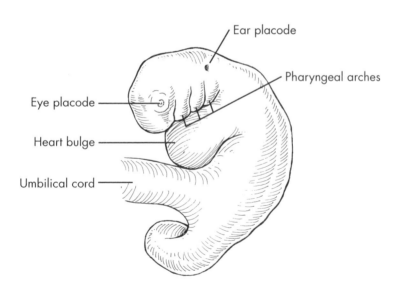

FIG. 3-1.   Lateral view of a 3- to 4-week-old embryo showing cardiac bulge, three pharyngeal arches, and a developing eye and ear.

For a better understanding of the structure of these pharyngeal arches it is necessary to look at a longitudinal section through the embryo, which is divided into equal halves (Fig. 3-2). Although Fig. 3-2 shows only the upper half of the embryo, you can see the foregut with the tube still closed at the top and bottom. Eventually, at about 4½ weeks, the upper end of the tube breaks down and connects with the primitive oral depression known as the **stomodeum** and forms the oral cavity and oral pharynx. At about 6 to 7 weeks, the bottom end of the tube breaks down and becomes the anal and urethral openings. The point in Fig. 3-2 where the foregut region and the stomodeum share a common wall is known as the **buccopharyngeal membrane.** This membrane is found in the location that will become the region between the palatine tonsils and an area about two thirds of the way back from the tip of the tongue. When the buccopharyngeal membrane breaks down at about 4½ weeks, the connection between the oral cavity and the digestive tract is established.

FACIAL DEVELOPMENT

The upper two pharyngeal arches, numbered with Roman numerals I and II, are also known respectively as the **mandibular** and **hyoid arches.** First, the mandibular arch begins to show growth from the upper surface of the posterior end of the arch, which will be the maxillary process. When that begins to happen, it can be subdivided into **mandibular processes** below and **maxillary processes** above (Fig. 3-3). The mandibular processes will form the mandible, and the maxillary processes will form the maxillae, the zygomatic bones of the cheek, and the palatine bones, which form the hard palate in the roof of the mouth. The maxillae also comprise the upper jaw.

In the anterior (frontal) view of a 3-week embryo, notice the forehead area, known as the **frontal prominence,** the stomodeum (primitive oral cavity), and the mandibular processes of the mandibular arch (Fig. 3-4). During the fourth embryonic week some changes can be seen. First, two small depressions form low on the frontal prominence; these are the **nasal pits,** the begin-

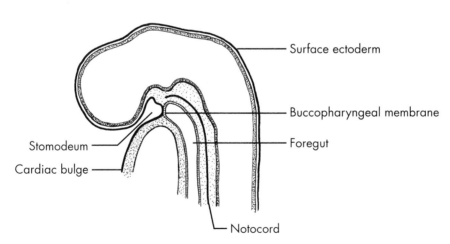

FIG. 3-2.   Longitudinal section through a 3-week embryo. Note the relationship between the stomodeum, the buccopharyngeal membrane, and the foregut.

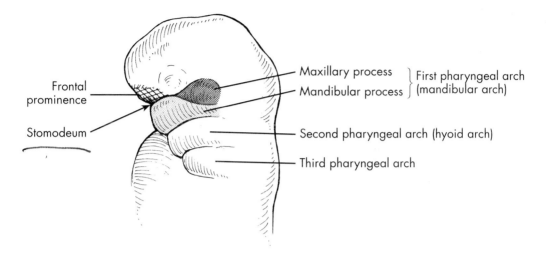

FIG. 3-3.   Lateral view of a 3-week embryo. Note the frontal prominence of the forehead region and the first three pharyngeal arches. Also observe that the mandibular arch is now divided into maxillary and mandibular processes.

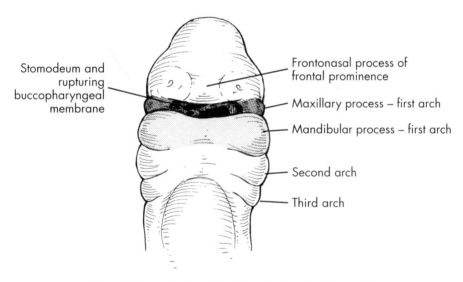

FIG. 3-4.   Frontal view of a 3-week embryo. Note that the maxillary process is barely visible.

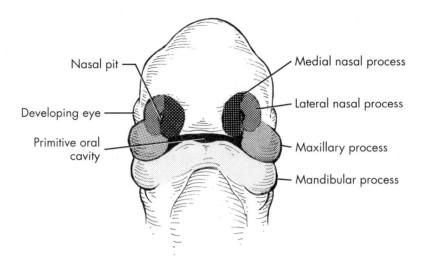

Nasal pit

Developing eye

Primitive oral cavity

Medial nasal process

Lateral nasal process

Maxillary process

Mandibular process

FIG. 3-5. Four-week embryo. The lower end of the frontal prominence has divided into medial and lateral nasal processes. Also there is forward growth of the maxillary process.

ning of the nasal cavities. The areas on either side of these nasal pits begin to form a ridge and become the **medial** and **lateral nasal processes** (Fig. 3-5). From the side of the head notice that the maxillary processes are starting to enlarge slightly and seem to be growing toward the midline. By the sixth week the two medial nasal processes have fused together and, along with the two maxillary processes, have formed the upper lip (Fig. 3-6). The lateral nasal process takes no part in forming the upper lip. It gets pushed up and out of the way. Also about this time the nasal pits deepen until they open into the primitive oral cavity at about 6 weeks (Fig. 3-7).

The medial nasal and maxillary processes begin to fill in the groove that lies between them. There is an increase in the connective tissue of the upper lip in the area of the groove, and the groove fills in and slowly disappears. This process is known as **migration.** If this migration fails, the tissues will be stretched and will break down as development continues, resulting in a separation between the medial nasal process and

maxillary process known as a **cleft lip.** If this occurs, it takes place by about the sixth embryonic week. If the two medial nasal processes do not fuse together, the result is a midline cleft of the upper lip referred to as a **hare lip** because it resembles the cleft in the upper lip of a rabbit.

PALATAL DEVELOPMENT

The formation of the palate or roof of the mouth involves the same processes: the right and left maxillary processes and the medial nasal processes. The medial nasal processes form a block of tissue that includes the area of the maxillary central and lateral incisors as well as a small V-shaped wedge of tissue lingual to these teeth back to the **incisive foramen.** This is known as the **primary palate** or **premaxilla** (Fig. 3-8). The medial nasal processes also help to form the nasal septum, the wall that divides the nasal cavity into right and left halves.

The remainder of the hard and soft palate develops from the maxillary processes. This action

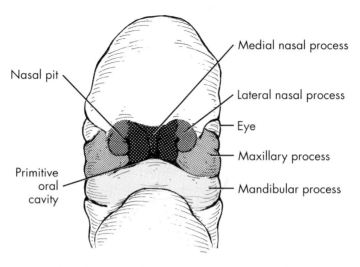

FIG. 3-6.   Six-week embryo. Medial nasal processes and maxillary processes are filling in the groove to form the upper lip.

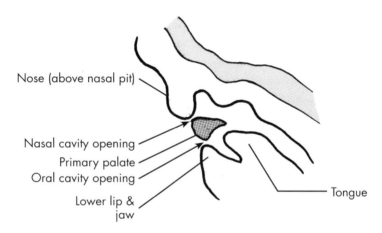

FIG. 3-7.   Sagittal section through the head at the nasal pit area during the sixth week of development showing the nasal pit opening into the primitive nasal cavity area. There is only one chamber for oral and nasal cavities at this time.

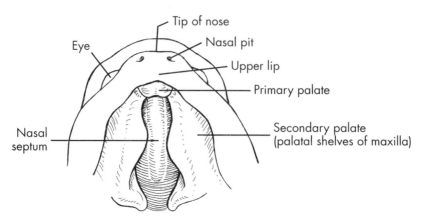

FIG. 3-8.   Inferior view of the primitive oral cavity of a 7-week embryo. Note the V-shaped growth of the primary palate (premaxilla) and the beginning growth of the palatal processes of the maxillae.

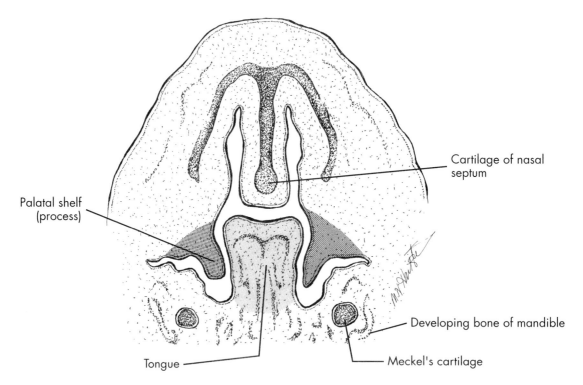

FIG. 3-9.   Frontal section of an 8-week embryo. The palatal processes are trapped beneath the tongue.

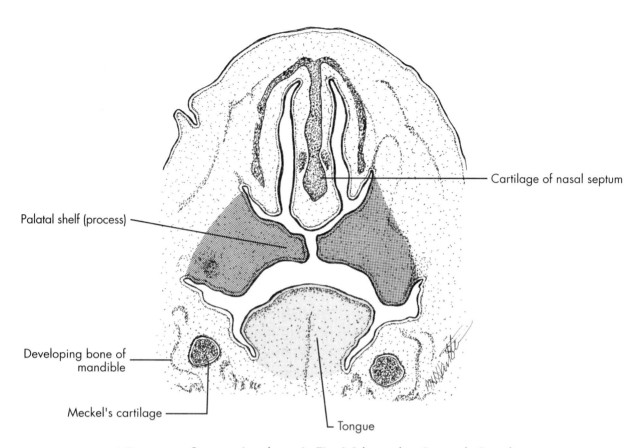

Cartilage of nasal septum

Palatal shelf (process)

Developing bone of mandible

Meckel's cartilage

Tongue

Fig. 3-10.   Same section shown in Fig. 3-9 but at late 8 or early 9 weeks. Note the downward movement of the tongue and the palatal processes now in a horizontal position contacting the nasal septum.

begins at about week 6½ to 7 with the growth of the medial nasal processes into the primary palate. Small ledges of epithelial-covered tissue start to grow inward from the maxillary processes and form the **palatal shelves** or the palatal processes of the maxillae. As they grow in, they tend to become trapped beneath the developing tongue (Fig. 3-9). However, at this time the face is growing in a downward and forward direction, and the tongue moves down, pulling out from between the palatal processes. The palatal

shelves move into a horizontal position and come into contact first with the primary palate and then, more posteriorly, with each other and the downward growing nasal septum (Fig. 3-10).

What occurs next is the breakdown of the contacting epithelial layers of the palatal shelves because of the influence of chemicals produced by the epithelial cells. When this happens, the connective tissue beneath the epithelium on either palatal shelf flows together and fuses. This process is referred to as **fusion.** However, if this

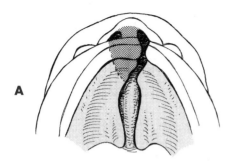
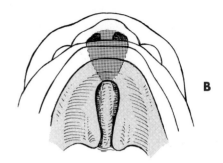

Fig. 3-11.   **A,** Cleft lip and palate formed during the seventh or eighth week. **B,** Cleft palate probably formed during the eighth or ninth week. Note the difference in the extent of the clefts.

area is viewed microscopically, one can see that not all of the epithelial cells break down; rather, a few of them remain embedded in the connective tissue. These cells are referred to as **epithelial rests.** It is possible that at a later time these clumps of epithelial cells will begin to multiply and form a sac of cells known as a **cyst,** which is generally filled with fluid. If the cyst develops along the fusion line of the two palatal shelves, it is in the midline of the palate and is known as a **median palatine cyst.** If it develops along the lines of fusion between the primary palate and the palatal shelves, it is known as a **globulomaxillary cyst.** This cyst lies between the maxillary lateral incisor and canine. It may grow and distort the tissues around it, possibly causing the teeth to be pushed out of alignment, and it generally should be removed.

The two maxillary processes fuse with the primary palate during the seventh to eighth week and then fuse with one another, first in the anterior region and then moving backward, like a zipper being zipped from front to back. This process is completed by about the eleventh week. If a **cleft palate** is going to develop, it will begin somewhere between the seventh and the eleventh week. If it occurs early, the entire palate will be open or cleft; if it happens near the eleventh

week, only the soft palate or the uvula will be affected (Fig. 3-11).

Cleft Lips and Palates

A combined cleft lip and palate occurs in about 1:700 births for whites in the United States. It is more frequent in Asians, at about 1:350, but lower in blacks, at about 1:1400. It is interesting to note that in clefts involving only the palate and not the lip the ratio is about the same for all races, 1:2500.

The two most common types of cleft lips are the unilateral and bilateral clefts. A unilateral cleft lip is the lack of connective tissue migration between one maxillary process and the fused medial nasal process. A bilateral cleft lip is the lack of connective tissue migration between both maxillary processes and the fused medial nasal process. This usually includes an outward protrusion of the midline of the lip and the primary palate, including bone (see Fig. 3-16, A and B, p. 56).

The cleft palate has similar terms. A unilateral cleft palate occurs when only one of the two palatal processes fuses with the nasal septum, resulting in an opening from the oral cavity into one side of the nasal cavity. A bilateral cleft palate exists when neither palatal process fuses with the opposing process or the nasal septum. This leaves an opening from the oral cavity into both sides of the nasal cavity (see Fig. 3-16, C). The unilateral cleft lip tends to be a parallel cleft, whereas the bilateral cleft palate tends to be a V-shaped cleft, widening at the posterior end.

The cleft lip can usually be treated surgically with good results. A cleft palate is also treated surgically as often as possible. Today the attempt by many is to get this surgery done by 18 months of age. One of the reasons for this is the fact that, if done at that early age, there is no negative recollection of the surgical treatment, and the patient is not usually traumatized by the surgery. The other is the fact that, if you wait too long and the child is interacting socially with other children or adults, the child may be teased about his or her appearance. In a recent lecture, a well-known pediatric plastic surgeon who treats cleft lips and palates and other **craniofacial deformities,** said that many people, when they see an individual with a facial deformity, associate the deformity with mental retardation or evil. This has a historical basis in a number of cultures. Of course, in most instances the deformities have no relationship to mental development, nor do they relate in any way to an evil type of personality. However, people can be cruel at times and may make fun of the individual, which can lead to psychosocial problems that can psychologically scar the affected individual for a long time. Performing a corrective operation at an early stage in life can help eliminate these problems.

After all that can be done surgically for the patient is done, and if there is still need for replacement of lost function, the maxillofacial prosthodontist may make an appliance to fill in any remaining gap in the roof of the mouth. Then a speech therapist can retrain the person in proper speech patterns.

There are some recent advances in craniofacial radiology that improve the effectiveness of treating craniofacial abnormalities. Traditionally in orthodontics we have regularly seen **lateral head films** or **cephalometric films.** We have also seen some **A-P** or **P-A films** that may be used to study various types of problem areas relating to teeth, sinuses, etc. Additionally, however, **CAT scans** or **MRI scans** are now being done with the aid of a computer and digitized information. A few years ago faculty from Washington University School of Medicine perfected a three-dimensional CAT scan. By feeding a consecutive series of scans into a computer, the resulting output is a picture that looks like a three-dimensional photograph of a bony skull, but is in reality a scan of the bony part of a human head without the soft tissues. With this technique any portion of the skull in any plane can be studied. It also allows a person performing surgery in cases of craniofacial abnormalities to take the computerized images, move them around, and come up with a picture of what the individual will look like after the surgery.

One final thing to consider in studying cleft lips and palates is the relationship between the timing of the occurrences and their potential causes. Earlier in the chapter we noted that a cleft lip develops at 3 to 6 weeks after fertilization, and the cleft palate starts at 6½ to 11 weeks after fertilization. There are hereditary factors involved in the development of clefts, and if clefts exist somewhere in a family lineage, they will occur with greater frequency in that family than in a family without that history. The other main factor is environmental; if a pregnant woman abuses various kinds of drugs, either legal or illegal, smokes heavily, drinks heavily, or is in an environment that may have potentially damaging pollutants in the air, her child may stand a greater risk of suffering birth defects such as clefts. It is also possible for a woman to expose herself to potentially harmful situations at a time when she is not yet aware that she is pregnant. Because cleft deformities develop so early, it is important that women of child-bearing age be cognizant of the dangers that might affect an unborn child.

OTHER STRUCTURAL DEVELOPMENT INSIDE THE PHARYNGEAL ARCHES

There are a number of important structures that develop from the pharyngeal arches. To understand these structures better, imagine a cut from left to right, down through the head and the pharyngeal arches (Fig. 3-12). If you remove the front half of the head and neck and view it from behind, you see a series of bulges with depressions between them (Fig. 3-13). The depressions on the neck surface are known as **pharyngeal grooves** or **clefts,** and the depressions on the inside are known as **pharyngeal pouches.** In Fig. 3-13 you can see each of the arches numbered. In each arch is a bar of cartilage, an artery, a cranial nerve, and mesodermal tissue. Additionally, specific bone, cartilage, and muscle structures will develop from each one of these arches. For example, the cranial nerve of the first arch is the fifth cranial nerve or **trigeminal nerve,** and the cranial nerve of the second arch is the seventh cranial nerve or the **facial nerve.** In later chapters on muscles of the head and neck you will read that the muscles of mastication are innervated by the fifth cranial nerve and the muscles of facial expression by the seventh cranial nerve. This tells you that the muscles of mastication arise from the first arch, and the muscles of facial expression arise from the second arch. Table 3-1 lists the pharyngeal arches, the cranial nerves involved with each arch, and the muscles, bones, and cartilages that arise from these arches.

Fig. 3-14 is a view of one side of the cut seen in Fig. 3-13. The upper groove forms the exter-

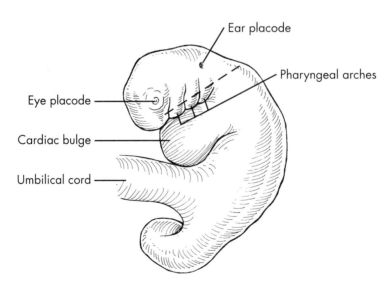

Fig. 3-12.   Duplicate of Fig. 3-1 with a dotted line marking a cut made from left to right through the pharyngeal arches.

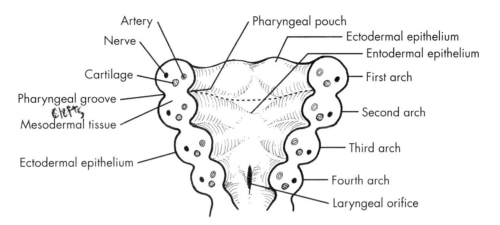

FIG. 3-13. Drawing of pharyngeal arches removed with the cut shown in Fig. 3-12 and viewed from behind showing four of the five arches. Notice external grooves and internal pouches. The *dotted line* separates the ectodermal epithelium above from the entodermal epithelium below.

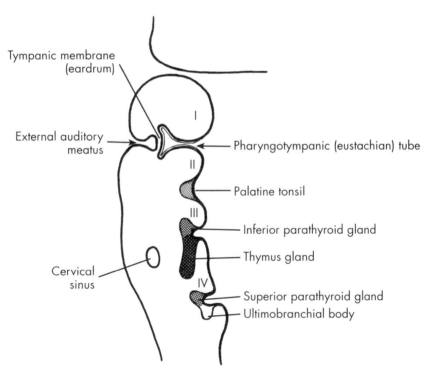

FIG. 3-14. Later view of one side of Fig. 3-13. All but the first external groove have been covered over. Notice other structures arising from pouches.

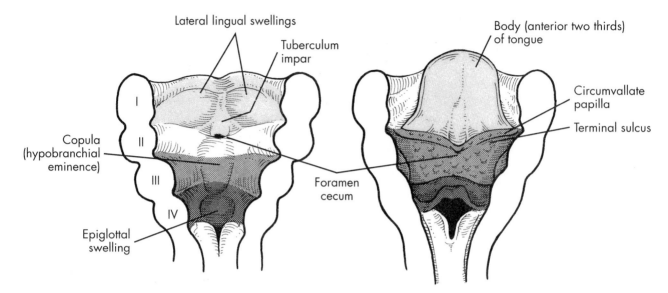

FIG. 3-15.   Various structures that go into the formation of the tongue and epiglottis.

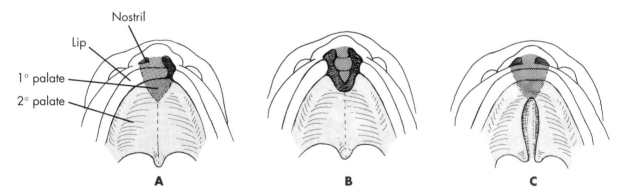

FIG. 3-16.   **A,** Unilateral cleft lip. **B,** Bilateral cleft lip. **C,** Bilateral cleft palate.

TABLE 3-1.   *Pharyngeal Arch Innervation and Arch Derivatives*

Arch	Cranial nerve(s)	Muscle(s)	Cartilage/bone
I	V	Muscles of mastication Mylohyoid Anterior digastric Tensor tympani (in ear) Tensor veli palatini	Malleus & incus bones
II	VII	Muscles of facial expression Posterior digastric Stylohyoid Stapedius (in ear)	Stapes Styloid process Lesser cornu of hyoid Upper body of hyoid
III	IX	Stylopharyngeus	Greater cornu of hyoid Lower body of hyoid
IV & VI	X (XI)	Muscles of larynx Muscles of pharynx Most muscles of soft palate	Cartilages of larynx

nal auditory meatus and one layer of the eardrum, while the upper pouch forms the inner layer of the eardrum (the primitive tympanic cavity, also known as the middle ear) and the **eustachian tube** or **auditory tube,** which leads into the back nose region or nasal pharynx. The second pouch forms the palatine tonsils, and the pouches below the palatine tonsils form some of the **endocrine glands,** such as the **parathyroid** and **thymus** glands. Looking at the middle portion of Fig. 3-15, one can see the region where the tongue and **thyroid gland** develop. In this view you can see a number of structures that go into making up the tongue, the basic ones being the **lateral lingual swellings,** the **tuberculum impar,** and the **copula.** You also can see a small depression in the middle of the tongue known as the **foramen cecum.** This is the point where the thyroid gland begins to develop and then migrates downward, eventually lying in the lower front neck region. The thyroid gland develops as any other gland develops. It starts out as a tube and grows downward with the glandular tissue developing at the

deep end of the tube. If for some reason the tube does not grow downward, the patient's thyroid gland instead forms into a big red lump at the back of the tongue and is known as a **lingual thyroid.** The thyroid gland is an endocrine gland and so eventually, after reaching its location in the neck, will lose its duct and become an endocrine gland. Sometimes it does not lose its duct system, and a thyroglossal duct remains as a source of cysts developing in the neck along the course of the duct. The timing for these structures varies somewhat, but their development takes place over several months.

One other important structure arises from this early oral cavity area. In the roof or top of the oral cavity is an upward growth of tissue that breaks loose from the oral cavity and comes into contact with a downward growth of tissue from the brain. This upward growth is known as **Rathke's pouch** and forms the anterior part of the **pituitary** gland and what is known as the pars intermedia or intermediate part of the gland. The downgrowth from the brain forms the posterior pituitary. This gland is the master control gland for many of the **hormones** of the body. For further information consult a text such as *Sandler/Langman's Medical Embryology* (see Unit II Suggested Readings).

Review Questions

1. What and when are the three embryonic stages of development?
2. During which embryonic weeks do the lips form?
3. What is the buccopharyngeal membrane, and when does it rupture?
4. Which processes form the upper lip?
5. Which processes form the hard and soft palates, and when do they form?
6. What are epithelial rests, and what might they do in later life?
7. What is a cyst, and if located in the bone of the jaw, what might it do?
8. What are unilateral and bilateral cleft lips and palates?
9. When do cleft lips and palates form?
10. What muscles arise from the first pharyngeal arch? What bones?
11. What pharyngeal arch do the muscles of facial expression arise from, and why do we know that?
12. What groups of muscles form from the IV and VI pharyngeal arches?
13. What is Rathke's pouch? Where does it come from, and what does it form?
14. What is a lingual thyroid, and why does it develop?
15. What are the differences in the mechanism between the development of the upper lip and the palate?

CHAPTER 4

DENTAL LAMINA AND ENAMEL ORGAN

OBJECTIVES
- To define dental lamina and indicate in what embryonic week it is first seen
- To define successional and vestibular laminae
- To describe bud, cap, and bell stages and the various layers found in each
- To describe dental papilla, dental sac, and their functions

DENTAL LAMINA

The first signs of tooth development are seen during the sixth embryonic week. At that time the embryonic **oral** (stratified squamous) **epithelium** begins thickening. As the epithelium thickens, it grows downward into the underlying connective tissue and does not create a visible ridge in the oral cavity at the time. This thickened oral epithelium is known as the **dental lamina.** It is a U-shaped thickening of the epithelium of the primitive oral cavity and is found in a position corresponding to the future arch-shaped arrangement of the upper and lower teeth (dental arch). This thickening does not begin all at once throughout the mouth but is first seen in the anterior midline, slowly spreading posteriorly toward the molar region

(Fig. 4-1). It takes only several weeks for this thickening to extend to the future position of the primary molars.

At about the eighth embryonic week starting at the midline and spreading posteriorly, there is a continued thickening in the dental lamina in 10 areas of the upper arch and 10 areas of the lower arch. These 20 localized thickenings correspond to the position of the future primary dentition and will form the enamel of the future teeth. However, the enamel could be affected by a condition called **ectodermal dysplasia,** in which there is poor development of structures arising from ectoderm, such as sweat, salivary, and sebaceous glands, skin, hair, and the enamel of teeth. It can also involve the white sclera of the eye, causing discoloration.

59

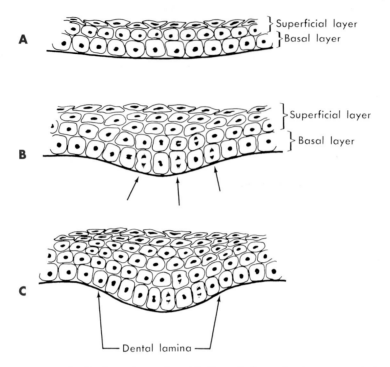

FIG. 4-1. **A,** Embryonic oral epithelium before development of dental lamina. Note the thickness of the superficial and basal layers of cells. Embryonic connective tissue lies beneath embryonic oral epithelium. **B,** Thickening of the superficial layer and multiplication of cells *(arrows)* in the basal layer. **C,** Further advancement in completed thickening of dental lamina.

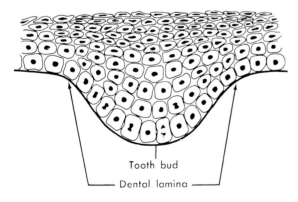

FIG. 4-2.   Bud stage. Note the further downward extension of the cells of the oral epithelium to form the bud. The stretching out of cells is still considered part of the dental lamina.

ENAMEL ORGAN

Bud Stage

The initial budding from the dental lamina at the 10 thickened areas in each arch is referred to as the **bud stage** (Fig. 4-2), the first stage in the development of the **enamel organ** that forms the enamel of the teeth. At first the buds look like blobs of cells from the dental lamina projecting deeper into the underlying connective tissue. The cells in the middle of the buds come from the outer or superficial layers of the oral epithelium, whereas the cells in the periphery of the bud come from the deep or basal layers of the oral epithelium. The buds seem to stretch out from the dental lamina as they grow. As development

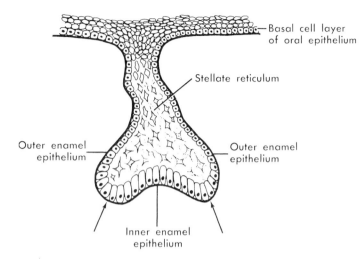

Basal cell layer of oral epithelium

Stellate reticulum

Outer enamel epithelium

Outer enamel epithelium

Inner enamel epithelium

FIG. 4-3.   Cap stage. Basal layer of the cells of the oral epithelium is continuous with the inner and outer enamel epithelium. Dividing points of IEE and OEE *(arrows)*. Stellate reticulum can be seen as a continuation of the superficial layers of the oral epithelium.

continues, the deepest parts of the buds become slightly concave. It is at this point that the developing enamel organ goes from the bud stage into the **cap stage.**

 Cap Stage

As the enamel organ moves into the cap stage it consists of the following three components: outer enamel epithelium (OEE), inner enamel epithelium (IEE), and stellate reticulum.

Outer enamel epithelium

The outermost part of the structure of the cap stage is the **outer enamel epithelium.** It is a direct continuation of the basal layer of oral epithelium. These are low columnar or cuboidal cells.

Inner enamel epithelium

The cells that outline the concavity in the deepest part of the cap stage compose the **inner enamel epithelium.** These cells are continuous with the OEE cells and also come from the basal layer of the oral epithelium.

Stellate reticulum

The cells between the IEE and the OEE compose the **stellate reticulum.** These cells origi-

nate from the superficial layers of the oral epithelium. Although they may resemble embryonic mesenchymal cells, they are really ectodermal cells, as are other parts of the enamel organ (Fig. 4-3). As the concavity of the cap grows more pronounced, enamel organ reaches the **bell stage.**

Bell Stage

The differentiation between the cap and bell stages is made when a fourth layer of epithelium, the **stratum intermedium,** appears in addition to the three already mentioned. The stratum intermedium comprises several layers of flattened squamous cells lying between the IEE and the stellate reticulum (Fig. 4-4).

As the development continues in the bell stage, two processes occur. First, the future outline or form of the crown of the tooth is determined by the way in which the cell layers expand as the enamel organ grows. Second, there are changes in the various cells, particularly the IEE cells, that will lead to the production of enamel (see also Chapter 5).

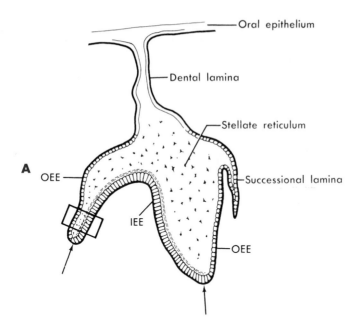

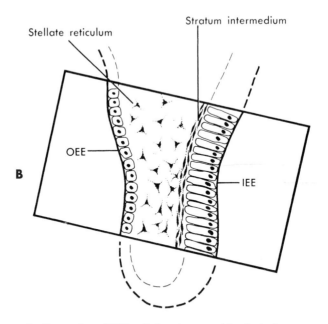

FIG. 4-4.   Bell stage. **A,** Concavity of IEE cells has increased in the bell stage. Successional lamina can be seen developing to the lingual side of the primary tooth. **B,** Enlargement of the boxed section of *A*. There are several layers of flattened cells, which are stratum intermedium, as well as IEE, OEE, and stellate reticulum.

Function of the Four Layers of the Enamel Organ

1. Basically the OEE can be considered a protective layer for the entire enamel organ. Later it will play a role in attaching the gingiva to the tooth.
2. The cells of the IEE elongate and change internally to become **ameloblasts,** which are responsible for actual enamel formation (see also Chapter 5).
3. The stellate reticulum functions as a cushioned protection for IEE cells and also plays some role in nourishment of the stratum intermedium by allowing vascular fluids to move between the loosely packed cells.
4. The cells of the stratum intermedium probably help provide nourishment for IEE cells. They are also producers of protein and may receive products from and provide products for the ameloblasts.

SUCCESSIONAL LAMINA

In the developing primary teeth the dental lamina develops an extension to the lingual side of each tooth (see Fig. 4-4). This extension is known as the **successional lamina.** Successional laminae go through a bud, cap, and bell stage just like the primary teeth and form the permanent incisors, canines, and premolars. The permanent molars develop from a posterior growth of the dental lamina and are nonsuccessional. The rate of formation will vary from tooth to tooth, with the permanent teeth developing at a much slower rate than the primary teeth.

VESTIBULAR LAMINA

The vestibular lamina is a thickening of oral epithelium in a facial or buccal direction from the dental lamina. This epithelium thickens, and then a clefting or splitting can be seen in the thickened area (Fig. 4-5). Eventually this cleft forms a groove that becomes the area of the mucobuccal or mucolabial fold in the future vestibule. If this vestibular lamina did not form, the vestibule would end at the level of the alveolar ridge, and denture construction would be very difficult or impossible.

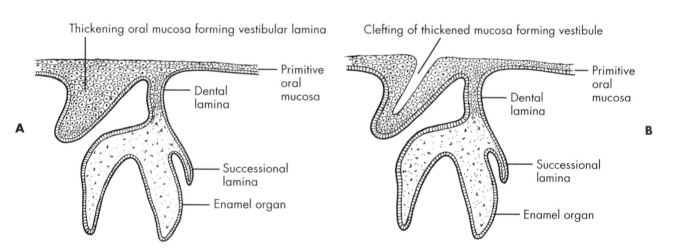

FIG. 4-5.   **A,** Thickened epithelium of future vestibule forming facial to the dental lamina. **B,** A cleft has developed in the vestibular lamina, and a vestibular fold has formed.

DENTAL PAPILLA AND DENTAL SAC

The **dental papilla** is a small area of condensed cells arising from mesoderm and located next to or deep to the IEE. It is first seen in the late bud stage and grows and becomes more pronounced as it goes through the bell stage. This structure forms the dentin and pulp of the tooth. As the development progresses from bud to bell stage, the cells of the dental papilla become more compact, and the area enlarges. It sits within the conical shape of the IEE cells and becomes very pronounced, bulging out from the enamel organ.

The nerves and blood vessels of the pulp formed by the dental papilla are first seen in the early stages of dental papilla development. They invade the early pulpal tissue, and as the rest of the tooth forms, the neural and vascular components of the pulp are already present.

The **dental sac** comprises several rows of flattened cells; they surround that part of the dental papilla not in contact with the IEE cells and also surround part of the enamel organ. Like the dental papilla, the dental sac also arises from mesoderm, and it forms the cementum of the tooth, the periodontal ligament, and some alveolar bone (Fig. 4-6).

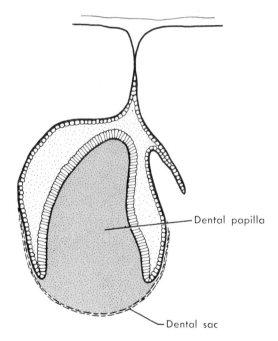

Dental papilla

Dental sac

FIG. 4-6. Condensed cells, which make up the dental papilla, as well as flattened layers of the dental sac, which surrounds part of the dental papilla and part of the enamel organ.

Review Questions

1. What is the first sign of tooth development, and when is it seen?
2. Oral epithelium is an example of what type of epithelial arrangement?
3. The enamel organ comes from what germ layer?
4. What are the stages of the enamel organ, and what general changes are taking place?
5. What is ectodermal dysplasia, and what is the significance of the origin of the enamel organ in relation to this pathologic condition? Aside from enamel, what other structures develop abnormally from this condition?
6. What are the four layers of the enamel organ as seen in the bell stage, and what is their function?
7. Define and describe the roles of the following:
    • Successional lamina
    • Vestibular lamina
    • Dental papilla
    • Dental sac

CHAPTER 5

ENAMEL, DENTIN, AND PULP

OBJECTIVES
- To discuss the changes in the inner enamel epithelial cells that allow them to become enamel-forming cells
- To discuss the interrelationship between enamel formation and dentin formation
- To describe the role of the dental papilla in the formation of the enamel organ and the shaping of the crown
- To describe the properties of enamel and the makeup of the enamel rod
- To understand the keyhole shape of the enamel rod and the direction of the hydroxyapatite crystals in different areas of the cross section of rod
- To define the following terms: *striae of Retzius, hypoplastic enamel, hypocalcified enamel, enamel lamellae, enamel tuft,* and *enamel spindle*
- To describe the properties and components of dentin
- To differentiate primary, secondary, and reparative dentin
- To define the following terms: *interglobular dentin, dead tracts, sclerotic dentin*
- To describe the components and age changes of pulp
- To describe and classify pulp stones

A CLOSE relationship exists between the formation of enamel, dentin, and pulp. Enamel develops from the enamel organ, which is derived from ectoderm, whereas dentin and pulp develop from the dental papilla, which is derived from mesoderm. The mesoderm of the dental papilla determines the shape of the developing crown of the tooth. Animal experiments have shown that if you transplant the dental papilla from an anterior tooth beneath the enamel organ of a posterior tooth, the posterior tooth will assume the shape of the anterior tooth from

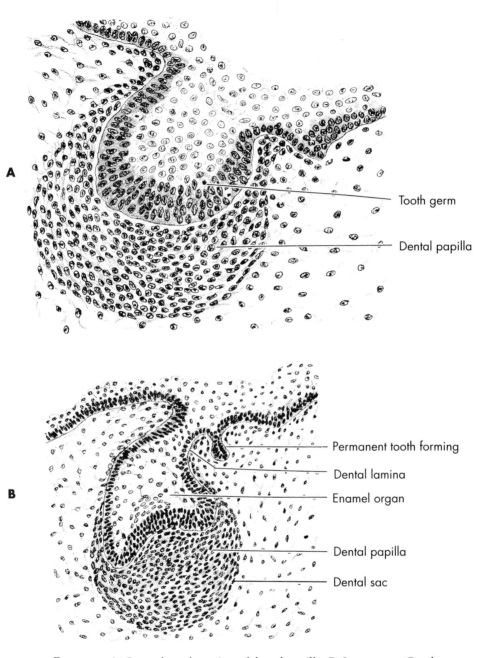

— Tooth germ

— Dental papilla

— Permanent tooth forming

— Dental lamina

— Enamel organ

— Dental papilla

— Dental sac

FIG. 5-1.   **A,** General condensation of dental papilla. **B,** Later stage. Conden-sation of the cells in dental papilla is more pronounced. (From Bevelander G: *Outline of histology,* ed 8, St Louis, 1979, Mosby.)

which the dental papilla came. Although there is an interrelationship between enamel and dentin, it is the dental papilla that has genetic control over tooth shape.

DENTAL PAPILLA

During the bud stage the cells of the embryonic connective tissue deep to the bud resemble large multipointed cells called *mesenchymal cells.* As the enamel organ goes into the cap stage, the mesenchymal cells adjacent to the cap become more rounded and condensed and are then called *dental papilla cells.* The enamel organ is also enlarging at this time (Fig. 5-1). This condensation continues into the bell stage, during which further changes occur. It is at this point that the relationship between enamel and dentin formation becomes more obvious. Following is a list of events that occur during their formation:

1. During the bell stage the inner enamel epithelial cells (IEE) become taller. They increase from 12 to 40 μm in length. These taller cells are then referred to as preameloblasts. As these cells enlarge, preparing to become secretory cells, their organelles are multiplying to prepare for this. We could expect to see more mitochondria and endoplasmic reticula, and a more obvious Golgi apparatus.
2. The peripheral cells of the dental papilla adjacent to the preameloblasts become low columnar or cuboidal cells and are called *odontoblasts* (Fig. 5-2).
3. The odontoblasts move away from the preameloblasts toward the center of the dental papilla and secrete a **matrix** of mucopolysaccharide ground substance and collagen fibers.
4. The secretion of this dentin matrix causes the preameloblast to change its polarity (the nucleus moves from the center of the cell to the end nearest the stratum intermedium). This is attributable to the change in the route of nourishment of the preameloblasts. Until

this time the nourishment had been going from the dental papilla directly to the adjacent cells. However, after the dentin matrix is laid down, it acts as a barrier between the dental papilla and the preameloblasts, and it becomes necessary for the preameloblasts to find a new route for nourishment. Vascular channels begin to penetrate the enamel organ through the outer enamel epithelium. Fluid nutrients pass to the stellate reticulum, the stratum intermedium, and then the preameloblasts. The nuclear shift of a preameloblast cell relates to the nucleus's need to be closer to the nutrient supply. With the change in polarity the cell is called an **ameloblast** and is ready to begin the secretion of enamel matrix.
5. The ameloblast lays down a matrix of mucopolysaccharide and organic fiber next to the dentin matrix, and the future **dentinoenamel junction** (DEJ) is formed. As the ameloblast secretes the matrix, it moves away from the dentin toward the outer enamel epithelium (OEE) (Fig. 5-3).
6. The dentin begins to lay down hydroxyapatite crystals and calcify (crystals begin growing).
7. The enamel begins to lay down hydroxyapatite crystals and calcify (crystals begin growing).

This process is identical for all developing teeth. It is seen first in developing anterior teeth and later in posterior teeth. It tends to be seen first in the mandibular arch slightly before the maxillary arch. Within any single tooth this type of interrelationship is first seen at the tip of the cusp of a tooth and later spreads toward the cervical line. As you look at a developing tooth, you may see enamel and dentin formation at the tip of a cusp, and yet near the cervical line the odontoblasts have not yet differentiated, and the cells of the enamel organ may still be at the IEE stage.

This development takes place in each tooth, whether primary or permanent. The permanent molars develop as a budding off of a posterior extension of the dental lamina, whereas the ante-

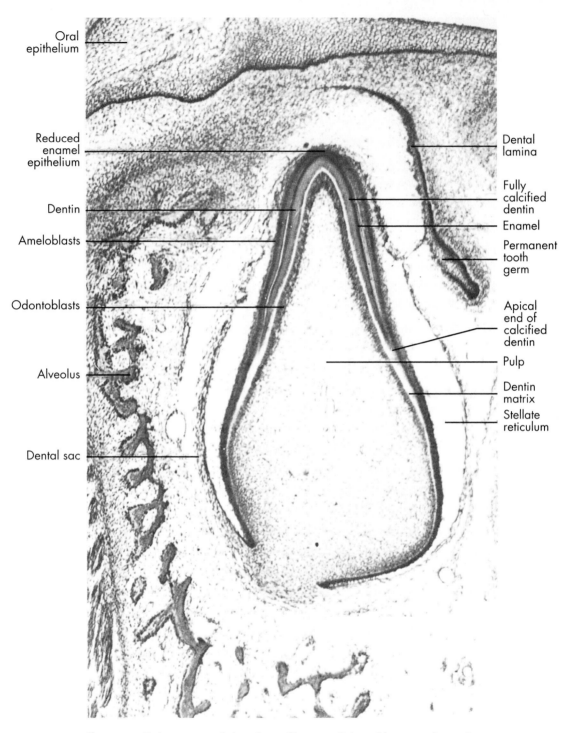

Oral epithelium

Reduced enamel epithelium

Dentin

Ameloblasts

Odontoblasts

Alveolus

Dental sac

Dental lamina

Fully calcified dentin

Enamel

Permanent tooth germ

Apical end of calcified dentin

Pulp

Dentin matrix

Stellate reticulum

FIG. 5-2. Enlargement of dental papilla area. Odontoblasts are becoming more columnar. Ameloblasts at the tip of cusps have met the outer enamel epithelium (OEE), forming reduced enamel epithelium. From Bevelander G: *Atlas of oral histology and embryology*, Philadelphia, 1967, Lea & Febiger.

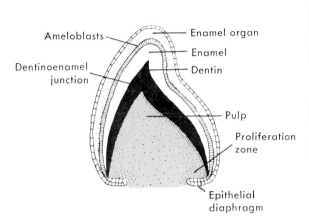

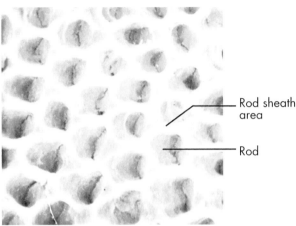

FIG. 5-3.   Beginning of dentinoenamel junction (DEJ) formation. Ameloblasts have already moved away from the DEJ in the upper section but not in the lower section. Modified from Bhaskar SN: *Orban's oral histology and embryology,* ed 10, St Louis, 1986, Mosby.

FIG. 5-4.   Rod sheath area, which surrounds the rod itself. From Bhaskar SN: *Orban's oral histology and embryology,* ed 10, St Louis, 1986, Mosby.

rior permanent teeth and the permanent premolars develop from a budding off of the dental lamina of the primary teeth developing in that position. Regardless of the tooth, the steps of development are always the same.

ENAMEL COMPOSITION

Enamel is the hardest structure of the body. It is generally white, but at times appears yellowish because of the reflection of the color of the underlying dentin. Enamel is about 96% inorganic in composition. This inorganic structure is composed of many millions of crystals of hydroxyapatite, the chemical formula of which is $Ca_{10}(PO_4)_6 \cdot (OH)_2$. The other 4% of enamel is composed of water and a fibrous organic material.

The enamel structure comprises two parts: the **rod sheath** and the **enamel rod.** The rod sheath outlines the rod and contains most of the fibrous organic substance (Fig. 5-4). However, the rod, which is made up of hydroxyapatite crystals, is the primary unit of enamel's structure. The rod is a column of enamel that runs all the way from the dentinoenamel junction to the surface

of the tooth. It is somewhat perpendicular to the dentinoenamel junction and to the surface of the crown (Fig. 5-5).

There is much debate about how the enamel rod develops. However, it is generally believed that at least three or four ameloblasts act together to form one enamel rod by laying down fibers and a matrix composed of a gluelike material called *ground substance* and depositing millions of hydroxyapatite crystals into the matrix.

The shape of enamel rods is also debatable. The enamel rods, which fit together tightly because of a cementing substance called *interrod,* are usually described as "keyhole shaped." However, they may have different appearances in various areas of enamel or because of species differences. For example, enamel rods have also been described as being round to oblong.

A "typical" enamel rod with the keyhole shape (Fig. 5-6, *A*) has a wide upper end and a narrowed bottom end. The reason for the different appearances of the upper and lower parts of the keyhole is that the crystals in those parts are oriented in different directions. When the amelo-

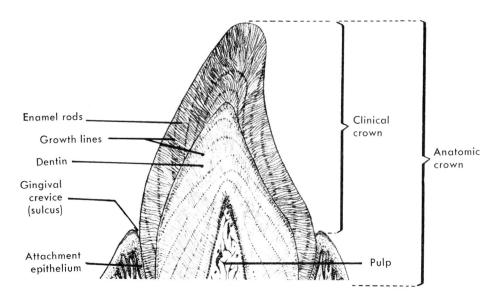

FIG. 5-5.   Notice the slight curvature of enamel rods and that the ends of the rods are perpendicular to the DEJ and outer surface of tooth. From Ham AW, Cormack D: *Histology,* ed 8, Philadelphia, 1979, JB Lippincott Co.

blasts produce the matrix and then deposit the crystals into the matrix, the secreting ends of the ameloblasts bulge outward in the direction of the DEJ. This asymmetrical bulge is called the *Tomes' process* of an ameloblast. Each ameloblast does not lie parallel to the long axis of the enamel rod but is canted at an angle. As the crystals are secreted, they emerge from the pointed part of the ameloblast in an arrangement perpendicular to the cell membrane. The result is that the crystals in the upper part of the keyhole are arranged in a pattern longitudinal to the long axis of the rod, while the crystals in the lower end are angled almost 60 degrees off of the long axis.

A cross section view of the rod shows the upper-end crystals cut vertically and the lower-end crystals cut at an angle, giving each area a distinct appearance. It was only with the advent of new microscopes and techniques that allowed study of individual crystals that there came an understanding of the differing descriptions of

enamel that had been described. Looking at the appearances of the enamel rods cut at different angles (Fig. 5-6, *B*) you can understand the controversy about enamel rod shapes.

DEVELOPMENT OF ENAMEL

As previously discussed, the ameloblasts begin to lay down a matrix and in a few days deposit millions of hydroxyapatite crystals into the small area of matrix. This is seen first at the tip of a cusp and then further toward the cervical line. It is important to remember that all the crystals that will ever be in that particular area of rod are laid down initially. This is referred to as the **mineralization stage** of enamel rod calcification (Fig. 5-7, *A*).

The second stage of calcification is called the **maturation stage** (Fig. 5-7, *B*). During this stage the crystals should grow in size until they are tightly packed together. The ameloblast produces the matrix and enamel at a rate of about 4 mm

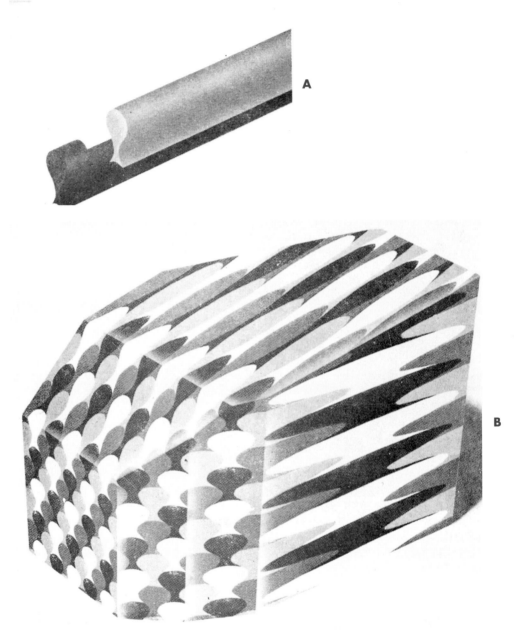

FIG. 5-6.   **A,** Three enamel rods. **B,** Groups of rods and their relation to one another. Notice how different cutting angles change appearance. (From Meckel AH, Griebstein WJ, Neal RJ: Structure of mature human dental enamel as observed by electron microscopy, *Arch Oral Biol* 10:775, 1965.)

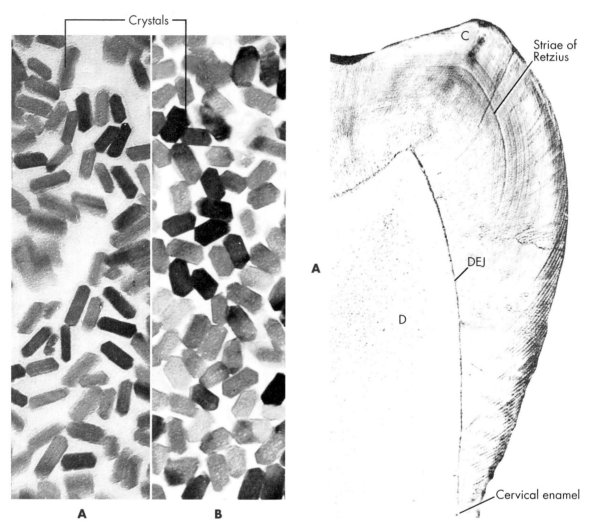

FIG. 5-7. **A,** Mineralization stage of calcification. Notice the spaces between crystals. **B,** Same magnification as *A* but showing maturation stage with crystal growth and increased density. (From Bhaskar SN: *Orban's oral histology and embryology,* ed 8, St Louis, 1976, Mosby.)

FIG. 5-8. **A,** Heavy black lines represent striae of Retzius. Notice their curving direction. *C,* cusp; *DEJ,* dentinoenamel junction; *D,* dentin. (From Provenza DV: *Fundamentals of oral histology and embryology,* ed 2, Philadelphia, 1972, JB Lippincott Co.)

Continued

per day. Every fourth day there seems to be a change in the development of the rod, and a brownish line develops in the enamel. These lines are called the **striae of Retzius** and curve outwardly and occlusally from the DEJ (Fig. 5-8). They can be seen in a longitudinal section of a tooth and can also be seen on the surfaces of a number of teeth. If you look at the labial surface of an anterior tooth you can see horizontal lines on the crown. These are known as **imbrication lines** and are surface manifestations of the striae of Retzius.

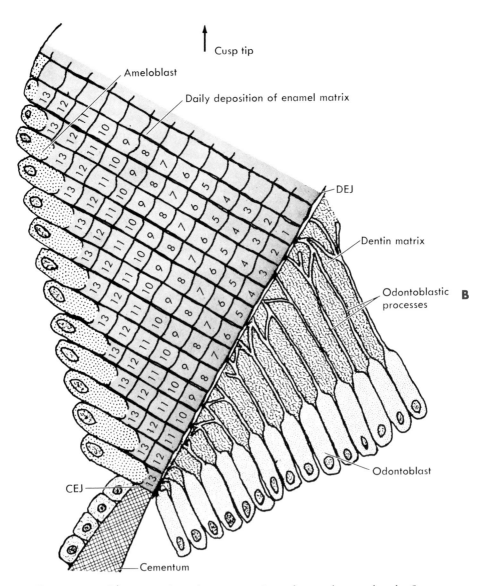

FIG. 5-8, cont'd.   **B,** Enlarged representation of several enamel rods. Segments are labeled according to the day of formation. Enamel formation is most advanced at the cusp tip. (*CEJ* = cementoenamel junction.)

FATE OF ENAMEL ORGAN

As the ameloblast moves away from the DEJ toward the OEE, it begins to compress the two layers in the middle—the stratum intermedium and the stellate reticulum. These two middle layers eventually lose their identity, and the ameloblasts contact the OEE (see Fig. 5-2). This is the signal for the ameloblasts to cease formation of enamel. The final job of the ameloblast is to lay down a protective layer over the enamel, called the **primary enamel cuticle** or **Nasmyth's membrane.** This membrane covers the crown and remains there for many months after eruption until worn away by toothbrushing and other abrasion. It is this membrane that is stained green or yellow in the newly erupted teeth of young children, particularly in the cervical one third of the crown. The stained membrane can be removed by polishing and the use of other instruments.

After the ameloblast produces the primary cuticle, it begins flattening out and blending with the outer enamel epithelial cells in what is called the **reduced enamel epithelium.** This reduced enamel epithelium produces an adhesive-like secretion called the **secondary enamel cuticle** or **epithelial attachment,** which functions to hold the gingiva to the tooth. This epithelium adheres to the tooth and is known as the **attachment epithelium.** It is found at the base of the gingival sulcus (see Chapter 7).

ABNORMALITIES OF ENAMEL

There are a number of enamel abnormalities. Some are readily seen with clinical examination, others are confirmed by radiographic examination, and still others are seen only by histologic examination of the sectioned tooth.

Hypocalcified Enamel

With **hypocalcified enamel,** spots or entire areas of the teeth appear white to whitish yellow in color. It is the result of insufficient growth of the enamel crystals or an insufficient number of crystals originally deposited in the matrix. If the crystals do not grow to full size during the maturation stage, they are not packed together tightly, and the enamel is less than 96% inorganic, causing hypocalcification or "soft teeth." Because the enamel is less dense than normal, it may decay more rapidly.

Hypoplastic Enamel

The density of **hypoplastic enamel** is generally normal, but the enamel is thin. The enamel will have a yellow to gray hue and may be seen radiographically as a thinner layer than normal enamel.

Enamel Lamellae

Cracks in the enamel caused by developmental problems or **trauma** are called **enamel lamellae.** The most common types are those caused by trauma. Clinically they appear as hairline cracks in the enamel and may extend all the way through the enamel and even into the dentin. The less common type of lamella is a developmental defect and is the result of one or more ameloblasts ceasing enamel production and thus leaving a space between other enamel rods, Providing a potential pathway through the enamel for bacteria. These are usually seen histologically and not clinically.

Enamel Tuft

A small area of hypocalcified enamel seen at the DEJ and extending about one fourth to one third of the way through the enamel is an **enamel tuft.** It is not seen clinically but only in a histologic section of tooth, and it has no great clinical significance. It is probably the result of early enamel formation at the DEJ not being complete and therefore a bit hypomineralized. There also seems to be a bit more organic constituent in this area of enamel.

Enamel Spindle

An **enamel spindle** is an **odontoblastic process,** a cellular extension of the odontoblast, that becomes trapped between ameloblasts in

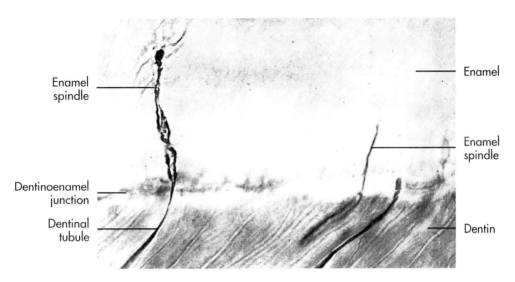

Enamel
spindle

Enamel

Enamel
spindle

Dentinoenamel
junction

Dentinal
tubule

Dentin

FIG. 5-9.   An enamel spindle or odontoblastic process extension crossing the DEJ and lying in enamel. (From Bhaskar SN: *Orban's oral histology and embryology*, ed 8, St Louis, 1976, Mosby.)

early development and thus ends up in the enamel (Fig. 5-9). It is seen only histologically. It may contribute to a minor extent to an area of slight hypersensitivity in young individuals, but this is more theoretic than clinical.

DENTIN COMPOSITION

Dentin is a hard yellowish substance. It is about 70% inorganic hydroxyapatite crystal; the remaining 30% is primarily organic, composed of collagen, mucopolysaccharide ground substance, and water. Dentin comprises the following three distinct areas (Fig. 5-10):

1. **Dentinal tubule**—A long tube, running from the DEJ or DCJ to the pulp. Each dentinal tubule contains an **odontoblastic process.**
2. **Peritubular dentin**—An area of higher crystalline content immediately surrounding the dentinal tubules.
3. **Intertubular dentin**—The bulk of the dentinal material.

These are all microscopic structures. Clinically, dentin appears to be solid.

FORMATION OF REGULAR DENTIN (PRIMARY DENTIN)

As the odontoblast begins to secrete dentin matrix at the future DEJ or dentinocemental junction, the cell begins to move toward the pulp. The odontoblast differs from the ameloblast in that it leaves part of the cell behind and secretes matrix around it. Through this process the cell wall stretches or lengthens so that part of the odontoblast stretches all the way from the DEJ or DCJ inward to the periphery of the pulp (Fig. 5-11). The secreted matrix from an odontoblast spreads peripherally until it meets with other dentin matrices and eventually calcifies and forms intertubular dentin. Later the odontoblastic process contained within the intertubular dentin shrinks in diameter, and the space that it formerly occupied is filled with a highly calcified dentin

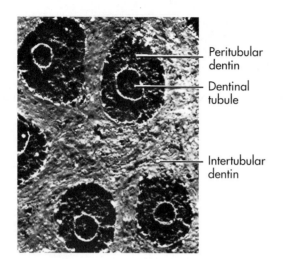

FIG. 5-10. Cross-sectional view of dentin. (From Bhaskar SN: *Orban's oral histology and embryology,* ed 8, St Louis, 1976, Mosby.)

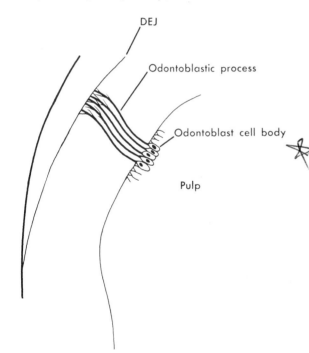

FIG. 5-11. Cell body of an odontoblast with an elongated odontoblastic process stretching from the DEJ to the pulp.

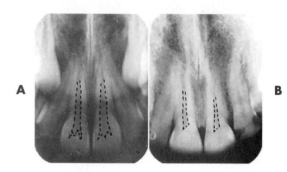

FIG. 5-12. Radiographs of a maxillary central incisor of, **A,** an 8-year-old, and, **B,** a 43-year-old. Notice the prominence of the pulp horns and chamber size of the 8-year-old pulp compared with the 43-year-old pulp.

known as peritubular dentin (see Fig. 5-10). When the tooth erupts into the oral cavity, the dentin that has formed by that time is known as **primary dentin** or regular dentin. Dentin continues to be formed as either secondary or reparative dentin.

FORMATION OF SECONDARY AND REPARATIVE DENTIN

Secondary Dentin

The layer formed inside the regular dentin and positioned closest to the pulp is **secondary dentin.** It starts forming about the time the tooth erupts and comes into contact with the opposing tooth. It is formed by the same odontoblasts that form the regular dentin. As the secondary dentin forms, it causes the overall size of the pulp chamber to decrease. This is most noticeable when comparing radiographs of newly erupted permanent maxillary central incisors with radiographs of the same teeth that have been erupted for a number of years (Fig. 5-12). Newly erupted teeth have large pulp chambers and prominent pulp horns. As secondary dentin formation proceeds, a decrease in the size of the pulp canals, chambers, and pulp horns occurs. It is this process of secondary dentin formation that allows metal crowns to be constructed on teeth after they have been erupted for a few years. If this formation did not take place, cutting tooth structure for the placement of crowns would tend to injure the large prominent pulp horns and pulp chambers of teeth.

Reparative Dentin

Reparative dentin is formed in response to local trauma and is located immediately beneath the area of trauma. The trauma may be one of several varieties: occlusal, mechanical, or chemical trauma.

Occlusal trauma is the condition that exists when one tooth or part of a tooth is subjected to more occlusal stress than normal. This usually relates to the cusp area of the tooth. The odontoblast layer beneath the cusp responds to the trauma by quickly producing dentin. This dentin has very few if any dentinal tubules, and under the microscope looks very dense and unorganized.

Mechanical trauma is usually the result of cavity preparations in the tooth. Cavity preparations generally extend through the enamel and into the dentin. For every square millimeter of dentin that is cut, there are 30,000 to 40,000 odontoblastic processes damaged. Most of this damage leads to the death of the odontoblasts in that area. These odontoblasts are replaced with reserve mesenchymal cells from adjacent pulpal tissue, which change into odontoblasts and produce reparative dentin.

Chemical trauma is usually brought about by the acids produced by the bacteria that cause dental caries. Chemical trauma is also sometimes produced by substances used in filling teeth if the cavity preparation has not been lined in some manner. Lining the cavity preparation protects the pulp from the chemicals used in restorations, and some of them also help soothe the pulpal tissue that has been damaged by the preparatory process.

It is possible to radiographically determine the type of trauma. Occlusal trauma results in reparative dentin being produced beneath the involved area, usually a cusp tip. Mechanical and chemical traumas are in areas where there has been decay or cavity preparations, such as occlusal grooves or cervical or interproximal areas (Fig. 5-13).

ABNORMALITIES IN DENTIN

There are several abnormalities found in dentin. Because dentin lies beneath either enamel or cementum, most of the more common abnormalities cannot be seen without sectioning the tooth and studying it with a hand lens or microscope.

Interglobular Dentin

During the process of calcification, some areas of poorly calcified dentin become entrapped. These poorly calcified areas are the **interglobular dentin.** They are found next to the DEJ in the crown and the dentinocemental junction in the root. The root interglobular dentin is generally called the **granular layer of Tomes.** They are of no real clinical significance.

Dead Tracts

Dentinal tubules that are empty because of the death of the odontoblasts that originally occupied them are known as **dead tracts.** These are not seen clinically, only microscopically. Because the tubules are empty they provide a pathway to the pulp for bacteria involved in decay. This means more rapid penetration of decay once it has reached the DEJ, and there is insufficient time for reparative dentin to be formed.

Sclerotic Dentin

A condition in which the dentinal tubules are filled with a dentin material is called **sclerotic dentin.** The cause of this is related to occlusal trauma or decay. The odontoblastic processes in the area of the trauma retract and begin secret-

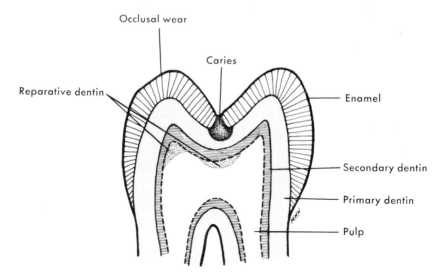

FIG. 5-13. Primary, secondary, and reparative dentin. Notice how the secondary dentin has decreased the size of the entire pulp chamber, whereas reparative dentin is formed only beneath traumatic areas, such as a carious region and an area of occlusal wear.

ing matrix substance, filling in the empty tubule. The odontoblasts may also degenerate, and the tubules of the degenerating odontoblasts are filled. This has also been referred to as **transparent dentin.**

PULP

As mentioned before, the pulp develops from the mesodermal tissue of the dental papilla. It will eventually consist of blood vessels, lymphatic vessels, nerves, fibroblasts, and collagen fibers, as well as other cells of connective tissue. As dentin grows inward, it compresses the inner tissue of the dental papilla. At this point, blood vessels, lymphatic channels, nerves, and connective tissue cells are very evident. Many of the mesenchymal cells become fibroblasts and begin forming collagen fibers (Fig. 5-14). The nerves of the pulp are primarily sensory and transmit only one type of sensation—pain. There are some au-

tonomic sympathetic nerves that innervate the smooth muscle cells in the walls of the blood vessels and cause them to constrict. This kind of reaction is important in vascular changes in the pulp caused by irritation to the tooth.

Young pulpal tissue is considered primarily cellular with a lesser concentration of fibers than older pulp. There are a number of cell types present. Aside from the fibroblasts there are macrophages, which will protect the pulp, and a large number of reserve mesenchymal cells. These mesenchymal cells are the kind we see in the dental papilla as the tooth starts to develop. They have the ability to form a number of different types of cells, including fibroblasts and odontoblasts. As the pulp ages, some of these cells are used to form odontoblasts to replace those that are damaged. (Although odontoblasts are an integral part of dentin, they are also the peripheral cells of the pulp [Fig. 5-15]). Some of them will change to fibroblasts and produce more colla-

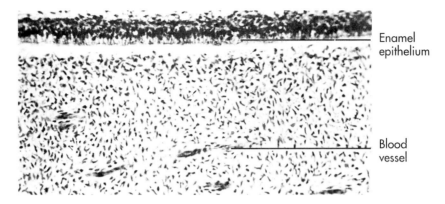

Enamel
epithelium

Blood
vessel

FIG. 5-14. Young pulp with mesenchymal cells and developing blood vessels. (From Bhaskar SN: *Orban's oral histology and embryology*, ed 8, St Louis, 1976, Mosby.)

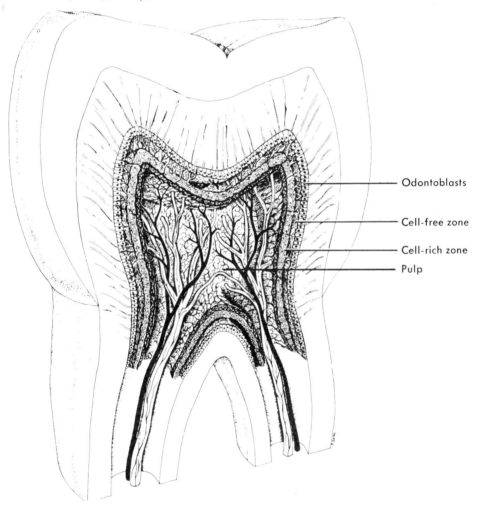

Odontoblasts

Cell-free zone

Cell-rich zone

Pulp

FIG. 5-15. Odontoblasts surrounding pulp as the outer layer. (From Bhaskar SN: *Orban's oral histology and embryology*, ed 8, St Louis, 1976, Mosby.)

gen. With the aging of the tooth, the pulp becomes smaller because of the production of secondary and reparative dentin and is less able to resist trauma because it loses its reserve cells, which explains why young people are less susceptible than adults to permanent pulpal damage.

ABNORMALITIES IN PULP

Pulp stones are the primary abnormality seen in pulp. They are small, circular, calcified areas found in the pulps of about 80% of older persons age 70 to 80 years. With such a high rate of occurrence it might be questionable to identify them as abnormalities, but they are considered a pathologic condition. There are several classifications of stones based on their origin and density. True pulp stones originate from odontoblasts and are very rare. False stones are the most common type and probably originate from dead cells with concentric layers of calcium phosphate around them. When studied under the microscope, a false stone resembles an onion cut in cross section. Another classification of stones is referred to as diffuse calcifications; they are very tiny calcified structures found in groups.

Pulp stones are also classified according to their location. Free pulp stones are found in the middle of the pulp. Attached pulp stones are those that have become attached to the dentin in the periphery of the pulp. Embedded stones are those that were attached to the dentin and became surrounded by secondary dentin (Fig. 5-16).

Pulp stones usually do not affect the health of the pulp. The pulp can have a number of stones and still be vital. They may be seen as small globular **radiopacities** on radiographs. The only problem that may occur would be in the endodontic treatment of a tooth with numerous pulp stones. The stones could make it difficult to remove pulpal tissue with reamers and files.

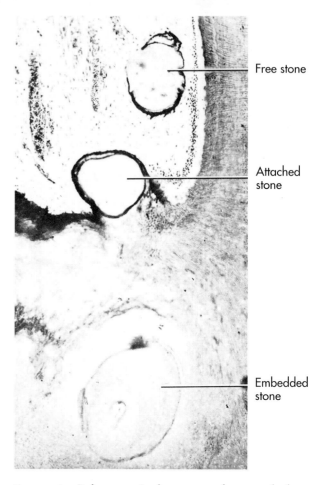

FIG. 5-16.   Pulp stones in three stages: free, attached, and embedded. (From Bhaskar SN: *Orban's oral histology and embryology,* ed 8, St Louis, 1976, Mosby.)

Labels in figure: Free stone; Attached stone; Embedded stone

Review Questions

1. How do inner enamel epithelial cells change to become preameloblasts?
2. How do preameloblasts change to become ameloblasts?
3. What is the interrelationship between enamel and dentin during formation?
4. What happens if enamel crystals do not grow to full size?

5. What is the orientation of crystals in the upper and lower parts of the keyhole-shaped enamel rod?

6. What is Nasmyth's membrane?

7. What are enamel lamellae?

8. What are the three distinct areas of primary dentin?

9. What is the difference between secondary dentin and reparative dentin in terms of composition and location?

10. What are dead tracts and sclerotic (or transparent) dentin?

11. What happens to the pulp as it grows older?

12. What are pulp stones?

13. How do pulp stones affect the health of the pulp?

CHAPTER 6

ROOT FORMATION AND ATTACHMENT APPARATUS

OBJECTIVES
- To discuss the role of the epithelial root sheath in root formation and dentin formation
- To describe the fate of the epithelial root sheath
- To describe the beginning of cementum formation, the two varieties, and where they are found
- To define and diagram alveolar bone and its components
- To define periodontal ligament and list its various groups and subgroups of fibers
- To briefly describe bone's reaction to pressure and tension and how this affects tooth movement

THIS CHAPTER deals with the formation of the root—how its form is determined and developed and the development of the cementum, periodontal ligament, and alveolar bone, collectively referred to as the **attachment apparatus.**

ROOT FORMATION

Root formation begins after the outline of the crown has been established but before the full crown is calcified. If you refer to Figs. 4-4 and 5-3 (bell stage), you will see that the point where the outer enamel epithelium (OEE) meets the inner enamel epithelium (IEE) is located at the deepest part of the enamel organ and is known as the **cervical loop.** There are no interposing layers of stellate reticulum or stratum intermedium here, which one would see higher in the crown. These layers of OEE and IEE, which make up the **epithelial root sheath (Hertwig's epithelial root sheath),** begin to undergo rapid **mitotic division** and grow deep into the underlying connective tissue—the beginning of root formation. It is important to keep in mind the relationship of the dental papilla and the dental sac to this growing epithelial root sheath. The dental papilla is on the inside, and

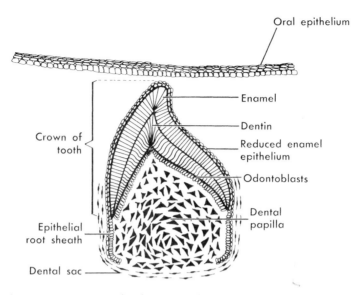

Oral epithelium

Enamel

Dentin

Reduced enamel
epithelium

Odontoblasts

Dental
papilla

Crown of
tooth

Epithelial
root sheath

Dental sac

FIG. 6-1. Beginning root development. The epithelial root sheath interposed between the dental papilla and the dental sac.

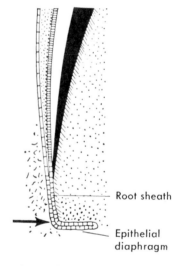

Root sheath

Epithelial
diaphragm

the dental sac is on the outside (Fig. 6-1). As the downgrowth continues, the tip of the epithelial root sheath turns horizontally inward; this turned-in portion is known as the **epithelial diaphragm** of the root sheath. The epithelial root sheath and epithelial diaphragm guide the shape and the number of roots.

Figs. 6-1 and 6-2 are two-dimensional representations of a three-dimensional object. To help you better understand this three-dimensionally, visualize a paper cup. The rim of the cup represents the cervical line of the tooth, and the side of the cup is the epithelial root sheath. If you cut a round hole in the bottom of the cup about two thirds the diameter of the cup and made a vertical cut through the middle, the horizontal bottom of the cup that remained would represent the epithelial diaphragm. The way in which this epithelial diaphragm continues to grow inward determines whether the tooth will have one, two, or three roots.

FIG. 6-2. The epithelial diaphragm is the horizontal component of the epithelial root sheath. Mitosis and growth of the root sheath take place at the point of the arrow. (From Bhaskar SN: *Orban's oral histology and embryology,* ed 8, St Louis, 1976, Mosby.)

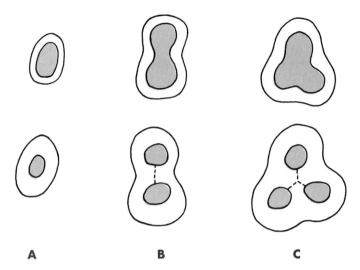

FIG. 6-3.   Inferior view of an epithelial diaphragm. **A,** The entire circumference of the epithelial diaphragm grows inward, and a single-rooted tooth will be formed. **B,** The epithelial diaphragm grows inward at two opposite areas and meets in the middle, forming a double-rooted tooth. **C,** The epithelial diaphragm grows inward at three areas and meets, forming a three-rooted tooth.

Changes continue to occur at the deep surface of the epithelial diaphragm. As the vertical epithelial root sheath grows longer, forming root length, the horizontal epithelial diaphragm continues to grow in toward the middle of the tooth. If the entire circumference of the diaphragm grows evenly, it will eventually form a single-rooted tooth. If two areas opposite one another grow inward more rapidly and meet, it will then separate into two columns of root formation to form a birooted tooth. If three areas grow inward to meet, a trirooted tooth will be formed (Fig. 6-3). In multirooted teeth, the point where the epithelial diaphragm meets is the bifurcation or trifurcation of the tooth.

ATTACHMENT APPARATUS

Dentinocemental Junction

Fig. 6-1 shows the relationship of the epithelial root sheath to the dental papilla and dental sac. As the root sheath grows from the cervical line deeper into the connective tissue, it influences the peripheral cells of the dental papilla to change into odontoblasts, similar to what happens in the crown of the tooth. The odontoblasts begin to secrete matrix and calcify. Once dentin begins to form next to the epithelial root sheath, cellular influence causes the root sheath to begin to break up. There is still some debate as to which cells cause this breakup. It may be the inside odontoblasts, or it may be the cells of the dental sac on the outside.

To envision this deterioration of the epithelial root sheath, imagine that the sheath is originally a solid wall of cells surrounding the developing tooth root. Later it becomes riddled with holes, like a piece of Swiss cheese. With the appearance of these holes there is no longer any barrier separating the odontoblasts and dentin on the inside from the cells of the dental sac on the outside. Some of the dental sac cells begin to change into cementoblasts, move through the holes, and begin to form cementum. This cementum is laid down against the previously formed dentin and establishes the dentinocemental junction (Fig. 6-4). Remember that the epithelial root sheath is perforated; therefore the cementoblasts that contact dentin are able to accomplish the transformation only in the areas where the sheath has broken up. While this occurs, the remaining root sheath cells pull away from the dentin, and the cementoblasts contact all of the dentin and establish the rest of the dentinocemental junction. Occasionally, some epithelial root sheath cells do not pull away and may become ameloblasts, forming small globs of enamel on the surface of the dentin. These are referred to as **enamel pearls** and are usually found in bifurcations and trifurcations of roots. Other defects occurring at this time may lead to the formation of **accessory root canals,** which make it difficult for a dentist to remove all pulpal tissue completely if the tooth has to be treated endodontically.

After they have broken up and moved away from the dentin, the remaining cells of the epithelial root sheath are found in the periodontal space next to the tooth and are called **epithelial rests of Malassez** or just epithelial rest cells. If these cells later begin dividing, they may lead to the formation of periodontal cysts in the jaws, similar in origin to the palatal cysts mentioned in Chapter 3.

Cementum

Cementum is a hard, yellowish substance covering the root of the tooth. It is composed of about 45% to 50% inorganic hydroxyapatite crystals, and the remaining 50% to 55% is organic components and water. As in most hard substances in the teeth, except for enamel, the organic component is primarily collagen fibers and mucopolysaccharide ground substance.

As cementum formation begins, it is first seen at the cervical line of the tooth, also called the cementoenamel junction. As cementum is laid down, it may assume three different relationships with the enamel of the crown. In about 60% of the cases the cementum overlaps the enamel, in 30% the cementum meets the enamel

at a sharp junction, and in the remaining 10% of the cases the cementum and enamel do not meet, thus leaving dentin exposed at the cervical line. Exposed dentin may make the tooth very sensitive in that area if the patient develops gingival recession (Fig. 6-5).

As the cementoblast begins laying down cementum, it functions in somewhat the same way as the ameloblast, moving away from the dentinocemental junction and secreting matrix behind it. This type of secretion results in **acellular cementum,** in which all of the cementoblasts remain on the surface rather than becoming trapped within the cementum. These surface cementoblasts not only initially build cementum but also aid in rebuilding cementum when it is damaged. This type of cellular arrangement is noted in the cervical two thirds of the root but not usually to any extent in the apical one third where another type of cementum arrangement takes place.

As root formation and therefore cementum formation proceeds from the cervical line to the apex of the root, the cementoblasts surround themselves and become entrapped as they are secreting matrix, similar to osteoblasts in bone formation. A histologic examination of the tissue reveals numerous entrapped cells, which are referred to as **cementocytes.** Because of these cells the tissue is described as **cellular cementum.** In the middle and apical third of the root, cellular cementum can be seen overlapping acellular cementum (Fig. 6-6). Because of the presence of the cementocytes, cellular cementum is more vital than acellular cementum and therefore more responsive to remodeling itself, albeit a slow process. However, to remain vital the entrapped cells within cellular cementum must be maintained. Therefore the cementocytes have long cellular processes that point toward the surface of the tooth. The overall nourishment comes from the blood vessels of the periodontium.

The cellular cementum at the apex of the root tends to increase in thickness with the passage of time and as a result of stress. This thickening is

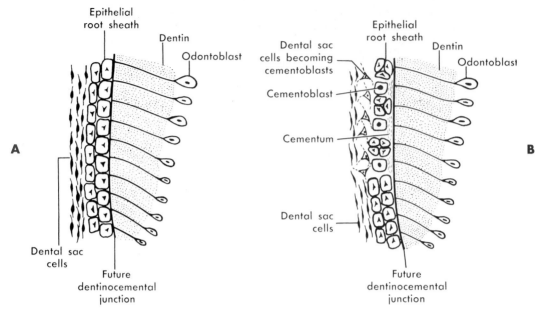

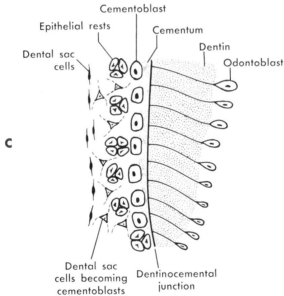

FIG. 6-4.   **A,** The epithelial root sheath separates dentin from the dental sac cells. **B,** The epithelial root sheath breaks up, and the dental sac cells become cementoblasts. **C,** The epithelial root sheath moves away from dentin, and the dentinocemental junction is formed.

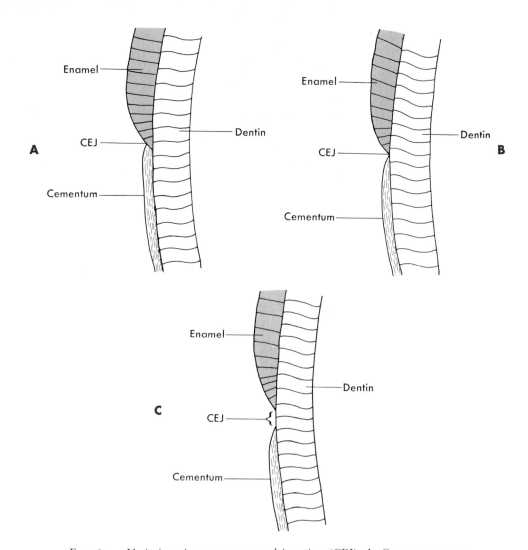

FIG. 6-5.   Variations in cementoenamel junction (CEJ). **A,** Cementum overlaps enamel. **B,** Cementum and enamel meet in a sharp junction. **C,** Cementum and enamel do not meet, and dentin is exposed.

called **hypercementosis** and in general causes no great problem to the tooth unless it becomes necessary to extract it. If so, the bulbous apex might make extraction a bit more difficult than usual, and it may be necessary to remove the bone around the tooth as it may be impos-

sible to spread the tooth socket wide enough (Fig. 6-7).

As mentioned before, the outer layer of cementum is lined with cementoblasts, which probably are capable of cementum formation throughout a person's life. As the **periodontal**

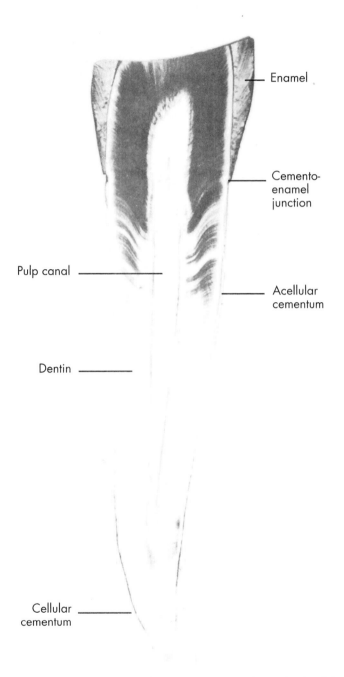

Enamel

Cemento-enamel junction

Pulp canal

Acellular cementum

Dentin

Cellular cementum

FIG. 6-6.   Acellular cementum is found on the cervical two thirds of the root. Cellular cementum covers the apical one third of the root, overlapping the acellular cementum near the middle. (From Bevelander G: *Atlas of oral histology and embryology,* Philadelphia, 1967, Lea & Febiger.)

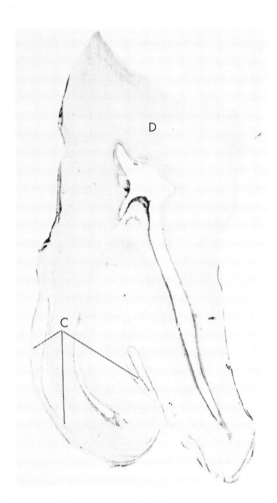

FIG. 6-7.   Hypercementosis. The apex of the root has become quite bulbous and can become trapped in the socket by cementum overgrowth as indicated by lines. (From Provenza DV: *Fundamentals of oral histology and embryology,* ed 2, Philadelphia, 1972, JB Lippincott Co.)

membrane or **ligament** forms from the middle of the layer of cells in the old dental sac, the ends of the periodontal fibers become surrounded by cementoblasts, whose secretion hardens around the ends of the fibers, attaching them to the cementum. The parts of the periodontal ligament embedded in cementum are known as **Sharpey's fibers.** They are the parts of the periodontal liga-

ment surrounded by cementum on the tooth side and alveolar bone on the opposite side in the wall of the tooth socket (Fig. 6-8).

Cementum resorption

The same cell that destroys bone, the osteoclast, may also destroy or resorb cementum, as well as dentin, which lies beneath it. Later in the chapter we will discuss bone resorption, which is the same type of reaction seen in cementum. However, resorption proceeds much slower in cementum because of a much lower metabolic rate. Therefore, cementum is not affected by trauma as quickly as bone is, an important consideration in orthodontic tooth movement.

Alveolar Bone

By definition **alveolar bone** or **alveolar process** is the bone of the upper or lower jaw that makes up the sockets for the teeth. The composition of dried bone varies, depending on whether it is young or adult bone. Adult bone is about 65% inorganic crystal, and the remaining 35% organic composition is about 89% collagen and 11% noncollagenous material. Alveolar bone originates by intramembranous development, as discussed in Chapter 2, and is mesodermal in origin, as are all types of connective tissue.

Alveolar bone is composed of three layers, as seen in cross section (Fig. 6-9, *A*). The layer of compact bone on the buccal or lingual surface is referred to as the **cortical plate** of bone. It is typical bone with a normal periosteum. The bone that forms the socket for the tooth is also a compact bone but does not have a normal periosteum. Although this is a compact layer, it contains numerous holes that allow for the passage of blood vessels, connecting the deeper part of the bone with the vessels of the periodontal space. This layer is called the **cribriform plate** or **alveolar bone proper.** Radiographically it is referred to as the **lamina dura.** The cribriform plate originates from the outer layer of the dental sac.

The tooth socket is constantly being remodeled, and additional bone, called **bundle bone,** is

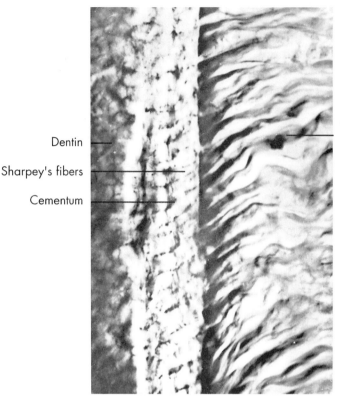

Dentin

Sharpey's fibers

Cementum

Fibers of periodontal ligament

FIG. 6-8. Sharpey's fibers. The ends of the periodontal ligament become entrapped in cementum, and these entrapped parts are called Sharpey's fiber. (From Bhaskar SN: *Orban's oral histology and embryology,* ed 8, St Louis, 1976, Mosby.)

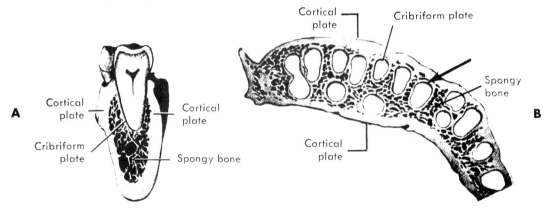

Cortical plate

Cribriform plate

Spongy bone

Cortical plate

A

Cortical plate

Cortical plate

Cribriform plate

Spongy bone

B

FIG. 6-9. Alveolar bone. **A,** A cross section view through a mandible. The cortical plate is on the buccal and lingual sides with the cribriform plate in the socket. Spongy bone is in between. **B,** A longitudinal horizontal section through a mandible. Notice the thickened lamina dura *(arrow).* This is caused by bundle bone being deposited on the cribriform plate. (From Bhaskar SN: *Orban's oral histology and embryology,* ed 8, St Louis, 1976, Mosby.)

laid down on the cribriform plate (Fig. 6-9, *B*). A thickened lamina dura, which can be seen in a radiograph, is caused by bundle bone being laid down on the cribriform plate. A thickened lamina dura in one or more teeth in a patient is frequently an indication of occlusal trauma to that tooth or teeth. Finally, in between the cortical plate and the cribriform plate is a layer of **spongy** or **cancellous bone.** This spongy bone is a bone marrow, as mentioned in Chapter 2.

Radiographically the cortical plate cannot be seen because it is only on the buccal and lingual sides of the socket; a radiograph will only show the cribriform plate, the spongy bone and the crest of bone that joins two sockets, called the interproximal **alveolar crest** of bone. The contours of this bony area are a good indicator of periodontal health (Fig. 6-10).

Like cementum, bone has embedded parts of the periodontal ligament within it also called Sharpey's fibers. However, a difference between

bone and cementum is that bone has a much higher metabolic rate than cementum. It is this difference that allows bone to change in response to stress; yet there is very little if any change in cementum because it is not so rapidly responsive.

Periodontal Ligament

The periodontal ligament also develops from the middle layer of mesodermal cells of the dental sac. This happens after the cementum has begun forming. As the dental sac cells begin to change, they first become fibroblasts, and the fibroblasts form collagen fibers. At first these fibers are arranged around the tooth and parallel with the root surface in the middle of the periodontal space. The fibers that are forming adjacent to cementum and alveolar bone are initially more obliquely oriented. Later they will band into groups of fibers that span the periodontal space. Some of the early arrangements of fibers are discussed in Chapter 7.

About the same time the fibers are forming, the other components of the periodontal ligament are also starting to appear, including blood vessels, lymphatic vessels, nerves, and various types of connective tissue cells. Unlike the nerves of the pulp, which can transmit only impulses of pain, the nerves of the periodontal space also have fibers that allow one to feel light touch and pressure and probably heat and cold. When biting down on something hard produces a sharp pain, it is the nerves of the periodontal ligament that are stimulated, not the pulp of the tooth. After a person has had root canal work done on a tooth, it is still possible to feel pain at times; however, this is not from the pulpal area but from the periodontal ligament. The blood vessels of the ligament space are branches of the same vessels that go to the pulp, but they also have branches that penetrate the holes in the wall of the cribriform plate and join with the vascular channels in the spongy part of the alveolar bone, while still others come from the gingival blood supply and anastomose or interconnect with these other vessels.

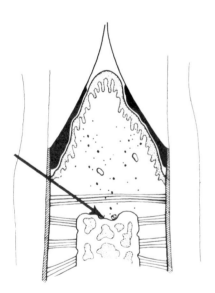

FIG. 6-10. Destruction of the alveolar crest. The blunted alveolar crest *(arrow)* is indicative of periodontal disease. (From Pawlak E, Hoag PM: *Essentials of periodontics,* ed 2, St Louis, 1980, Mosby.)

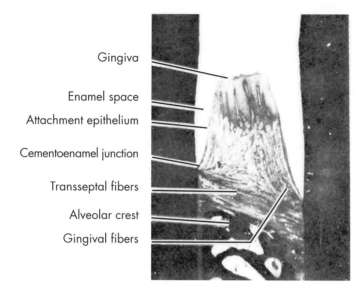

Gingiva

Enamel space

Attachment epithelium

Cementoenamel junction

Transseptal fibers

Alveolar crest

Gingival fibers

FIG. 6-11.   Gingival and transseptal fibers. The transseptal fibers go from the cementum of one tooth to the cementum of an adjacent tooth. The gingival fibers extend from the cementum up into the gingiva. The circular gingival fibers (cut in cross section) circle the tooth in free gingiva. (From Bevelander G: *Outline of histology,* ed 7, St Louis, 1971, Mosby)

As the fibers of the ligament form, they begin to arrange themselves in a definite pattern. When the fibers reach their final arrangement, they are descriptively arranged into three groups: **gingival fibers, transseptal fibers,** and **alveolodental fibers.**

1. Gingival fibers
   a. Gingival fibers—run from the cementum into the free and attached gingival area; tend to support gingiva
   b. Circular gingival fibers—run around the tooth in free gingiva and hold gingiva against the tooth
2. Transseptal fibers—run from the cementum of the interproximal portion of one tooth, across the alveolar crest of bone, to the cementum of the interproximal portion of the adjacent tooth; function is to hold the teeth in interproximal contact (Fig. 6-11)
3. Alveolodental fibers—run from cementum to alveolar bone (Fig. 6-12)

   a. Alveolar crest group—runs from cementum, slightly apical to the alveolar crest of bone; helps resist horizontal movements of teeth
   b. Horizontal group—runs from the cementum horizontally to the alveolar crest; helps resist horizontal movement
   c. Oblique group—runs from the cementum coronally into the alveolar bone; main fiber group for resisting occlusal stresses
   d. Apical group—runs from the apex of the tooth into the adjacent alveolar bone; resists forces trying to pull the tooth from its socket
   e. Interradicular group—found only on multirooted teeth; runs from the alveolar crest of the bone between the roots of the tooth to adjacent cementum; resists the forces trying to remove the tooth

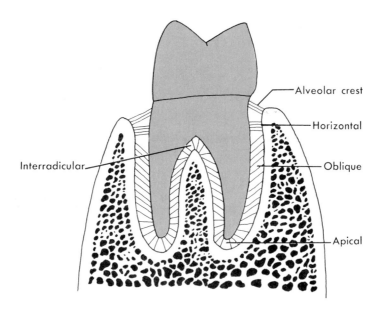

FIG. 6-12. Diagram showing the five groups of alveolodental fibers. In single-rooted teeth there would be no interradicular fibers.

STRUCTURAL OVERVIEW

A look at the total periodontal space and all of its associated structures shows on one side the cementum of the tooth with cementoblasts lying on its surface. The ends of the periodontal ligament (Sharpey's fibers) are embedded in the cementum lying perpendicular to the surface. Close to the surface of the tooth amid the periodontal fibers are small clumps of epithelial cells, the epithelial rests of Malassez. On the other side of the periodontal space is the cribriform plate, the compact bony layer that is perforated in many places. Additional bone has been laid down as bundle bone, and there is a thickening of the lamina dura. Here also are the embedded Sharpey's fibers of the periodontal ligament. Various types of nerve fibers are also found within this periodontal space. Additionally there are fibroblasts, macrophages, various blood cells, and numerous open areas wherein one can see the well-developed pattern of blood vessels.

BONE REMODELING IN TOOTH MOVEMENT

What happens when a tooth is lost? Many times the tooth posterior to the missing tooth will tilt forward into the unoccupied space. This phenomenon has been referred to as *mesial drift*. The same type of movement can be accomplished in orthodontic tooth movement. Because each tooth fits into a socket, it is necessary to change the shape of that socket if the tooth is to be moved. In most tooth movement the tooth does not move bodily but tilts on an axis. This rotational point on a tooth is located about two thirds of the way down the root. If a tooth tilts mesially (Fig. 6-13), bone is resorbed on the cervical two thirds of the mesial side and the apical one third of the distal side. This resorption is a result of the tooth putting pressure on the alveolar bone in these areas, causing reduced blood flow, which results in the formation of osteoclasts, cells that destroy bone. Also as the tooth

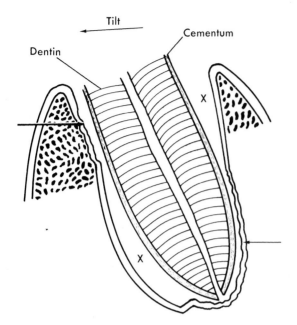

FIG. 6-13. Mesial drift. The tooth is tilted mesially, and bone is destroyed at the areas marked X, areas once occupied by tooth.

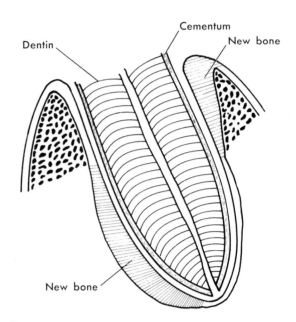

FIG. 6-14. Remodeling of bone. Hash marks indicate new bone formation after tooth movement.

moves, there is tension on the periodontal fibers in the apical one third of the mesial side and the cervical two thirds of the distal side. This tension causes bone to build new bone, and the socket fills in at the area once occupied by the tooth's root (Fig. 6-14).

Why does the bone change and remodel and the cementum usually does not? Remember that cementum has a low metabolic rate, whereas bone metabolism is much higher. Because of this, the bone reacts more quickly to stress and can remodel itself before the stress on the cementum causes any destruction. If a tooth is moved too fast in orthodontic treatment, it is possible that the fibers attaching the tooth to bone will be torn out of their attachment; before they can be reembedded, the tooth could conceivably loosen and be lost.

Review Questions

1. The epithelial root sheath develops from what earlier structures?
2. What happens to the epithelial root sheath after root dentin starts to form?
3. What are epithelial rests, and what might happen to them later in life?
4. What three structures do cells of the dental sac form?
5. What are the two types of cementum, and where are they found on the root?
6. What are Sharpey's fibers?
7. What are the layers of alveolar bone?
8. What is the lamina dura? What does it mean clinically if it is thickened?
9. What are the various periodontal fiber groups, and what are their functions?
10. What is mesial drift?
11. What causes bone resorption and apposition (remodeling)?

CHAPTER 7

ERUPTION AND SHEDDING OF TEETH

ACTIVE TOOTH ERUPTION

The term *active tooth eruption* implies the emergence of a crown into the oral cavity. In general, however, the term refers to the total life span of the tooth, from the beginning of crown development until the tooth is lost or the individual dies. This eruptive process is usually divided into three stages, and although there may be some difference in the terminology, they refer to the same mechanism.

Preeruptive Stage

The **preeruptive stage** begins as the crown starts to develop. Recall that dental lamina formation—bud, cap, and bell stages, as well as the calcification of the crown—takes place in the connective tissue beneath the oral epithelium. During this time the bone of the maxilla or mandible surrounds the developing primary tooth in a U-shaped crypt or beginning socket (Fig. 7-1).

The eruptive movement associated with the preeruptive stage is of two varieties—spatial and

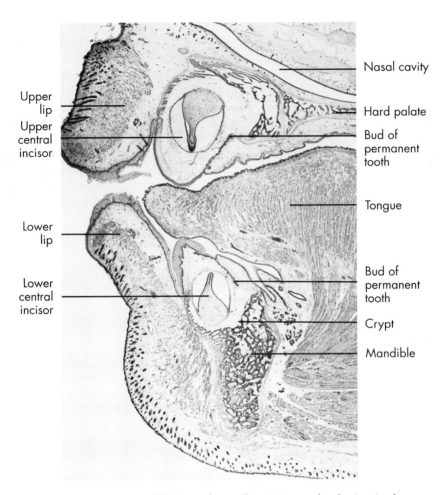

Upper lip

Upper central incisor

Lower lip

Lower central incisor

Nasal cavity

Hard palate

Bud of permanent tooth

Tongue

Bud of permanent tooth

Crypt

Mandible

Fig. 7-1.   Primary mandibular and maxillary incisors developing in the recess or crypt of the bone, which forms a socket. The depth of the crypt builds up from osteoclastic activity at its base and increases in height to form future alveolar bone. (From Bhaskar SN: *Orban's oral histology and embryology,* ed 8, St Louis, 1976, Mosby.)

excentric. In spatial movement the crown develops while the bottom of the socket fills in with bone, pushing the crown toward the surface. There is also a similar facial movement that accompanies jaw growth. In excentric or off-center growth the crown of a tooth does not grow in a perfectly symmetrical pattern. As the crown enlarges, it grows more in one area than in another,

and so the tooth seems to be moving because the center of the tooth is shifting. This can be visualized by blowing up a small round balloon to a diameter of 3 to 4 inches. Put a mark on the center of the balloon and continue to blow it up to a diameter of 8 to 10 inches. Again mark the center of the balloon. Because the balloon walls may not be of equal thickness, one area may expand more than another. Thus the center of the balloon moves from the original marking. This same principle can be applied to the developing crown. It appears to have moved because the center point of the developing crown has shifted. This is the activity of the preeruptive stage. It involves crown growth and some movement toward the surface while the crypt is developing.

Eruptive Stage

The **eruptive stage** or **prefunctional eruptive stage** begins with the development of the root. In Chapter 6 the development of the root and Hertwig's epithelial root sheath were discussed. The root develops in a crypt of bone. As it begins forming, osteoclasts temporarily may deepen the crypt by resorbing bone at the bottom to accommodate for the increase in root length. While the root continues to lengthen, the tooth begins to move toward the surface of the oral cavity. As it approaches the oral cavity, the alveolar bone is growing to keep pace with it. However, in time the tooth moves faster than the growing alveolar bone and approaches the surface of the oral epithelium and breaks into the oral cavity.

The crown of the tooth is surrounded by reduced enamel epithelium. As the tooth moves to the surface, this reduced enamel epithelium moves with it until it compresses the connective tissue and causes it to disintegrate. The reduced enamel epithelium then contacts the oral epithelium, and these two layers fuse into one layer—the **united oral epithelium.** The tooth breaks through this layer and emerges into the oral cavity. It is believed that this breakdown of epithelium is caused by an enzyme probably produced by the reduced enamel epithelium. This stage continues until the erupting teeth meet the opposing teeth.

For both primary and secondary dentition tooth movement in the eruptive stage tends to be occlusal and facial, more facial in the anteriors than in the posteriors. When we think about the pathway for the secondary teeth we have to take into consideration their mechanism for development. As discussed in Chapter 4, the succes-

sional lamina buds off the dental lamina and forms a permanent tooth at its end, still partially attached by the successional lamina. As the permanent tooth becomes surrounded by bone, the attachment of the successional lamina forms a small canal in the bone known as the **gubernacular canal.** If you look at the mandible of a five-year-old child, you will see small openings in the alveolar bone just lingual to the primary teeth. This is the gubernacular canal, and under normal circumstances the erupting permanent tooth will follow the pathway of the gubernacular canal to reach the surface.

Posteruptive Stage

The **posteruptive stage** begins when the teeth come into occlusion and continues until they are lost or death occurs. This posteruptive stage functions in several ways. First, as the mandible continues to grow and increase the space between the maxilla and mandible, the teeth will continue to erupt to maintain a balance in the arches. Second, as the teeth wear occlusally because of prolonged masticatory stress and wear, they will continue to erupt to maintain tooth contact. Third, because there is slight interproximal wear, there will be a slight mesial eruptive force that keeps the teeth in contact. This mesial drifting can be caused, particularly in the mandible, to unerupted third molars that are pushing against the second molars; however, there is a physiologic mesial drift inherent to teeth. Both of these circumstances are referred to as mesial drift. Finally, if an opposing tooth is lost, the tooth may continue to erupt in what is generally referred to as **supraeruption.** (Some authorities still consider this as a part of the eruptive stage.) Supraeruption can cause serious problems in the replacement of the missing tooth, because it makes it difficult to establish the normal occlusal plane.

CAUSES OF ERUPTION

What causes tooth eruption? What are the forces involved? Much research has been done concerning this question, but much more still needs to be done. Recently published articles from the United States and New Zealand have focused on a number of theories. Following are some of the discussions and thoughts.

Root Elongation

It has been said that the increase in root length, or root elongation, forces the tooth into the oral cavity. However, several things would tend to disprove this. Experiments have been done in which Hertwig's root sheath has been destroyed and root growth has been stopped or inhibited, yet the tooth has still erupted. Teeth have had their roots cut and a pin placed through the apical section, but the occlusal portion continues to erupt. On the other hand, third molars have grown roots to full length, but the teeth have not erupted. It seems that root elongation by itself is not required for tooth eruption, but probably has a relationship to the process.

Alveolar Bone Formation and Changes

It has been said that alveolar bone growth, tooth development, and eruption are interdependent mechanisms. The alveolar process forms in areas where teeth are developing and is deficient in areas where teeth fail to develop. Alveolar bone changes involve both formation and resorption, and these metabolic events are dependent on the presence of the various parts of the dental sac or **dental folicle.** The dental sac plays a role in the formation of cementum of the root, the periodontal ligament, and alveolar bone. The presence of the outer layers of the enamel organ also are important in assisting with the osteoclastic activity and soft tissue destruction necessary for the crown to move up through the bone and soft tissue. This cycle of bone development is rhythmic both in the crest and crypt of the alveolar bone—instances of osteoblastic activity followed by osteoclastic activ-

ity or inactivity. In multirooted teeth the interradicular bone seems to have a fairly significant role in the eruptive process, according to some researchers.

Periodontal Ligament

Even though the periodontal ligament is less involved in tooth eruption than was once believed, it still has a role to play, probably more so toward the end of eruption than at the beginning. Earlier theories of the periodontal ligament having contractile properties in some of its fibers is now a thing of the past in most of the literature. There does still appear to be a remodeling of the intertwining of periodontal fibers in later tooth eruption that is part of the process, but teeth without roots have been shown to erupt in the absence of the periodontal ligament.

Vascular Pressure in Dental Tissues

It has been known for a long time that there are vascular pressures present in pulpal tissues as well as in the periodontal ligament. There is also reasonable agreement that the function of the periodontal ligament as a "shock absorber" for teeth is a result of these vascular pressures. These pulsating blood pressures not only enhance cellular activity but seem to have a direct eruptive role. However, it is difficult to assess, because removal of all fluid pressures would mean the elimination of oxygen and other nutrients from the developing teeth.

The Role of the Tooth Itself

The tooth plays little if any role in eruption, because developing teeth have been surgically removed and replaced by metal or silicone implants into the dental sac, and these implants have erupted.

The question is yet to be answered as to the actual factors in tooth eruption. It is obvious from the information presented above that tooth eruption is definitely multifactorial. Much research is being focused on the biochemistry and cell and molecular biology aspects of the subject, and it seems that these disciplines will begin to provide more and more answers.

SHEDDING OF PRIMARY DENTITION

As mentioned before, the 20 permanent teeth that follow the primary teeth develop as offshoots of the primary dental lamina. Recall that the anterior permanent teeth develop apically and lingually to the primary teeth (Fig. 7-2), whereas the permanent premolars develop between the roots of the primary molars (Fig. 7-3). Regardless of its position, the fact that the permanent tooth is there and is in the eruptive stage means that the permanent tooth is moving toward the surface and putting pressure on the root of the primary tooth. It is believed that this

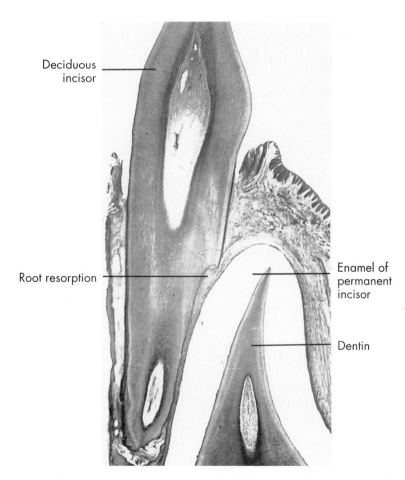

FIG. 7-2. A permanent anterior tooth lying lingual and apical to its deciduous predecessor, causing resorption of that tooth. (From Bhaskar SN: *Orban's oral histology and embryology,* ed 8, St Louis, 1976, Mosby.)

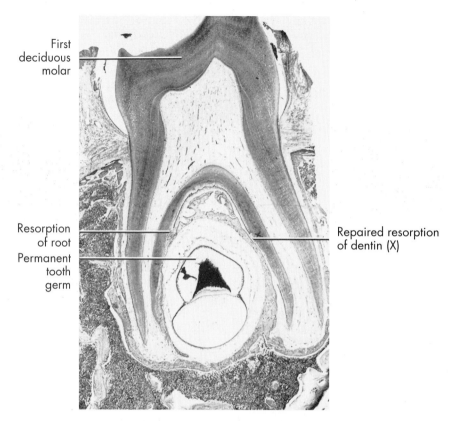

First deciduous molar

Resorption of root

Permanent tooth germ

Repaired resorption of dentin (X)

FIG. 7-3.   Notice the position of the permanent posterior tooth lying between the roots of the primary tooth. (From Bhaskar SN: *Orban's oral histology and embryology,* ed 8, St Louis, 1976, Mosby.)

pressure causes osteoclasts to form and begin resorbing the primary tooth root. This resorption is intermittent and not constant. This is the usual manner in which resorption occurs, but there may be other factors involved. Although most primary teeth would be retained if a permanent tooth did not develop, it is still possible to see a primary tooth undergo root resorption in the absence of a permanent tooth and a primary tooth retained in the presence of a permanent tooth. Therefore, although the pressure of a

developing tooth is a major factor in resorption of primary teeth, it is not the only factor; there is a focus on the role of the enamel organ of the erupting tooth in the whole process.

RETAINED PRIMARY TEETH

There are several reasons why primary teeth are retained beyond their normal time for **exfoliation.** Here we are not really considering a general delayed eruption that you may see in some

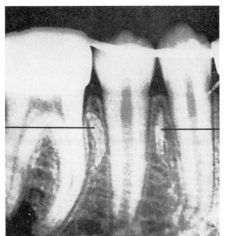

Root remnant of deciduous tooth

Root remnant of deciduous tooth

FIG. 7-4.   Radiograph shows remnants of the roots of a deciduous molar still embedded in bone because of a lack of resorption. (From Bhaskar SN: *Orban's oral histology and embryology,* ed 8, St Louis, 1976, Mosby.)

patients because of retarded growth patterns, but rather the cases in which one or two teeth are retained well beyond the expected period of time for them to be lost.

The reasons for this are several. First, there may be no permanent successor, and the tooth remains. Second, there may be **ankylosis** of the primary tooth, a condition in which the alveolar crest of bone fuses in the cervical area with the cementum of a resorbing root. Although virtually all the root may have been resorbed, the tooth remains firmly in place, preventing the permanent tooth below from erupting. This may remain that way for years, and yet when the ankylosed tooth is removed the permanent tooth will generally begin to erupt. The last reason for a retained primary tooth is that the permanent tooth does not erupt in its normal position and therefore does not cause resorption of the primary tooth root or roots, and the tooth remains. This is frequently seen in the anterior mandibular area, where the permanent teeth erupt apically, rather than apically and labially. In these cases, both sets of anterior teeth will be seen.

Another problem associated with the shedding of primary teeth is unresorbed root fragments. This condition is usually but not always associated with a malaligned primary or permanent tooth. If the root tip of a primary tooth is not in the path of eruption of a permanent tooth, the cervical portion of the root may be resorbed, leaving the apical part still embedded in the jaw (Fig. 7-4). The fragments may remain there for some time and eventually may work their way to the surface and be removed. These retained root tips are seen in radiographs from time to time.

The time schedule of eruption and shedding is varied. In general, the posterior teeth go through a slower process than the anterior teeth do. Not only does the length of time for eruption vary, but also its beginning or ending time varies from one person to another. There is a range for normal eruption time, and only when this period is exceeded is there cause for concern (see Chapter 24).

Review Questions

1. What is active eruption, and how long does it last?
2. What are the three stages of active tooth eruption? When do they begin and end?
3. What is supraeruption?
4. What are some of the theories of tooth eruption, and is there a most likely cause?

5. What causes the breakdown of the united oral epithelium as the tooth breaks through and erupts?
6. What is the position of the permanent teeth in relation to their deciduous predecessors?
7. What is ankylosis? What problems may it cause? How is it treated?
8. Give three causes of retained primary teeth.

CHAPTER 8

ORAL MUCOUS MEMBRANE

DIVISIONS OF MUCOUS MEMBRANE

The lining of the oral cavity is referred to as *oral mucosa* or *oral mucous membrane*. It is a stratified squamous epithelial arrangement that runs from the margins of the lips posteriorly to the area of the tonsils. Although this same epithelium is found posterior to this point, there it is part of the oral pharynx and not the oral cavity. Behind the tonsils and in the posterior throat wall it would be referred to as *pharyngeal mu-* *cosa*. Oral mucous membrane is divided into three categories:

1. **Specialized mucosa**—mucosa on the upper surface or **dorsum of the tongue** (discussed in detail in Chapter 9)
2. **Masticatory mucosa**—comprises the gingiva and hard palatal tissue; undergoes trauma or compression during mastication
3. **Lining mucosa**—all other areas of oral mucosa

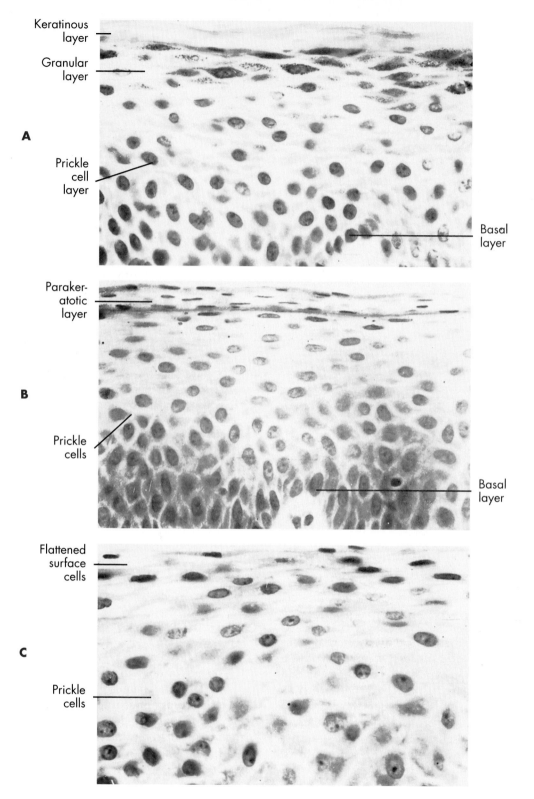

Keratinous
layer

Granular
layer

A

Prickle
cell
layer

Basal
layer

Paraker-
atotic
layer

B

Prickle
cells

Basal
layer

Flattened
surface
cells

C

Prickle
cells

FIG. 8-1. For legend, see opposite page.

FIG. 8-1.   **A,** Keratinized epithelium. Notice the thick layer at the top without any sign of nuclei. These are dead cells. **B,** Parakeratinized epithelium. Although nuclei are present even at the top, there are fewer than in nonkeratinized epithelium, and they appear flattened and shriveled. **C,** Nonkeratinized epithelium. Nuclei are obvious even at the top. (From Bhaskar SN: *Orban's oral histology and embryology,* ed 8, St Louis, 1976, Mosby.)

Mucous membrane is composed of stratified squamous epithelium and connective tissue. Stratified squamous epithelium can have various characteristics on its surface (Fig. 8-1) depending on whether it is keratinized, parakeratinized or nonkeratinized.

1. **Keratinized**—On its surface are layers of dead cells without nuclei. This layer is generally called the *stratum corneum.* The stratum granulosum layer beneath the corneum is relatively evident at this stage of keratinization. As keratinization increases, there tends to be an increase in the thickness of the stratum spinosum as well.

2. **Parakeratinized**—On its surface are some dead cells without nuclei and some apparently dying cells with slightly shriveled nuclei. The stratum granulosum is not quite as evident as in the keratinized mucosa.

3. **Nonkeratinized**—Cells on the surface all tend to have nuclei that appear fairly healthy and normal. The stratum granulosum is missing in this type of mucosa.

The lining mucosa is nonkeratinized to parakeratinized under most circumstances. The basal layer of cells rests on the underlying connective tissue with a basement membrane in between these two components. Although this underlying connective tissue contains some well-developed collagen fibers, it is still loose enough to allow the overlying epithelium to be fairly movable. Also allowing for this mobility is the way in which the epithelium and the connective tissue interdigitate with one another.

As seen in Fig. 8-2, there is a definite interdigitation between the epithelium and the connective tissue. In this illustration the ridges appear to interdigitate between the two; however, looking at a three-dimensional representation (Fig. 8-3), you can see that there are not only ridges of connective tissue but also pegs of connective tissue projecting up into the epithelium. The length of these ridges and connective tissue pegs determines how tightly the epithelium attaches to the underlying connective tissue and therefore how movable the epithelium is. The connective tissue is attached to underlying bone in some areas or to fatty or muscle tissue in other areas.

The lining mucosa tends to have poorly developed epithelial-connective tissue interdigitations and therefore is rather movable on the underlying tissue. This degree of mobility is influenced as well by the attachment of the connective tissue to the type of tissue lying beneath it. The lining mucosa includes the mucosa of the cheeks, lips, soft palate, floor of the mouth beneath the tongue, undersurface or ventral surface of the tongue, and the alveolar mucosa, which is the movable tissue immediately apical to the gingiva.

MASTICATORY MUCOSA

Masticatory mucosa is the mucosa of the gingiva and hard palate. During mastication, food is forced off the teeth and onto the gingiva around the necks of the teeth. The pressure of the food on this tissue causes it to become parakeratinized or keratinized. Food in the hard-palate area and the slight pressure of the tongue

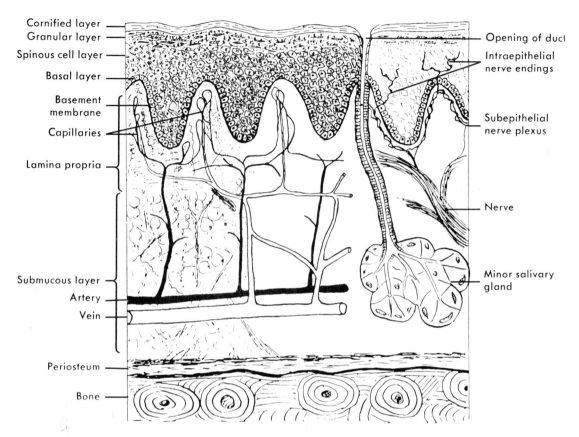

Cornified layer
Granular layer
Spinous cell layer
Basal layer
Basement membrane
Capillaries
Lamina propria
Submucous layer
Artery
Vein
Periosteum
Bone

Opening of duct
Intraepithelial nerve endings
Subepithelial nerve plexus
Nerve
Minor salivary gland

FIG. 8-2.   Epithelium-connective tissue junction in a two-dimensional representation. Notice the interdigitation of the ridges or pegs of each tissue layer. (From Bhaskar SN: *Orban's oral histology and embryology*, ed 8, St Louis, 1976, Mosby.)

rubbing on the palate also cause this area to become parakeratinized or keratinized, depending on the amount of trauma.

The gingiva is divided into two regions, the **free gingiva (marginal gingiva)** and the **attached gingiva.** These two regions combine to form the peak of gingiva that extends coronally between the teeth, which is known as the **interdental papilla** (Fig. 8-4). The function of the interdental papilla is to prevent food from impacting interproximally beneath the contact area of the teeth and setting up an irritation that could eventually lead to periodontal disease. The part of the inter-

dental papilla that is apical to the contact area and connects the facial and lingual interdental papilla is known as the **col** and is nonkeratinized. If there is drifting of the teeth, or if Class II restorations are done without properly restoring the contact area, then the col will become irritated. At first the trauma may cause bleeding, but later it will likely become parakeratinized or possibly even keratinized. If the proper contact areas are restored, there will be a slow return to nonkeratinized epithelium.

Looking closely at the teeth and gingiva, you will find that there is a very shallow groove or

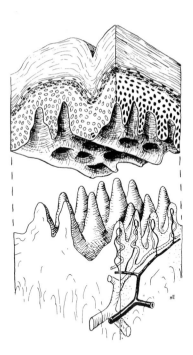

FIG. 8-3. In a three-dimensional representation connective tissue pegs can be seen projecting up from ridges into the epithelium. (From Elias H et al: *Human microanatomy,* ed 4, Philadelphia, 1978, FA Davis Co.)

sulcus around the tooth. The average depth of this sulcus measured with a periodontal probe is about 2 mm (Fig. 8-5). The stratified squamous epithelium that lines this sulcus is nonkeratinized, and at the bottom of the sulcus the epithelium is continuous with the cells that attach to the tooth, known as the **attachment epithelium (junctional epithelium)**. In cases of periodontal disease the sulcus deepens either as a result of the free gingiva swelling or the attachment epithelium breaking down or moving farther apically on the tooth. The extent of the free gingiva is usually readily seen because there may be a shallow groove on the gingival surface that corresponds to its depth. This is called the *free gingival groove.*

The interdental papilla is an extremely important part of the gingiva. In a healthy state it fills the area between the teeth up to their contact areas and prevents food from becoming lodged or impacted between the teeth during mastication. It is also one of the first areas involved in periodontal disease, becoming swollen and blunted. As this happens, the lack of original contour causes it to be further irritated during mastication, and the problem becomes more complicated. For this reason it is an important area to study and check for swelling, blunting, reddening, and so on, as disease indicators.

The remainder of the gingiva is called the *attached gingiva.* Its name is derived from the fact that it is tightly attached to the underlying connective tissue and bone (see Fig. 8-4). In a healthy state the gingiva usually has a stippled or dimpled appearance. This is caused by the connective tissue fibers attaching epithelium to the underlying bone. In periodontal disease one of the first signs of gingival problems is a loss of stippling. This is initially caused by swelling or **edema** of the gingival tissues. The normal color of this gingiva is pink, but in the diseased state it might become reddish, whitish, or have ulcerations or outgrowths of the mucosa.

Where the attached gingiva meets the **alveolar mucosa** there is a change in color and a loss of stippling because the epithelium is not attached tightly to the bone. The alveolar mucosa is more reddened by the underlying blood vessels and thinness of the epithelium of the mucosa.

In the maxillary arch the lingual gingiva does not change into alveolar mucosa but is directly continuous with the masticatory mucosa of the hard palate. This palatal mucosa is generally the area of thickest mucosa in the oral cavity and the most likely to be keratinized.

In this area of masticatory mucosa the interdigitations between connective tissue and epithelium are long and narrow and therefore help make the epithelium very adherent and relatively immovable (Fig. 8-6). It is within this connective tissue that the blood vessels, nerves, small salivary glands, and some fatty deposits are found.

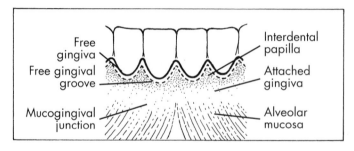

FIG. 8-4.   Free gingiva and the free gingival groove, which divides the free gingiva from attached gingiva. Notice the stippled appearance of the gingiva compared with the alveolar mucosa. (Modified from Pawlak E, Hoag PM: *Essentials of periodontics,* ed 2, St Louis, 1980, Mosby.)

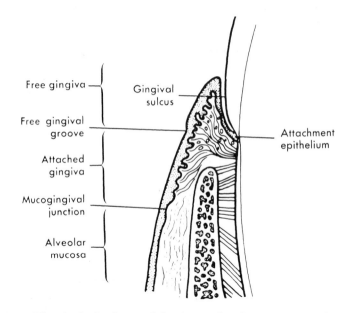

FIG. 8-5.   The gingival sulcus and the tissues that form it. Notice the area of attachment epithelium at the bottom and the free gingival groove that marks the depth of the sulcus. (From Pawlak E, Hoag PM: *Essentials of periodontics,* ed 2, St Louis, 1980, Mosby.)

LINING MUCOSA

Following are descriptions of the various areas of lining mucosa and their different appearances. Some of these have already been discussed earlier in the chapter.

a. Alveolar mucosa—Runs from the gingiva to the area of the mucobuccal or mucolabial fold; has already been discussed.

b. Buccal mucosa—If the buccal mucosa, the mucosa of the cheek, is constantly traumatized by chewing, it will become thickened and keratinized in a line corresponding to the occlusal surfaces of the teeth. There are many

Epithelium

Connective
tissue

Submucosa

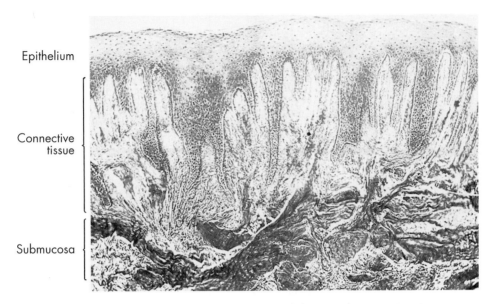

FIG. 8-6. Long interdigitations between epithelium and connective tissue. These make masticatory mucosa immovable. (From Bhaskar SN: *Orban's oral histology and embryology,* ed 8, St Louis, 1976, Mosby.)

pathologic conditions that produce whitish lesions of the cheek mucosa. Most of them are rather harmless, whereas others may be very serious. Sebaceous glands are frequently found in the buccal mucosa.

c. Labial mucosa—Trauma to mucosa of the lip may cause some thickening as in the cheek, but more frequently will cause trauma to a minor salivary gland and cause a blisterlike lesion known as a **mucocele.**

d. Col has already been discussed.

e. Gingival sulcus has already been discussed.

f. Mucosa of the soft palate—A mucosa of about the same thickness as the buccal and labial mucosa, although not as easily traumatized. There are times when the connective tissue of the soft palate is excessive and causes **sleep apnea,** a condition in which the patient not only snores and wakes up tired in the morning, but also ceases breathing for more than 20 seconds numerous times each hour. They never get into a deep sleep and thus are tired in the morning.

g. Sublingual gingiva and ventral surface of tongue—These areas are very well protected from trauma. The epithelium is very thin, and if it is traumatized by something sharp, there may be a laceration or at least severe irritation to the mucosa.

SUBMUCOSA

The **submucosa** is the connective tissue beneath the mucosa that contains blood vessels and nerves and also helps determine the mobility of the mucosa by the length of its connective tissue ridges and pegs. It is not present in all areas of the oral cavity, but when it is it tends to increase the mobility of the mucosa on top of it. If a submucosa is present, it tends to contain fatty tissue, minor salivary glands, or both. There is very little if any submucosa in the gingiva and anteromedial hard palate. In these areas the mucosa is tightly attached to the periosteum of the underlying bone.

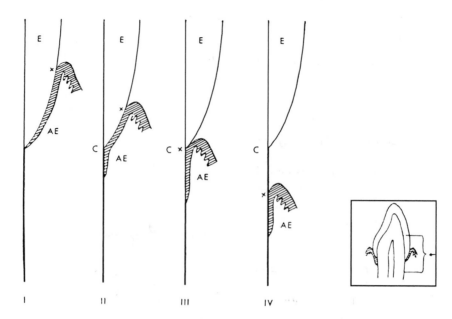

Fig. 8-7.   Four stages of passive eruption. *X*, base of sulcus; *AE*, attachment epithelium; *C*, cementum; *E*, enamel.

PASSIVE ERUPTION

In Chapter 7 we discussed active eruption and how the tooth breaks through the mucosa and into the oral cavity. There is also a process known as **passive eruption** in which the attachment epithelium moves from the crown of the tooth apically. Remember that as the tooth breaks through into the oral cavity the attachment epithelium is formed from the reduced enamel epithelium. This is frequently referred to as the **primary attachment epithelium.** Later the primary attachment epithelium is replaced by a **secondary attachment epithelium,** which arises from the basal layer of the epithelium in the free gingiva. Passive eruption is generally broken down into the following four stages (Fig. 8-7).

Stage I—The attachment epithelium at the base of the gingival sulcus rests entirely on enamel. The more recent the eruption, the

more incisally or occlusally it may be located.

Stage II—The attachment epithelium is primarily on enamel with a bit on cementum. This may be a relatively long stage.

Stage III—The attachment epithelium extends from the cementoenamel junction (CEJ) onto cementum. This may also be a relatively long stage.

Stage IV—The attachment epithelium is entirely on cementum apical to the CEJ.

There is no specific timing for the process of passive eruption, and it may never reach stage IV, which is considered by some as pathologic and is generally referred to as gingival recession.

The attaching of epithelium to tooth is an extremely active process. The cells that provide for this attachment are replaced every 3 to 5 days, and this rapid turnover aids in the repair of early gingival or periodontal disease. With proper dental prophylaxis there can be significant improvements in attachment epithelium in a week or slightly more.

CHANGES IN ORAL MUCOSA

Sometimes the tissue of the oral cavity deviates from its normal color; it may appear quite reddish or whitish. Epithelial cells have no color themselves, but they may take up pigments produced by the body and carry them to the surface. It is this carried pigment that gives differential colors to the skin. The redness of the mucosa comes from the oxygen-carrying pigment in the blood, known as *hemoglobin*. These blood vessels are located immediately beneath the mucosa in the connective tissue, and the reflection of the blood through the epithelium imparts a red color to the mucosa. When the mucosa is excessively red, this is the result of inflammation—the blood vessels beneath the mucosa expand and bring more blood to the area to fight the causative irritation. In a pathologic condition you will find that redness is one of the primary signs of inflammation. How then can the epithelium appear whitish? Is it because there is less blood beneath the epithelium? It generally is the result of irritation of the mucosa, which causes the cells to multiply faster and the epithelium to become thicker, a condition similar to the development of a callus. When it becomes thicker, the tissue becomes more **opaque,** and the blood does not show through easily; therefore the tissue is whiter than normal. Looking at thickened, whitish mucosa, you can see histologically that the thickened layers are the stratum spinosum and the stratum corneum. This, of course, is a keratinized epithelium.

It cannot be stressed too strongly that the oral mucosa is a very important indicator for both the oral and general health of the person. The color, tone, and contours of the tissue are extremely important health indicators. Study these tissues carefully—they will provide much important information.

Review Questions

1. What are the three divisions of the oral mucosa, and where are they located?
2. What are the three variations of stratified squamous epithelium?
3. What are the changes in layers evident in these variations?
4. What determines the mobility of the mucosa?
5. What are the general causes of change in mucosal color?
6. What structures can be found in the submucosa?
7. What is the average depth of the gingival sulcus?
8. What is the function of the interdental papilla?
9. What is the col, and when may it be damaged?
10. What is the descriptive term used for normal gingival appearance?
11. Describe the relationship of the attachment epithelium to the tooth in the four stages of eruption.

CHAPTER 9

THE TONGUE

OBJECTIVES
- To describe the formation of the tongue as it relates to the germ layers and its pharyngeal arches of origin
- To discuss the difference between extrinsic and intrinsic muscles of the tongue
- To describe briefly how tongue movement is accomplished
- To describe the papillae of the tongue and their function
- To describe the kinds of changes seen on the tongue that indicate health problems

DEVELOPMENT OF THE TONGUE

As discussed in Chapter 3, there are a number of bars of tissue found on the anterior surface of the developing embryo that are referred to as *pharyngeal arches*. The first pharyngeal arch is the mandibular arch, the second is the hyoid arch, and the remainder are numbered III, IV, and VI (V disappears). Just above the first arch and extending down behind all the arches is a hollow tube, the digestive tract. Before the end of the fourth embryonic week, this tube is closed off at the upper end by the buccopharyngeal membrane, which separates the upper end or foregut from the primitive oral cavity or stomodeum. The epithelium anterior to the buccopha-

ryngeal membrane develops from the outer germ layer or ectoderm. The tube behind the buccopharyngeal membrane develops from the inner germ layer or entoderm. At about $4\frac{1}{2}$ weeks the buccopharyngeal membrane ruptures, but the epithelium in that area still comes from two distinct germ layers. It is at this point that the tongue starts to develop as a swelling that arises out of the back part of the pharyngeal arches (Fig. 9-1). This swelling develops from the future floor of the mouth. The epithelial covering of the tongue develops from ectoderm and entoderm— the anterior two thirds from ectoderm and the posterior one third from entoderm. The tongue is basically a sac of epithelium filled with mus-

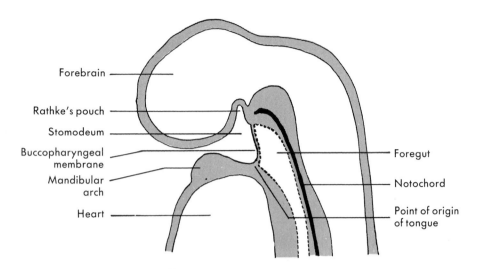

Forebrain

Rathke's pouch

Stomodeum

Buccopharyngeal
membrane

Mandibular
arch

Heart

Foregut

Notochord

Point of origin
of tongue

FIG. 9-1.   An anteroposterior section through an embryo. The mandibular or first pharyngeal arch is marked, and others are below it partially covered by the heart. The tongue arises from an area at the lower end of the buccopharyngeal membrane. (From Bhaskar SN: *Orban's oral histology and embryology*, ed 8, St Louis, 1976, Mosby.)

cles. These muscles arise from the middle germ layer of the embryo, known as *mesoderm.*

Each pharyngeal arch is associated with a particular cranial nerve; Chapter 19 on the nervous system discusses from which pharyngeal arch the various parts of the tongue develop. If you refer back to Chapter 3 you will find that the anterior two thirds of the tongue develop from two lateral lingual swellings and a midline tuberculum impar. These are both from the first arch. The posterior one third of the tongue develops from the copula (hypobranchial eminence) and the third arch. The root of the tongue and epiglottis develops from the epiglottal swelling of the fourth arch.

TONGUE MUSCLES

As mentioned before, the tongue is an epithelial sac filled with muscles and connective tissue. These muscles can be controlled willfully and are generally referred to as *skeletal muscle* or *voluntary striated muscle.* They are divided into two

groupings: **intrinsic** and **extrinsic** muscles. Those that start and end wholly within the tongue are referred to as intrinsic muscles and include the four following groups:

1. Superior longitudinal group—runs from front to back (anterior to posterior) and lies near the dorsum of the tongue
2. Inferior longitudinal group—also runs anterior to posterior but lies near the bottom or ventrum of the tongue
3. Transverse group—runs from side to side
4. Vertical group—runs from top to bottom (dorsal to ventral)

What happens when the muscles in these groups contract? Keep in mind the direction of the muscle fibers and imagine the tongue as an oblong balloon with a constant volume. If the longitudinal group of fibers contracts, the tongue is shortened. Shortening the tongue makes it thicker and wider. If you contract the group that runs transversely, the tongue may get a little thicker and longer. Contract the vertical group, and the tongue may get wider and longer. Try to picture what would happen if you contracted two of these groups at the same time.

Along with the intrinsic muscles in the tongue are groups of muscles that originate outside the tongue and run into it. These are the extrinsic muscles. The extrinsic muscles of the tongue actually are more directly related to gross anatomy than oral histology, but because they affect intrinsic muscle action, they should be mentioned here. There are four pairs of muscles, left and right. The **hyoglossus** runs from the lateral sides of the **hyoid** bone up into the lateral borders of the tongue and pulls the lateral edges or borders of the tongue down onto the floor of the mouth (see Fig. 13-6). The **styloglossus** runs from the styloid process down and forward into the lateral borders of the tongue and blends with the hyoglossus. The styloglossus pulls the tongue backward and slightly up. The **palatoglossus** runs from the anterior soft palate down and slightly forward into the lateral borders of the tongue (see Fig. 16-1). It elevates the posterior part of the tongue and pulls it slightly backward. The **genioglossus** originates from the superior **genial tubercles** on the midline of the mandible and inserts into the midline of the tongue from the tip to the base (see Fig. 13-6). It aids in protrusion or depression of the tongue.

PAPILLAE

The tongue is covered with stratified squamous epithelium. The ventral surface of the tongue has very thin epithelium, but the upper surface has thick parakeratinized to keratinized epithelium. Scattered throughout this epithelium on the uppermost surface are four types of elevated structures known as papillae.

Circumvallate or Vallate Papillae

One type of papilla is **circumvallate** or **vallate papillae**, a V-shaped row of circular raised papillae. There are about 13 elevations in the V, which is located about two thirds of the way back on the tongue with the point of the V facing backward. This row anatomically divides the anterior two thirds of the tongue from the posterior one third and marks the area that develops from different pharyngeal arches with different nerve supplies (see also Chapter 19.) Under a microscope vallate papillae appear to rest in troughs, and they have many tiny **taste buds** all around their lateral surfaces (Fig. 9-2). These taste buds are made up of many cells supporting several small hairlike nerve endings that perceive taste (Fig. 9-3). Small salivary glands are located beneath these papillae, and they serve to wash the papillae clean, making them ready to perceive new tastes. These are the Ebner's glands.

Fungiform Papillae

The anterior two thirds of the tongue have tiny, round, raised spots. In younger persons these spots frequently appear redder than the area around them. These are the **fungiform papillae**. There are taste buds in these papillae similar to those in the vallate papillae, only located on the upper surface instead of the side (Fig. 9-4, *A*).

Filiform Papillae

The remainder of the anterior two thirds of the tongue is covered with tiny pointed projections of parakeratinized to keratinized epithelium known as **filiform papillae** (Fig. 9-4, *B*). They have no taste function and probably only provide tactile sensation or the ability to know that there is something on the tongue. In cats they are well developed, and you can feel the rough surface of these papillae when a cat licks your hand. Sometimes the epithelia on these papillae grow very long and trap between them food and pigments originating from oral bacteria and food. When these papillae are very long, the condition is called **hairy tongue**. Other times the epithelia of these papillae are lost, and the surface in that area becomes very smooth. This is referred to as *glossitis*, and it occurs in a number

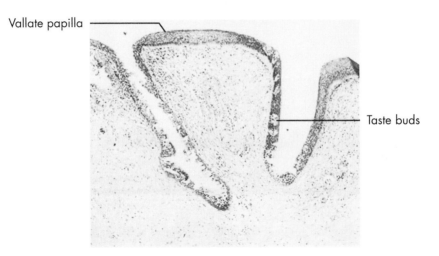

Vallate papilla

Taste buds

FIG. 9-2. Large vallate papilla in a trough, with light-colored taste buds along its side. (From Bhaskar SN: *Orban's oral histology and embryology,* ed 8, St Louis, 1976, Mosby.)

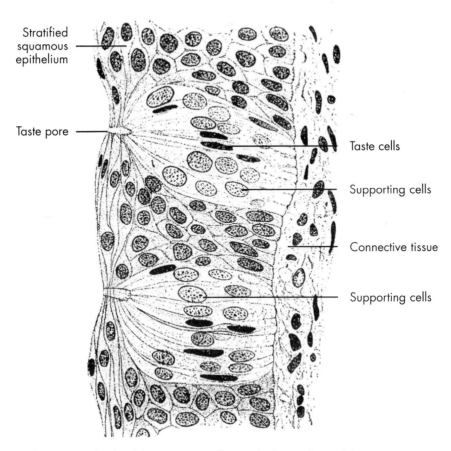

Stratified squamous epithelium

Taste pore

Taste cells

Supporting cells

Connective tissue

Supporting cells

FIG. 9-3. The hairlike receptors of taste buds are located in taste pores. (From Bhaskar SN: *Orban's oral histology and embryology,* ed 8, St Louis, 1976, Mosby.)

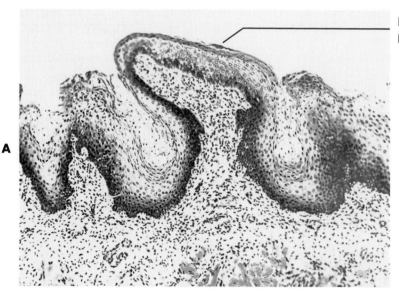

Fungiform
papillae

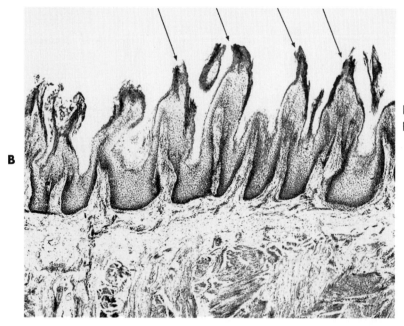

Filiform
papillae

FIG. 9-4. **A,** Fungiform papillae. Although taste buds are not visible in fungiform papillae, they are present in small numbers. **B,** Filiform papillae. (From Bhaskar SN: *Orban's oral histology and embryology,* ed 8, St Louis, 1976, Mosby.)

of disease processes, one of which is vitamin deficiencies.

Foliate Papillae

If you grasp the tip of the tongue with a piece of gauze and pull it out and to the side, you will see a roughened lateral surface back in the region of the vallate papillae. In lower forms of animals this area is another set of well-developed papillae with many taste buds, known as the **foliate papillae.** In humans these are not so well developed and contain fewer taste buds than those in animals.

The posterior lateral border of the tongue where the foliate papillae are located is an area that can become irritated and reddened. It is also an area where oral cancer can begin but be obscured because of the location and folds of tissue. It is therefore an important area to check in oral examinations (Fig. 9-5).

Another area that should be mentioned is a region near the midline on the dorsum of the tongue just behind the vallate papillae, known as the **lingual tonsils.** This is lymphoid tissue similar to the palatine tonsil and provides a defense mechanism for infection in that area. Infection in this part of the tongue will involve the lingual tonsils, and they will become reddened and enlarged. Therefore this is an important clinical indicator of potential problems (see Fig. 9-5).

The tongue as a whole is a good indicator of the patient's overall health, as is the gingival tissue. These areas should be carefully studied when a patient is being examined.

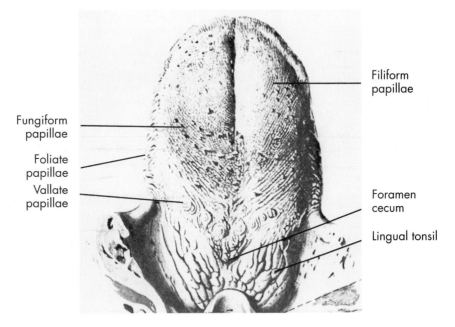

FIG. 9-5.   Overall view of a tongue showing large lingual tonsils on the posterior and the roughened area of foliate papillae on the side. (From Bhaskar SN: *Orban's oral histology and embryology,* ed 8, St Louis, 1976, Mosby.)

Review Questions

1. How many different germ layers form the entire tongue?
2. What is the difference between extrinsic and intrinsic muscles?
3. How are various tongue movements and shapes accomplished?
4. Name the papillae of the tongue, where they are located, and what their functions are.
5. What two kinds of cells do you see in a taste bud?
6. What kinds of changes can you see in the tongue that relate to the health of a person?

CHAPTER 10

SALIVARY GLANDS

OBJECTIVES
- To describe the components of a salivary gland
- To describe the duct system of a salivary gland
- To describe the arrangement of the cells of a mixed salivary gland
- To describe how saliva is formed and modified before secretion
- To describe the functions of saliva

IN THIS chapter we will attempt to describe only the histology of salivary glands. For the description of size, location, and function of these glands, refer to Chapter 18.

COMPONENTS OF A SALIVARY GLAND

As discussed in Chapter 2, salivary glands arise from a cord of epithelium growing into the underlying connective tissue, and the cord later forms a tube. At the end of this tube a cluster of secretory cells forms, and these clusters, which look like bunches of grapes, will have endpieces that are either round or tubelike.

Acini

The secretory endpieces are known as **acini**. There are two kinds of acinic cells, **mucous acini** and **serous acini**. Although these cells form a grapelike or tubular endpiece, in cross section they are described as **pyramidal cells** (Fig. 10-1). The outer edge or base of the cells rests on a basement membrane between the cells and the connective tissue. Within this connective tissue are the nerves and blood vessels necessary for the various aspects of cellular activity. The apex of the cells faces the center of the tube or grapelike structure. The base of the cells is surrounded by connective tissue, and partially surrounding each secretory acinus is a **myoepithelial cell** (Fig. 10-2). This cell has long cellular projections that make it look like a squid. It also has the ability to contract like a muscle. Hence the prefix *myo* meaning muscle. These projections surround the acinus, and when the myoepithelial cell contracts, it squeezes the acinus and aids in the se-

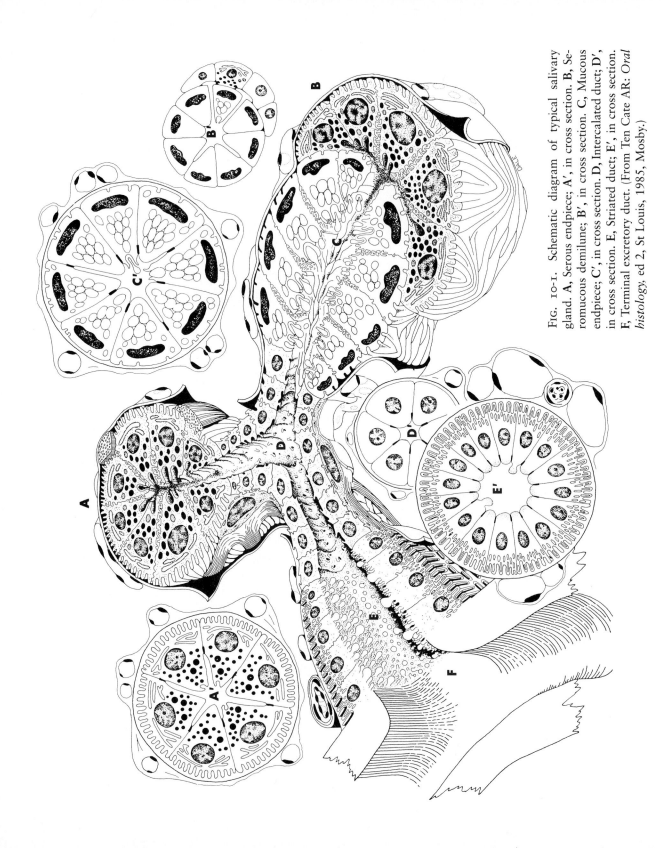

FIG. 10-1. Schematic diagram of typical salivary gland. A, Serous endpiece; A', in cross section. B, Seromucous demilune; B', in cross section. C, Mucous endpiece; C', in cross section. D, Intercalated duct; D', in cross section. E, Striated duct; E', in cross section. F, Terminal excretory duct. (From Ten Cate AR: *Oral histology*, ed 2, St Louis, 1985, Mosby.)

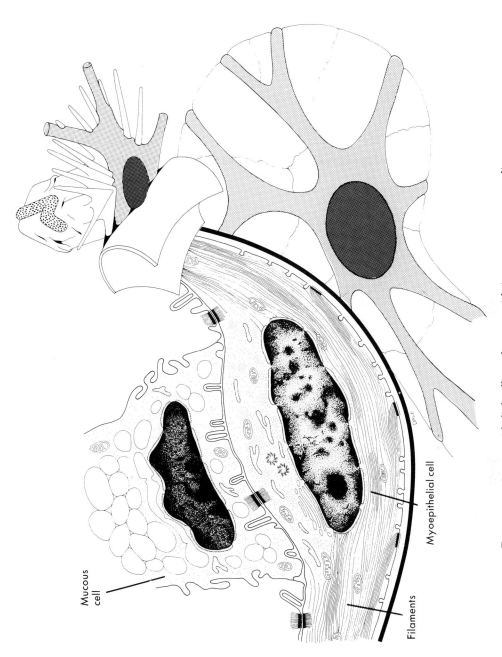

Mucous
cell

Myoepithelial cell

Filaments

FIG. 10-2.   A myoepithelial cell can be seen with its processes surrounding
an acinus.

cretion of saliva that has accumulated in the hollow center of the acinus and helps move it out the duct system. All types of acini—mucous, serous, and seromucous—secrete their products through the process of merocrine secretion.

Mucous acini

A **mucous** secretion is slightly viscous because of the production of several mucins. Although its product is 99% water, it does have a number of inorganic ions, such as sodium, potassium, and chloride, and very minor amounts of **amylase,** a carbohydrate-splitting enzyme that begins to break down starches into long-chain sugars. It probably also has some proteins that aid in inhibiting caries and periodontal disease. A mucous acinus is more tubular and has a larger **lumen** than a serous acinus, and the cell membranes can more easily be seen at adjacent sides of the cells. The nucleus of a mucous cell is usually very flat and lies against the basal part of the cell, and the cell itself is pyramidal in shape. The apical end of these cells appears frothy under the light microscope. In the electron microscope one can see a great number of mucous droplets that stain very poorly and so give an empty, frothy appearance.

Serous acini

The makeup of serous acinus secretions is similar to that of mucous acini, only without the mucins; a **serous** secretion is a thinner, more watery secretion. A serous acinus is the primary source of amylase. The secretory granules stain deeply, the lumen is very small and difficult to see, and the adjacent cell membranes are not easily seen. A serous cell is also pyramidal in shape. The nucleus is round and is close to the base of the cell.

Seromucous acini

In glands that have both mucous and serous components you can see the separate types of acini, and you can also see them joined together as mixed or **seromucous acini.** In a seromucous acinus, the mucous cells form a tubelike structure, and on the end of the tube a group of se-

rous cells forms into a half-moon cluster. These are referred to as **serous demilunes.** As the term **seromucous** suggests, these acini produce both mucous and serous secretions (see Fig. 10-1).

Connective Tissue Capsule

A salivary gland is surrounded by a connective tissue capsule. The connective tissue not only surrounds the gland but also sends partitions into the gland carrying nerves and blood vessels with it and dividing the gland into lobes and smaller units called lobules (Fig. 10-3).

Duct System

Salivary glands have varying numbers of lobules, depending on their size, and as just mentioned, each lobule is surrounded by connective tissue. There is a series of different kinds of ducts, some of them within the lobule, some between the lobule, and some outside of the gland leading to the surface of the oral cavity.

Intralobular ducts

Within the lobule are two kinds of ducts that by location are classified as **intralobular ducts,** meaning "within the lobule."

Intercalated ducts. **Intercalated ducts** are very small intralobular ducts that directly drain the acini. The cells in these ducts are not much taller than their nuclei. In some glands the ducts are long and easily seen, whereas in others they are short and rarely seen. These intercalated ducts carry the secretions, unchanged, to the next set of ducts within the lobule.

Striated (secretory) ducts. Intralobular **striated ducts** are so named because the bases of the cells within these ducts appear to be striped. The basal cell membrane has infoldings in which mitochondria become trapped. These mitochondria can be stained, causing a striped appearance. These ducts are also called *secretory* because, as the salivary fluid passes through them, their content is modified. Water and various substances such as sodium, potassium, chloride, and other ions are reabsorbed and then secreted out of the

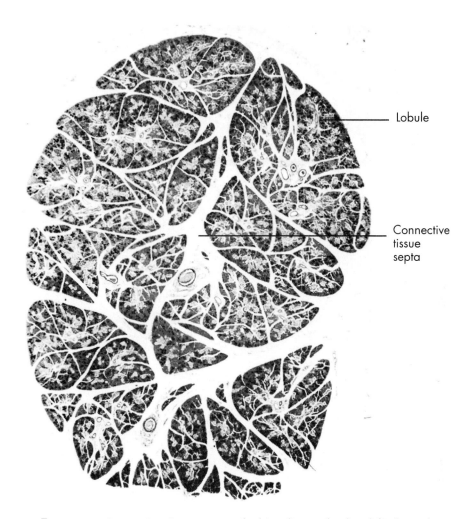

Lobule

Connective
tissue
septa

FIG. 10-3.   Connective tissue surrounds this salivary gland and further subdivides it into lobules.

basal end of the cell where they are picked up again by the capillaries and lymphatic vessels. This function is important because it conserves water and electrolytes (see Fig. 10-1).

Interlobular ducts

Interlobular ducts lie within the connective tissue between lobules of the gland. Some of these are striated like the striated intralobular ducts, but most of them are nonstriated and large. These nonstriated ducts are generally referred to as **excretory ducts.** These ducts do not modify the salivary secretions but simply carry them out of the gland and to the surface tissues of the oral cavity (Fig. 10-4).

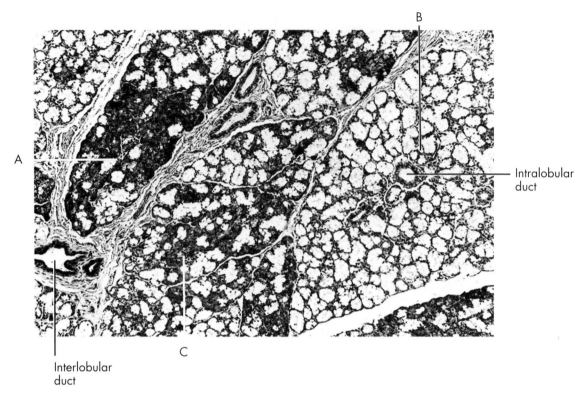

FIG. 10-4.   Both intralobular and interlobular ducts. *A,* Mostly serous lobule; *B,* Mostly mucous lobule; *C,* Lobule fairly even in mucous and serous
acini.

CONTROL OF SECRETIONS

Secretory control comes from the **autonomic nervous system,** particularly the parasympathetic nervous system (see Chapter 19). The control of secretion is tied to chewing, taste, and smell. Each of these is capable of modifying the amount and consistency of the salivary secretions.

FORMATION OF SALIVA

Saliva is formed within the endoplasmic reticulum of individual cells. If you remember from Chapter 2, the control of production within the endoplasmic reticulum comes from the DNA in the nucleus via the varying types of RNA. The future saliva is packaged by a membrane within the Golgi apparatus and moves out into the cytoplasm of the mucous or serous acini. The apical end of the cell accumulates these granules of future saliva, when the gland is stimulated by the parasympathetic nervous system, the granules move to the apical cell membrane, fuse with it, release their substance into the center of the acini. From there the secretion moves out through the intercalated ducts into the striated, intralobular ducts and the extrinsic ducts opening into the oral cavity.

As it passes through the striated ducts, there

are active changes in the fluid content. Water is pulled out of the lumen of the duct, through the striated duct, and into the capillaries lying at the base of the cells of the duct. At the same time there is conservation of electrolytes and secretion of potassium and bicarbonate. The fluid within the duct becomes more concentrated. Depending on the type of secretion, the amount of amylase will vary and be available to begin the breakdown of starches before further breakdown in the stomach and duodenum. There are also immunoglobulins in the saliva as well as antibacterial lysozymes that protect the body from bacteria. The saliva also acts as a Ph buffer, which plays a role in resistance to decay if it is working properly.

FUNCTION OF SALIVA

Basically, saliva functions to help prepare the bolus of food so that it can be swallowed more easily. It also may play a role in dehydration. If there are not enough body fluids, saliva production will be decreased, and the mouth will become dry, a stimulus to drink more water. As was just mentioned, saliva also acts as a Ph buffer, and the immunoglobulins and lysozymes within saliva play a role in protection of the body.

Review Questions

1. What are acini, and what are three types? Describe their appearance.
2. What is a myoepithelial cell, and what is its function?
3. Define the following and their function:
   a. Intercalated duct
   b. Striated duct
   c. Secretory duct
   d. Excretory duct
   e. Intralobular duct
   f. Interlobular duct
4. What are serous demilunes?
5. What controls the secretion of salivary glands?
6. What enzyme is found in saliva, and what does it do?
7. What is the function of saliva?

TEST

1. Small localized growths of bone on the buccal cortical plate are known as
   a. torus mandibularis
   b. exostoses
   c. torus palatinus
   d. both a and c above
   e. None of the above
2. What are Fordyce granules?
   a. abnormal minor salivary glands
   b. excessive numbers of salivary glands
   c. misplaced sebaceous glands
   d. abnormal hair follicles
   e. none of the above
3. What is the location of the fovea palatinae?
   a. in the posterior lateral palate over the opening of the greater palatine foramen
   b. in the anterior palate over the incisive foramen
   c. on either side of the posterior nasal spine
   d. between the anterior and posterior tonsillar pillars
   e. none of the above
4. The space between the left and right palatine tonsils is known as what?
   a. anterior pillars
   b. posterior pillars
   c. palatoglossal folds
   d. fauces
   e. none of the above
5. If denture flanges are overextended, which of the following muscles may cause displacement of the lower denture?
   a. styloglossus
   b. hyoglossus
   c. mylohyoid
   d. all of the above
   e. none of the above
6. With the mouth open wide, which of the following may impinge upon the vestibule?
   a. mandibular condyle
   b. lingual frenum
   c. torus mandibularis
   d. coronoid process
   e. none of the above
7. Which of the following structures may cause a diastema?
   a. maxillary lingual frenum
   b. mandibular lingual frenum
   c. maxillary labial frenum
   d. mandibular labial frenum
   e. all of the above
8. Which of the following is *not* a cell organelle?
   a. nucleus
   b. glycogen
   c. endoplasmic reticulum
   d. Golgi apparatus
   e. all are organelles
9. The skin and mucosa of the oral cavity are an example of _____ epithelium.
   a. simple squamous
   b. simple columnar
   c. transitional
   d. stratified squamous
   e. pseudostratified squamous
10. Which of the following would *not* be classed as connective tissue?
    a. bone
    b. cartilage
    c. collagen
    d. tendon
    e. ligament
    f. all are connective tissue

11. Which of the following is *not* a granulocyte blood cell?
    a. neutrophil
    b. lymphocyte
    c. basophil
    d. eosinophil
    e. all are granulocytes
12. Which of the following muscle tissues is classified as striated voluntary muscle?
    a. cardiac
    b. skeletal
    c. smooth
    d. a and b
    e. b and c
    f. a, b, and c
13. The smallest functioning unit of a skeletal muscle is the
    a. myofibril
    b. sarcomere
    c. Z line
    d. myofiber
    e. intercalated disk
14. The protective sheath around a nerve cell is known as a _____ sheath.
    a. dendrite
    b. axon
    c. myelin
    d. cellulin
    e. none of the above
15. In the development of the germ layers in the embryo, where does the mesoderm come from?
    a. comes from ectoderm
    b. comes from entoderm
    c. may come from ectoderm or entoderm
    d. comes from the membranes surrounding the embryo
    e. none of the above is correct
16. The type of epithelium found in the urinary bladder and urethra is
    a. simple cuboidal or columnar
    b. stratified squamous
    c. pseudostratified columnar
    d. stratified columnar
    e. none of the above

17. One of the most important and abundant cells in irregular connective tissue is the
    a. reticulocyte
    b. fibroblast
    c. elastocyte
    d. macrophage
    e. basal cell
18. The developmental period of the embryo is
    a. 0-2 weeks
    b. 3-8 weeks
    c. 8-12 weeks
    d. 12-36 weeks
19. The upper lip develops from the
    a. medial nasal process
    b. lateral nasal process
    c. maxillary process
    d. mandibular process
    e. a and b
    f. b and c
    g. a and c
    h. none of the above
20. The upper lip forms by a process of _____, while the palate forms by a process of _____.
    a. elongation, migration
    b. migration, fusion
    c. fusion, elongation
    d. none of the above
21. The premaxilla comes from the
    a. lateral nasal process
    b. medial nasal process
    c. mandibular process
    d. maxillary process
    e. none of the above
22. The buccopharyngeal membrane breaks down during the _____ embryonic week.
    a. second
    b. third
    c. fourth
    d. fifth
23. The critical time for facial development is _____ weeks.
    a. 2-5
    b. 3-6
    c. 5-9
    d. 7-10

24. The critical time for palatal development is _____ weeks.
    a. 2-6
    b. 3-7
    c. 5-9
    d. 7-11
25. There are _____ pharyngeal arches that develop
    a. two
    b. three
    c. four
    d. five
26. Cleft lips occur about once in every _____ births among U. S. whites.
    a. 300
    b. 800
    c. 1500
    d. 7000
    e. 10,000
27. Which of the following are *not* a part of an early pharyngeal arch?
    a. cartilage
    b. bone
    c. nerve
    d. blood vessel
    e. mesodermal tissue
28. The first signs of tooth development are seen in the _____ week.
    a. fourth
    b. sixth
    c. tenth
    d. twelfth
    e. none of the above
29. The first stage of the enamel organ is the _____ stage.
    a. cap
    b. bell
    c. bud
    d. incisive
    e. none of the above
30. The beginning of the bell stage occurs when the _____ appears.
    a. outer enamel epithelium
    b. stellate reticulum

c. stratum intermedium
d. inner enamel epithelium
e. none of the above
31. Which of the following *does not* arise from the dental sac?
    a. dentin
    b. cementum
    c. periodontal ligament
    d. they all arise from it
32. The ameloblast arises from the
    a. dental papilla
    b. inner enamel epithelium
    c. outer enamel epithelium
    d. stellate reticulum
    e. none of the above
33. Enamel is about _____ hydroxyapatite crystals.
    a. 30%
    b. 70%
    c. 95%
    d. 5%
34. The last thing the ameloblast produces is the
    a. primary enamel cuticle
    b. Nasmyth's membrane
    c. reduced enamel epithelium
    d. secondary enamel cuticle
    e. a and b
35. What shape are ameloblasts?
    a. round
    b. hexagonal
    c. keyhole shaped
    d. flat
    e. both a and b above
36. Cracks in the enamel are known as
    a. enamel spindles
    b. enamel tufts
    c. imbrication lines
    d. enamel lamellae
    e. none of the above
37. Dentin is about __ crystal in composition.
    a. 10%
    b. 30%
    c. 50%
    d. 70%

e. none of the above

38. Dentin formed beneath an area of decay is known as _____ dentin.
    a. mantle
    b. circumpulpal
    c. primary
    d. reparative
    e. secondary
    f. none of the above

39. Pulp develops from
    a. dental papilla
    b. mesenchyme
    c. pulp stones
    d. dental sac
    e. a and b
    f. none of the above

40. When odontoblasts die they are replaced by
    a. adjacent odontoblasts
    b. fibroblasts
    c. mesenchymal cells
    d. cementoblasts
    e. none of the above

41. Cementum is about _____ inorganic crystals.
    a. 10%
    b. 30%
    c. 50%
    d. 70%
    e. 90%

42. Hertwig's root sheath comes from
    a. enamel organ
    b. dental papilla
    c. dentin
    d. dental sac
    e. none of the above

43. If osteoclasts in the periodontal space destroy cementum and dentin, what kind of cell do you think will repair the dentin?
    a. osteoblast
    b. odontoblast
    c. cementoblast
    d. fibroblast
    e. none of the above

44. At the cementoenamel junction, cementum overlaps enamel about _____ of the time.

a. 10%
b. 20%
c. 30%
d. 60%
e. 90%

45. Which of the following is *not* a true statement concerning Sharpey's fibers?
    a. They are found in cementum.
    b. They are found in dentin.
    c. They are found in alveolar bone.
    d. They are the embedded portion of the periodontal ligament.
    e. All of the above are true statements.

46. Cellular cementum is usually found
    a. at the cementoenamel junction
    b. in the cervical third of the root
    c. in the middle third of the root only
    d. in the apical third of the root

47. Which of the following is *not* found originally as alveolar bone is forming?
    a. bundle bone
    b. cribriform plate
    c. spongy bone
    d. cortical plate
    e. They are all an original part of alveolar bone.

48. Which of the following alveolodental fibers would resist the forces of mastication?
    a. apical
    b. horizontal
    c. oblique
    d. alveolar crest
    e. none of the above

49. In active tooth eruption, the "eruptive" stage begins when
    a. crown formation begins
    b. root formation begins
    c. tooth erupts into the oral cavity
    d. root formation is completed
    e. none of the above

50. In tooth eruption, the normal path of eruption is
    a. occlusal and facial
    b. occlusal and lingual

c. apical and facial
d. apical and lingual
e. straight occlusally

51. The most probable cause of tooth eruption is
    a. growth of pulpal tissue
    b. root growth
    c. bone growth in socket
    d. changes within periodontal ligament
    e. none of the above

52. The permanent molars develop
    a. between the roots of the primary molars
    b. between the roots of the premolars
    c. apical and lingual to primary molars
    d. lingual to primary molars
    e. none of the above

53. Attached gingiva is an example of
    a. specialized mucosa
    b. lining mucosa
    c. masticatory mucosa
    d. b and c
    e. none of the above

54. Specialized mucosa is found
    a. on the hard palate
    b. on the soft palate
    c. on the dorsum of the tongue
    d. on the mucosa of the cheek
    e. a and b
    f. in none of the above

55. What kind of epithelium would you find in the gingival sulcus?
    a. simple squamous
    b. simple cuboidal
    c. stratified squamous
    d. pseudostratified columnar
    e. none of the above

56. The height of the free gingiva is generally the same height as the
    a. attached gingiva
    b. alveolar mucosa
    c. gingival sulcus
    d. interdental papilla

57. Which of the following papillae of the tongue have *no* taste buds on them?
    a. filiform
    b. fungiform

c. vallate (circumvallate)
d. foliate
e. all have taste buds

58. The intrinsic muscles of the tongue run
    a. front to back
    b. top to bottom
    c. side to side
    d. all of the above
    e. none of the above

59. Which of the following muscles would pull the lateral borders of the tongue downward?
    a. styloglossus
    b. genioglossus
    c. geniohyoid
    d. palatoglossus
    e. none of the above

60. Hairy tongue is an elongation of the
    a. fungiform papillae
    b. filiform papillae
    c. circumvallate papillae
    d. foliate papillae
    e. none of the above

61. The ducts in salivary glands that carry the secretions directly out of the acini are the _____ ducts.
    a. interlobular
    b. excretory
    c. striated
    d. intercalated
    e. none of the above

62. The enzyme found in saliva that splits starches into long-chain sugars is
    a. peptidase
    b. sucrase
    c. amylase
    d. protease
    e. none of the above

63. Intralobular ducts are surrounded by
    a. connective tissue
    b. blood vessels
    c. other ducts
    d. acini
    e. none of the above

64. Striated salivary ducts
    a. aid in conserving water

b. aid in conserving electrolytes
c. modify the saliva
d. all of the above
e. none of the above

65. Which of the following statements *is not* true about intercalated ducts?
   a. Their nucleus is as high as the cell.
   b. They are interposed between acini and striated ducts.
   c. They modify the salivary content as it passes through.
   d. They may be short or long ducts.
   e. The above statements are *all* true.

Suggested Readings

Avery JK: *Essentials of oral histology and embryology: a clinical approach,* St Louis, 1992, Mosby.

Berkovitz EDZ, Holland GM, Moxham BJ: *Color atlas and textbook of oral anatomy, histology, and embryology,* ed 2, St Louis, 1992, Mosby.

Berkowitz S: *The cleft palate story,* Carol Stream, Ill, 1994, Quintessence.

Bevelander G: *Outline of histology,* ed 8, St Louis, 1979, Mosby.

Bevelander G: *Atlas of oral histology and embryology,* Philadelphia, 1967, Lea & Febiger.

Bhaskar SN: *Orban's oral histology and embryology,* ed 11, St Louis, 1991, Mosby.

Carlson BM: *Human embryology and developmental biology,* St Louis, 1994, Mosby.

Larsen WJ: *Human embryology,* New York, 1993, Churchill Livingstone.

Melfi R: *Permar's oral embryology and microscopic anatomy: a textbook for students in dental hygiene,* ed 9, Baltimore, 1993, Williams & Wilkins.

Moss-Salentijn L, Hendricks-Klyvert M: *Dental and oral tissues: an introduction,* ed 3, Baltimore, 1990, Williams & Wilkins.

Provenza DV: *Oral histology: inheritance and development,* ed 2, Philadelphia, 1976, Lea & Febiger.

Sadler TW: *Langman's medical embryology,* ed 7, Baltimore, 1995, Williams & Wilkins.

Ten Cate AR: *Oral histology, development, structure and function,* ed 3, St Louis, 1989, Mosby.

UNIT III

HEAD AND NECK ANATOMY

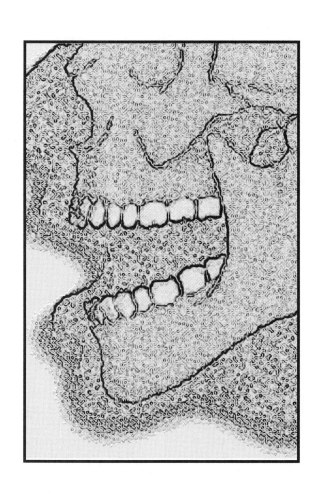

Chapter 11

Osteology of the Skull

OBJECTIVES
- To name the bones of the neurocranium and the viscerocranium
- To identify the various bones and sutures as seen from anterior, lateral, posterior, inferior, and interior views of the skull
- To name the openings, foramina, and canals as seen from the aforementioned views
- To describe the boundaries of the three cranial fossae and what lies within them
- To describe the pterygoid processes of the sphenoid bone and their components
- To describe in detail the various parts and landmarks of the maxillae
- To describe in detail the various parts and landmarks of the mandible
- To describe where growth takes place in the maxillae and mandible to allow for increase in arch length

THE BONES of the skull play several different roles. They surround the brain and protect it from injury, and also form the facial skeleton and participate in the growth process of the jaws, which in turn controls whether a patient has a malocclusion (improper relationship of the teeth and jaws) and whether there is balance between the mid face and lower face.

This chapter will present the more important bones of the skull and their landmarks. However, the discussion is certainly not all inclusive.

Excluding the three small **ossicles** (the malleus, incus, and stapes in each ear, which aid in hearing), there are 22 bones that make up the skull. Some of these are single, and some are paired bones. They are grouped into two categories: one group surrounds the brain, and one group forms the face.

The following eight bones make up the **neurocranium,** the bones surrounding the brain:

frontal bone (single)
sphenoid bone (single)
ethmoid bone (single)
occipital bone (single)
temporal bones (paired)
parietal bones (paired)

Of these eight, the sphenoid and ethmoid are difficult to visualize because they cannot easily be seen in their entirety on the surface of the skull. The ethmoid is primarily located in the facial area of the nose, but because a small part of it surrounds the brain, it is classified as part of the neurocranium.

The 14 bones that make up the **viscerocranium,** the bones of the face, include the following:

mandible (single)
vomer (single)
nasal bones (paired)
lacrimal bones (paired)
zygomatic bones (paired)
inferior nasal conchae (paired)
palatine bones (paired)
maxillae (paired)

Instead of considering the bones around the brain and of the face as two completely separate groups, this chapter will present various views of the skull and study the relationships of the bones to one another. Refer back to the groupings just listed, as necessary.

Several terms that are used in the following chapters should be introduced. One of the first terms you will come across is **suture,** which is a joining together of two or more bones. Two other key terms are **foramen** and **canal.** A foramen is a short tubelike opening through bone, and a canal is a long tubelike opening through bone.

VIEWS OF THE SKULL

Anterior View

In the anterior or frontal view of an adult skull (Fig. 11-1), the area from the eyes up to the top of the skull is made up of the frontal bone. The area below the eyes down to the occlusal plane between the upper and lower teeth comprises the paired zygomatic or cheekbones and the paired maxillae. The nasal bones form the bridge of the nose, and the lower jaw is formed by the single mandible. The inner or medial corner of the eye cavity (**orbit**) contains a small lacrimal bone. Within the nasal cavity the vertical **nasal septum** is composed of the vomer and the perpendicular plate of the ethmoid bone. The inferior nasal conchae are found in the lower, lateral portions of the nasal cavity. More details of the bones of the nasal cavity are discussed in Chapter 12.

If you look back into the orbit, in the medial wall you can see the orbital portion of the ethmoid bone and the **lesser** and **greater wings of the sphenoid** forming the superior orbital fissure in the posterior part of the orbit. The roof of the orbit is formed primarily by the orbital plate of the frontal bone, the lateral wall of the orbit is primarily zygomatic bone, and the floor of the orbit is primarily the maxilla and some of the zygomatic bone. In Fig. 11-1 note that the rim of the orbit is formed from equal parts of the frontal, zygomatic, and maxillary bones. At the lateral edges of the skull some parts of the parietal and temporal bones are visible, as well as the greater wing of the sphenoid.

Lateral View

From a side or lateral view, parts of the following bones can be seen: the frontal, zygomatic, maxilla, mandible, nasal, lacrimal, a small bit of the ethmoid bone in the medial wall of the orbit, the greater wing of the sphenoid, the temporal with its squamous, mastoid, and zygomatic portions, the parietal, and the occipital. Fig. 11-2 shows jagged suture lines separating one bone from another. It may be difficult to see

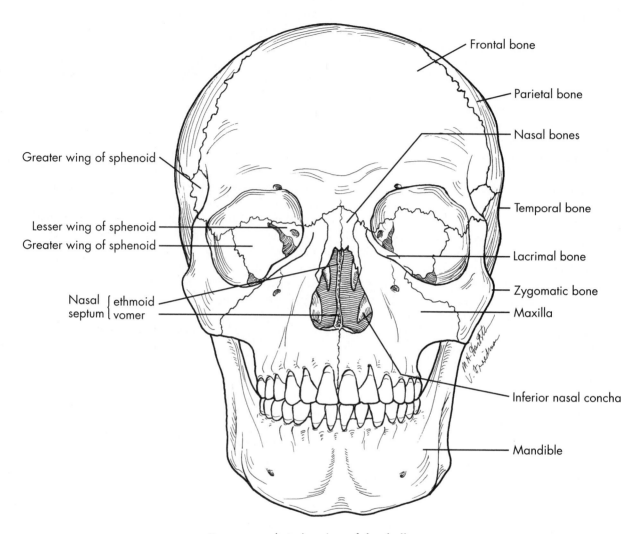

FIG. 11-1.   Anterior view of the skull.

some of them, but it is more important to be able to visualize the relationship of one bone to another rather than to differentiate every single suture.

Inferior View

The most difficult view of the skull for the beginning student of anatomy is the inferior view. There are numerous points or landmarks of

study, and it is difficult to see the suture lines between the bones in many instances. Nevertheless, in the anterior region illustrated in Fig. 11-3, the hard palate, which is formed by the **palatal processes of the maxillae** and the **palatal processes of the palatine bones,** is visible. Just behind and above the palate a small portion of the vomer bone can be seen forming the lower part of the nasal septum. Just behind that and running the

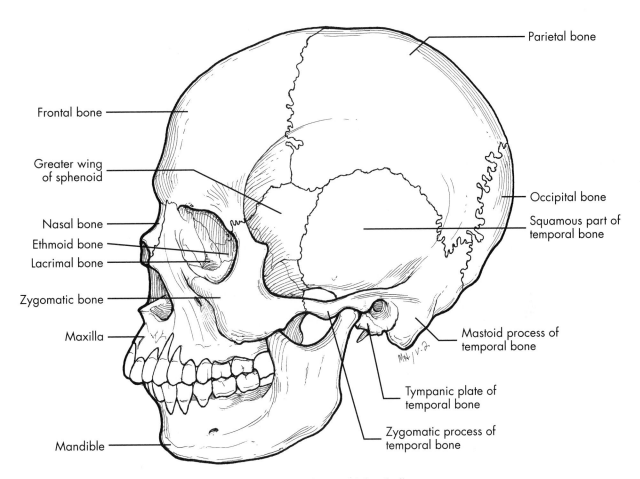

FIG. 11-2.   Lateral view of the skull.

full width of the skull is the sphenoid bone, which is discussed in greater detail later in this chapter. It is difficult to see the suture line between the sphenoid and the occipital bones because it disappears when a person is about 18 years of age. The area marked by the dashed line in Fig. 11-3 is known as the **sphenoccipital synchondrosis.** This is a major area of endochondral bone formation, which is an important factor in the development of facial profiles and types of malocclusions. From this view, portions of the zygomatic bones, the temporal bones, and

just a tiny portion of the posterior part of the parietal bones can also be seen.

Interior View

There is one other view of the skull that should be considered, and that is a view of the inside of the skull with the top removed (Fig. 11-4). Much of the front of the skull is formed by the frontal bone; however, there is a small area near the midline in the front that is part of the ethmoid bone with its crista galli and cribriform plate. Immediately behind these bones is

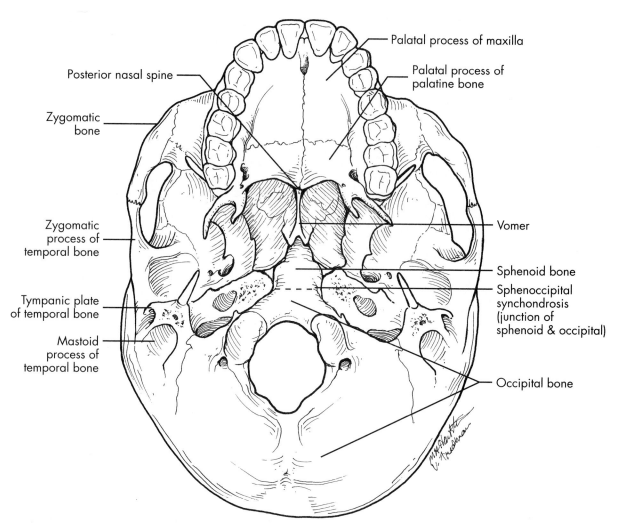

Posterior nasal spine

Zygomatic bone

Zygomatic process of temporal bone

Tympanic plate of temporal bone

Mastoid process of temporal bone

Palatal process of maxilla

Palatal process of palatine bone

Vomer

Sphenoid bone

Sphenoccipital synchondrosis (junction of sphenoid & occipital)

Occipital bone

FIG. 11-3.   Inferior view of the skull.

the sphenoid bone with its greater and lesser wings, and behind and lateral to it are the temporal and parietal bones. The occipital bone lies posterior to this.

LANDMARKS OF THE SKULL

Now let us reexamine the same views of the skull, this time concentrating on the landmarks

rather than on the arrangement of the bones. Again, not every point of study on these views will be named but only those most important for consideration at this stage in your studies.

Anterior View

In Fig. 11-5 you can again see that the rim of the orbit is formed by the frontal, zygomatic, and maxillary bones. The **supraorbital notch** or

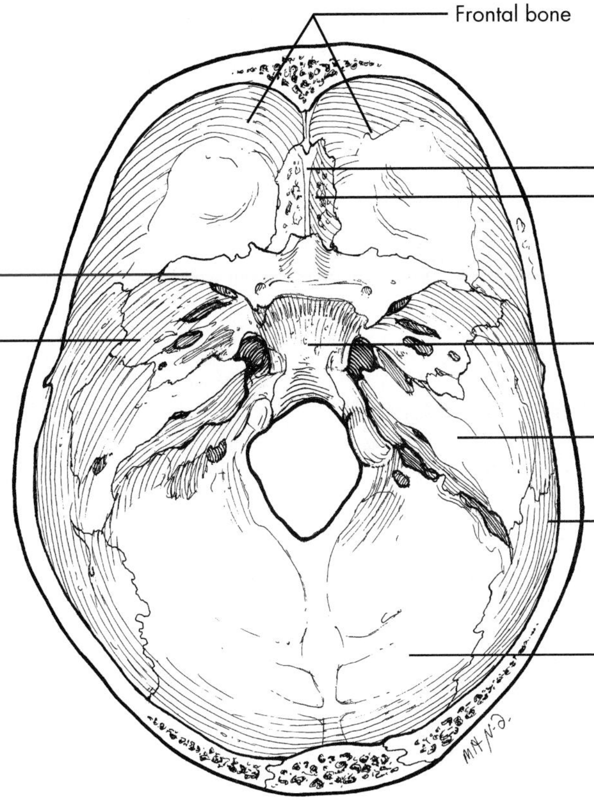

FIG. 11-4. Floor of the cranial cavity with the top of the skull removed.

foramen is seen in the upper rim of the orbit in the frontal bone. The nerve and blood supply to the forehead come through this opening. Toward either side at the top you can see a part of the **coronal suture,** also called the **frontoparietal suture.** A few sutures, such as the coronal, have special names, but most of them are named by the two bones they join. In Fig. 11-5 you can also see the **nasal** or **piriform aperture.** Below the orbit, in the maxillae, are the **infraorbital foramina,** which transmit the infraorbital vessels and nerves to the upper lip, lower eyelid, and side of the nose; you can also see the **intermaxillary suture.** The **canine eminence** is the ridge of bone over the maxillary

canine. The depressions in the maxillae, just above the canines, are the **canine fossae.** The alveolar processes are the areas in the maxillae and the mandible that form the sockets for the teeth. You can also clearly see the **mental foramen** in the mandible. Through this foramen pass the mental nerves and vessels to the chin, lower lip, and facial anterior gingiva of the mandible.

Within the orbit are the **superior** and **inferior orbital fissures,** the **optic foramen,** and parts of the greater and lesser wings of the sphenoid. You can also see the lacrimal bone and the orbital plate of the ethmoid bone, which forms most of the medial wall of the orbit.

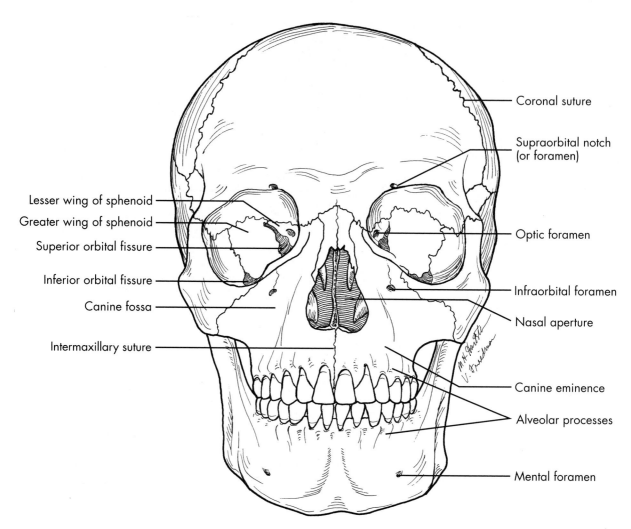

Coronal suture

Supraorbital notch (or foramen)

Lesser wing of sphenoid

Greater wing of sphenoid

Superior orbital fissure

Inferior orbital fissure

Canine fossa

Intermaxillary suture

Optic foramen

Infraorbital foramen

Nasal aperture

Canine eminence

Alveolar processes

Mental foramen

FIG. 11-5. Anterior landmarks of the skull.

Lateral View

In Fig. 11-6 you can see the coronal suture as well as the **lambdoid suture** or the **parietooccipital suture.** The lambdoid suture forms an inverted V, only half of which can be seen from the lateral view. The area outlined by the dotted line is the **temporal fossa** and is made up of areas of the frontal, parietal, sphenoid, and temporal bones. Within the temporal fossa, between the squamous part of the temporal bone and the parietal bone, is the **squamosal suture.** This is an interesting suture in that most suture joints butt up against one another, whereas the squamosal

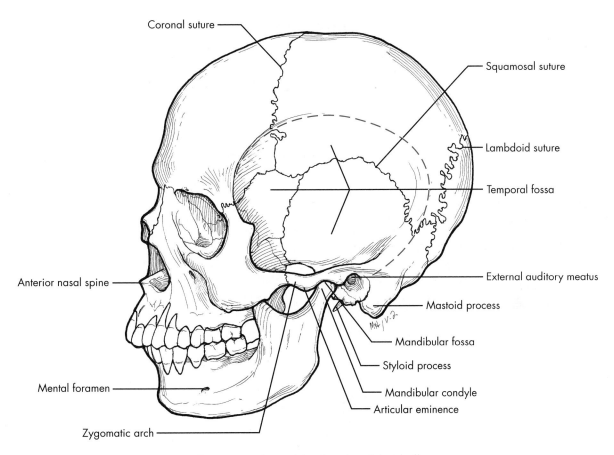

FIG. 11-6.   Lateral landmarks of the skull.

suture is an overlapping suture. There are some who believe that some temporomandibular joint (TMJ) problems are the result of slippage in this suture, and they attempt to manually manipulate the suture to relieve TMJ pain. The **mastoid process** is the projection on the temporal bone just behind the **external auditory meatus** or outer ear canal. The mastoid process serves as the insertion point for the sternocleidomastoid muscle. Projecting forward from the temporal bone and joining with the zygomatic bone is the **zygomatic arch.** This arch is made up of the zygomatic process of the temporal bone and the temporal pro-

cess of the zygomatic bone. The **mandibular fossa,** which articulates with the **mandibular condyle,** is found in this area. Just anterior to the mandibular fossa is the **articular eminence** of the temporal bone. However, these two structures are possibly better seen in an inferior view of the skull. Below and medial to the ear area is a small projection, the **styloid process,** for the attachment of some muscles of the neck region.

Inferior View

Again, the most difficult view is that of the inferior portion of the skull, seen in Fig. 11-7.

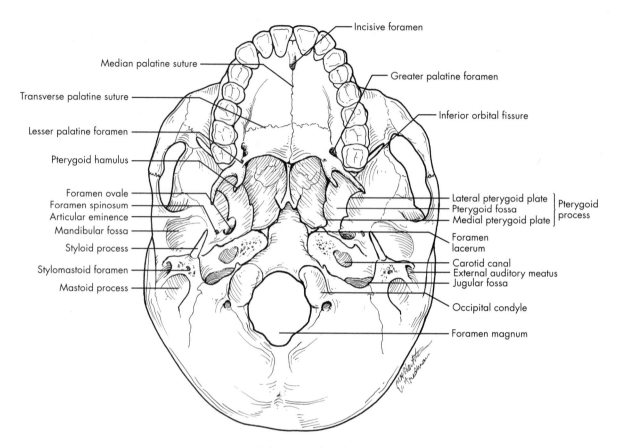

FIG. 11-7. Inferior landmarks of the skull.

In the palatal region you can see the **incisive foramen, median palatine suture,** and **transverse** palatine or **palatomaxillary suture.** In the posterolateral portion of the hard palate you can also see the **greater palatine foramina.** There are **lesser palatine foramina** just posterior to the greater. Just behind that are the **pterygoid hamuli** or **hamular processes** of the medial pterygoid plate.

In Fig. 11-7 you can also see the **pterygoid processes** of the sphenoid bone, which include the **medial** and **lateral pterygoid plates** and the **pterygoid fossa** between them. Just lateral to that area, still in the sphenoid bone, is the **fora-**men ovale. Posterior to the foramen ovale is the **foramen spinosum,** which transmits the **middle meningeal artery,** the major blood supply to the coverings of the brain and frequently a source of severe headaches. Posterior to these structures are the openings for the internal carotid arteries, the **carotid canals.** Medial to the foramen ovale and foramen spinosum is the **foramen lacerum,** an opening in the floor of the carotid canal, which in life is filled with cartilage.

Grouped together are the styloid processes, mastoid processes, and **stylomastoid foramina,** from which exits the facial nerve to the muscles of facial expression. The mandibular fossae of

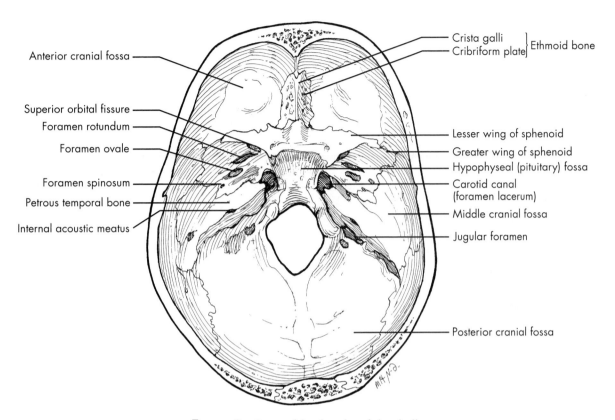

FIG. 11-8. Internal landmarks of the skull.

the TMJ and the articular eminence just anterior to it can also be seen from an inferior view, as well as the **jugular fossae** or **foramina** and the **occipital condyles.** Although there are many more points of study in this view, it is probably sufficient to be familiar with those mentioned.

Interior View

Internally you can see the **crista galli,** which serves as an attachment for part of the dura mater layer covering the brain, and the **cribriform plate,** which is the passageway for the **olfactory nerve** or nerves of smell from the nasal cavity to the brain. Both are parts of the ethmoid bone. Just behind this are the greater and lesser wings of the sphenoid extending from the body of the

sphenoid. From the lesser wing of the sphenoid anterior to the frontal bone is the **anterior cranial fossa,** which houses the frontal lobe of the brain. In the body of the sphenoid is a depression called the **hypophyseal fossa,** in which lies the master control gland of the body, the pituitary gland. Also in the sphenoid are the foramen ovale and **foramen rotundum,** where the nerves to the lower and upper teeth leave the skull. You can also see the foramen spinosum and, by looking down through the anterior end of the carotid canal, the foramen lacerum. The large opening toward the posterior of the skull is the **foramen magnum** of the occipital bone. Just lateral to this the jugular foramen and the **internal acoustic meatus** can be seen (Fig. 11-8). Above the internal acoustic meatus is the crest of the **petrous temporal bone,** which houses the middle and internal ear. From this crest forward to the lesser wing of the sphenoid is the **middle cranial fossa,** which houses the temporal lobe of the brain. From the crest of the petrous temporal bone back to the posterior of the skull is the **posterior cranial fossa,** which houses the brain stem (pons and medulla) and the cerebellum.

A brief view of the top of the skull reveals the coronal and lambdoid sutures; running between them is the **sagittal** or **interparietal suture.** You can also see parts of the frontal, temporal, parietal, and occipital bones (Fig. 11-9).

MAJOR BONES OF THE SKULL

Sphenoid

As has been discussed, the sphenoid is composed of a body, greater and lesser wings, and paired pterygoid processes. Within the body is one of the pairs of **paranasal sinuses,** the **sphenoid sinuses.** The areas of greatest interest are the pterygoid processes, which project down from the body of the sphenoid, just behind the maxillae. Each process has two thin walls of bone that project backward, the medial and lateral pterygoid plates. Projecting down from the medial pterygoid plate is the hamulus or hamular process, which plays a role in the function of

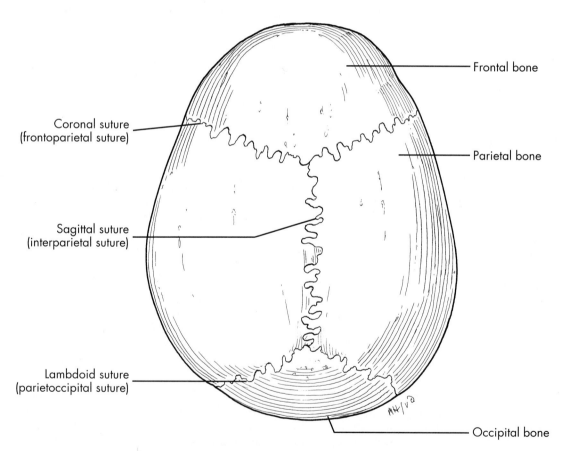

Frontal bone

Parietal bone

Coronal suture
(frontoparietal suture)

Sagittal suture
(interparietal suture)

Lambdoid suture
(parietoccipital suture)

Occipital bone

FIG. 11-9.   Superior view of the skull.

a muscle of the anterior soft palate. The area between these plates is a depression known as a pterygoid fossa. From the fossae and the lateral pterygoid plates originate two pairs of mastication muscles, which move the jaw (Fig. 11-10). Between the maxillae and the pterygoid processes is an opening into an area behind and below the eye known as the *pterygopalatine fossa* (Fig. 11-11). Major nerves and blood vessels to the oral and nasal cavities and midface branch in this area.

Maxillae

Processes

The maxillae consist of a body and four processes in each bone. The frontal process and the zygomatic process are the projections of the maxilla that meet the frontal and zygomatic bones, respectively; between these processes the bone forms about one third of the rim of the orbit. The third process is the alveolar process of the maxilla, which forms the sockets for the upper teeth. The fourth is the horizontal palatine process of the maxilla, which together with its counterpart forms most of the hard palate.

Maxillary sinuses

Within the bodies of the maxillae are the **maxillary sinuses,** the largest and possibly most troublesome of the paranasal sinuses. As you will study in radiology, the maxillary sinuses are quite large, forming a very thin wall of bone between the roots of the maxillary posterior teeth and the sinus spaces themselves. Infections in the sinuses may affect the teeth, and, conversely, in-

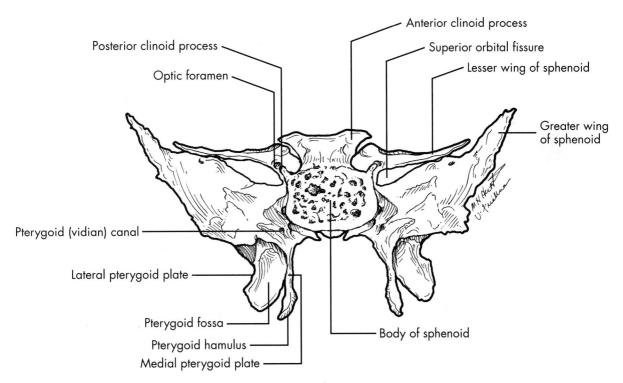

FIG. 11-10. Posterior view of the sphenoid bone. Notice the pterygoid processes and their components.

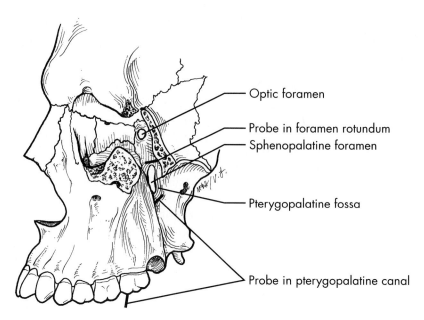

FIG. 11-11.   In this lateral view zygomatic bone has been removed to better show the opening between the maxilla and the pterygoid process (pterygo-maxillary fissure), which leads into the pterygopalatine fossa.

fections in the teeth may affect the sinuses (see Chapter 12).

Lateral view

Fig. 11-12 is a lateral view of a maxilla. Here you can see the body, as well as the alveolar, zygomatic, and frontal processes. You can also see how the maxilla forms half of the opening of the nasal cavity. At the lower end of the nasal cavity, in front, is the **anterior nasal spine.** This is a radiographic landmark frequently used in lateral head films for orthodontics. In the alveolar process you can see how the anterior teeth and sometimes the premolars cause bulgings known as **alveolar eminences** in the bone. Above the canine the canine fossa can be seen, and in the upper end of that fossa area, the infraorbital foramen. If you look behind the third molar region, you see the posterior bulging of bone; this is known as the **maxillary tuberosity.** In this area blood vessels and nerves enter the bone to supply the posterior teeth and part of the maxillary sinus. It is also the area where much of the growth of the maxillae takes place. This growth causes the maxillary bones to become longer in an anteroposterior direction. Insufficient growth usually means inadequate room for the third molars to erupt and an upper jaw that may be shorter than it should be, possibly causing the mandible to appear to be more forward than it is and causing an apparent Class III occlusion. Growth of these bones and therefore of the upper face takes place not only at that point but also between the palatine processes, between the frontal bone and the maxillae, and between the zygomatic bones and the maxillae.

Inferior view

Fig. 11-13 is an inferior or palatal view of the maxillae. Notice the median palatine suture line, which accounts for lateral palatal growth, and also the incisive foramen in the anterior region.

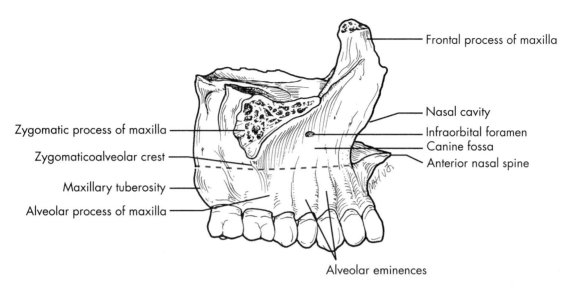

FIG. 11-12.   Lateral view of the maxilla. Little room is available for the third molars to erupt at this point. Division between the body of the maxilla and the alveolar process *(broken line)*.

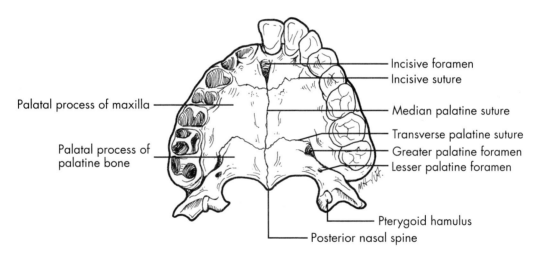

FIG. 11-13.   Inferior or palatal view of the maxillae and part of the palatine bone. The incisive suture tends to disappear in older persons.

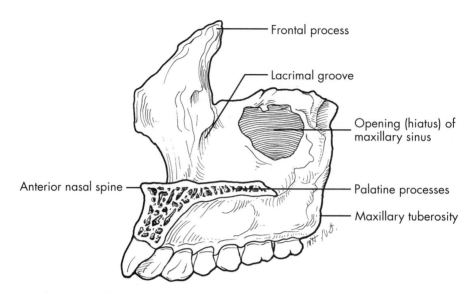

FIG. 11-14.   Medial view of the maxilla. Notice the thickness of the hard palate separating the oral cavity from the nasal cavity. The opening in this illustration is exceedingly larger than normal. Many times there are two or more smaller openings.

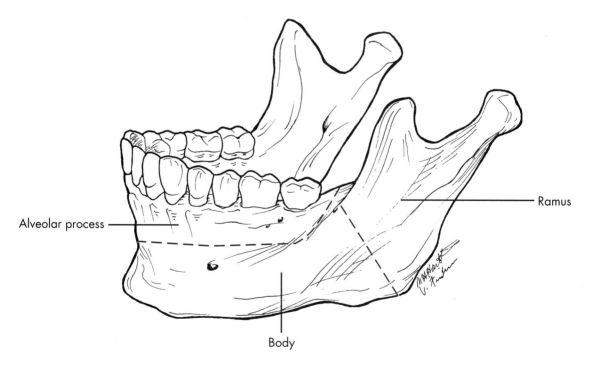

FIG. 11-15.   Lateral view of the mandible. Its three components are separated by broken lines.

Also visible are the palatine bones that form the posterior part of the hard palate. Between the maxilla and the palatine bone is the transverse palatine suture.

Medial view

A medial view of the maxilla from the nasal cavity shows several landmarks already mentioned, but primarily shows the opening into the nasal cavity of the maxillary sinus (Fig. 11-14). The opening is known as the **hiatus** or the **ostium of the maxillary sinus** and varies considerably in size. The smaller the opening, the more likely the sinus will become clogged from nasal congestion. In this view you can also see the **lacrimal groove,** which runs down from the inner-corner of the eye. This is the source from which tears flow into the nose, accounting for the runny nose that occurs when a person is crying.

Mandible

The mandible is a single bone made up of three parts: the horizontal body, with the alveolar process on top of it, and the vertical portion of bone known as the ramus. Generally there is considered to be one body and one alveolar process, but two rami in a mandible (Fig. 11-15).

Lateral view

In Fig. 11-16 you can see landmarks of the mandible. The tip of the chin area is called the **mental protuberance.** Just posterior is the mental foramen, from which the blood vessels and nerves for the lower lip and chin emerge. This foramen is just about at a position that divides the body of the mandible below from the alveolar process above it. The point where the inferior border of the mandible turns upward is the mandibular angle. This is the dividing line between the body and the ramus. On the inferior border of the body of the mandible, just anterior to the angle, you can see or feel an indention. This is where the facial artery and vein cross the mandible. This is a pressure point to slow bleeding in cuts of the face (see Chapters 17 and 18). Moving up along the posterior border of the ramus, we come to the condyle of the mandible, which

articulates with the temporal bone to form the TMJ. The slightly narrowed area just beneath the condyle is known as the **condylar neck.** In front of the condyle, the depression in the ramus is called the **coronoid notch** or **mandibular notch.** Just anterior to this notch is the **coronoid process,** which is the attachment for one of the muscles of mastication, the temporalis. The anterior border of the ramus ends in the **external oblique line,** which shows up as a radiopacity on posterior periapical or pantographic radiographs.

Growth of the mandible takes place in several areas. First the alveolar process and body increase in width and height. The lengthening of the mandibular arch takes place by bone being added to the posterior border of the ramus and taken away from the anterior border. If there is insufficient growth, there may be no room for the normal eruption of mandibular third molars.

Medial view

Fig. 11-17. About midway up the ramus is the **mandibular foramen,** where the nerves and blood vessels for the lower teeth and lip enter the mandible. Just in front of the foramen and running forward and down is the **mylohyoid line,** the attachment for the mylohyoid muscle. Below the mandibular foramen is the mylohyoid groove for the passage of the mylohyoid nerve and vessels to the mylohyoid and anterior digastric muscles. Toward the anterior part of that line are two depressions in the bone, one above the line and one below it. These are the **sublingual** and **submandibular fossae.** The sublingual and submandibular salivary glands lie in these depressions. The area immediately behind the third molars is referred to as the **retromolar triangle.** You may hear more of this in conjunction with denture construction and landmarks. The lateral margin of this triangle is the external oblique line, and the medial margin of this triangle is the internal oblique line.

Posterior view

(Fig. 11-18). Right at the midline are two small, grouped projections, one above and one

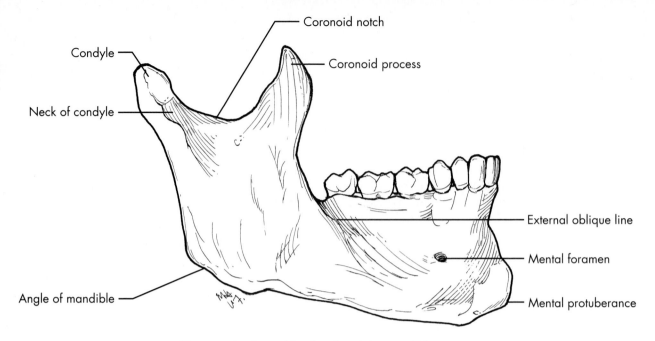

FIG. 11-16.   Lateral landmarks of the mandible.

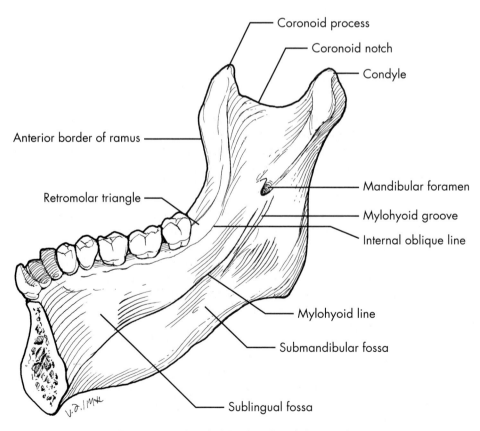

FIG. 11-17.   Medial landmarks of the mandible.

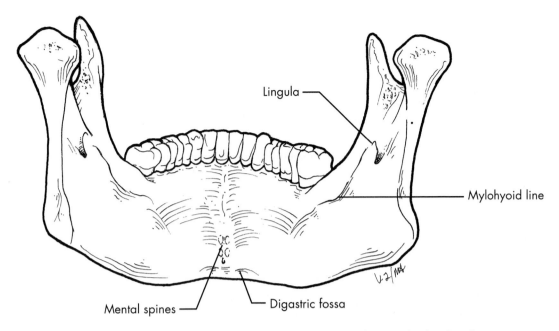

FIG. 11-18.   Posterior view of the mandible. Notice the genial tubercles, digastric fossae, and lingulae, which could not be easily seen on the medial view of the mandible.

below. These are the superior and inferior **genial tubercles** or **mental spines,** attachments for muscles that aid in tongue movement and swallowing. Just below these projections at the inferior border of the mandible are the **digastric fossae,** also points of attachment for the anterior digastric muscle. The last landmark is the **lingula,** which means "little tongue." The lingula is a projection of bone that partially covers the opening of the mandibular foramen. This is a point of attachment for the **sphenomandibular ligament,** whose location and size may at times affect the success of the anesthetic injections in the area.

From time to time, review this chapter on the osteology of the skull. You will find a great deal of correlation between this material and your radiology studies. A thorough knowledge of osteology will make you a better practitioner of radiologic techniques and will benefit the patient you are radiographing.

Review Questions

1. How many bones form the skull?
2. How are the bones subdivided?
3. Define the following:
   a. Suture
   b. Foramen
   c. Canal
   d. Fossa
   e. Alveolar process
4. Which bones form the hard palate?
5. What would be another name for each of the following sutures?
   a. Coronal
   b. Sagittal
   c. Lambdoid
6. Where is the largest of the paranasal sinuses?
7. Name the area immediately behind the maxillary third molars.

8. What are the divisions of the mandible?
9. Name the major landmarks of the maxillae and mandible.
10. Discuss growth of mandibular and maxillary arch length.
11. What are the parts of the sphenoid bone, and where is the sphenoid sinus?

12. What bones make up the rim of the orbit?
13. What part of what bone divides the anterior and middle cranial fossae, and what one divides the middle and posterior cranial fossae?

CHAPTER 12

Nose, Nasal Cavity, and Paranasal Sinuses

OBJECTIVES
- To define the terms *nose, nasal cavity,* and *paranasal sinuses*
- To understand the anatomy of the nose, nasal cavity, and paranasal sinuses
- To describe the function of the nasal cavity, nasal epithelium, and paranasal sinuses
- To discuss the anatomic relationship of the maxillary sinus and the maxillary teeth
- To describe the relationship of maxillary teeth to the maxillary sinus in infections of either one

NOSE AND NASAL CAVITY

External View

The nose and nasal cavity are a complex arrangement of hard and soft tissues. The nose is that portion of the nasal complex that protrudes outward from the skeletal component. The nose, or more properly, the external nose, is attached superiorly to the nasal bones and inferiorly to the anterior nasal spine. Each protruding lateral margin is known individually as a wing of the nose, or an **ala.** The external nose is divided in half by the cartilaginous part of the nasal septum, which is the wall that divides the nasal complex into right and left halves (Fig. 12-1). If you look at a skull, you will see that the nasal aperture, the anterior most portion of the nasal cavity, is somewhat pear shaped.

Internal View

Peering inside the nasal cavity you can see the nasal septum. Additionally, the lateral walls of the nasal cavity have three shelves called *nasal conchae* that project in toward the septum. The superior portion of the bony nasal cavity has small holes that open into the anterior cranial fossa through the cribriform plate of the ethmoid bone to transmit the olfactory nerves from the nose up to the brain.

The septum is formed from the vomer bone and a portion of the ethmoid bone as well as the

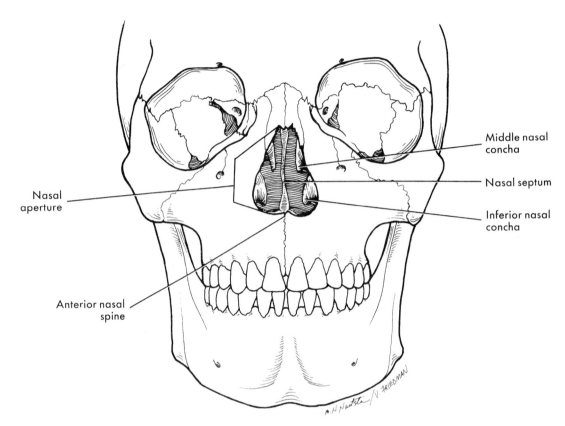

FIG. 12-1.   Anterior view of a skull showing the nasal aperture, nasal septum, and nasal conchae.

fibrocartilaginous part of the septum (Fig. 12-2). The inferior portion or floor of the cavity is formed from the bones of the hard palate, which are the palatal processes of the maxillae and the horizontal portion of the palatine bones. The most complicated portion of the nasal cavity is its lateral walls. The upper half to two thirds of the lateral wall of the cavity is formed from parts of the ethmoid bone. It consists of the wall and two shelflike structures known as the **superior** and **middle nasal conchae.** The lower part of the lateral walls are formed by portions of the maxillae. At the point where the maxillae and the

ethmoid bone meet in the lateral wall there is a third medial projection, which is a separate bone itself, known as the *inferior nasal concha* (Fig. 12-3).

As you reach the posterior part of the nasal septum, you come to an area known as the **choana,** or **posterior nasal aperture.** Posterior to this is the nasal pharynx, which is discussed in Chapter 16. The posterior-superior part of the nasal cavity is composed of a portion of the body of the sphenoid bone where it meets the ethmoid bone and is known as the **sphenoethmoidal recess.** Visualizing this from a sagittal

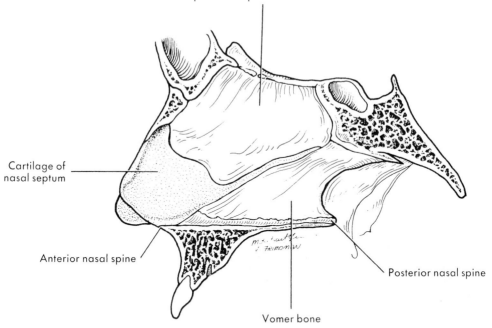

Perpendicular plate of ethmoid bone

Cartilage of nasal septum

Anterior nasal spine

Posterior nasal spine

Vomer bone

FIG. 12-2. Sagittal section showing the nasal septum and its components.

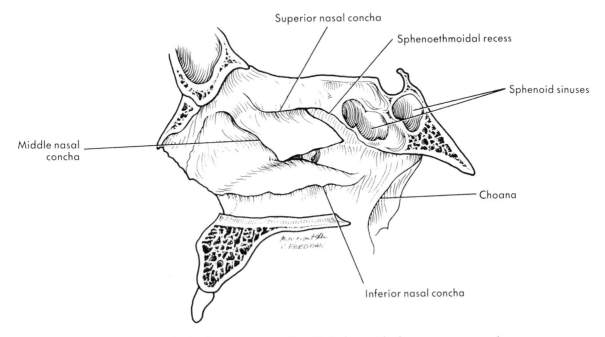

Superior nasal concha

Sphenoethmoidal recess

Sphenoid sinuses

Middle nasal concha

Choana

Inferior nasal concha

FIG. 12-3. Sagittal section, as in Fig. 12-2, but with the septum removed, showing the lateral nasal wall and bony conchae.

view of a skull, the sphenoidal sinus is below the pituitary fossa. With the advent of fiber optics and microscopic instruments, surgery on tumors of the pituitary gland can be performed by going through the nasal cavity, into the sphenoid sinus, and cutting away the roof of that sinus, thereby gaining access to the pituitary gland from below and operating on it without having to go through the skull.

Epithelial Lining

Recall from Chapter 2 on epithelial tissues that there is one type of epithelium known as pseudostratified columnar epithelium with goblet cells. This epithelial tissue is usually called **respiratory epithelium** because it is primarily found in the respiratory tract. (You should be aware by now that the nasal cavity is the beginning of the respiratory tract or system.) The epithelium has many hairlike projections known as *cilia* that move in a synchronized beating pattern toward the anterior portion of the nasal cavity. The tiny goblet cells secrete a sticky mucous substance onto the cilia, trapping contaminants as they enter the nasal cavity and moving them toward the front where they are removed by blowing the nose; during sleep this mucus may flow backward as postnasal drip. For this mechanism to be successful it is important to have as much surface area as possible in the nasal cavity. The conchae help accomplish that.

The epithelium in the roof of the nasal cavity and coming down onto the upper surface of the superior concha and upper nasal septum is modified and has nerve fibers that perceive odors. This is called **olfactory epithelium.**

PARANASAL SINUSES

Location

You now should have a clearer picture in your mind of the nasal cavity. To visualize it even better, you would be helped by studying a skull that has been specially prepared by being split along the midline. This would give you a greater ap-

preciation of the complexity of the structure. Studying this area more closely, you would see that there are a number of openings into the nasal cavity from other areas. Most of these openings are from compartments or cavities of various sizes known as the **paranasal sinuses.** There are four pairs of these sinuses: two ethmoids, two frontals, two maxillaries, and two sphenoids. These sinuses are not easily seen at first; we must first locate the nasal conchae. These conchae on either side of the nasal cavity are there for several reasons, one of them being to increase the surface area for the respiratory epithelium, which, as mentioned earlier, acts as a filter for incoming air.

The area of the lateral nasal wall sheltered underneath each concha is known as the **meatus** of each concha. The **inferior meatus** is beneath the inferior nasal concha and has one small opening, which is the opening of the nasolacrimal duct. This duct carries tears from the corner of the eye into the nasal cavity. The middle meatus lies beneath the middle nasal concha. Here there is a crescent-shaped opening called the **hiatus semilunaris,** which means a half-moon–shaped opening. In this area there are a number of other openings, which will be discussed shortly. There is a bulbous ridge above the hiatus semilunaris called the **ethmoid bulla.** The **superior meatus** lies beneath the superior concha and is the smallest meatus (Fig. 12-4).

Frontal Sinuses

The paired **frontal sinuses** are located in the frontal bone just above the orbital cavity; these vary in size from person to person. They frequently cross the midline and may be partially located on the opposite side. These sinuses drain into the very anterior end of the hiatus semilunaris. Infections in these sinuses cause pressure and pain just above the eye.

Sphenoid Sinuses

The paired **sphenoid sinuses** are located in the body of the sphenoid bone just underneath the

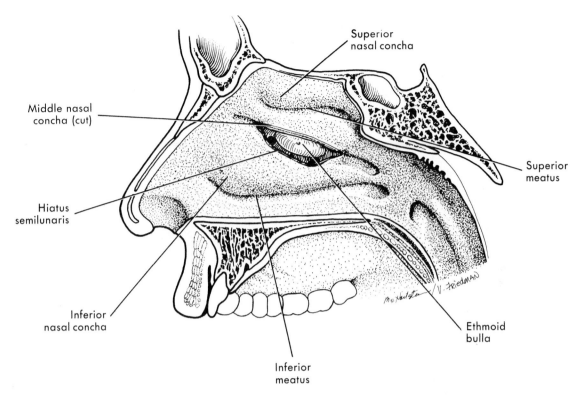

FIG. 12-4.   Same view as in Fig. 12-3 but covered with nasal mucosa. The middle concha has been partially removed to show the hiatus semilunaris and the ethmoid bulla in middle meatus.

pituitary fossa, which is located in the middle cranial fossa. These sinuses also cross the midline. They open into the highest and most posterior part of the nasal cavity—the sphenoethmoidal recess. Infections in the sphenoid sinuses cause pressure and a congested feeling that is hard to localize but is deep in the midline of the head.

Ethmoid Sinuses

The **ethmoid sinuses** are frequently called **ethmoid air cells** because they are not single-paired sinuses like the other paranasal sinuses but are subdivided into numerous small compartments. These clusters of air cells are further di-

vided into anterior, middle, and posterior ethmoid air cells.

Anterior ethmoids

The anterior ethmoids are located in the lateral wall of the nasal cavity at the base of the middle nasal concha. These air cells open into the hiatus semilunaris just posterior-inferior to the opening for the frontal sinus.

Middle ethmoids

The middle ethmoids are also located in the base of the middle nasal concha, just behind the anterior air cells. They are also located within the ethmoid bulla. These may have a couple of openings, one on the ethmoid bulla and another possibly in the hiatus semilunaris.

Posterior ethmoids

The posterior ethmoid air cells are located in the base of the superior nasal concha and open into the superior meatus.

Sinus infections in the ethmoid sinuses are difficult to treat because of the small compartments. When infected, they give a feeling of congestion and aching within the nasal cavity area.

Maxillary Sinuses

The maxillary sinuses are the largest of the paranasal sinuses and open into the posterior end of the hiatus semilunaris through one or more openings. At birth the maxillary sinus in each maxilla is the size of a small pea. As growth takes place, each sinus continues to expand and occupy greater proportions of the body of the maxilla. In young adults the maxillary sinus occupies an area from just posterior to the maxillary canine back to the area of the third molar in an anteroposterior direction. In a superior-inferior direction it would extend from the floor of the orbital cavity inferiorly to the point where it might extend down around the root tips of the maxillary posterior teeth (Fig. 12-5). The maxillary sinus may develop compartmental walls, but generally all of them are connected by large openings. If you look at the location of the opening for the maxillary sinus in the middle meatus region and compare it with its location on the medial wall of the sinus, you will find that this opening is almost two thirds of the way up the medial wall (see Fig. 12-5). You can appreciate the significance of trying to drain a cavity through an opening that is near the top of the space. Several things come into play here, the first being that everybody's maxillary sinus is different. Sometimes there is more than one opening in each sinus, sometimes the opening or openings are very small, and sometimes they are very big. During a nasal infection there is swelling in the nasal mucosa. If the maxillary sinus has a very small opening or openings, they may swell shut as a result of the mucosal swelling. If there is already infection in the sinus, it continues to multiply, and the fact that the sinus is now

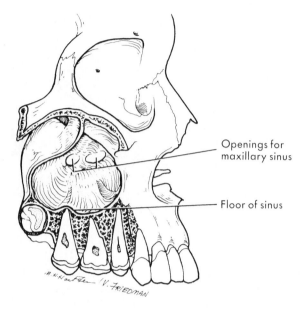

Openings for maxillary sinus

Floor of sinus

FIG. 12-5.   Lateral view of the facial part of a skull with the lateral wall of the maxillary sinus removed, showing the relationship of the floor of the sinus to the maxillary roots of the teeth. The opening of the maxillary sinus from the nasal cavity can be seen two thirds up the medial wall of the sinus.

a warm, closed space causes it to act like an incubator for the microorganisms causing the infection. As the infection increases in severity, there is increased pressure in the maxillae. Tilting the head forward causes the pressure to increase because the fluid produced by the infection flows forward against the anterior wall of the sinus. The use of nasal sprays frequently gives some temporary relief, but then the cavity eventually clogs again. If there is some opening of the sinus, tilting the head to one side while lying down may allow for some drainage from the opposite side or the high-side sinus. When this clogging happens repeatedly, an ear, nose, and throat (ENT) specialist sometimes punches a hole from the inferior meatus into the medial wall of the maxillary sinus near its base and enlarges it until it effects good drainage and a decrease in maxillary sinus infections.

FUNCTION OF SINUSES

Historically there have been several functions discussed in regard to the sinuses. Probably the most popular was that they warmed the air as it passed into the respiratory system. Later studies showed that the flow of air into and out of these sinuses is actually very minimal. The general belief now is that the hollow cavities of the nasal sinuses function to lighten the overall bone weight.

CLINICAL PROBLEMS

Aside from the problems mentioned regarding the maxillary sinus, there are also dental considerations relating to this structure. The same nerves that supply the maxillary posterior teeth also supply the maxillary sinuses. These are sensory nerves carrying different types of messages to the brain. In everyday life these nerves are constantly sending messages to the brain from the maxillary teeth. Biting down on a piece of bone or a seed, for example, causes results in a painful stimulus being sent to the brain. That same nerves to the teeth also have fibers from the maxillary sinuses, but the sinuses seldom send messages to the brain. As a result, the brain gets used to interpreting everything that travels along those nerves as a message from the teeth. However, during a maxillary sinus infection, the sinuses also send messages along the same nerves. The brain correctly interprets these messages as pain; however, it incorrectly interprets the pain as coming from the tooth because that is where all the messages came from in the past.

When this occurs, the individual usually contacts the family dentist and complains about a rather severe toothache. When that patient is examined, no apparent signs of any caries are found, there are no periodontal pockets, and the tooth is only mildly sensitive to percussion. A **periapical** radiograph shows no periapical lesion and no interproximal caries, although at times

there may be a cloudiness appearing in the maxillary sinus. This is usually a sign of fluid buildup. Pulp testing appears to be normal.

Where do we go from here? There could be things that are many times undetectable, such as a cracked tooth, but we need to explore one other option before proceeding with any other tests or treatment. We need to go back to the medical and dental history form and check for a history of sinus infections. If the history form in your office does not have that category, then question the patient concerning sinus infections, especially recent sinus problems. If the patient confirms a problem with sinus infections, then the patient should be referred to a physician for treatment. This will usually take care of the problem unless it recurs after medical treatment. Under such circumstances further evaluation must be done.

Another area of concern is the relationship of the floor of the sinus to the teeth. In a number of instances the floor of the sinus dips down around the tip of one or more roots of the posterior teeth. Under some circumstances it is possible that a periapical infection of a tooth may involve the sinus. It is also possible that the sinus may dip between the roots of a maxillary molar. If that molar has roots that are **dilacerated** (curved because of disturbances in development) and it needs to be extracted for any reason, use reliable radiographs to assess the situation. It is embarrassing and negligent treatment if, without radiographs of the region, one proceeds to extract a molar tooth and finds that besides the extracted tooth a part of the maxillary sinus floor was also extracted. Generally, a tooth with dilacerated roots needs to have the roots sectioned and removed one at a time to minimize the possibility of a fracture of the sinus floor.

When maxillary teeth are extracted and healing takes place, there is a tendency for the maxillary sinus to enlarge into the area formerly occupied by the posterior maxillary roots and impacted third maxillary molars. This means that the thickness of bone in the maxillary tuberosity and alveolar ridge up to and sometimes including the canine region may be very thin and has to be evaluated in deciding what type of treatment to use to replace the teeth with a **prosthetic appliance.**

Evaluation and treatment need to go beyond the teeth and involve other areas or systems of the patient. This is just one more reason why the members of the dental team need to know more about the total evaluation of the patient.

Review Questions

1. Which bones or structures form the nasal septum?
2. What bones would we find in the lateral wall of the nasal cavity?
3. What is a meatus?
4. What is the function of respiratory epithelium?
5. What opens into the:
    a. Inferior meatus?
    b. Middle meatus?
    c. Superior meatus?
    d. Sphenoethmoidal recess?
6. Where specifically is the olfactory epithelium found?
7. Why, anatomically, may maxillary sinuses create problems with sinus infections and with maxillary posterior teeth extractions?
8. Why may a maxillary sinus infection seem to be coming from the teeth?

Chapter 13

Muscles of Mastication, Hyoid Muscles, and Sternocleidomastoid and Trapezius Muscles

Objectives

- To describe the origin, insertion, action, and nerve and blood supply of the muscles of mastication
- To categorize the muscles according to their roles in elevation, depression, protrusion, retrusion, and lateral excursion
- To describe the functions of the sternocleidomastoid and trapezius muscles and their roles in referred pain to various areas, including the temporomandibular joint
- To name the suprahyoid and infrahyoid muscles and their roles in mandibular movement, swallowing, and phonation

Because this is the first of three chapters dealing with muscles and their functions, it seems appropriate to mention briefly some terms relevant to this subject. In general as one reads about muscles there are five terms that are constantly seen: *origin, insertion, action, nerve supply,* and *blood supply.* Because nerve supply and blood supply are self-explanatory, we will be primarily concerned with the first three. The **origin** of a muscle is generally considered to be the end of the muscle that is attached to the least movable structure. The **insertion** of a muscle is the other end of the muscle, which is attached to the more movable structure. The **ac**tion is the work that is accomplished when the muscle fibers contract. If you are familiar with the action of a muscle but are not sure which end is the origin or the insertion, keep in mind that, in general, the insertion moves toward the origin when the muscle is contracted. Likewise, if you know the direction of the muscle fibers, you can usually deduce the action by imagining the insertion moving toward the origin and picturing what happens. Keep in mind that there may at times be more than one function to a particular muscle because either end of a muscle can function as an insertion if the other end is fixed or because there may be different fiber directions within the muscles and different groups of fibers being called into function, thereby creating different actions.

MUSCLES OF MASTICATION

The muscles of **mastication** are four pairs of muscles attached to the mandible and primarily responsible for elevating, protruding, retruding, or causing the mandible to move laterally. They develop from the first (mandibular) pharyngeal arch, which is also responsible for the development of some of the bony facial structures. Because they develop from this arch, they are inner-vated by the nerve of the first arch, the fifth cranial nerve (trigeminal nerve). More specifically, the muscles are innervated by the third part of the fifth nerve, which is called the mandibular division or V_3. The blood supply to these muscles comes from the maxillary artery, which is a branch of the external carotid artery. Blood vessels and nerves are further discussed in Chapters 17 and 19.

Masseter Muscle

The **masseter muscle** is probably the most powerful of the muscles of mastication. It takes its origin from two areas on the zygomatic arch.

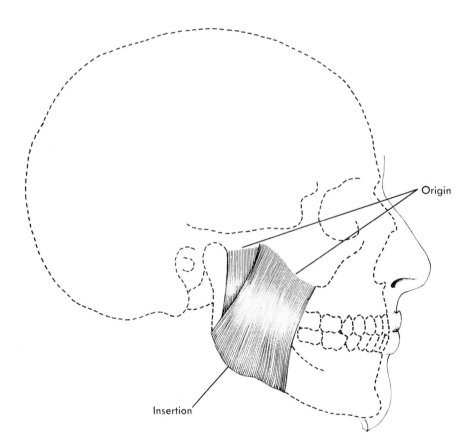

FIG. 13-1. Lateral view of a skull. Shows that the origin of the masseter muscle is from the zygomatic arch. Fibers run down and slightly back to insert into the angle of the mandible.

The superficial head originates from the inferior border of the anterior two thirds of the zygomatic arch. The deep head arises from the inferior border of the posterior one third of the zygomatic arch and the entire medial side of the zygomatic arch. The fibers of the superficial head run down and slightly back to be inserted into the angle of the mandible on the lateral side. The deep head has vertically oriented fibers. When the masseter muscle contracts, it elevates the mandible, closing the mouth (Fig. 13-1).

Temporal Muscle

The **temporal muscle**, frequently called the **temporalis muscle**, has a very wide origin from the entire temporal fossa and the fascia covering the muscle. The anterior fibers run almost vertically, but the posterior fibers run in a more horizontal direction over the ear. All of these fibers insert into the coronoid process of the mandible and sometimes run down the anterior border of the ramus of the mandible as far as the third molar (Fig. 13-2). If the entire muscle contracts, the

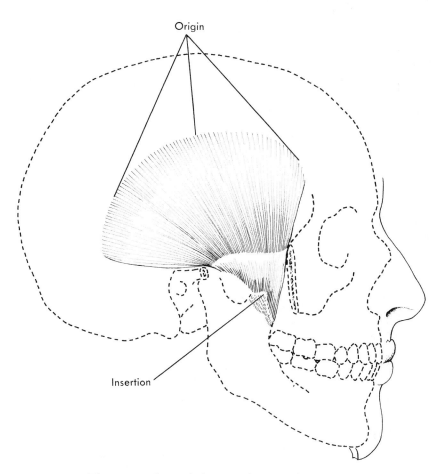

FIG. 13-2.   The temporal muscle has a wide origin from the temporal fossa. Notice the vertical, inclined, and horizontal muscle fibers, which insert primarily on the medial side and the tip of the coronoid process.

overall action pulls up on the coronoid process and elevates the mandible, closing the mouth. If only the posterior fibers are contracted, the result is a horizontal pulling of the coronoid process in a posterior direction. This pulls the mandible backward, which is referred to as *retruding the mandible.*

Medial Pterygoid Muscle

In studying the origin of the **medial pterygoid muscle,** it is probably best to examine a model of the skull while reading the description. The muscle has two origins. The larger and major origin is from the medial side of the lateral pterygoid plate and the pterygoid fossa as well as a tiny area of the palatine bone at the lower end of the medial and lateral pterygoid plates. This area is called the *pyramidal process* of the palatine bone. The smaller origin is just anterior to that area, coming from the maxillary tuberosity just behind the third molar. All of the fibers run down and slightly posteriorly and laterally to be inserted into the angle of the mandible on the medial side. This is just opposite the masseter insertion on the lateral side. When the muscle contracts, the resulting action is elevation of the mandible and closing of the mouth (Fig. 13-3).

Lateral Pterygoid Muscle

The **lateral pterygoid muscle** also has two separate origins. The smaller, superior origin or head arises from the area called the *infratemporal crest* of the greater wing of the sphenoid bone. The larger, inferior origin or head arises from the lateral side of the lateral pterygoid plate. This is just opposite the origin of the medial pterygoid muscle. The fibers from both origins of the lateral pterygoid muscle run horizontally in a posterior direction. Some of the fibers from the superior head penetrate the capsule of the temporomandibular joint (TMJ) and insert into the anterior border of the disc of the joint. The remainder of the fibers from that origin and the fibers of the inferior head insert into the neck of the condyle on the anterior and medial side (see Fig. 13-3).

The lateral pterygoid muscle has several actions. The inferior head pulls the condyle forward and helps protrude and depress the mandible. The disc is also brought forward because of its attachment to the condyle. When both left and right inferior heads function, the mandible is protruded and depressed. If only one lateral pterygoid is contracted, there will be lateral excursion to the opposite side of the contracted muscle. The superior head of the lateral pterygoid functions primarily in the action of biting or what is sometimes called the power stroke. It functions to guide the posterior movement of the disc and condyle as it goes back to a centric position (see Fig. 13-3).

HYOID MUSCLES

We have just discussed the muscles that accomplish virtually all jaw movements except strong depression of the mandible or opening the mouth and some retrusion of the mandible. These actions are accomplished by muscles in the neck called the **hyoid muscles.**

The hyoid muscles are so named because they attach to or are associated with the hyoid bone in the neck. The hyoid is a horseshoe-shaped bone suspended beneath the mandible, with the open end of the horseshoe pointed posteriorly (Fig. 13-4). It is unusual in that it articulates with no other bone; its only connection with other bones is by muscles. These muscles are divided into two groups—those above the hyoid are called **suprahyoid muscles,** and those below are called **infrahyoid muscles.**

Suprahyoid Group
Digastric muscle

The **digastric muscle** has a relatively unusual arrangement of fibers, with muscle fibers at either end and a collagenous tendon in the middle. Classically, it has been described as having an origin at either end with an insertion in the middle. For the sake of clearer understanding, it might be best to say that its origin is at the digastric notch just medial to the mastoid process behind the ear. The

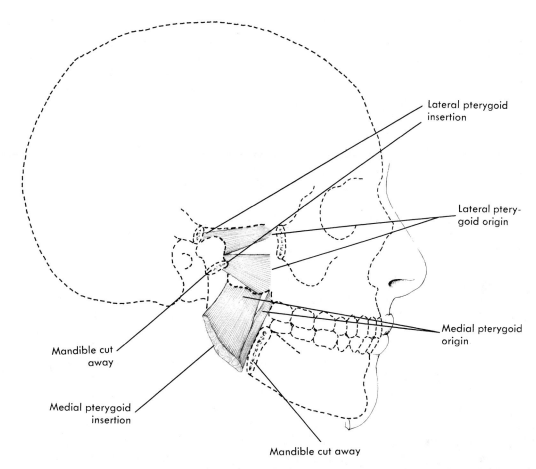

Lateral pterygoid
insertion

Lateral ptery-
goid origin

Medial pterygoid
origin

Mandible cut
away

Medial pterygoid
insertion

Mandible cut away

FIG. 13-3. Lateral view of a skull showing the origins of the lateral pterygoid muscle from the infratemporal crest and pterygoid plate, with fibers inserting into the disc and neck of the condyle. Notice the medial pterygoid
muscle originating from the pterygoid area, as well as a small origin from the
maxillary tuberosity. Insertion onto the medial side of the angle of the mandible is also visible.

fibers run forward and down to the area of the intermediate tendon, which attaches to the hyoid
bone by a tendinous loop through which it can
slide. From here the muscle fibers extend forward
and slightly up to be inserted into the digastric
fossa on the inferior surface of the mandible at the
midline (Figs. 13-5 and 13-6).

The action of this muscle is twofold. By contracting it can create a backward pull on the

mandible, thus retruding it. If the jaw is
clenched, contraction of the muscle elevates the
hyoid bone and lifts up on the larynx or voice
box. It can also aid in pulling the mandible
down if the infrahyoid muscles pull the hyoid
bone down.

The digastric muscle is also unusual in that it
has two nerves supplying it. The anterior part of
the muscle is supplied by the third part of the tri-

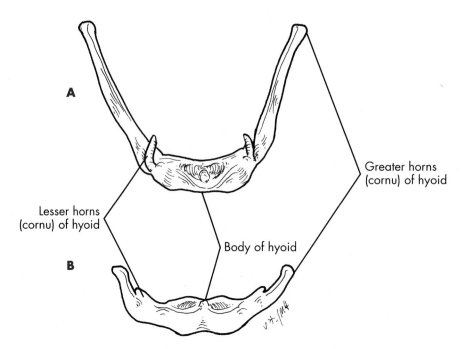

A

Greater horns
(cornu) of hyoid

Lesser horns
(cornu) of hyoid

Body of hyoid

B

FIG. 13-4.   Hyoid bone. **A,** Superior view. **B,** Anterior view. This bone articulates with no other bone but is attached to other bones entirely by muscles.

geminal nerve (V_3), and the posterior part is supplied by the facial nerve (VII).

Mylohyoid muscle

The **mylohyoid muscle** forms what is called the *floor of the mouth.* The muscle originates from the mylohyoid line on the medial surface of each side of the mandible, running down and inserting into the hyoid bone. The left and right muscles also fuse together in the midline of the neck. This type of fusion is known as a **raphe.** The action is related to the depression of the mandible or the elevation of the hyoid bone. The nerve supply is the mylohyoid branch of V_3 (trigeminal). The blood supply is a branch of the inferior alveolar artery (see Figs. 13-5 and 13-6).

Geniohyoid muscle

The **geniohyoid muscle** originates from the inferior genial tubercle or mental spine on the lingual surface of the mandible at the midline. It lies deep to the mylohyoid muscle, running down and back to insert into the hyoid bone by the midline. It also acts as a depressor of the mandible or elevator of the hyoid bone. Its nerve supply comes from the first cervical nerve in the neck. The blood supply is a branch of the lingual artery (Fig. 13-7).

Stylohyoid muscle

The **stylohyoid muscle** takes its origin from the styloid process of the base of the skull. The muscle runs down and forward to insert into the posterior part of the hyoid bone. At its insertion on the hyoid bone the muscle splits and part of the posterior portion of the digastric muscle passes through it. The action of the muscle is to pull the hyoid bone back and up. The nerve supply is a branch of the facial nerve (VII), which also supplies the posterior belly of the digastric muscle. The facial and occipital

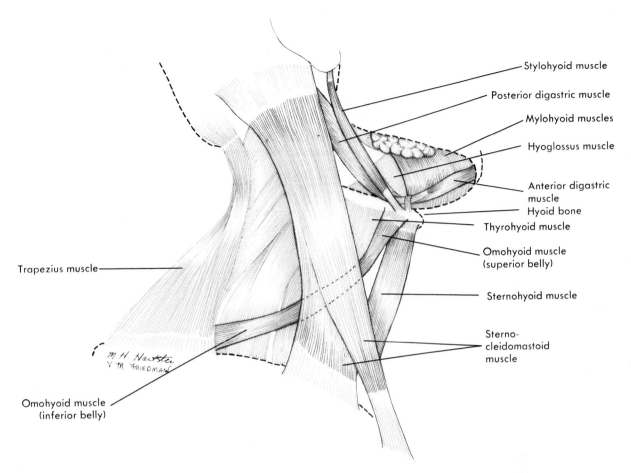

FIG. 13-5.   Lateral view of the neck showing the digastric muscle suspended above the hyoid bone and attaching to it by a ligamentous loop. Mylohyoid and stylohyoid muscles are also visible above the hyoid bone, and omohyoid, thyrohyoid, and sternohyoid muscles are visible below the hyoid bone. Also, the large sternocleidomastoid muscle covers a large area on the side of the neck.

arteries provide its blood supply (see Figs. 13-5 and 13-6).

Infrahyoid Group

Omohyoid muscle

The two muscular bellies of the **omohyoid muscle** are separated by an intermediate tendon. One of the bellies arises from the upper border of the scapula (shoulder blade), and the other from the hyoid bone. The two bellies are joined by an intermediate tendon beneath the **sternomastoid (sternocleidomastoid) muscle** in the side of the neck. When the muscle contracts, it pulls the hyoid bone down. The nerve supply comes from the second and third cervical nerves, and the blood supply from the lingual and superior thyroid arteries (see Figs. 13-5 and 13-6).

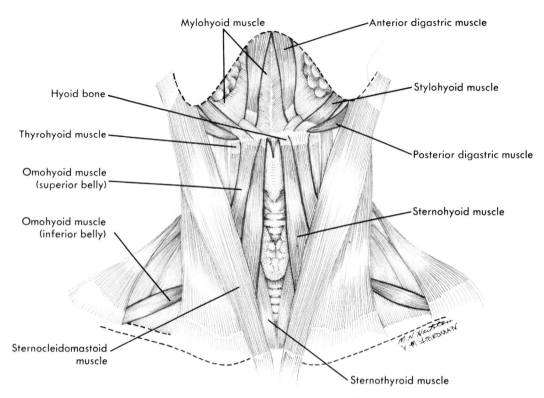

Mylohyoid muscle

Anterior digastric muscle

Hyoid bone

Thyrohyoid muscle

Omohyoid muscle (superior belly)

Omohyoid muscle (inferior belly)

Stylohyoid muscle

Posterior digastric muscle

Sternohyoid muscle

Sternocleidomastoid muscle

Sternothyroid muscle

FIG. 13-6. Anterior and inferior view of the mylohyoid muscle. Left and right muscles fuse in the midline and form a slinglike arrangement that forms the mouth floor. You can also see the anterior view of the digastric, stylohyoid, sternohyoid, sternothyroid, and sternocleidomastoid muscles.

Sternohyoid muscle

The **sternohyoid muscle** takes its origin from the upper border of the manubrium of the sternum. It runs up to be inserted into the front part of the body of the hyoid bone. When the muscle contracts, it pulls the hyoid bone down. Its nerve supply is from the second and third cervical nerves. Its blood supply is the lingual and superior thyroid arteries (see Figs. 13-5 and 13-6).

Sternothyroid muscle

The **sternothyroid muscle** arises from the upper part of the sternum, running up to be inserted onto an oblique line on the side of the thyroid cartilage of the larynx. It is not easily seen

because the sternohyoid muscle tends to lie superficial to it. When the muscle contracts, it pulls the larynx down. The nerve supply comes from the second and third cervical nerves. The blood supply is from the superior thyroid artery (Fig. 13-8). (Also see Fig. 13-6.)

Thyrohyoid muscle

The **thyrohyoid muscle** originates from the oblique line on the lateral side of the thyroid cartilage, which serves as the insertion of the sternothyroid muscle. The fibers run up to be inserted into the hyoid bone. When the muscle contracts, it either lifts the thyroid cartilage and raises the **larynx** or helps depress the hyoid bone. The first

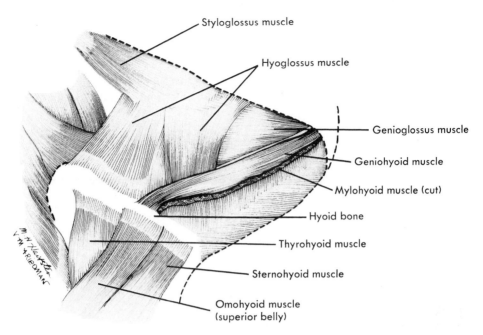

FIG. 13-7. With the mylohyoid muscle cut away, the geniohyoid muscle extends from the genial tubercles of the mandible down to the hyoid bone.

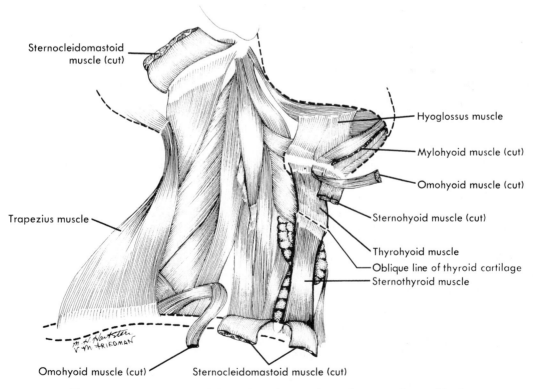

FIG. 13-8. Lateral view of the neck with several muscles cut and turned back (reflected). Notice the extent of the sternothyroid and thyrohyoid muscles.

cervical nerve provides the nerve supply, and the superior thyroid artery is the blood supply (see Figs. 13-5 and 13-8).

MOVEMENTS OF THE JAW AND LARYNX

Following is a brief description of the movements accomplished by the muscles of mastication and the hyoid muscles.

Mandibular Protrusion

Lateral pterygoid muscles acting together produce mandibular **protrusion.**

Mandibular Retrusion

The posterior or horizontal fibers of the temporal muscle, as well as the digastric muscle, accomplish **retrusion** of the mandible.

Lateral Excursion of the Mandible

One of the lateral pterygoid muscles acting by itself accomplishes **lateral excursion.** If the left lateral pterygoid muscle contracts, the left condyle is pulled forward and the mandible will move to the right. Contraction of the right lateral pterygoid muscle accomplishes the opposite movement. While the one lateral pterygoid is contracting, the opposite elevators of the mandible hold the other condyle in place (Fig. 13-9).

Elevation of the Mandible

The medial pterygoid, masseter, and temporal muscles accomplish **elevation.**

Depression of the Mandible

The **depression** of the mandible is accomplished by the inferior head of the lateral pterygoid muscle plus the hyoid muscles. It is important to know that this includes the suprahyoid and infrahyoid muscles. If the mandible is to be depressed, it is important that the infrahyoid muscles contract and pull down on the hyoid bone. Once the hyoid bone is stabilized or held

down from below, contraction of the suprahyoid muscles can aid in pulling the mandible down. These muscles influence the inferior head of the lateral pterygoid muscle to accomplish depression of the mandible.

Laryngeal Movements

The larynx moves up and down in swallowing and phonation. For this to be accomplished, certain muscles must contract. Before continuing, try this demonstration. Place your fingers lightly on the larynx and swallow. What happens? The larynx moves up and under the shelter of the **epiglottis,** which moves back over the laryngeal opening so that anything being swallowed would pass over the laryngeal opening and enter the esophagus. Actually most of this action is accomplished by the tongue moving the food in the mouth back and pushing back on the epiglottis. If this action did not take place, you could choke when trying to swallow food. The hyoid bone is pulled slightly up by the contraction of the suprahyoid muscles. The thyrohyoid muscle then contracts, elevating the thyroid cartilage of the larynx and, along with the contraction of the muscles attached to the epiglottis and the backward movement of the tongue, moves the epiglottis over the opening of the larynx, allowing the swallowed material to enter the esophagus (Fig. 13-10).

This by no means covers all the muscles in the neck area, but it does include those most intimately involved in mandibular and laryngeal movements, providing a better understanding of some of the controls of mastication and swallowing (**deglutition**).

STERNOCLEIDOMASTOID MUSCLE

In an extraoral examination of a patient, it is necessary to press or palpate beneath the posterior border of the sternocleidomastoid muscle to check for enlargement of the lymph nodes lying against the internal jugular vein in the neck. This muscle also is involved in referred pain.

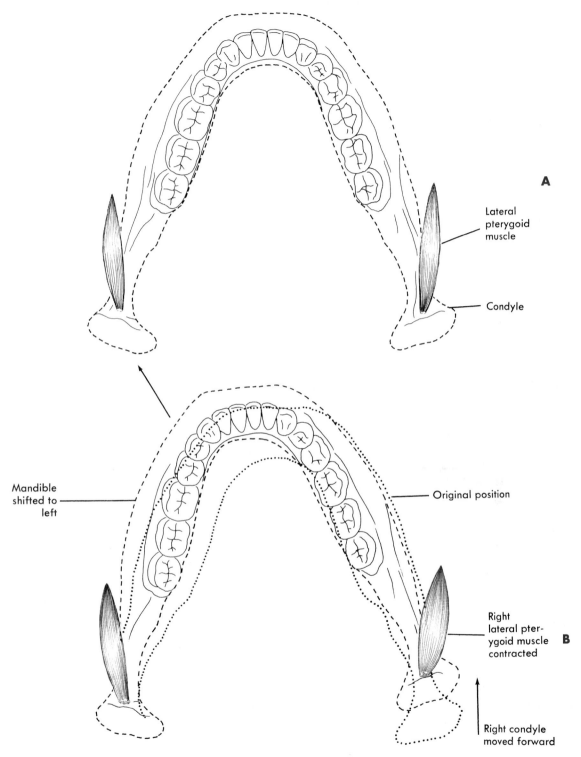

Lateral pterygoid muscle

Condyle

A

Mandible shifted to left

Original position

Right lateral pterygoid muscle contracted

B

Right condyle moved forward

FIG. 13-9. **A,** Superior view of the mandible in rest position showing the condyles and lateral pterygoid muscles. **B,** The right lateral pterygoid muscle has contracted, pulling the condyle on that side forward. The mandible swings to the opposite side, as shown by the *dashed line* and *arrow.*

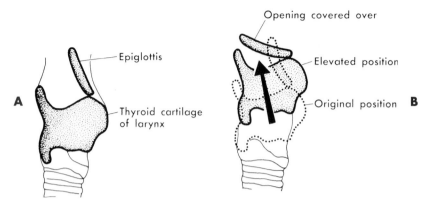

FIG. 13-10. **A,** Thyroid cartilage of the larynx and epiglottis is suspended in part from the hyoid bone. **B,** As the suprahyoid muscles are contracted along with the thyrohyoid muscle, the larynx is elevated and the epiglottis moves back and down to cover the laryngeal opening.

The sternocleidomastoid muscle has its origin in the upper border of the sternum and the medial one third of the clavicle or collarbone. The muscle runs up and back on the side of the neck to insert into the mastoid process of the temporal bone. The action of the muscle is involved in tilting and rotating the head. It is innervated by the eleventh (XI) cranial nerve (accessory nerve), and its blood supply is a branch of the external carotid artery (see Figs. 13-5 and 13-6).

TRAPEZIUS MUSCLE

The **trapezius muscle** takes its origin from the external occipital protuberance on the occipital bone and from the bony ridges, the superior nuchal lines, running lateral from that. It also has origin from spinous processes of cervical and thoracic vertebrae. Its insertion is into the spine of the scapula, the acromion process of the scapula, and the lateral one third of the clavicle. Its function is to **adduct** and elevate the scapula, as well as slightly rotate it (see Figs. 13-5 and 13-8). The shrugging of the

shoulders is a major function of the trapezius muscle. Work such as typing at an improper height can cause pains in the trapezius from holding the arms in a raised position while doing the work.

The sternomastoid and trapezius muscles can involuntarily contract under tension or in conjunction with migraine headaches. Some malocclusions can also cause such spasms. Because these muscles have some of their sensory nerve supply from the second, third, and fourth cervical nerves, they are in close approximation to the lower part of the trigeminal nerve nucleus in the upper spinal chord. This can at times cause pain to emanate from the area of the temporomandibular joint (TMJ). Many people have come to dental offices complaining of TMJ pain. When nothing could be found within the joint or associated muscles, the sternomastoid and/or trapezius muscle was anesthetized, and the pain in the joint disappeared. This illustrates the importance of considering all muscles, even the muscles of mastication, when diagnosing problems of the area of the TMJ.

Review Questions

1. How can you distinguish the origin of a muscle from the insertion?
2. Describe the action of a muscle.
3. Define or describe the following terms in relation to mandibular movements:
   a. Elevation
   b. Protrusion
   c. Retrusion
   d. Depression
   e. Lateral excursion of the mandible
4. Name the muscles involved in creating the actions mentioned in question 3.
5. What does the fact that the anterior belly of the digastric muscle is innervated by the trigeminal nerve while the posterior belly is innervated by the facial nerve tell you about the embryologic origin of the muscle?
6. Which muscles or general groups of muscles affect the movements of the larynx?
7. What is found beneath the sternomastoid muscle?
8. What is referred pain, and what muscles can refer pain to the TMJ?
9. Which suprahyoid and infrahyoid muscles are innervated by cervical nerves as opposed to cranial nerves?

CHAPTER 14

TEMPOROMANDIBULAR JOINT

OBJECTIVES
- To diagram and label a sagittal section of the temporomandibular joint (TMJ)
- To define the role of a synovial cavity
- To describe the two movements of the TMJ as the mouth opens and know where these movements take place
- To describe the role of the superior posterior elastic lamina, the inferior posterior collagenous lamina, and the superior and inferior heads of the lateral pterygoid muscle as the jaw goes through its various functional movements
- To define disc derangement, subluxation, bruxism, and TMJ sounds
- To discuss probable causes of TMJ pain

STRUCTURE

As the name indicates, the **temporomandibular joint** (TMJ) is the articulation between the temporal bone and the mandible. A joint is a joining together of two bones, and there are a number of joint types. A suture of the skull is one type of joint that we have already studied (see Chapter 11), and the TMJ is another type because it is a joint in which the surface of one bone moves over the surface of another.

Actually, the TMJ is two joints that move and function as one. It is also a bilateral or two-sided joint in that the mandible is fused at the midline so the left and right joints are interrelated in their movements. In Chapter 11 you learned the osteology or the system of bony parts of the TMJ. Fig. 14-1 shows the mandibular fossa, posterior tubercle, and articular eminence of the temporal bone, as well as the condyle of the mandible. Between these two bones you can see a small fibrous pad of dense collagen tissue called the **articular disc.** The upper surface of the disc is concavoconvex to match the contours of the mandibular fossa and articular eminence,

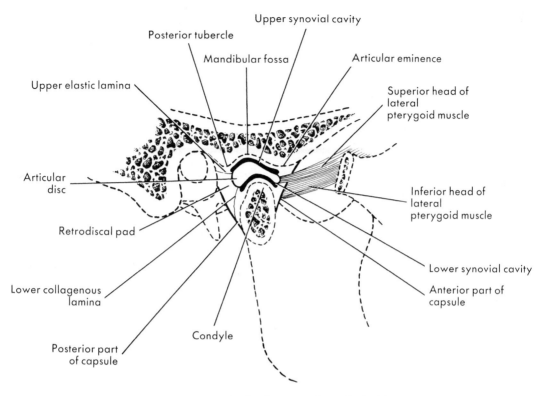

FIG. 14-1.   Longitudinal section through the TMJ.

whereas the lower surface of the disc is concave to match the contour of the condyle. Fig. 14-1 shows that the articular disc is thickest at its posterior end, it is thinnest at its middle, and there is a slight increase in thickness at its anterior end. The thick posterior area is called the *posterior band,* the thin middle area is called the *intermediate zone,* and the slightly thicker anterior area is called the *anterior band.* Above and below this disc are small saclike compartments called **synovial cavities.** Part of the tissue lining these cavities is an epithelium that secretes a few drops of lubricating liquid called **synovial fluid,** which allows the surfaces to rub over one another without irritation.

The entire TMJ is surrounded by a thick fi-

brous capsule. The lateral side of this capsule is thickened between the articular tubercle and the lateral pole of the condyle. This thickened area is the **temporomandibular ligament.** This ligament prevents the condyle from being displaced too far inferiorly and posteriorly and provides some resistance to lateral displacement (Fig. 14-2).

The articular disc is attached both medially and laterally to the poles of the condyle (Fig. 14-3). Anteriorly it is attached to some fibers of the superior head of the lateral pterygoid muscle. These fibers penetrate the capsule and insert into the disc. The area posterior to the disc is the **retrodiscal pad.** This is an area of relatively loose connective tissue in which is located much of the blood and nerve supply to the joint. Running

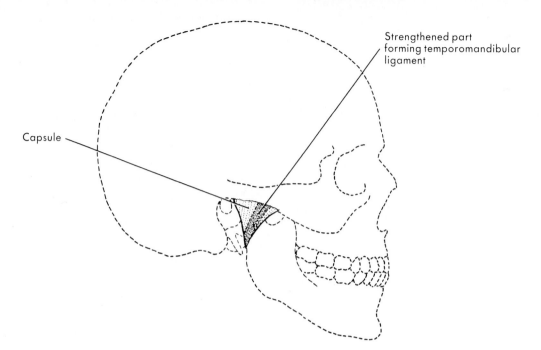

Capsule

Strengthened part
forming temporomandibular
ligament

FIG. 14-2. The capsule surrounding the entire TMJ. The capsule is strengthened on the deep side of the lateral surface by the temporomandibular ligament, which helps prevent lateral, posterior, and inferior movement of the condyle out of the fossa.

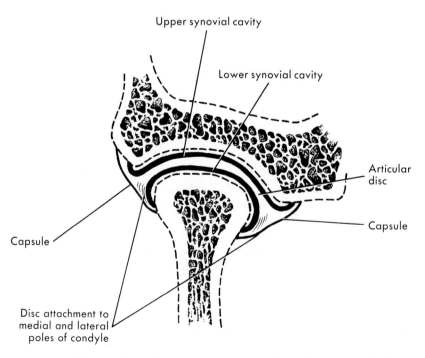

Upper synovial cavity

Lower synovial cavity

Articular
disc

Capsule

Capsule

Disc attachment to
medial and lateral
poles of condyle

FIG. 14-3. From left to right, a frontal section through the condyle, disc, capsule, and fossa. The disc fibers curve down to insert into the poles of the condyle.

from the posterior upper part of the disc is an elastic lamina or tissue layer that lies above the retrodiscal pad and inserts into the posterior upper end of the TMJ capsule where it attaches to the tympanic plate of the temporal bone. Running from the posterior lower border of the disc is a collagenous lamina that lies below the retrodiscal pad and attaches the posterior neck of the condyle, where the capsule attaches to it (see Fig. 14-1).

MOVEMENT

The TMJ has two distinct types of movement: a rotational movement and a gliding movement along an inclined plane. This is frequently called a *hinge and sliding joint* or a *gliding joint*. As the teeth begin to separate (the first few millimeters) there is a rotational movement in the lower synovial cavity between the disc and the condyle below. The reason for the rotational movement is the posterior elastic lamina. As the condyle begins rotating the disc wants to move anteriorly with it because it is attached to the poles of the condyle. However, the elastic lamina pulls posteriorly on the disc, and the disc and condyle rotate on one another. As the jaw opens farther the rotational movement continues, but there is also an additional anterior gliding movement along the posterior slope of the articular eminence. This gliding movement takes place between the disc and the temporal bone above. The forward movement is caused by contraction of the inferior head of the lateral pterygoid muscle (Chapter 13). The condyle and disc move forward until they reach just slightly anterior to the crest of the articular eminence.

If the jaw moves slowly back into a centric relation, the superior head of the lateral pterygoid controls the posterior movement of the disc by controlling the release of its contraction and by balancing the posterior pull exerted by the elastic lamina. The lower posterior collagenous lamina prevents the elastic lamina and disc from being pulled too far forward, thereby preventing injury.

During chewing, the mandible is depressed by the hyoid muscles, and the lateral pterygoid muscle pulls forward and down. As this depression takes place, the lateral pterygoid muscle opposite the chewing side pulls forward even more, causing the mandible to move into a lateral excursion to the chewing side. As you begin the power stroke and elevate the mandible and begin to bite down on a thick piece of food placed between the teeth on the chewing side, the condyle on that side will be in a position where the condyle, disc, and temporal bone are in contact with one another. However, on the nonchewing side, as you continue to bite down, the condyle, disc, and temporal surfaces will be pulled slightly apart. This makes the nonchewing side of the joint somewhat unstable, which could cause the surfaces to bounce against one another and possibly injure the structures. However, this does not happen because the superior head of the lateral pterygoid muscle contracts, pulling the disc forward. In doing so it moves the thicker posterior part of the disc forward, which fills the space created by the surfaces moving slightly apart and so balances and stabilizes the joint on that side. With continued contraction, the posterior fibers of the temporalis on the nonchewing side contract, pulling back on the coronoid process and therefore pulling the condyle posteriorly, causing the occlusal surface of the mandibular teeth to grind the food as the mandible moves from lateral excursion back into a more centric position. By slowly relaxing its contracted fibers, the upper head of the lateral pterygoid controls the posterior movement of the disc with a posterior pull from the superior elastic lamina, and a smooth closing movement takes place.

PROBLEMS ASSOCIATED WITH THE TMJ

There are myriad problems associated with the TMJ, and in many cases there is disagreement over how these problems should be treated. The following discussion presents some of these problems and their possible causes. It is quite likely that you will see many of these cases in the office, where they will be either treated or referred elsewhere for treatment.

Pain in the TMJ Area

Many patients complain of pain in the region of the TMJ. If radiographic studies show a normal TMJ and there does not seem to be any pain upon palpation of the area, the possibility of referred pain should be considered (see Chapter 13). Referred pain is a condition in which sensory messages, seemingly coming from the area of the TMJ, are actually traveling to the brain from other regions of the body. Many of these pains come from spasms in neck muscles and from the muscles of mastication. Many times muscle relaxants or physical therapy allow these muscles to relax and subsequently relieve the pain. In Chapter 19 you will study the cranial nerves. Four of these nerves—the V, VII, IX, and X—supply sensory areas around the ear. Involvement with these nerves may cause pain that seems to come from the TMJ. Pain in the TMJ may also come from malocclusion, caused by shifting, wear, or loss of teeth. (It should be pointed out here, in reference to pain originating in the disc, that the central portion of the disc has no nerve supply, which is why one can wear a hole through the disc and not know it. The medial and lateral attachments of the disc to the condyle and anterior and posterior attachments are in areas that have nerve supply, and injury to those areas will cause significant pain.)

Internal Problems of the TMJ

TMJ sounds

Many patients complain of a popping, clicking, or grinding in the TMJ yet have no other symptoms, such as pain. The popping or clicking noise may occur when the disc is pulled too far forward in the opening movement. The thick posterior band of the disc gets caught between the head of the condyle and the articular emi-

nence. It then pops forward and is displaced too far anteriorly. It may also pop posteriorly from its trapped position. Many times the dentist is not able to hear the clicking or popping without the aid of a stethoscope. Sometimes by palpating the joint as popping occurs, a jumping movement of the condyle can be felt as the disc pops forward. If this only happens on one side, you can frequently see the movement by standing in front of patients and observing whether the mandible moves in a straight downward movement or whether it shifts to one side and then moves back to the midline during opening. Many times these problems can be treated with ultrasound, physical therapy, or a plastic splint, similar to a nightguard. The grinding sound may come from adhesions in the synovial membranes of the joint, arthritic changes, or possibly perforations of the disc. It can also be treated by ultrasound, although it may recur.

Disc derangement

The cause of TMJ sounds may also be the result of a type of disc derangement. In constant anterior displacement of the disc, there may be permanent damage to the components of the disc. The posterior laminae may be torn and the disc permanently displaced anteriorly. Also, the medial or lateral attachments of the disc to the poles of the condyle may be torn. If this happens, the tear is usually to the lateral pole attachment. Both of these circumstances will probably require surgery, and the surgery tends to be fairly successful in the proper hands.

Subluxation

A condition in which a person opens his or her mouth too wide and is not able to close it again or in which closing it causes a popping back into position is called **subluxation**. This happens when the condyle glides too far forward and moves too far anterior to the height of the articular eminence (Fig. 14-4). When the patient tries to close, the condyle cannot move back because the muscles are trying to pull up and back and the articular eminence does not allow the condyle to move back. If a patient cannot close, place

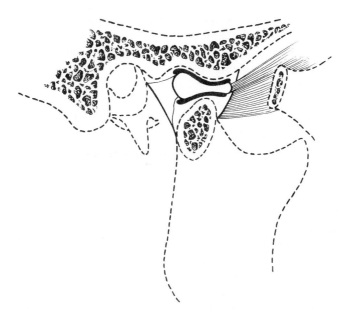

FIG. 14-4.   The condyle has ridden forward to the height of eminence. If it moves further forward, it may become trapped and unable to move back because of contour. It therefore has to be pushed down, or depressed, before it can be eased back into its normal position.

your thumbs on the occlusal surface of the mandibular posterior teeth with the index fingers beneath the inferior border of the mandible and pushing down while at the same time guiding the jaw slowly back into its posterior position. It is advisable to wrap your thumbs in gauze so that they are protected in case the patient closes down on them. In general, there are several reasons for subluxation. One is the depth of the condylar fossa and the height of the articular eminence. Another is the position of the capsule around the joint, a factor that controls the amount of contraction of the lateral pterygoid muscle. This problem can be treated by surgically decreasing the height of the articular eminence.

Bruxism

Many people grind their teeth; this is called **bruxism.** Most of the time this is done during sleep, although it does occur sometimes during waking hours. Over a long period it may wear down the teeth, but a more immediate result is a very tired and sore TMJ. Much of this tenderness has to do with the muscles of mastication tiring, yet it is the joint that seems to ache. One of the methods of treatment is to make a plastic nightguard to cover the upper teeth. To a great extent this eliminates the excessive wear on the teeth and the tenderness of the teeth from stress on the periodontal ligament. Others might be treated with tranquilizers to relieve the tension that may contribute to the bruxism.

Arthritis and other pain in the TMJ

The TMJ is also subject to such conditions as **arthritis** and the pain that results from it. **Cortisone** may relieve the arthritis, but the pain can still be a major problem. Other patients have a grinding sensation in the joint. Authorities contend that this is caused by excessive wear of the disc in the joint so that there is no longer a smooth gliding movement within the synovial cavities. This explanation seems very reasonable, because the TMJ is a stress-bearing joint, and too much stress may cause it to wear out early in life and cause problems. However, there are reports of people who have had both condyles fractures so severely that they had to be removed surgically, and the patients have continued to function well without a real joint, which tells us that not enough is known about the TMJ and that it is more complicated than was formerly believed.

Over the years a patient may wear away some of the occlusal surfaces of teeth and begin to experience pain in the TMJ. Many times, simply rebuilding the teeth to their original height with crowns and onlays eases the pain. Most authorities agree that most of the problems in these cases rest not in the joint itself but in the muscles of mastication, other head and neck muscles, and the occlusion of the teeth. With changes in the relationship of the jaws caused by tooth wear, the muscles of mastication are no longer in their normal relaxed position. Therefore they might tend to go into **spasm** and cause pain.

Review Questions

1. What is a synovial cavity, and what is its function?
2. Describe the TMJ capsule and ligament.
3. What are the two TMJ movements? Where and when do they occur?
4. Describe the roles of the posterior laminae and the lateral pterygoid muscle in mastication.
5. What are some causes of TMJ pain?
6. What may cause TMJ sounds?
7. What is a disc derangement?

MUSCLES OF FACIAL EXPRESSION

THE TERM *facial expression* in the chapter title may be a bit misleading because the muscles included in this chapter are located around the ears, scalp, neck, eyes, nose, and mouth. However, although some of them are not located in an area normally thought of as the face, they are located in areas that can physically display some kind of emotion or attentiveness. All of these muscles are innervated by the seventh (VII) cranial nerve (facial). Although most of the muscles are mentioned, only the muscles around the oral cavity are discussed in great detail. These are the muscles you will be most concerned with in the dental office, and they are responsible for some functions related to speech and mastication.

EARS

The muscles around the ears are not well developed in humans. However, in lower forms of animals, they are better developed, and the ears can be easily moved and repositioned to better catch sounds. There are three pairs of ear muscles (Fig. 15-1).

Anterior Auricular Muscle

The **anterior auricular muscle** arises from connective tissue of the scalp in front of the ear and runs posteriorly into the anterior part of the ear. The action of this muscle pulls the ear slightly forward.

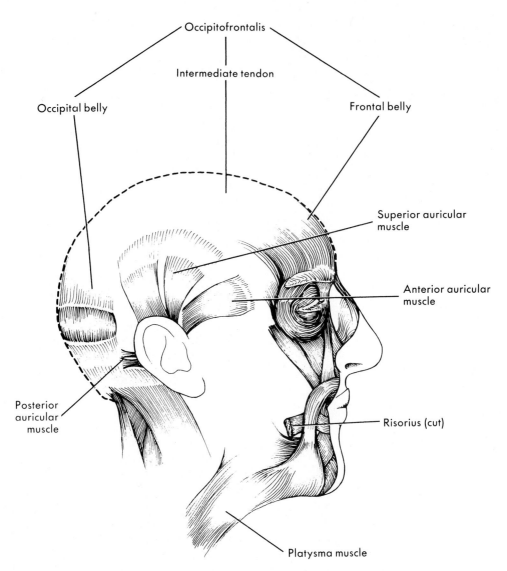

Occipitofrontalis

Intermediate tendon

Occipital belly

Frontal belly

Superior auricular muscle

Anterior auricular muscle

Posterior auricular muscle

Risorius (cut)

Platysma muscle

Fig. 15-1.   Three groups of auricular muscles around the ear. There are two bellies of the occipitofrontalis with the intermediate tendon.

Superior Auricular Muscle

The **superior auricular muscle** arises from connective tissue of the scalp above the ear, and the fibers run down and insert into the upper part of the ear. The action of this muscle raises the ear.

Posterior Auricular Muscle

The **posterior auricular muscle** arises from the **superior nuchal line** of the occipital bone and the mastoid area. The fibers run forward to insert into the posterior part of the ear. The action of this muscle pulls the ear back. This is probably the best developed of the ear muscles.

SCALP

The muscles of the scalp allow for its mobility both forward and backward.

Occipitofrontalis (Epicranius)

The **occipitofrontalis (epicranius)** is a paired muscle with groups of fibers in front and back connected by a broad flat band of **fascia**. The anterior and posterior groups of muscle fibers take their origin from connective tissue of the scalp. This kind of attachment allows for either forward or backward movement of the scalp. The forward movement results in a frown or a squint, and the backward movement raises the forehead skin as in surprise (see Fig. 15-1).

NECK

You may wonder how a muscle in the neck can show facial expression. However, pulling down the corners of the mouth as in a grimace is partly accomplished by the platysma muscle in the neck.

Platysma

There is some disagreement as to which end of the **platysma** is the origin and which is the insertion. The upper end of the fibers attaches to the inferior border of the mandible, near the angles of the mouth and the skin of the face in that area. They pass down in a broad flat sheet to end in the skin of the chest area just below the clavicle. The muscle lies just below the skin of the neck; thus it moves the skin over the neck quite noticeably when it contracts, pulling the corners of the mouth down or the skin of the upper pectoral region up.

EYES

Several muscles located around the eyes close the eyes and move the eyebrows (Fig. 15-2).

Orbicularis Oculi

Although the Latin term **orbicularis oculi** may prove problematic for some, by studying it carefully you can infer its meaning. The term *orbicularis* relates to the word *circular*, and it is easy to understand how the orbicularis oculi circles the eye.

There are two parts to the orbicularis oculi. The part that encircles the eye is the orbital part. It attaches to the skull at the medial and lateral edges of the orbit. The muscle fibers in the eyelid comprise the palpebral part. Their fibers also attach at the medial and lateral corners of the orbit. The action of the orbicularis oculi closes the eyelids and contracts the skin around the eye. Another muscle in this area, which has its origin at the back of the orbit and inserts into the upper eyelid, is the **levator palpebrae superioris** muscle. As the term *levator* indicates, this muscle raises the upper eyelid. It is supplied by the III cranial nerve (oculomotor nerve) and is considered a muscle of the orbit because it is not innervated by the facial nerve.

Corrugator

The **corrugator** runs from the bridge of the nose up and lateral to the lateral part of the eyebrow. It pulls the eyebrow medially and down, as in a frown.

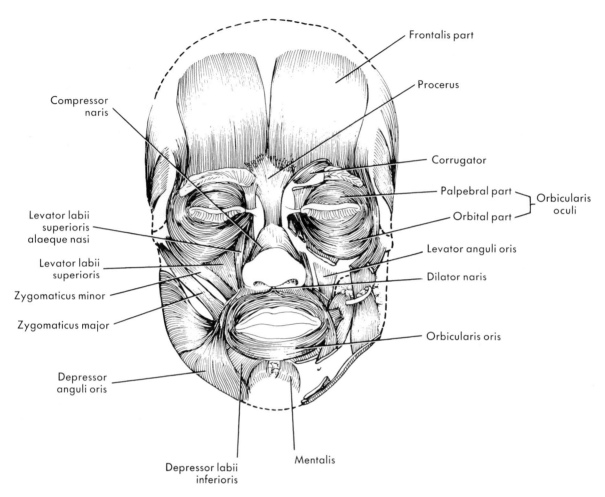

FIG. 15-2.   Muscles of the eye, nose, and mouth.

Procerus

From the bridge of the nose the fibers of the **procerus** extend up into the medial end of the eyebrow. They pull the eyebrow at the medial end down as in a frown or as in a squint.

NOSE

The muscles of the nose primarily circle the opening of the nostrils (see Fig. 15-2). The nasalis is the muscle that opens and closes the nostrils. It is composed of two parts.

Dilator Naris

The **dilator naris** pulls down on the nostrils, causing them to flare or dilate.

Compressor Naris

The **compressor naris** causes the nostrils to close or compress.

MOUTH

The muscles grouped around the mouth influence expression and speech and aid in mastication. The pressure of these muscles on the teeth helps hold the teeth in alignment if the pressures are normal. Abnormal pressures caused by cheek biting, lip biting, and lip compression may cause them to move out of alignment (see Fig. 15-2).

Orbicularis Oris

The **orbicularis oris** circles the oral cavity in the tissue of the lip. It has some bony attachment at the anterior nasal spine and at the midline above the chin. The fibers circle the lip like a purse string, and all the muscles surrounding the lips interlace with them. The action of the muscle is to close and compress the lips.

Levator Labii Superioris

The **levator labii superioris** elevates the upper lip. Its origin is just beneath the lower rim of the orbit. The fibers run down to be inserted into the fibers of the orbicularis oris of the upper lip, midway between the center of the lip and each corner of the mouth.

Zygomaticus Minor

The **zygomaticus minor** is a small muscle from the area of the zygomatic bone. The fibers run down and forward and insert into the orbicularis oris just lateral to the levator labii superioris. It also raises the upper lip, though it is usually a very poorly developed muscle and therefore does not exert great influence in this function.

Zygomaticus Major

The **zygomaticus major** is the larger muscle originating from the zygomatic bone. Its origin is lateral to the zygomaticus minor on the most prominent portion of the cheek and runs down and forward to insert into the orbicularis oris at the angle of the mouth. Its action is to elevate the corners of the mouth, as in a smile.

Levator Anguli Oris

The **levator anguli oris** lies deep to the levator labii superioris, the zygomaticus major, and the zygomaticus minor. It originates from the maxilla, just below the infraorbital foramen. The fibers run down and laterally to blend into the orbicularis oris at the corners of the mouth. This muscle pulls the angles of the mouth up and toward the midline.

Depressor Labii Inferioris

The origin of the **depressor labii inferioris** is the area beneath the angles of the mouth and just above the inferior border of the mandible. The fibers run up and medially to insert into the fibers of the orbicularis oris toward the middle of the lower lip. This muscle pulls the lower lip down as in a pout.

Depressor Anguli Oris

The origin of the **depressor anguli oris** is from the same general area as that of the depressor labii inferioris, and the fibers of the former partly overlap the latter. From the origin, the fibers run up and converge to blend into the orbicularis oris at the angle of the mouth. This muscle pulls the corners of the mouth down. Many of these fibers appear to be a continuation of the fibers of the platysma.

Mentalis

The **mentalis** originates on the anterior surface of the mandible just beneath the lateral incisors. The fibers run down and toward the midline, where some even cross to meet the muscle on the opposite side, terminating with insertion into the skin of the chin. When the muscle contracts, it pulls this skin up.

Buccinator

The **buccinator** is probably the most important of the muscles of the mouth (Fig. 15-3). Although it is a muscle of facial expression, it also plays a role in mastication. The muscle originates from a fibrous band (the **pterygomandibu-**

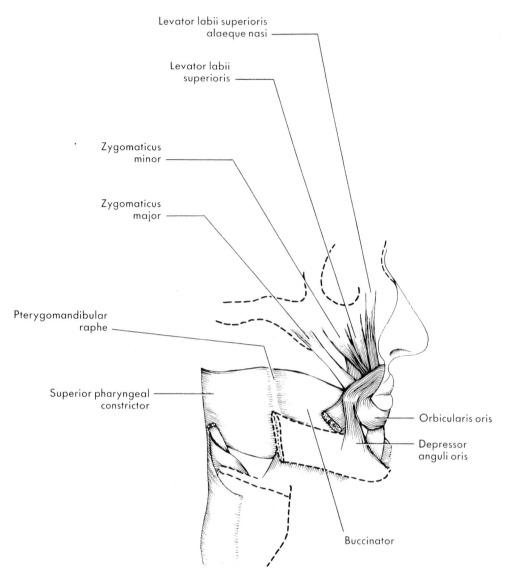

Levator labii superioris
alaeque nasi

Levator labii
superioris

Zygomaticus
minor

Zygomaticus
major

Pterygomandibular
raphe

Superior pharyngeal
constrictor

Orbicularis oris

Depressor
anguli oris

Buccinator

FIG. 15-3. Muscles of the mouth.

lar raphe), which runs from the pterygoid hamulus on the inferior portion of the medial pterygoid plate down to the medial surface of the mandible near the posterior part of the mylohyoid line. The pterygomandibular raphe con-

nects the anterior part of the **superior constrictor muscle** of the pharynx with the posterior part of the buccinator.

The buccinator also originates from the buccal alveolar bone of the maxillary molars and from the corresponding area of the mandibular molars. From these two bony origins and from the pterygomandibular raphe, the fibers of the buccinator run anteriorly, making up the musculature of the cheek. The fibers insert into the orbicularis oris at the corners of the mouth. When the muscle contracts, it pulls the corners of the mouth back and compresses the cheek. During chewing, the food is crushed and ground between the molars. As the food is squeezed out from the occlusal surfaces, some of the food is pushed onto the tongue and the remainder is deposited into the buccal vestibule. The food on the tongue can be pushed back up onto the occlusal surface by the action of the tongue. The food that is forced out into the vestibule is pushed back up onto the occlusal surfaces in part by the contraction of the buccinator muscle.

The buccinator muscle is frequently referred to as an *accessory muscle of mastication* because of the help it provides in chewing food. A person with facial muscle paralysis would have difficulty chewing food. It would pile up in the buccal vestibule because the buccinator muscle could not force it back up onto the occlusal surfaces.

Risorius

The **risorius** is a small muscle that arises from the soft tissue near the angle of the mandible. It runs forward on the surface of the buccinator and inserts into the corner of the mouth. It aids in smiling but is usually very poorly developed. It also is an apparent continuation of the posterior fibers of the platysma muscle (see Fig. 15-1).

Review Questions

1. Describe or name the head and neck locations of the muscles of facial expression.
2. Which nerve innervates the muscles of facial expression?
3. Of all the muscles of facial expression, which one is the most important for mastication? Why?
4. Describe where the following muscles enter the orbicularis oris muscle, the direction from which they enter, and their function:
   a. Levator labii superioris
   b. Zygomaticus minor
   c. Zygomaticus major
   d. Levator anguli oris
   e. Depressor labii inferioris
   f. Depressor anguli oris
   g. Buccinator

CHAPTER 16

SOFT PALATE
AND PHARYNX

OBJECTIVES
- To describe the origins, insertions, actions, and nerve supplies of the muscles of the soft palate and pharynx
- To describe the interrelationship of all of these muscles in chewing, swallowing, and speech

THE MUSCLES of the soft palate and **pharynx** are intricate in their arrangement and interrelationship. They share some common boundaries with the upper end of the digestive and respiratory systems and are important in the production of speech sounds. The soft palate forms the posterior end of the roof of the mouth. The pharynx has three components: the upper part, the nasal pharynx, is located at the posterior end of the nasal cavity; the middle part, the oral pharynx, is the back throat wall; and the lower part, the laryngeal pharynx, is below the tongue where the digestive and respiratory systems branch into their respective parts, the esophagus and larynx.

SOFT PALATE

There are five pairs of muscles in the soft palate. These muscles help move the soft palate up and back to contact the posterior throat wall and seal off the nasal cavity from the oral cavity and also to narrow the space between the two palatine tonsils. This space is called the *fauces* and is used in swallowing.

Palatoglossal Muscle

If you open the mouth and look at the tonsils on the side of the throat wall, you will see that there is a vertical fold of tissue in front of and behind each tonsil. These are called the *anterior* and *posterior faucial pillars* or the *palatoglossal* and *palatopharyngeal folds,* respectively. Beneath the palatoglossal fold is the **palatoglossal muscle.** It originates from the posterior end of the hard palate and the anterior end of the soft palate. The fibers run downward, laterally, and forward to insert into the posterior and lateral part of the tongue. When the palatoglossal muscle contracts, it pulls the sides of the tongue up and back, pulls the soft palate down on the lateral edges, and narrows the space between the left and right faucial pillars. The nerve that supplies this muscle is a part of the eleventh (XI) cranial nerve running with branches of the tenth (X) cranial nerve (Figs. 16-1 and 16-2).

Palatopharyngeal Muscle

The posterior faucial pillar is formed by the **palatopharyngeal muscle.** It originates from the posterolateral part of the soft palate and runs downward and laterally to insert into the pharyngeal constrictor muscle and the thyroid cartilage of the larynx. When it contracts, it narrows the fauces and elevates the pharynx. The nerve supply is also the eleventh and tenth cranial nerves (Figs. 16-1 to 16-3).

Muscles of Uvula

The uvula is the small fold of tissue that hangs down in the throat from the posterior part of the soft palate. It is formed by two small bands of muscle that originate from the posterior end of the hard palate and run back and down in the soft palate to form that structure. When the **muscle of the uvula** contracts, it shortens and broadens the uvula and changes the contour of the posterior end of the soft palate so that it adapts to the posterior throat wall when it is moved up against it. This muscle is also innervated by the eleventh and tenth cranial nerves (see Fig. 16-3).

Levator Veli Palatini

The **levator veli palatini** elevates the posterior end of the soft palate. It originates from the pe-

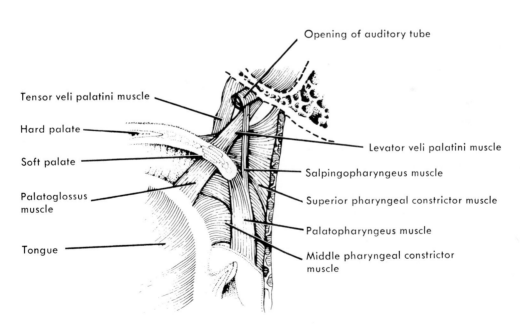

Opening of auditory tube

Tensor veli palatini muscle

Hard palate

Soft palate

Palatoglossus muscle

Tongue

Levator veli palatini muscle

Salpingopharyngeus muscle

Superior pharyngeal constrictor muscle

Palatopharyngeus muscle

Middle pharyngeal constrictor muscle

FIG. 16-1.   View of the lateral throat wall looking from the midline. Mucosa has been removed and various muscles can be seen. Palatoglossal and palatopharyngeal muscles form anterior and posterior pillars, respectively; the palatine tonsil would lie between them.

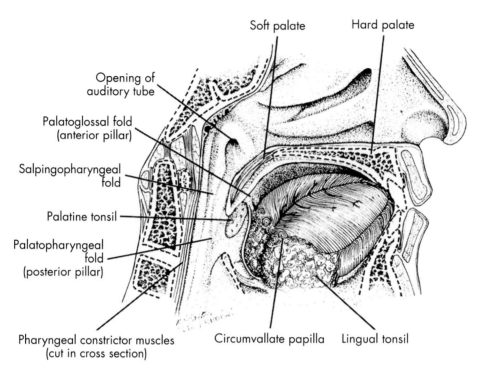

Soft palate   Hard palate

Opening of
auditory tube

Palatoglossal fold
(anterior pillar)

Salpingopharyngeal
fold

Palatine tonsil

Palatopharyngeal
fold
(posterior pillar)

Pharyngeal constrictor muscles   Circumvallate papilla   Lingual tonsil
(cut in cross section)

FIG. 16-2.   View of the lateral throat wall similar to Fig. 16-1 but with mucosa in place. Anterior and posterior pillars can be seen, as can the opening of
the auditory tube in the nasal pharynx; the fold caused by the salpingopharyngeal muscle runs down from it.

trous part of the temporal bone just anterior
to the carotid canal and from the medial wall
of the cartilagenous part of the auditory canal
or tube, which lies in the lateral wall of the
nasal pharynx. The fibers run downward and
slightly medially into the posterior part of the
soft palate. When the muscle contracts, it pulls
the posterior end of the soft palate up and back
to contact the posterior pharyngeal (throat)
wall. It also functions to help open the auditory tube if it is edematous and closed. The
nerve supply to this muscle is also the eleventh and tenth cranial nerves (Figs. 16-1, 16-2,
and 16-4).

Tensor Veli Palatini

The last of the muscles of the soft palate is the
tensor veli palatini. This muscle takes its origin
from an area near the base of the medial pterygoid plate, where it meets the body of the sphenoid bone, as well as from the lateral wall of the
cartilage of the auditory tube. The fibers run
downward and forward to pass around the lateral side of the hamular process on the medial
pterygoid plate; as they pass around the hamular
process, they turn medially and insert into the
posterior edge of the hard palate and the anterior portion of the soft palate. As the name indicates, contraction of the muscle slightly tenses

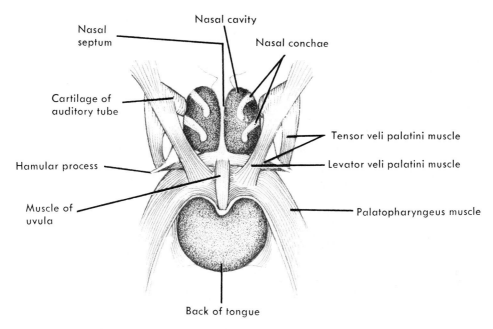

Nasal cavity

Nasal septum

Nasal conchae

Cartilage of auditory tube

Tensor veli palatini muscle

Levator veli palatini muscle

Hamular process

Muscle of uvula

Palatopharyngeus muscle

Back of tongue

FIG. 16-3.   Posterior view of the muscles of the soft palate. The pharyngeal constrictor muscles have been removed, and the view is from behind the throat. Notice especially how the levator veli palatini runs directly downward into the soft palate, whereas the tensor veli palatini runs downward and forward around the lateral side of the hamular process and then turns medially into the soft palate. You can see how shortening of this muscle would tense the soft palate.

the anterior portion of the soft palate. Because there is very little tensing achieved, it functions more to open the auditory tube when it is closed. The nerve supply to this muscle is the third part of the fifth (V) cranial nerve and is usually denoted V_3 (see Figs. 16-1, 16-3, and 16-4).

PHARYNX

Pharyngeal Constrictors

The pharynx has two groups of muscles associated with it—one group that constricts the pharynx and another group that elevates and dilates the pharynx. There are three pairs of pha-

ryngeal constrictors, all of which insert into a midline tendon in the posterior throat wall known as the **median raphe.** These three muscles overlap one another in their insertion into this raphe (Fig. 16-5).

Superior pharyngeal constrictor muscle

The **superior pharyngeal constrictor muscle** originates in the lower part of the medial pterygoid plate and its hamular process, from the mandibular alveolar process on the lingual side just above the mylohyoid line, and from a tendinous band called the *pterygomandibular raphe* that runs between these two areas. These points of origin are the same as for the buccinator

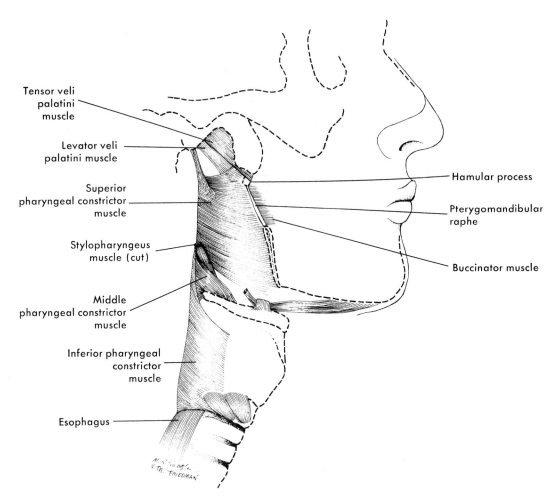

FIG. 16-4.   Lateral view of the pharyngeal constrictor muscles. Above them you can see the tensor and levator veli palatini running downward into the soft palate.

muscle discussed in Chapter 15. The buccinator muscle runs forward, whereas the superior pharyngeal constrictor runs backward to insert into the base of the skull just in front of the foramen magnum and into the median raphe. As the muscle passes posteriorly, its fibers fan out upward and downward. When the muscle contracts, it constricts the upper part of the pharynx and is able to force the contents of the pharynx

downward. The muscle is supplied by the tenth and eleventh cranial nerves (see Figs. 16-4 and 16-5), which make up what is known for most of these muscles as the **pharyngeal plexus of nerves.**

Middle pharyngeal constrictor muscle

The **middle pharyngeal constrictor muscle** takes its origin from the posterior, upper part of the hyoid bone and from the stylohyoid liga-

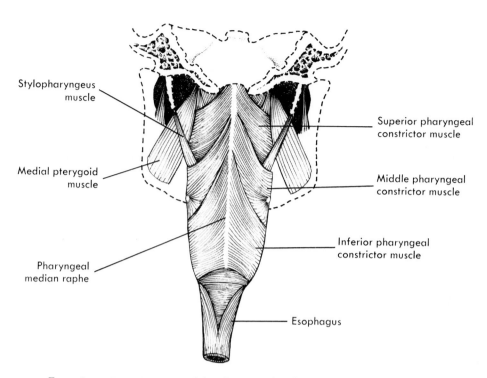

Stylopharyngeus
muscle

Superior pharyngeal
constrictor muscle

Medial pterygoid
muscle

Middle pharyngeal
constrictor muscle

Inferior pharyngeal
constrictor muscle

Pharyngeal
median raphe

Esophagus

FIG. 16-5.   Posterior view of the pharyngeal wall. You can see overlapping of
the pharyngeal constrictor muscles and the position of the stylopharyngeal
muscle running down into them.

ment. The fibers run backward, fanning out and
overlapping the superior constrictor muscle
above and underlying the inferior constrictor below as it inserts into the median raphe. When the
muscle contracts, it also constricts the pharyngeal opening and forces the food down toward
the esophagus. This muscle is also supplied by
the tenth and eleventh cranial nerves (see Figs.
16-4 and 16-5).

Inferior pharyngeal constrictor muscle

The **inferior pharyngeal constrictor muscle**
takes its origin from the posterior part of the
thyroid cartilage of the larynx. The fibers run
backward, overlying the middle pharyngeal constrictor, and insert into the median raphe. The
lowest of these fibers blend in with the upper

part of the wall of the esophagus so that contraction of this muscle also constricts the lower end
of the pharynx and forces the food into the
esophagus, which then continues the movement
of the food toward the stomach. The nerve supply to this muscle is also the tenth and eleventh
cranial nerves (see Figs. 16-4 and 16-5).

Pharyngeal Elevators and Dilators

The second group of muscles in the pharynx
aids in elevating and dilating the pharynx.

Palatopharyngeal muscle

Although the palatopharyngeal muscle has
already been listed as a muscle of the soft palate, you can see from its action that it also has
the ability to elevate the pharynx. This action

is necessary to receive the food that is to be swallowed.

Stylopharyngeal muscle

The **stylopharyngeal muscle** takes its origin from the base of the styloid process on the medial side. It then runs downward and medially to enter the pharyngeal constrictors between the superior and middle constrictor to blend in with some fibers of the palatopharyngeal muscle, which then insert into the lateral pharyngeal wall and the thyroid cartilage of the larynx. Contraction of the muscle causes dilation and elevation of the pharynx. This is the primary dilator of the pharynx. The nerve supply to this muscle is the ninth cranial nerve (see Fig. 16-5).

Salpingopharyngeal muscle

The **salpingopharyngeal muscle** takes its origin from the end of the auditory tube in the lateral wall of the nasal pharynx. The fibers run downward to blend in with the palatopharyngeal muscle and the lateral pharyngeal wall. Contraction of the muscle primarily lifts the pharyngeal wall in the act of swallowing, as does contraction of the other muscles just listed. The nerve supply to this muscle is the tenth and eleventh cranial nerves (see Figs. 16-1 and 16-2).

ACTIONS

Speech

When we speak, we pull the soft palate up and back to contact the posterior pharyngeal wall. This is accomplished primarily by the levator veli palatini and the muscle of the uvula. If the soft palate is unable to adapt well to the posterior pharyngeal wall, the speech will have a nasal sound. A common example of this occurs when a person has enlarged adenoids (pharyngeal tonsils), which are in the posterior pharyngeal wall just where the soft palate contacts it. These enlarged adenoids give the voice a definite nasal tone. For another example, if there is a large open contact region, as occurs in a cleft palate, the voice may be unintelligible.

Swallowing

While we are considering the act of swallowing, let us look at what precedes it and follow it through to completion, using the example of meat. Meat is incised by the anterior teeth and ground up by the posterior teeth. While this happens, the meat is also being mixed with saliva. When it reaches the proper consistency, it is shaped into a ball of food by the teeth, cheeks, and tongue; this ball is referred to as a **bolus of food.**

The bolus is placed on the tongue, the tongue moves up and back, and the bolus is shifted onto the posterior part of the tongue and moved back into the oral pharyngeal area. As the tongue moves up and back, the muscles of the soft palate raise the posterior end of the soft palate to contact the posterior pharyngeal wall and narrow the fauces so that they press tightly to the sides of the tongue, sealing off the back part of the tongue and the oral pharynx from the front part of the tongue and the oral cavity.

If we look at the action of the pharyngeal muscles in this swallowing process, we see that the elevators and dilators of the pharynx lift and widen the pharynx to accommodate the bolus of food that has just been moved back into the oral pharynx. Next the constrictors compress the upper part of the oral pharynx and push the food down into the laryngeal pharynx. As this happens, some of the pharyngeal muscles elevate the thyroid cartilage of the larynx with assistance from the thyrohyoid and a number of muscles. This allows the epiglottis to help shelter the laryngeal opening from food moving into it, and the food moves down into the upper end of the esophagus. The upper half of the esophagus is also a voluntary skeletal muscle, and a person can willfully move the food about halfway down the esophagus before the further movement is taken over by involuntary smooth muscle, which creates wavelike constrictions of the digestive tube known as **peristaltic contractions.** At one time or another we have all moved too much food into the esophagus too quickly and have felt as if it was stuck halfway down. In essence this is true because we can move the food only that far voluntarily; then it has to stop and wait for the involuntary peristaltic waves to take it the rest of the way; these waves proceed at a much slower rate than the voluntary waves of contraction that we can create.

Review Questions

1. What are the muscles of the soft palate that narrow the fauces, and what other actions can they accomplish? Describe their origins and insertions.
2. Which muscles of the pharynx aid in elevation and dilatation of the pharynx? Which nerves supply them?
3. Name the origins and insertions of the pharyngeal constrictors as well as their nerve supply.
4. What creates nasal sounds in a person's speech?
5. What muscle closes off the oral pharynx from the nasal pharynx in speech and what is its nerve supply?
6. List the sequence of events that take place when food is masticated and swallowed.
7. Why do we sometimes feel as if food is caught halfway down our throats?

Chapter 17

Arterial Supply and Venous Drainage

Objectives
- To trace the blood from the time it returns from the body to the heart, out, and back until it returns again from the overall body
- To trace the blood supply from the heart to all areas of the oral cavity, including the teeth
- To trace the venous drainage from the teeth and oral cavity back to the heart
- To define hematoma
- To discuss the possible problems associated with a posterior superior alveolar injection

A STUDENT of anatomy should have a clear picture of the blood flow to and from the body. Blood enters into the right atrium of the heart from the body. From the right atrium it travels through the right atrioventricular valve (tricuspid valve) to the right ventricle. The right ventricle pumps it out through the pulmonary valve into the **pulmonary artery** and then to the lungs. There it picks up oxygen and returns to the left atrium of the heart through paired **pulmonary veins** on each side. From the left atrium, blood passes through the left atrioventricular valve (bicuspid or mitral valve) to the left ventricle, and the left ventricle pumps it out through the aortic valve into the **aorta.** From the aorta, the blood flows through the thorax and abdomen. In the pelvis the aorta ends as paired common iliac arteries. The common iliacs split into internal and external iliac arteries. The internal iliacs mainly supply the pelvis and nearby areas, while the external iliacs continue as femoral arteries down into the leg. Internal, external, and common iliac veins bring blood back from those regions until it reaches the abdomen, where the veins become the inferior vena cava, which returns blood to the right atrium.

Within the head and neck are many blood vessels, each with numerous branches. In this chapter we will concentrate on those vessels that supply and drain the teeth and oral cavity, starting with the heart and tracing the blood into the head and neck and then back to the heart again.

ARTERIAL SUPPLY

The pathways to the right and left sides of the head and neck are slightly different. On the right side the **brachiocephalic artery** (*brachio* meaning "arm"; *cephalic* meaning "head") branches off of the arch of the aorta. Coming off of the brachiocephalic artery are the right subclavian artery to the right arm, and the right **common carotid artery** to the right side of the head. The left common carotid artery comes directly off the arch of the aorta on the left side, and the left subclavian artery comes off of the arch of the aorta lateral to the left common carotid artery.

Common Carotid Artery

In the neck on both sides the common carotid artery runs within the **carotid sheath,** along with the internal jugular vein and the vagus nerve, and lies beneath the sternocleidomastoid muscle, which runs along the side of the neck. At about the level of the larynx, the common carotid divides into the **external carotid** and the **internal carotid arteries.**

The internal carotid artery has no branches in the neck but goes up to enter the skull. Once inside the skull, it branches to supply the eyes, the brain, and some limited regions of the coverings of the brain (Fig. 17-1).

Unlike the internal carotid artery, the external carotid artery has a number of branches in the neck, as shown in Figs. 17-1 and 17-2. However, we will consider in detail only the **facial, lingual,** and **maxillary arteries.**

Facial artery

The facial artery ascends the side of the neck, runs deep to the submandibular gland, and crosses the lower border of the mandible just in front of the angle of the mandible. (You can feel a small depression on the lower border of the mandible. This is where the facial artery and vein cross the mandible, and it is a pressure point for facial bleeding.) After crossing the mandible, the artery travels across the face, ending near the inner corner of the eye as the angular artery. On its way, it supplies blood to the skin and muscles of facial expression. It also sends branches to the upper and lower lips and to the sides of the nose.

Lingual artery

The lingual artery branches off the external carotid artery below the facial artery. The lingual artery then travels forward and deep, going beneath the hyoglossus muscle of the tongue and ending in three branches: the dorsal lingual artery to the deep posterior part of the tongue, the deep lingual artery to the deep anterior part of the tongue, and the sublingual artery to the ventral surface of tongue and floor of the mouth. The lingual artery supplies the tongue and the tissue in the floor of the oral cavity. If you have ever cut your tongue, you know that there is a well-developed blood supply within this tissue, which is completely supplied by the lingual artery (Fig. 17-3). Quite frequently the lingual and facial arteries come off the external carotid as one branch and then split. This branch is referred to as the *linguofacial trunk.*

Maxillary artery

The maxillary artery, along with the superficial temporal artery, is a terminal branch of the external carotid artery. It diverges from the external carotid at the level of the neck of the condyle on its deep surface. There are about 15 branches of this artery, but in our discussion we will only be concerned with a little more than half of them. In general, this artery supplies the muscles of mastication, the teeth, the oral and nasal cavities, the coverings of the brain, and several smaller areas (Fig. 17-4).

From its beginning where it branches off the external carotid artery, the maxillary artery runs forward in an area known as the **infratemporal fossa,** where it crosses the surface of the lateral pterygoid muscle to enter the **pterygopalatine fossa** behind and below the eye.

Infratemporal fossa branches. The more important branches of the maxillary artery in the infratemporal fossa are the **inferior alveolar, mental, temporal, masseteric, pterygoid, middle meningeal,** and **buccal branches** (see Fig. 17-4).

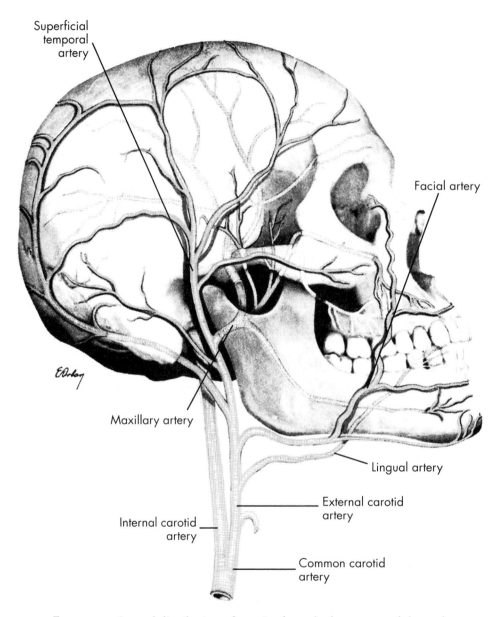

Superficial
temporal
artery

Facial artery

Maxillary artery

Lingual artery

External carotid
artery

Internal carotid
artery

Common carotid
artery

FIG. 17-1.   General distribution of arteries from the lower part of the neck up through the skull area. (From DuBrul EL: *Sicher's oral anatomy,* ed 7, St Louis, 1980, Mosby.)

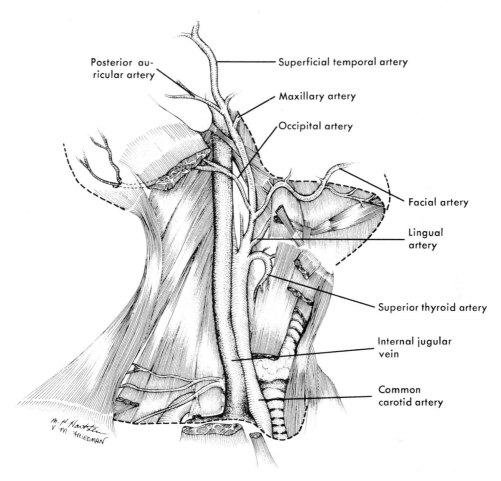

FIG. 17-2. Branches of the external carotid artery.

Inferior alveolar branch. The inferior alveolar branch runs down to enter the mandibular foramen and runs in the mandibular canal. It sends off branches to each of the mandibular teeth, their periodontal ligaments, and to the bone. In the premolar region the inferior alveolar artery sends off a small branch called the **mental artery,** which exits from the mandible through the mental foramen. It supplies the buccal gingiva and mucosa from the premolars to the incisors and also supplies the mucosa of the lower lip.

Temporal branches. Two temporal branches arise from the maxillary artery to supply the temporal muscle—an anterior and a posterior deep temporal artery.

Masseteric branch. The masseteric branch comes off the maxillary artery and runs laterally through the coronoid notch of the ramus, entering the deep surface of the masseter muscle to supply it with blood.

Pterygoid branches. There may be one or more pterygoid branches, which extend to the

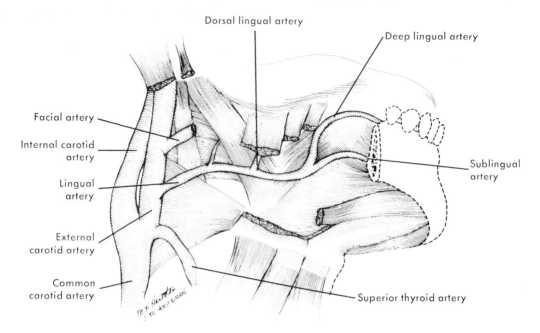

FIG. 17-3.   Lingual artery branches that supply blood to the tongue.

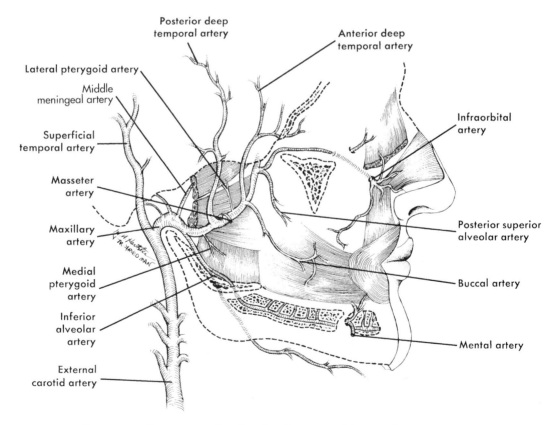

FIG. 17-4.   Cut-away section showing the origin of the maxillary artery from the external carotid artery just medial to what would be the neck of the condyle. Most branches of the maxillary artery can be seen.

medial and lateral pterygoid muscles. Their course and direction vary.

Middle meningeal artery. The middle meningeal artery comes off the maxillary, generally opposite the inferior alveolar artery, and runs up through the foramen spinosum to be the major blood supply to the meninges of the brain.

Buccal branch. The buccal branch runs down and forward to supply the mucosa of the cheek and the buccal mucosa and gingiva of the maxillary and mandibular posterior teeth (see Fig. 17-4).

Pterygopalatine fossa branches. At the ante-rior part of the infratemporal fossa the maxillary artery reaches the pterygopalatine fossa, entering it through the **pterygomaxillary fissure,** the opening between the maxillary tuberosity and the pterygoid process of the sphenoid bone. The pterygopalatine fossa lies behind and slightly below the orbital cavity. From there, branches divide into five general directions: backward to the nasal pharynx, down to the palate, medially into the nasal cavity and eventually to the anterior palatal area, laterally to the maxillary tuberosity, and forward into the infraorbital area of the face (Figs. 17-4 and 17-5).

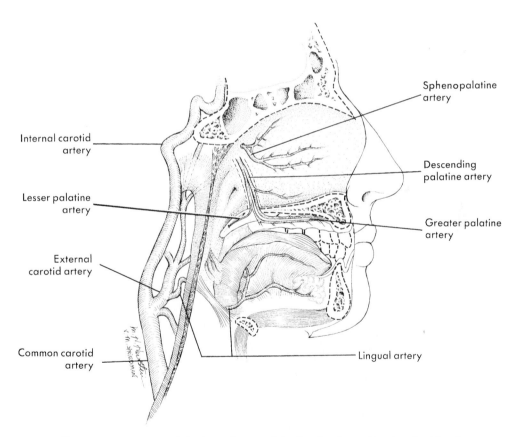

FIG. 17-5.   Section of the lateral part of the hard palate, showing the blood supply to the hard and soft palates and to the nasal cavity area.

Descending palatine artery. The **descending palatine artery** extends down from the maxillary artery to the posterior hard palate through the pterygopalatine canal. There it splits into two branches—the **lesser palatine artery,** which supplies the soft palate, and the **greater palatine artery,** which travels forward along the lateral part of the hard palate to supply the palatal mucosa and maxillary lingual gingiva. These vessels emerge into the palatal area through the lesser and greater palatine foramina respectively (see Fig. 17-5).

Posterior superior alveolar artery. The **posterior superior alveolar artery** comes out of the pterygopalatine fossa through the pterygomaxillary fissure, descends onto the maxillary tuberosity, and enters the bone behind the third molar. From there it supplies blood to all the maxillary posterior teeth and to part of the maxillary sinus, as well as to some branches that do not enter bone but rather supply the posterior buccal mucosa of the upper posterior teeth (Figs. 17-4 and 17-6).

Pterygopalatine (sphenopalatine) artery. The **pterygopalatine (sphenopalatine) artery** comes off the maxillary artery and runs medially through the sphenopalatine foramen into the nasal cavity, supplying most parts of the nasal cavity. It finally emerges from the incisive foramen to anastomose with the greater palatine artery (see Fig. 17-5).

Infraorbital artery. The **infraorbital artery** is the end part of the maxillary artery. From its location in the floor of the orbital cavity, it sends a branch, the **anterior superior alveolar artery,** down into the bone in front of the maxillary si-

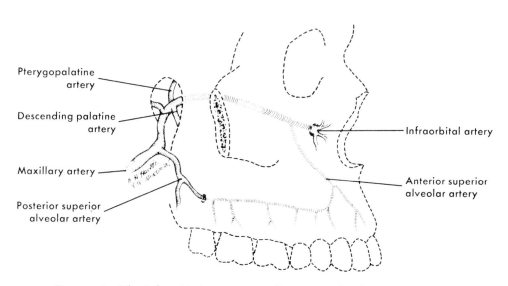

FIG. 17-6. The infraorbital artery extending across the floor of the orbit, with the anterior superior alveolar artery branching off and supplying the anterior teeth and possibly the premolars. The anterior and posterior superior alveolar arteries anastomose with one another.

nus, supplying the maxillary anterior teeth. It also anastomoses with the posterior superior alveolar artery in the wall of the sinus. The remainder of the infraorbital artery emerges through the infraorbital foramen onto the face and supplies the upper lip and its mucosa, maxillary labial gingiva, lower eyelid, and sides of the nose (see Figs. 17-4 and 17-6).

VENOUS DRAINAGE

Now that we have studied how blood reaches the head and neck, and in particular the oral cavity, we will examine the return of the blood to the heart. In general, veins follow the same pathways as arteries do and in most instances have the same names. For this reason the majority of discussion in most anatomic texts is devoted to the blood supply, or arteries, and focuses less on the veins.

Jugular Veins

In the head and neck the names of the veins vary slightly from those of the arteries. Instead of internal and external carotid veins, they are designated as **internal** and **external jugular veins.** The internal jugular vein drains the entire brain area and passes out of the skull through the jugular foramen. The internal jugular, in general, drains much of the area from in front of the ear to the front of the face through veins that correspond to arteries—for example, the facial, lingual, and part of the superficial temporal veins.

The maxillary vein is formed by an intertwining network of veins known as the **pterygoid plexus of veins.** These veins are so close to the maxillary tuberosity that there is a risk of piercing them if the angulation of the needle is incorrect during a posterior superior alveolar nerve block. When this happens, blood escapes into the tissue spaces and a **hematoma** occurs, a swelling and discoloration of the area that tends to upset the patient. In general, the application of moist heat will help dissipate the swelling and discoloration after initial use of cold packs.

The superficial temporal vein and the maxillary vein form the **retromandibular vein** (*retro* meaning "behind"). The retromandibular vein divides into a posterior and an anterior retromandibular vein. The posterior retromandibular vein joins with the posterior auricular vein to form the external jugular vein. The external jugular vein ends by emptying into the subclavian vein, which drains part of the temporal, maxillary, and posterior auricular areas. The anterior retromandibular vein joins with the facial vein and forms the common facial vein, which enters the internal jugular vein. The common facial vein then drains part of the superficial temporal and maxillary area as well as the facial region (Figs. 17-7 and 17-8).

Many times either the posterior or anterior branch of the retromandibular vein is missing. This causes more blood to shunt to either the external or internal jugular vein, causing differences in the sizes of these two veins.

The external jugular veins empty into the **subclavian vein** from the arm. This vein joins the internal jugular vein, forms the brachiocephalic vein, and flows into the **superior vena cava** and on into the heart. The supply to and from the head and neck is then complete, and the blood can flow out to the lungs again.

Clinical problem

Another point of interest is the area at the bridge of the nose, near the inner corner of the eye. Untreated infections in this area may spread through the superior ophthalmic veins into a venous sinus near the base of the brain called the *cavernous sinus,* where the infection may remain and stagnate. This condition can cause serious damage if left untreated and may even cause death.

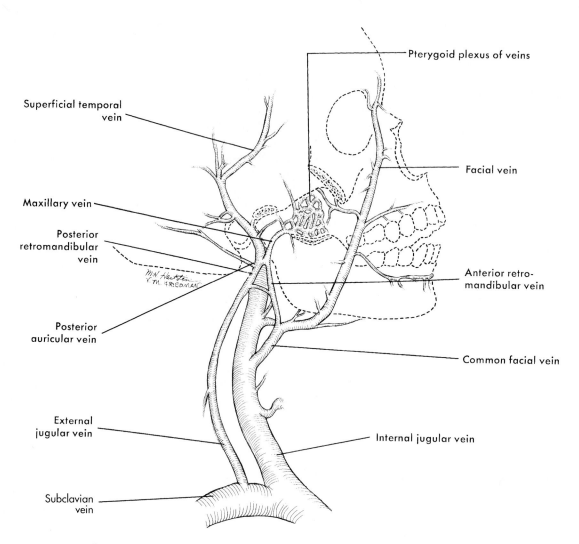

Pterygoid plexus of veins

Superficial temporal
vein

Facial vein

Maxillary vein

Posterior
retromandibular
vein

Anterior retro-
mandibular vein

Posterior
auricular vein

Common facial vein

External
jugular vein

Internal jugular vein

Subclavian
vein

FIG. 17-7.   General drainage areas of the internal and external jugular veins. The retromandibular vein connects the internal and external jugular veins and distributes blood between them.

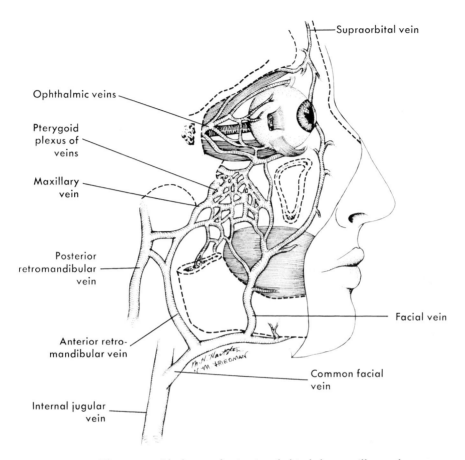

FIG. 17-8.   The pterygoid plexus of veins just behind the maxillary tuberosity. It may be injured during injection of that area of maxillary molars.

Review Questions

1. Trace blood from the time it first enters the heart until it gets back to the heart.
2. How does blood get from the heart into the head and neck?
3. What are the two divisions of the common carotid artery?
4. Which branches of the external carotid artery supply all the teeth and oral cavity?
5. Where does the blood supply to the muscles of mastication originate?
6. Name the individual vessels that supply all areas of the oral cavity.
7. What is the major vein that drains most of the head and neck?
8. What is the pterygoid plexus of veins, and what is its significance?
9. Trace the pathway of the venous blood from the neck back to the heart.
10. What happens to the jugular veins if either the anterior or posterior retromandibular vein is missing?

CHAPTER 18

SALIVARY GLANDS

OBJECTIVES
- To describe the difference between major and minor salivary glands
- To name and locate each of the major and minor glands
- To classify each of the glands according to its type of secretion
- To describe the function of saliva

As YOU may recall from Chapter 2, the glands of the body are classified in a number of ways. Salivary glands are classed as exocrine, merocrine, compound tubuloalveolar, serous, mixed, or mucous. They are also divided into major salivary glands, which are the three pairs of large glands, and minor salivary glands, which are found throughout the oral cavity.

MAJOR SALIVARY GLANDS

The major salivary glands are three pairs of glands that produce the bulk of the fluid in the mouth. This fluid is saliva, which mixes with food to make it easy to swallow and begins to break down starches into smaller carbohydrate units; further food breakdown takes place in the stomach. Saliva also keeps the mucosa in the oral cavity from drying out and aids in swallowing and speech (review Chapter 10 for the other functions of saliva). The three gland pairs are the parotid, the submandibular, and the sublingual.

Parotid Gland

The **parotid gland** is located on the surface of the masseter muscle, behind the ramus of the mandible and on the medial side of the ramus (Chapter 11). It is composed of many grapelike clusters of cells, which secrete into a system of tubes leading to the oral cavity. If you look at the cells of the secretory part of the gland through a microscope, you will see that the cells are all the same type—they produce a thin, watery secretion referred to as *serous secretion*. Although these glands are the largest of the salivary glands, the pair of them produce only about 25% of the total resting salivary volume. Fig. 18-1 shows the location of the gland. You can see that the duct leading from the gland travels anteriorly across the masseter muscle (Chapter 13) and pierces the buccinator muscle (Chapter 15) to open into the oral cavity opposite the maxillary second molar. Mumps is a viral infection of the parotid gland and possibly other glands, which causes pain when the gland secretes. Thus for a person with mumps, eating is sometimes quite painful because it causes stimulation of the gland.

Submandibular (Submaxillary) Gland

The **submandibular (submaxillary) gland** provides about 60% to 65% of the total resting salivary volume. It is called a mixed gland because it has serous and mucous cells in it. Mucous secretion is thicker and stickier than serous secretion, and although almost two thirds of the cells in the submandibular gland are serous, the mucous component results in a slightly viscous secretion. The gland is located below and toward the posterior part of the **body of the mandible** (Chapter 11). Place your finger on the **inferior border of the mandible** and run it back toward the **angle of**

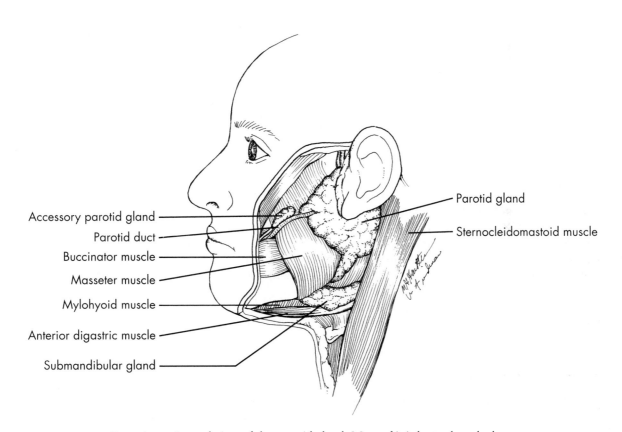

Accessory parotid gland

Parotid duct

Buccinator muscle

Masseter muscle

Mylohyoid muscle

Anterior digastric muscle

Submandibular gland

Parotid gland

Sternocleidomastoid muscle

FIG. 18-1.   Lateral view of the parotid gland. Most of it is located on the lateral side of the mandible and masseter muscle, wrapping around the back of the mandible also. The duct pierces the buccinator muscle as it opens into the oral cavity.

the mandible. As you near the angle, you will feel a slight depression in the inferior border where the facial artery and vein cross the mandible. If you move your finger medially from that point, you will feel a lump in the neck; that is the submandibular gland. The gland is wrapped around the mylohyoid muscle in the neck (Chapter 13). Most of the gland lies on the superficial side, and part of it lies on the deep side of the muscle in the posterior and lateral floor of the mouth. The duct extends from the deep part of the gland and runs forward in the floor of the mouth to open onto a small elevation called the *sublingual caruncle*. This is located at the base of the lingual frenum, the fold of tissue that attaches the tongue to the floor of the mouth (Figs. 18-2 and 18-3).

Sublingual Gland

The **sublingual gland** is the smallest of the three pairs of glands and contributes only 10% of total salivary volume. It is composed of mostly mucous cells with some serous cells; therefore, the secretion of this gland is even more viscous than that of the submandibular gland. It is located in the anterior floor of the mouth next to the mandibular canines. It has one major duct, which opens with the submandibular duct, and several smaller ducts, which open in a line along the fold of tissue beneath the tongue known as the *sublingual fold* (see Figs. 18-2 and 18-3). This gland is surrounded by minor sublingual glands, which are discussed later in this chapter.

All of these glands should be palpated in intraoral and extraoral examinations of the patient, and any enlargement of these glands should be further investigated. Sometimes, when a patient has lost all the teeth and there has been a loss of most of the mandibular ridge of bone, the sublingual gland will appear to bulge up into the floor of the mouth when the mouth is opened wide. This is not unusual and is no cause for alarm as long as the new denture replacing the lost teeth does not press on the gland.

MINOR SALIVARY GLANDS

The minor salivary glands have a similar structure to the major glands but are much smaller and have less branching. The primary differences between the two classifications are size, the number of secretory units or acini, and the number of ducts. The function of the minor glands is not to produce saliva for mixing with food, but rather to secrete minor amounts of saliva onto the surface to keep the mucosa moist. Some of these glands are pure serous cells, most are pure mucous cells, and the rest of them are mixed but mostly mucous. They do not have a long duct system; thus there are many clusters of these glands throughout the mouth, each with its own duct opening. They are located labially, buccally, palatally, glossopalatally, and lingually.

Labial Glands

In the upper and lower lips, opening onto the inner surface, are the **labial glands.** These are mixed glands but mostly mucous. You can see them in a mirror by pulling the lip out and looking at its inner surface, where they are present beneath the epithelium. This is also a good place to see the distribution of duct openings. Gently pull your lower lip out while standing in front of a mirror and dry off the inner surface with a tissue. Now pull the lip tight and watch for tiny drops of moisture to appear on the lip surface. These drops indicate the location of the labial gland ducts.

Buccal Glands

On the inner cheek region are the **buccal glands.** They are similar to the labial glands, differing only in location.

Palatine Glands

Located in the soft palate and in the posterior and lateral parts of the hard palate are the **palatine glands.** They are pure mucous glands in nature. Because there are no minor salivary glands in the anterior part of the hard palate to keep it

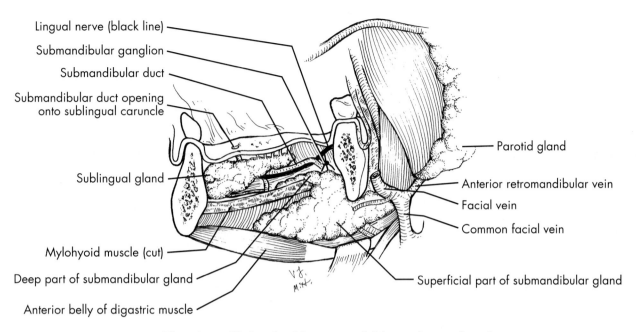

Lingual nerve (black line)
Submandibular ganglion
Submandibular duct
Submandibular duct opening onto sublingual caruncle
Sublingual gland
Mylohyoid muscle (cut)
Deep part of submandibular gland
Anterior belly of digastric muscle

Parotid gland
Anterior retromandibular vein
Facial vein
Common facial vein
Superficial part of submandibular gland

FIG. 18-2. The submandibular gland has a superficial part that can be palpated and a deep part from which the duct runs forward to the sublingual caruncle. *Dotted line*, path of duct.

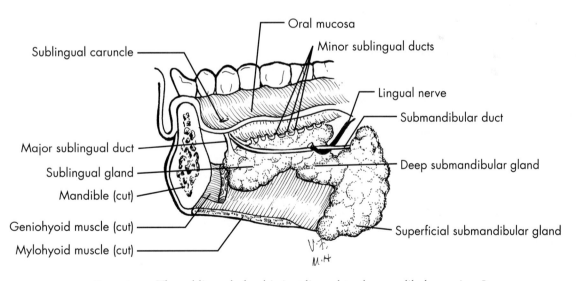

Sublingual caruncle
Major sublingual duct
Sublingual gland
Mandible (cut)
Geniohyoid muscle (cut)
Mylohyoid muscle (cut)

Oral mucosa
Minor sublingual ducts
Lingual nerve
Submandibular duct
Deep submandibular gland
Superficial submandibular gland

FIG. 18-3. The sublingual gland is just lingual to the mandibular canine. It has one major duct, which joins with the submandibular gland and many minor ducts, which open into the sublingual fold.

moist, the drying effect tends to cause the epithelium there to be more keratinized than in the posterior and lateral parts of the hard palate.

Glossopalatine Glands

Continuing from the posterior lateral parts of the palate down into the anterior fold of tissue in front of the palatine tonsil, you will find the **glossopalatine glands.** These are also pure mucous glands.

Lingual Glands

The **lingual glands** are divided into several groups.

Anterior lingual glands

These glands are found near the tip of the tongue and open onto the under or ventral surface. They are mostly mucous in nature.

Lingual glands of von Ebner

Lingual **glands of von Ebner** are pure serous glands located beneath the vallate papillae and opening into the trough around the gland. These glands function to wash off the taste buds so that they can perceive new tastes.

Posterior lingual glands

The posterior lingual glands are located around the lingual tonsils on the posterior third of the tongue. They are pure mucous glands in nature.

Sublingual glands

Although these are not usually listed separately, the sublingual glands are small individual glands that surround the major sublingual gland. They open into a row of ducts running back along the sublingual fold in the floor of the mouth. They are mainly mucous.

All these glands, whether major or minor, are controlled by the **autonomic nervous system.** To be specific, the **parasympathetic nervous system** within the autonomic nervous system is the main stimulus for salivation. Although the sympathetic nervous system does not itself play a major role in salivation, it does control blood flow, which is important in saliva production. Stimulation of the sympathetic nervous system decreases the flow of blood to the glands and slows the production of saliva. The smell of food or the presence of something in the mouth, even something without a pleasant taste, will start the glands secreting. Even chewing on plain paraffin can cause secretion. There are a number of medications that can cause overstimulation or understimulation of these glands, and a history of the patient's medications will help you understand why there may be more or less saliva in the mouth than you would normally expect and how the consistency might be different. You should also realize that "normal" amounts of saliva vary considerably from one person to another. Saliva also is affected by dehydration. If the body does not contain enough water, the salivary glands will stop saliva production in an effort to conserve water, causing the patient to have a dry mouth.

Review Questions

1. What are the major salivary glands, and where do their ducts open? What is their function?
2. What are the minor salivary glands, and where do their ducts open? What is their function?
3. What is the function of saliva as discussed in this chapter?

Chapter 19

Nervous System

Objectives
- To name the basic components of the nervous system
- To describe the general makeup of a spinal nerve
- To describe how a sensory impulse causes a motor response
- To name the twelve cranial nerves and their general function
- To describe the components and general function of the autonomic nervous system
- To name the specific branches of the trigeminal nerve and which areas of the face, teeth, and oral cavity each branch supplies
- To describe the nerves and areas involved in general and special sensation of the tongue
- To discuss the nerves and pathways involved in parasympathetic innervation to major salivary glands

The nervous system has many functions that it performs routinely. It relays messages from distant parts of the body that let the brain know exactly what is happening in each part. The brain may file the information in its memory for future reference or it may react immediately to that message. The brain coordinates and sends out messages that cause muscles to contract, stimulates glands to secrete, regulates numerous functions, and performs many of these tasks without true consciousness on our part. To accomplish all this the nervous system has to have tremendous organization and potential. It has both. Some authorities have theorized that we normally use only 10% of our mental capacity. There are clearly more cells in the brain

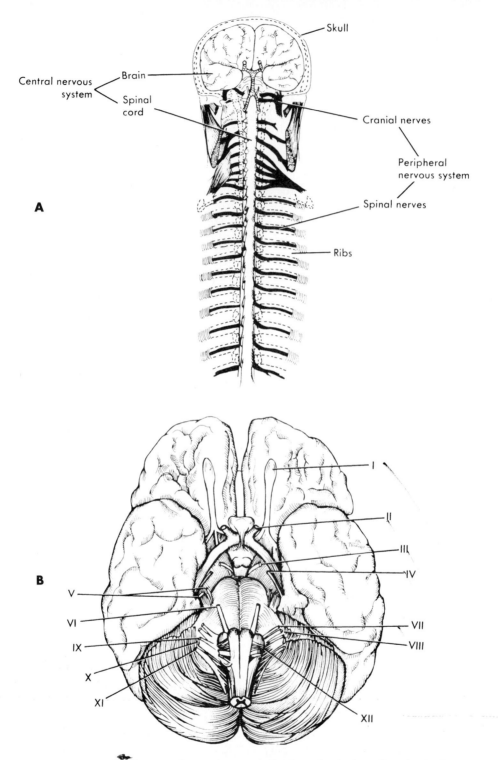

Fig. 19-1. **A,** The central nervous system (brain and spinal cord) and spinal segments and a few cranial nerves of the peripheral nervous system. **B,** Inferior view of the brain, showing the origin of 12 pairs of cranial nerves. (Modified from Goss CM: *Gray's anatomy of the human body,* ed 29, Philadelphia, 1973, Lea & Febiger.)

than we could ever use, and sometimes when there is brain damage, these unused cells can be called on to reestablish damaged pathways.

The nervous system is divided into two major categories: the **central nervous system,** consisting of the brain and spinal cord, and the **peripheral nervous system,** which comprises all nerves that extend outward from the brain and spinal cord (Fig. 19-1).

Remember from Chapter 2 that a neuron or group of neurons transmits a message or impulse in only one direction. Therefore, it is necessary to have both sensory and motor nerves, or more accurately, sensory and motor neurons. A nerve is actually a bundle of neurons, some of which are sensory and some of which are motor. These neurons are what enable messages to travel to and from the brain. Most nerves have both motor and sensory neurons, although some nerves may be either pure motor or pure sensory.

CENTRAL NERVOUS SYSTEM

The brain and spinal cord are made up of neurons that are either motor or sensory, but they are only part of the chain. Imagine you have caught your finger in a desk drawer. You feel pain and quickly pull your finger out of the drawer. Neurologically, a pain receptor or free nerve ending in the finger has picked up the message and carried it to the spinal cord. A second neuron has carried the message up the spinal cord to the lower parts of the brain, and a third neuron has taken it to the surface of the brain, where it was recognized as pain. The pain was interpreted by the brain, and past experience told the brain to remove the finger from the drawer so that it would no longer be crushed. A motor message then left the brain and traveled down the spinal cord, and a second motor neuron carried the message out of the spinal cord and along a peripheral nerve to muscles that pulled the finger out of the drawer (Fig. 19-2).

The nervous system also builds in a shortcut to this system known as a **reflex arc.** This short-

cut takes place in the spinal cord between the sensory neuron, as it enters the spinal cord, and the motor neuron, as it leaves the spinal cord. There is a shorter neuron, called the *intercalated neuron,* that runs between the two neurons and carries the message from the sensory side to the motor side without it having to go to the brain. The action is actually accomplished before the person thinks about it. Touch a hot stove, and what happens? You usually pull your hand away before you actually realize it is hot or before you consciously tell yourself to remove your hand from the stove (Fig. 19-3).

The brain and spinal cord are only a part of the sensory chain. The spinal cord and brain are the center of nervous activity, but they cannot perform alone. They need the contributions of the peripheral nervous system.

PERIPHERAL NERVOUS SYSTEM

The peripheral nervous system is traditionally grouped into three components: **spinal nerves, cranial nerves,** and the **autonomic nervous system.**

Spinal Nerves

The spinal nerves extend from the spinal cord to distant parts of the body. These nerves generally have both motor and sensory neurons in them. There are 31 pairs of spinal nerves: 8 in the **cervical** or neck region; 12 in the **thorax** or chest region; 5 in the **lumbar** or lower back region; 5 in the **sacral** or hip region; and 1 in the **coccygeal** or tailbone region (Fig. 19-4). These nerves are distributed by region from the neck to the toes. Several of the cervical nerves innervate some of the hyoid muscles that depress the mandible and raise the larynx.

Typical spinal nerves look like Fig. 19-3. The central speckled area of the spinal cord is known as **gray matter.** This gray matter is made up of the cell bodies of both motor and sensory neurons, which are arranged in the shape of a butterfly in the central area of the spinal cord. The

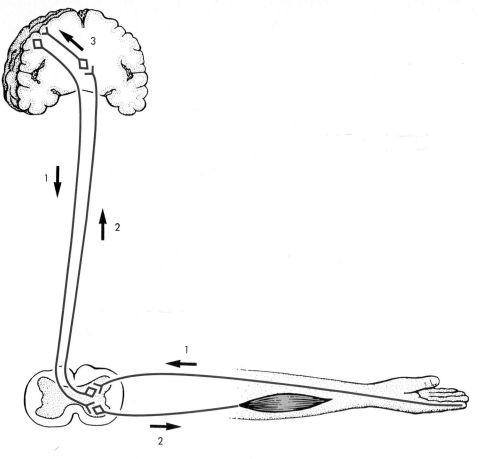

FIG. 19-2. Multiple neurons at various levels necessary to complete a conscious sensorimotor reaction.

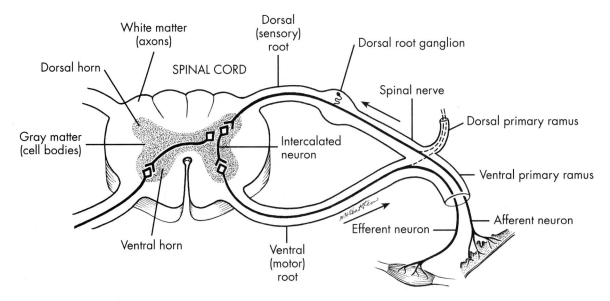

FIG. 19-3. A reflex arc. A message travels into the spinal cord and out again without reaching the brain.

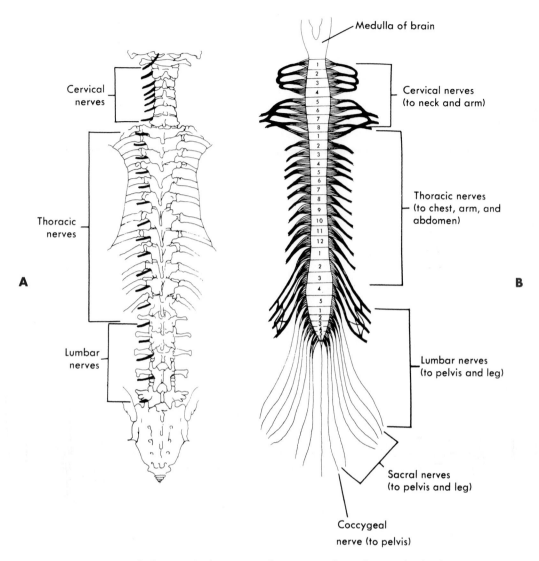

FIG. 19-4. **A,** Some spinal nerves as they emerge from the vertebral column. **B,** General arrangement of spinal nerves as they are grouped by regions. (Modified from Chusid JG, McDonald JJ: *Correlative neuroanatomy and functional neurology,* ed 17, Los Angeles, 1979, Lange Medical Publications.)

area around the gray matter is referred to as **white matter** and is made up of myelinated axons of both motor and sensory neurons. The spinal nerve has a **dorsal root,** which is the sensory root. The dorsal root has a **dorsal root ganglion,** which is a collection of cell bodies of the sensory neurons entering the spinal cord at that level. There is also a **ventral root,** which is the motor root. The point where the dorsal and ventral roots meet is the beginning of the **spinal nerve,** and at that point the spinal nerve contains both motor and sensory neurons. The spinal nerve then divides into a small **dorsal primary ramus** and a larger **ventral primary ramus.** Both of these primary rami are mixed motor and sensory nerves. The dorsal primary ramus carries sensation from the skin in a narrow band at the midline of the back, probably only a few inches wide, and also supplies the back muscles that lie immediately next to the vertebrae in the back. There are only a couple of dorsal primary rami that we can easily identify as nerves, and those are purely the sensory parts of the dorsal rami. The ventral primary rami are what we normally see as nerves in the body.

These nerves may be subject to damage in a number of ways. They exit from the spinal canal in the spinal vertebrae through intervertebral foramina. These foramina are formed as two semicircular openings, one from the vertebra above and one from the vertebra below. Damage to the vertebral discs between the vertebrae, or their slow compression with age may cause pinching of the spinal nerve at that level. Sometimes this causes some pain and/or numbness and possibly some muscle weakness. If this condition is not corrected, the nerve will deteriorate from the damaged area out to its peripheral ending. If the pinched nerve is relieved by surgery, there is a chance that there may be regrowth out from the area of damage and thus reestablishment of function. The nerves within the spinal cord do not regenerate well and damage to the spinal cord is usually permanent. Much work is going on today to find a way to stimulate regrowth of nerves in the spinal cord and brain.

Cranial Nerves

The cranial nerves attach directly to the brain. There are 12 pairs of these nerves, each with a separate function. When referring to these nerves, it is proper to use Roman numerals.

I, **olfactory nerve**—Sensory; provides special sense of smell from the nose to the brain.

II, **optic nerve**—Sensory; provides special sense of sight from the eye to the brain.

III, **oculomotor nerve**—Motor; supplies most of the muscles that move the eye in different directions and one that raises the upper eyelid; parasympathetic innervation to the eye to cause the pupil to contract and the lens to change shape and become more rounded for close vision.

IV, **trochlear nerve**—Motor; supplies one of the muscles that moves the eye downward and laterally.

V, **trigeminal nerve**—Motor and sensory; sensory innervation from all the teeth, the oral cavity, the anterior two thirds of the tongue, the maxillary sinus, the nasal cavity, and most of the skin of the front part of the face and head; motor innervation to the muscles of mastication, a soft palate muscle (tensor veli palatini) as well as the **tensor tympani muscle** of the middle ear. This is the most important nerve for our consideration and will be covered in greater detail later.

VI, **abducens nerve**—Motor; supplies one of the muscles that moves the eye laterally.

VII, **facial nerve**—Motor and sensory; motor innervation to the muscles of facial expression, the stylohyoid and posterior belly of the digastric muscle, as well the stapedius muscle of the middle ear; parasympathetic innervation to the submandibular and sublingual salivary glands, and the lacrimal gland of the eye (autonomic); sensory innervation from some areas behind the ear, and taste from the anterior two thirds of the tongue.

VIII, **statoacoustic nerve**—Sensory; for hearing and balance (equilibrium).

IX, **glossopharyngeal nerve**—Motor and sensory; motor innervation to one of the muscles the pharynx and the stylopharyngeus; parasympathetic innervation to the parotid salivary gland; sensory innervation to the posterior one third of the tongue for taste, as well as general sensation such as pain, pressure, heat, and cold; also provides sensation to most of the mucosa of the pharynx and to a small area of the skin of the ear.

X, **vagus nerve**—Motor and sensory; motor innervation to the muscles of the pharynx and larynx and most of the muscles of the soft palate; parasympathetic innervation controls most of the smooth muscle of the body, cardiac muscle, and many of the glands of the body; sensory innervation from the skin around the ear and taste and general sensation from the root of the tongue and epiglottis.

XI, accessory (spinal accessory) nerve—Motor; supplies the **trapezius muscle** and the sternomastoid muscle in the neck. Some parts of this nerve run with the vagus nerve and supply most of the soft palate, larynx, and pharynx muscles. Many of the muscles attributed to the vagus supply actually come from XI.

XII, hypoglossal nerve—Motor; supplies most of the intrinsic and extrinsic muscles of the tongue except the palatoglossus, which is supplied by X(XI) nerve.

AUTONOMIC NERVOUS SYSTEM

Before we continue with a more detailed description of some of these cranial nerves, a brief discussion of the autonomic nervous system and its function is necessary. This system is also called the *automatic nervous system* because it is not willfully controlled. The system has motor and sensory fibers; the motor fibers supply smooth and cardiac muscle and glands, and the sensory fibers carry what is called visceral sensation. This is sensation from the various viscera or organs of the body, as well as from the mucous membrane from the tonsils on down the digestive and respiratory tracts. Much of this visceral sensory pain is not well-isolated pain but pain of a more diffuse nature.

The autonomic system has two parts: the **sympathetic system,** also known as the **thoracolumbar outflow** or the "fight-or-flight mechanism," and the **parasympathetic system,** also known as the **craniosacral outflow.** Each of these components innervates all parts of the body, and therefore each organ generally has a sympathetic and a parasympathetic nerve supply. These systems are **antagonists,** which means they have opposite actions.

Consider the action of the sympathetic nervous system. If someone frightens you, the sympathetic nervous system is stimulated and you might find that the following things happen: your heart beats very fast and strong because of the release of **adrenalin** (or **epinephrine**); you become pale, and your skin feels cold and clammy from shutdown of the surface capillaries; and you feel a knot in your stomach from the shutdown of the blood supply to the digestive tract. All of this blood is being shunted to the skeletal muscles of the body; your heart beats faster, and you are breathing faster so that you are getting more oxygen into the body, which then goes to the muscles. The adrenalin helps with the actions of the heart and lungs and enables the body to meet stressful situations. You may also find that your mouth becomes dry from the shutdown of salivary glands, and the pupil of your eye dilates to let in more light so you can better see the situation that has caused the stress. This reaction is referred to as the *fight-or-flight mechanism.*

Stimulation of the parasympathetic nervous system and the resultant actions tend to be the opposite of those of the sympathetic nervous system. The sympathetic nervous system is referred to as the *vegetative system* because it relates to the process of digestion. Stimulation of this system slows down the heart and respiration, increases blood flow to the digestive system, and stimulates secretion of the glands of the body, including the salivary glands.

Where do the terms *craniosacral* and *thoracolumbar* come from? Parasympathetic fibers come off the brain with nerves III, VII, IX, and X and off the spinal cord at the sacral levels (S2 to S4); thus the name *craniosacral outflow* (Fig. 19-5). As you look at the functions of the cranial nerves, note the parasympathetic functions of nerves III, VII, IX, and X. The tenth nerve has virtually no parasympathetic function that affects the head and neck, but it affects structures within the thorax and abdomen. The sympathetic system comes off the spinal cord at the 12

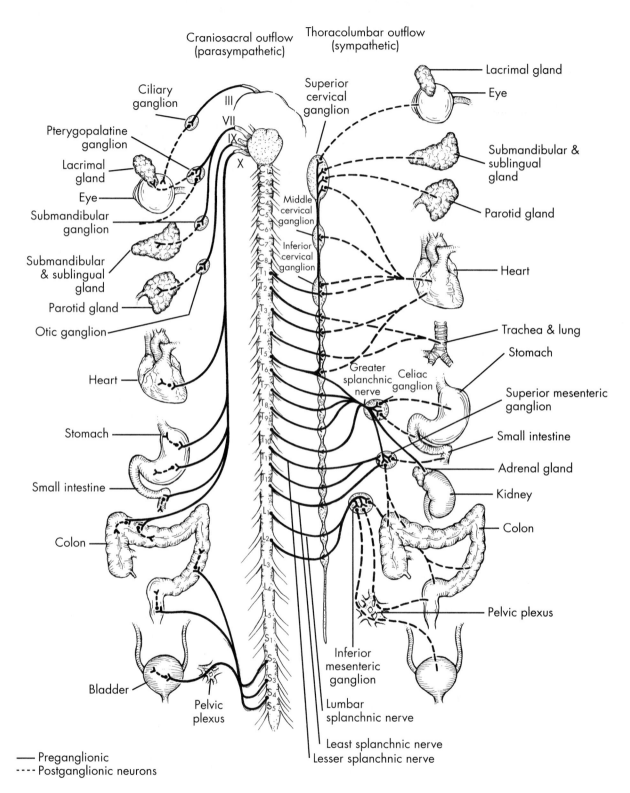

FIG. 19-5. Various levels of origin of the autonomic nervous system and some areas it supplies.

thoracic levels (T1 to T12) and the first 2 lumbar levels (L1 and L2); thus the name *thoracolumbar outflow.* The sympathetic nerves get to the head by running upward in a chain from the upper thoracic levels and then breaking off to run along the surfaces of the carotid arteries to virtually every part of the head. Sympathetic fibers also go back into the spinal nerves at all levels and run to the blood vessels, sweat glands, and smooth muscles, all of which are innervated by sympathetic fibers only.

The autonomic nervous system is a two-neuron system; there is a **preganglionic** and a **postganglionic neuron.** As the names indicate, these neurons synapse in a **ganglion,** which is an accumulation of cell bodies of the postganglionic neurons outside the central nervous system. There are a number of parasympathetic ganglia associated with the trigeminal nerve and one with the oculomotor nerve.

NERVES TO THE ORAL CAVITY AND ASSOCIATED STRUCTURES

Trigeminal Nerve (Cranial Nerve V)

The trigeminal nerve has three main branches, usually denoted as the **ophthalmic division (V_1),** the **maxillary division (V_2),** and the **mandibular division (V_3).** The first two divisions of the trigeminal nerve are purely sensory. One of the overall functions of these three divisions is the innervation of the skin of the anterior face and head region. Fig. 19-6 shows where each of these three divisions supplies the face. Note that it does not supply the skin over the angle of the mandible. That area is supplied by the **greater auricular nerve** or the cervical plexus of the neck.

Ophthalmic division (V_1)

The ophthalmic division of the trigeminal nerve leaves the skull through the superior orbital fissure and enters the orbital cavity. It has three major branches, one of which is the **frontal**

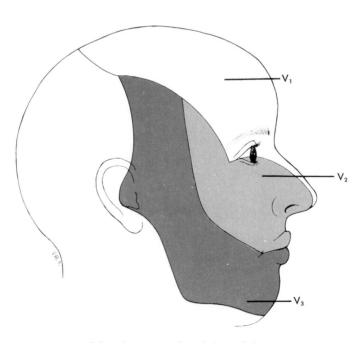

FIG. 19-6.   Areas of distribution on facial skin of the three divisions of the trigeminal nerve.

nerve. The frontal nerve travels forward in the roof of the orbit and breaks into two branches: the supraorbital nerve and the supratrochlear nerve. The **supraorbital nerve** emerges through the supraorbital notch and supplies the skin above the eye and up into the forehead. The **supratrochlear nerve** supplies the skin of the upper medial corner of the eye (Fig. 19-7). Another major branch of the ophthalmic division is the **lacrimal nerve,** which carries sensory responses from the skin above the lateral eye area and the lacrimal gland. The third major branch of the ophthalmic division is the **nasociliary nerve,** which sends **anterior** and **posterior ethmoidal nerve** branches into the nasal cavity and sends an **infratrochlear nerve** to the inferior, medial corner of the eye. One of the ethmoid branches, the anterior ethmoid, also has a branch that comes out onto the skin of the nose as an **external nasal nerve.**

Maxillary division (V$_2$)

The maxillary division of the trigeminal nerve exits from the skull through the foramen rotundum and lies in the pterygopalatine fossa behind and below the eye. The branches follow the same kind of distribution pattern as the maxillary artery does—that is, to the upper teeth and oral cavity, the nasal cavity, and the skin of the cheek and temporal region. These branches have basically the same names and pathways as the arterial supply to that area has, thereby giving you some idea of their distribution. In the pterygopalatine fossa the maxillary division divides into the following branches.

Posterior superior alveolar nerve. The **posterior superior alveolar nerve** emerges laterally from the pterygopalatine fossa through the pterygomaxillary fissure and travels along the posterior portion of the maxillary tuberosity. It supplies the maxillary buccal gingiva of the pre-

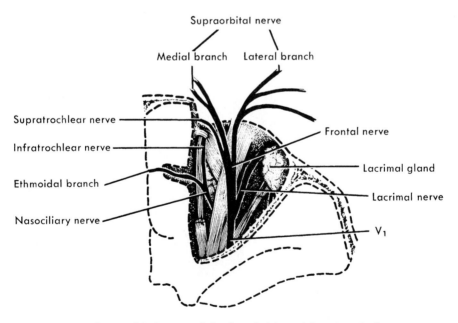

FIG. 19-7. Supraorbital nerve of the first division of the trigeminal nerve as it comes out through the supraorbital notch to supply the skin of the forehead.

molars and molars. It then enters the bone to supply the second and third maxillary molars and usually the distobuccal and lingual roots of the first maxillary molar. It also supplies part of the maxillary sinus (Fig. 19-8).

Sphenopalatine nerve. The **sphenopalatine nerve** branch comes off the maxillary division, goes through the sphenopalatine foramen, and supplies the lateral walls of the nasal cavity via **superior lateral nasal nerves.** It then goes up and comes down and forward across the nasal septum and leaves the nasal cavity through the incisive foramen as the **nasopalatine nerve** in the anterior palate, where it supplies the lingual gingiva adjacent to the maxillary central and lateral incisors (Fig. 19-9).

Pterygopalatine nerves. There are nerves that descend from the maxillary and that are known as the pteryg nerves. These nerves connect the **pterygopalatine ganglion** with the maxillary nerve. This ganglion is a parasympathetic ganglion that is supplied via the **greater petrosal nerve,** a preganglionic nerve from VII. The postganglionic nerve coming out of the ganglion travels in the zygomatic nerve to provide parasympathetic innervation to the lacrimal gland. There is also a sympathetic nerve, the **deep petrosal nerve,** which passes through the ganglion and distributes to glands (Figs. 19-8, 19-10, and 19-11).

Descending palatine nerve. The **descending palatine nerve** runs off the pterygopalatine gan-

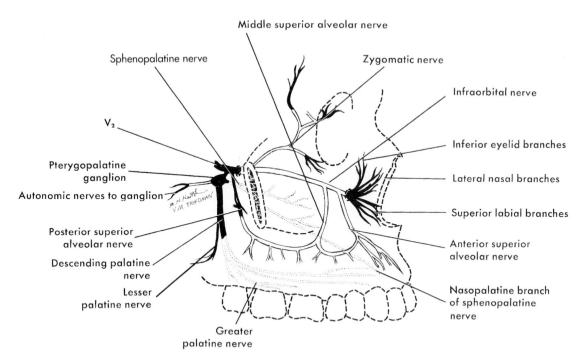

FIG. 19-8. General distribution of the maxillary division of the trigeminal nerve. The posterior superior alveolar nerve can be seen coming off the main trunk of V$_2$, and the middle and anterior superior alveolar nerves can be seen coming off the infraorbital nerve.

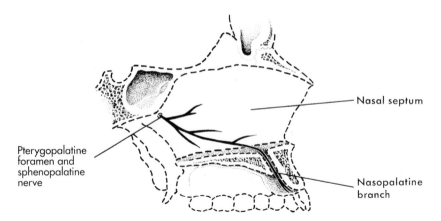

FIG. 19-9.   The sphenopalatine nerve enters the nasal cavity and one branch, the nasopalatine branch, goes down the nasal septum and out through the incisive foramen to the anterior palatal mucosa.

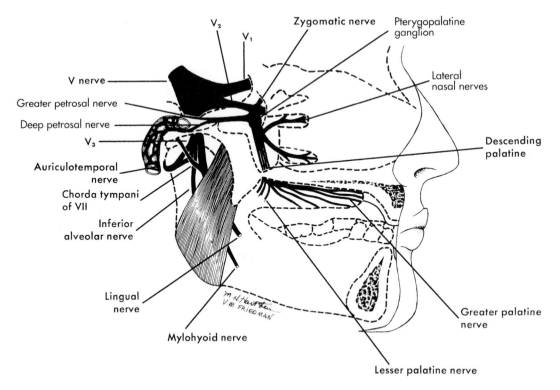

FIG. 19-10.   Partial diagram of V_2 and V_3. Notice the descending palatine nerve and its greater and lesser palatine branches going to the hard and soft palates, respectively.

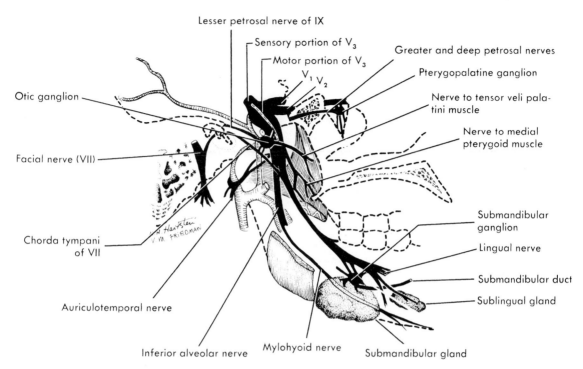

FIG. 19-11.   The third (mandibular) division of the trigeminal nerve and the facial nerve. Notice especially the chorda tympani connecting the facial nerve to V₃. This is a medial view.

glion straight down to the posterior part of the hard palate. There it separates into two branches: the **lesser palatine nerve,** which supplies the soft palate, and the **greater palatine nerve,** which supplies all the mucosa of the hard palate except the small area supplied by the nasopalatine branch of the sphenopalatine nerve. The greater palatine nerve extends along the lateral portion of the hard palate; the greater and lesser palatine nerves enter the palatal areas through the greater and lesser palatine foramina (see Figs. 19-8 and 19-10).

Zygomatic nerve. The **zygomatic nerve** comes off of the maxillary division, goes up into the orbit, and exits to supply the skin over the cheek and temple. It also carries postganglionic fibers from the pterygopalatine ganglion to pro-

vide parasympathetic innervation to the lacrimal gland.

Infraorbital nerve. The **infraorbital nerve** runs forward in the floor of the orbit to exit onto the face through the infraorbital canal and foramen. It supplies the skin of the nose, the lower eyelid, the skin and mucosa of the upper lip, and the maxillary labial gingiva. While in the floor of the orbit, it sends two branches down to supply the rest of the maxillary teeth. The first branch to come off as the nerve travels forward is the **middle superior alveolar nerve,** which lies in the wall of the sinus to supply the premolars and usually the mesiobuccal root of the maxillary first molar. This nerve also supplies part of the maxillary sinus. The **anterior superior alveolar nerve** extends down, anterior to the wall of the sinus, to supply the maxillary anterior teeth (see Fig. 19-8).

There are other branches of the maxillary division that go back to supply the area of the nasal pharynx.

Mandibular division (V$_3$)

The mandibular division of the trigeminal nerve leaves the skull through the foramen ovale, traveling downward. As it leaves the skull, it enters an area known as the infratemporal fossa, adjacent to the pterygoid muscles of mastication. It then breaks off into anterior and posterior divisions.

Anterior division. The anterior division breaks off into a number of branches. There are about five motor nerves for the muscles of mastication: two to the temporal muscle and one each to the masseter muscle and the medial and lateral pterygoids. The last branch of the anterior division is the buccal nerve.

Buccal nerve. The **buccal nerve** spreads out on the surface of the buccinator muscle and then penetrates the muscle. The lowest of its branches is frequently referred to as the **long buccal nerve** and lies in the posterior portion of the mandibular mucobuccal fold. There it supplies the buccal mandibular gingivae up to the mental foramen. The remainder of the buccal nerve supplies the skin and mucosa of the cheek and most of the maxillary buccal gingivae (Fig. 19-12).

Posterior division. The posterior division of the mandibular division of the trigeminal nerve has three major sensory branches and one motor branch.

Lingual nerve. The **lingual nerve** is one of the largest branches of the mandibular division. It supplies sensation to the floor of the mouth, the lingual mandibular gingivae, and the anterior two thirds of the tongue. Not too far below the foramen ovale, the lingual nerve is joined by a branch from the seventh cranial nerve (facial), known as the **chorda tympani.** This small branch of nerve VII has parasympathetic (secretomotor) fibers to supply the submandibular and sublingual salivary glands and also carries special sensory fibers of taste perception from the anterior two thirds of the tongue. Thus in the floor of the mouth, where the lingual nerve is located, there are actually fibers from nerve V and from nerve VII all wrapped together looking like one nerve. This juxtaposition also means that when the lingual nerve is inadvertently anesthetized during an injection of the lower teeth, the patient not only loses general sensation but also loses taste sensation in the anterior two thirds of the tongue. Just above the submandibular gland, the **submandibular ganglion** is suspended from the lingual nerve. This parasympathetic ganglion is part of nerve VII to supply the submandibular and sublingual salivary glands (see Fig. 19-11). These parasympathetic fibers come from the chorda tympani.

Inferior alveolar nerve. The **inferior alveolar nerve** primarily serves the lower teeth, although it has a small motor branch called the **mylohyoid nerve,** which supplies the mylohyoid muscle and the anterior belly of the digastric muscle. Just beyond the point where the mylohyoid nerve branches off, the inferior alveolar nerve enters the mandible through the mandibular foramen and supplies all the lower teeth and the periodontal ligaments of those teeth (Fig. 19-13). Between the mandibular premolars a small branch known as the **mental nerve** comes out laterally through the mental foramen to supply the mucosa of the lip and labial gingiva in the anterior mandible area. It also supplies the skin of the lower lip and chin. This accounts for numbing of the lower lip and chin during anesthetization of the lower teeth because they are all innervated by the same nerve.

Auriculotemporal nerve. The **auriculotemporal nerve** runs backward to supply the area above and in front of the ear. Lying on the medial surface of the mandibular division, just below the foramen ovale, is the **otic ganglion,** and coming off of the ganglion are regular motor fibers to the tensor veli palatini and the tensor tympani muscle. There is also a preganglionic nerve, the **lesser petrosal nerve** from IX, which

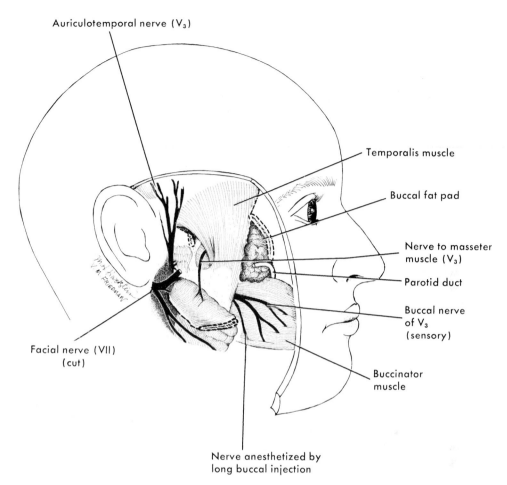

Auriculotemporal nerve (V₃)

Temporalis muscle

Buccal fat pad

Nerve to masseter muscle (V₃)

Parotid duct

Buccal nerve of V₃ (sensory)

Facial nerve (VII) (cut)

Buccinator muscle

Nerve anesthetized by long buccal injection

FIG. 19-12. The buccal and auriculotemporal nerves are the sensory branches of V_3.

comes down from the brain through the foramen ovale and synapses in the otic ganglion. Postganglionic fibers travel with the auriculotemporal nerve and provide parasympathetic innervation to the parotid gland (see Figs. 19-10 through 19-14).

Facial Nerve (Cranial Nerve VII)

Most of the facial nerve exits the brain through the stylomastoid foramen behind the ear. It comes forward and is found within the substance of the parotid gland. Inside the gland it separates into a number of branches to provide motor innervation to the muscles of facial expression. The distribution of these branches varies from person to person, but there generally is a temporal, a zygomatic, one or more buccal, a mandibular, and a cervical branch (Fig. 19-15). The cervical branch supplies the platysma muscle in the neck. Before the nerve enters the

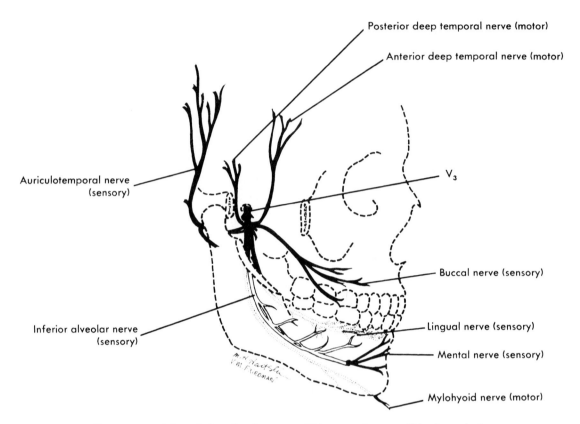

FIG. 19-13.   The inferior alveolar nerve (V$_3$) enters the mandible through the mandibular foramen, and the mental nerve branches off of it in the premolar region. The auriculotemporal nerve extends back over the ear.

parotid gland, a small nerve branches to the skin behind the ear, the auricular muscles, and the stylohyoid and posterior digastric muscles. While the facial nerve is still inside the skull, a branch extends through the middle ear and out of the skull as the chorda tympani. As mentioned earlier, this nerve carries parasympathetic (secretomotor) fibers to the submandibular and sublingual glands and special taste fibers from the anterior two thirds of the tongue. Again, these fibers run in the same bundle with the lingual nerve (see Figs. 19-11 and 19-15). Remember that the facial nerve also sends off a branch, the greater petrosal nerve, that goes to V$_2$ to carry

parasympathetic innervation to the lacrimal gland.

Glossopharyngeal Nerve (Cranial Nerve IX)

The glossopharyngeal nerve exits the skull along with the vagus and accessory nerves through the jugular foramen. It then sends one branch to a pharyngeal muscle, the stylopharyngeus, and branches to the mucosa of the constrictor muscles of the pharynx, which accomplish swallowing. There is also a branch that goes to the posterior one third of the tongue to supply both general sensation and taste to that region.

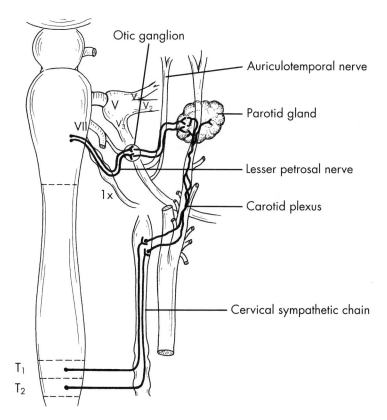

FIG. 19-14.   The lesser petrosal nerve of the ninth cranial nerve joins the auriculotemporal nerve just below the foramen ovale and travels with it back to the parotid gland. Notice how the branch of the ninth cranial nerve joins the otic ganglion. (Modified from Goss CM: *Gray's anatomy of the human body,* ed 29, Philadelphia, 1973, Lea & Febiger.)

As was indicated before, the lesser petrosal branch of nerve IX goes to provide parasympathetic innervation to the parotid gland (see Figs. 19-11, 19-13, and 19-14).

Vagus Nerve (Cranial Nerve X)

The vagus nerve affects more areas of the body than any of the other cranial nerves. It sends fibers down to the heart, lungs, kidneys, and most of the digestive tract. Its branches to the pharynx, larynx, and tongue are of the greatest importance to our discussion. The vagus sends a small branch to the base of the tongue, where it innervates the base of the tongue and the epiglottis. This branch carries general sensation and has a few taste fibers. There are two branches that go to the larynx—the superior and the inferior laryngeal (or recurrent laryngeal) nerves. These provide general sensation and motor activity to the muscles of the larynx. There is also a motor branch to the muscles of the soft palate and pharynx. All of these are accompanied by the cranial portion of nerve XI, which actually is be-

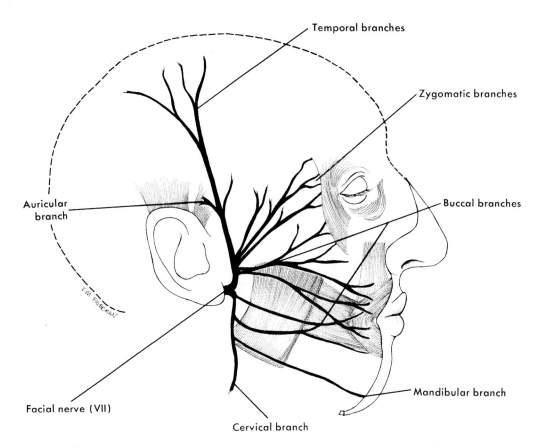

FIG. 19-15.   Branches of the facial nerve that supply the muscles of facial expression.

lieved to supply most of the above-mentioned structures.

Review Questions

1. What are the subdivisions of the nervous system?
2. What are the parts of a spinal nerve, and what are the two parts seen in a cross section of the spinal cord?
3. What happens when the sympathetic nervous system is stimulated?
4. What happens when the parasympathetic nervous system is stimulated?
5. Name the twelve cranial nerves and their general functions.
6. Which nerves carry parasympathetic fibers?
7. Which nerves supply each of the teeth in the mouth?
8. Name the nerves supplying each area of oral mucosa.

9. Name the nerve supply to the major salivary glands and describe their pathway to the glands.

10. Which nerve is responsible for the sensation of taste to the anterior two thirds of the tongue?

11. If the seventh cranial nerve was damaged emerging from the brain, what glands would have their functions affected?

12. If the parotid gland had a tumor and had to be removed, what nerve might be affected and what could be the result?

LYMPHATICS AND SPREAD OF DENTAL INFECTION

LYMPHATIC SYSTEM

The lymphatic system is a part of the overall lymphoid system of the body and a component of the immune system of the body. It is an accumulation of tiny channels or tubules with small **nodular** structures called **lymph nodes** interconnecting them. The system functions by returning fluids to the bloodstream from the various tissues of the body. A filtrate of the blood plasma flows out of the capillaries into the surrounding tissues, where it becomes extracellular fluid. It is eventually picked up by the lymphatic vessels or tubules. The extracellular fluid, now referred to as *lymphatic fluid,* flows through tubules, then through nodes, back through tubules, and possibly through some more nodes. It finally empties into the venous system at the junction of the internal jugular and subclavian veins in the root of the neck and travels back to the heart. This kind of fluid circulation repeats itself continually. The lymph nodes act as filters for the fluids, and the lymphocytes produced within the lymph nodes combat infections that might spread through the lymphatic channels. Most tissues, including the pulp of the teeth, have lymph vessels in them. The distribution of these vessels has been well determined, and this information can be used as a diagnostic tool in the study of oral infections and as a means of slowing the spread of cancers.

Distribution Pattern

We will now examine the distribution pattern of these channels and nodes and discover how they relate to the head and neck area. Fig. 20-1 shows some of the major groups of nodes in the head and neck. The nodes are grouped together into small clusters, which are all interconnected by channels. Each group drains fluids from certain structures or tissue areas, which explains why lymph nodes are involved in combating infections in areas of the body. A sore throat, for example, can be followed by tenderness in the neck and finally a tender lump in that area. In

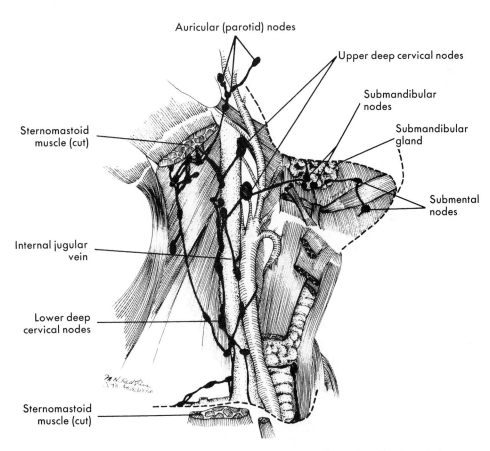

FIG. 20-1.   Locations of some of the major groups of lymph nodes that drain the head and neck. The retropharyngeal group is not visible because of its location behind the throat. The deep cervical chain lies on the internal jugular vein beneath the sternomastoid muscle, which has been removed in this view.

such an instance the infection from the throat has spread through the lymph channels until reaching the first lymph node or group of lymph nodes. The lymphocytes in the node have begun to combat the infection and also have started to multiply, causing the node to become enlarged and tender. If the infection is successfully combated in that node, it will subside; however, if the infection is great, it may spread through that lymph node or nodes and on to the next node or group of nodes.

Submental nodes

A very small accumulation of nodes, the **submental nodes,** is found beneath the chin. The lymphatic channels from the mandibular incisors, the tip of the tongue, and the midline of the lower lip and chin drain into these nodes. Any infection in these areas would generally cause some tenderness and enlargement of the nodes. These nodes tend to drain into the submandibular nodes or directly down and across the neck to the lower deep cervical nodes.

Submandibular nodes

The **submandibular nodes** are found grouped around the submandibular gland near the angle of the mandible. The easiest way to locate the gland and the nodes is to place a finger on the inferior border of the mandible near the angle. Run the finger back and forth until you feel the depression in the inferior border of the mandible. This is the point at which the facial artery and vein cross the inferior border. Just medial to this depression is the submandibular gland, and the submandibular lymph nodes are grouped around it.

The areas that drain into these nodes are all of the maxillary teeth and the maxillary sinus, with the exception of the maxillary third molars; the mandibular canines and all mandibular posterior teeth, with the possibility that the mandibular third molars may not drain here; the floor of the mouth and most of the tongue; the cheek area; the hard palate; and the anterior nasal cavity. As mentioned before, the submental nodes also

drain into these nodes. Any infections in these areas tend to cause enlargement and tenderness of the submandibular nodes. This condition is referred to as **lymphadenopathy.**

Upper deep cervical nodes

The **upper deep cervical nodes** are located on the lateral surface of the internal jugular vein and lie just beneath the anterior border of the sternomastoid muscle, about 2 inches below the ear. A number of other nodes drain into this group—the submandibular nodes, the nodes behind the back throat wall, known as the **retropharyngeal nodes,** the parotid nodes in front of the ear and the parotid gland, and others. This is the group affected when you have a particularly sore throat. When a throat infection begins, the first group of nodes involved are the retropharyngeal nodes because they are behind the throat wall. Because it is impractical to palpate these nodes, generally the next group of nodes that are involved in a throat infection, the upper deep cervical nodes, are the first to be noticed. Many people who have sore throats first notice the tenderness in the upper deep cervical nodes. The upper deep cervical group also drains the third molar regions, the base of the tongue, the tonsillar area, the soft palate, and the posterior nasal cavity region. Therefore, tenderness in the upper deep cervical nodes without a sore throat should cause you to look in a number of areas to discover the source of the infection.

Lower deep cervical nodes

The **lower deep cervical nodes** are also found on the lateral surface of the internal jugular vein and beneath the anterior border of the sternomastoid muscle. These nodes are located about 2 inches above the clavicle. They drain the upper deep cervical nodes and many of the nodes at the back of the neck, frequently referred to as *occipital nodes,* as well as some glands in the anterior neck. From the lower deep cervical nodes the lymphatic fluid drains into the junction of the subclavian and internal jugular veins.

NODE GROUPS AFFECTED BY DISEASE

The terms **primary nodes, secondary nodes,** and **tertiary nodes** are often used in discussions about infections and cancer, both of which spread through lymphatic channels. These terms refer to the groups of nodes that are affected in a disease process. If an infection is not stopped by the first (primary) group of nodes, it will spread to the second (secondary) group. If it is not stopped there, it may spread to the third (tertiary) group. One node or group of nodes can be primarily involved in one source of infection, and the same group of nodes can be secondarily or tertiarily involved in another source of infection. Look at the upper deep cervical nodes (see Fig. 20-1). An infection of the third molars may involve these nodes first—they would be the primary group involved. If the infection were in a first molar, the initial sign of infection would be in the submandibular nodes; if it were not successfully combated there, it would spread secondarily to the upper deep cervical nodes. Infections originating in the middle of the lower lip would spread first to the submental nodes, secondarily to the submandibular nodes, and then to the upper deep cervical nodes, which in this instance would be tertiary nodes of involvement. Keep in mind that in infections, any group of nodes may overcome the infection if it is not too severe, and the infection may go no further.

An understanding of this concept is necessary to comprehend the spread of oral cancer. Each group of nodes acts as a resistance barrier against the spread of cancer. The nodes slow the spread, and if the cancer is detected early enough, it can be treated more successfully. Once the infection or the cancer reaches the lower deep cervical nodes and passes through them, it enters the bloodstream, moving directly into the heart and then throughout the body. With this in mind, it is easy to understand why cancer on the tip of the tongue does not result in as high a **mortality rate** as does cancer that begins further back on the tongue or in the throat. The tip of the tongue generally drains through four groups of nodes before it enters the bloodstream and spreads throughout the body, whereas cancer in the posterior portion of the tongue or in the throat travels to the upper deep cervical nodes, on to the lower deep cervical nodes, and into the bloodstream. In that area there are only two groups to stop the spread of the disease. When cancer is detected, knowing the location of the cancer and having a knowledge of the nodes involved allows the surgeon to do a biopsy of the next group of nodes in the chain to see if there is cancer in them. If they are free of cancer, that can be a good sign that the cancer has not spread any further and generally means a more favorable prognosis for the patient.

SPREAD OF INFECTION IN FASCIAL SPACES

Another way through which infections may spread is through **fascial spaces.** Although infection spread through fascial spaces is much less common, it displays much more dramatic clinical symptoms. The spaces between muscle and tissue layers are referred to as fascial layers or planes, and infections may spread here. You may have seen a patient with a large swollen jaw or with a swollen area beneath the eye. In this situation the infection of dental origin is not spreading through small lymphatic channels but has broken out of the bone around the tooth and is spreading between the tissue or muscle layers.

This kind of infection spread will follow certain predictable pathways, depending on its location. In general, dental infections start in the maxillae or mandible at the apex of a tooth or in the periodontal space around a tooth. Most periodontal space infections cause a swelling of the gingival or mucosal tissue within the oral cavity. Infections at the apices of the teeth cause swelling in one of two directions: buccal or lingual. Most buccal swellings also lead to a swelling in the vestibule of the oral cavity. This swelling is sometimes referred to as a *gumboil*. The infection comes to a pointed head, breaks through the mucosa, and drains into the oral cavity. If a mandibular infection spreads not in the buccal but in the lingual direction, it will travel to the tissue spaces in two specific areas—above the mylohyoid muscle in the floor of the mouth, or beneath the mylohyoid muscle in the tissue beneath the chin—depending on its point of origin.

How can one predict where the infection will go? Refer to Fig. 11-17, a medial view of the body of the mandible, and picture the lengths of the roots of the individual teeth. Look at the mylohyoid line on the mandible and notice its location relative to the apices of the roots. You can see that, in general, the apices of the mandibular molar teeth are inferior to the mylohyoid line, whereas the premolars and the anterior teeth have the apices of their roots above the mylohyoid line. Therefore, a molar infection will tend to break out of the bone below the mylohyoid line and spread to the space beneath the chin, referred to as the *submental space*. Infections of the premolars and the anterior teeth will tend to break out of bone above the mylohyoid line and spread to the spaces in the floor of the mouth, referred to as the *sublingual space*.

Infection spreading into the sublingual space causes a swelling into the floor of the mouth. If it spreads into the submental space, it will cause a swelling beneath the chin, sometimes referred to as **Ludwig's angina.** These infections continue to spread by gravity if not treated. Whether above or below the mylohyoid muscle, as they spread down and back, they reach the posterior end of the mylohyoid muscle. Both kinds of infection eventually reach the side of the neck next to the pharynx, which is referred to as the **lateral pharyngeal** or **parapharyngeal space.** This causes swelling on the side of the neck if left untreated. From here the infection may spread around the pharynx to its posterior border, which is referred to as the **retropharyngeal space,** and from there to the **posterior mediastinum,** which is in the back of the chest or thoracic cavity. If the infec-

tion reaches this point, the person may die within a short period of time. With the advent of antibiotics, these infections are not so frequently seen as they were in the past, but can occasionally still be found.

The importance of this section is not to be able to completely describe or define the boundaries of these spaces or **potential spaces,** but to understand how the origin or location of the original infection determines the pathway it will follow and the potential outcome if left untreated.

OTHER MAXILLARY INFECTIONS

Maxillary infections react slightly differently because of the anatomic features of the area. If the infection does not open into the maxillary buccal vestibule or onto the palate, it may spread toward three areas—the nasal cavity, the maxillary sinus, or the soft-tissue spaces of the cheek or the area below the eye. The area involved is related to the tooth involved. A swelling below the eye is usually related to infection from an anterior tooth, usually the maxillary canine, whereas swelling in the cheek is usually related to infection in a posterior tooth. Although it is possible for infection to spread to the nasal cavity or maxillary sinus, it is rather rare. These maxillary infections around the eye or cheek can also spread to the lateral pharyngeal space and from there to other areas.

Review Questions

1. What is the function of lymph nodes?
2. What are the major groups of lymph nodes in the head and neck?
3. Name the structures that drain primarily into each group of lymph nodes.

4. What are fascial spaces?
5. Where may fascial space infections eventually end up if left untreated, and how serious could this be?
6. Submental space infections come from which group of teeth?

7. Swelling below the eye would come from infection in which teeth?
8. What group of nodes would first be noticed as being painful in a throat infection?

UNIT III

TEST

1. Excluding the ear ossicles, there are _____ bones in the skull.
   a. 8
   b. 14
   c. 12
   d. 18
   e. none of the above
2. The nasal septum is formed by the _____ bone.
   a. sphenoid
   b. ethmoid
   c. vomer
   d. maxilla
   e. a and b
   f. b and c
3. Which of the following bones is *not* a part of the neurocranium?
   a. sphenoid
   b. ethmoid
   c. temporal
   d. frontal
   e. occipital
   f. All are a part of the neurocranium.
4. The mental foramen is in the
   a. body of the maxilla
   b. ramus of the mandible
   c. alveolar process of the mandible
   d. alveolar process of the maxilla
   e. none of the above

5. The posterior nasal spine is a part of the _____ bone.
   a. nasal
   b. maxilla
   c. mandible
   d. palatine
   e. none of the above
6. Which of the following statements is **true** concerning the greater wing of the sphenoid?
   a. It can be seen from a lateral view of skull.
   b. It can be seen from an internal view of skull.
   c. It can be seen in the orbit.
   d. both a and b above
   e. both a and c above
   f. all of the above
7. The sagittal suture may also be called the
   a. frontotemporal suture
   b. parietofrontal suture
   c. interparietal suture
   d. parieto-occipital suture
   e. none of the above
8. In which of the following bones would you find the external auditory meatus?
   a. the mastoid bone
   b. the temporal bone
   c. the occipital bone
   d. both a and c above
   e. none of the above
9. The hiatus semilunaris is found in the
   a. sphenoethmoidal recess
   b. superior meatus
   c. middle meatus
   d. inferior meatus
   e. none of the above
10. Which of the following opens into the inferior meatus?
    a. frontal sinus
    b. maxillary sinus
    c. anterior ethmoid sinus
    d. nasolacrimal duct
    e. all of the above

11. Which of the following teeth would *not* be found in proximity to the floor of the maxillary sinus?
    a. maxillary first molar
    b. maxillary lateral incisor
    c. maxillary first premolar
    d. maxillary third molar
    e. They would all be close to the floor of the sinus.

12. The opening of the maxillary sinus into the nasal cavity is found
    a. in the floor of the sinus
    b. in the roof of the sinus
    c. two thirds of the way up the lateral wall
    d. two thirds of the way up the medial wall
    e. none of the above

13. The ethmoid bulla is found in the
    a. inferior meatus
    b. superior meatus
    c. sphenoethmoidal recess
    d. middle meatus
    e. none of the above

14. What is the most superior-anterior opening in the hiatus semilunaris?
    a. opening of frontal sinus
    b. opening of nasolacrimal duct
    c. opening of anterior ethmoid air cells
    d. opening of maxillary sinus
    e. none of the above

15. The region where the nasal cavity becomes the nasal pharynx is known as the
    a. choana
    b. sphenoethmoidal recess
    c. posterior nasal aperture
    d. both a and b above
    e. both a and c above
    f. all of the above

16. The temporalis muscle is a(n) _____ of the mandible.
    a. depressor
    b. elevator
    c. protrudor
    d. retrudor
    e. a and c
    f. b and d

17. Which of the following is *not* an origin of the medial pterygoid muscle?
    a. maxillary tuberosity
    b. pterygoid fossa
    c. medial wall of the lateral pterygoid plate
    d. lateral wall of the medial pterygoid plate

18. Which of the following muscles most directly affects TMJ movement?
    a. temporalis
    b. masseter
    c. medial pterygoid
    d. lateral pterygoid

19. The muscles of mastication are innervated by the _____ cranial nerve.
    a. V
    b. VII
    c. IX
    d. X
    e. none of the above

20. The muscle most directly affecting elevation of the larynx is the _____ muscle.
    a. sternohyoid
    b. sternothyroid
    c. thyrohyoid
    d. mylohyoid
    e. digastric

21. Which of the following muscles is capable of depressing and/or retruding the mandible?
    a. temporal
    b. digastric
    c. mylohyoid
    d. lateral pterygoid
    e. none of the above

22. Which of the following is *not* an infrahyoid muscle?
    a. sternohyoid
    b. omohyoid
    c. mylohyoid
    d. thyrohyoid
    e. They are *all* infrahyoid muscles.

23. Which of the following statements is *not* true about the sternomastoid and trapezius muscles?
    a. They both can move the head significantly in different directions.

b. They both are innervated by the same nerve.

c. Spasms in either muscle can refer pain to the TMJ.

d. They both have similar insertions.

e. *All* of the above are true.

24. The disc of the TMJ is attached laterally and medially to the
    a. medial pterygoid muscle
    b. lateral pterygoid muscle
    c. poles of the condyle
    d. retrodiscal pad
    e. none of the above

25. The posterior collagenous lamina functions to
    a. pull the disc back
    b. pull the disc forward
    c. keep the disc from being pulled too far back
    d. keep disc from being pulled too far forward
    e. none of the above

26. The temporomandibular ligament is found in the
    a. posterior part of the capsule
    b. medial part of the capsule
    c. anterior part of the capsule
    d. lateral part of the capsule

27. Pain in the area of the TMJ coming from other areas is known as _____ pain.
    a. myofascial
    b. referred
    c. false
    d. none of the above

28. Dislocation of the TMJ is referred to as
    a. protraction
    b. retrusion
    c. subluxation
    d. depression
    e. none of the above

29. When the disc of the TMJ is deranged, it is usually
    a. immobile
    b. displaced posteriorly
    c. displaced anteriorly
    d. none of the above

30. The posterior elastic lamina functions to
    a. pull the disc backward
    b. pull the disc forward
    c. keep the disc from being pulled too far forward
    d. keep the disc from being pulled too far backward
    e. none of the above

31. The muscles of facial expression are innervated by the _____ cranial nerve.
    a. V
    b. VII
    c. IX
    d. X
    e. XI

32. The buccinator shares a common origin with the _____ muscle.
    a. orbicularis oris
    b. superior pharyngeal constrictor
    c. uvula
    d. levator veli palatini
    e. none of the above

33. Which of the following muscles plays a role in smiling?
    a. levator labii superioris
    b. depressor labii inferioris
    c. zygomatic major
    d. mentalis
    e. orbicularis oris

34. Which of the following muscles plays a direct role in keeping the food on the occlusal surfaces during mastication?
    a. orbicularis oris
    b. orbicularis oculi
    c. zygomaticus major
    d. mentalis
    e. none of the above

35. Which of the following groups of muscles of facial expression is most poorly developed?
    a. eye
    b. ear
    c. mouth
    d. scalp
    e. neck

36. Which of the following muscles would play a major role in a frown?
    a. nasalis
    b. orbicularis oculi
    c. corrugator
    d. orbicularis oris
    e. none of the above

37. Which of the following muscles plays a major role in pouting?
    a. procerus
    b. zygomaticus minor
    c. depressor anguli oris
    d. depressor labii inferioris
    e. none of the above

38. Which of the following palatal muscles is innervated by the fifth cranial nerve?
    a. uvula
    b. palatopharyngeus
    c. palatoglossus
    d. levator veli palatini
    e. tensor veli palatini

39. The stylopharyngeus muscle _____ the pharynx.
    a. elevates
    b. dilates
    c. depresses
    d. pulls forward
    e. a and b

40. Which of the following muscles pulls the soft palate into contact with the posterior pharyngeal wall?
    a. uvula
    b. palatopharyngeus
    c. palatoglossus
    d. levator veli palatini
    e. none of the above

41. Which of the following muscles would help move the bolus of food upward and backward to the oral pharynx?
    a. palatoglossus
    b. palatopharyngeus
    c. levator veli palatini
    d. tensor veli palatini

42. Which of the following would help to open the auditory tube if it was closed because of edema?
    a. palatoglossus
    b. styloglossus
    c. uvula
    d. levator veli palatini
    e. all of the above
    f. none of the above

43. Which of the following muscles would narrow the fauces in swallowing?
    a. levator veli palatini
    b. palatoglossus
    c. tensor veli palatini
    d. salpingopharyngeus
    e. all of the above

44. Which of the pharyngeal constrictors takes its origin from the thyroid cartilage?
    a. superior constrictor
    b. middle constrictor
    c. inferior constrictor
    d. both a and b above
    e. both b and c above
    f. none of the above

45. Which of the following arteries supplies blood to the oral cavity?
    a. lingual
    b. maxillary
    c. palatal
    d. mental
    e. They all do.

46. Which of the following are branches of the internal carotid artery?
    a. lingual
    b. maxillary
    c. superficial temporal
    d. facial
    e. all of the above
    f. none of the above

47. The blood supply to the muscles of mastication is from the _____ artery.
    a. mental
    b. facial
    c. lingual
    d. maxillary
    e. superficial temporal

48. The vein that may be injured in anesthesia of the posterior superior alveolar nerve is the
   a. retromandibular vein
   b. pterygoid plexus of veins
   c. facial vein
   d. temporal vein
   e. none of the above

49. If the posterior retromandibular vein is absent on one side, which of the following statement(s) is(are) true?
   a. The external jugular vein will be smaller than normal.
   b. The internal jugular vein will be larger than normal.
   c. All blood from the maxillary vein will enter the common facial vein.
   d. both a and b above
   e. both b and c above
   f. all of the above

50. If the posterior superior alveolar artery were blocked, how would blood get to the maxillary molars?
   a. via the greater palatine artery
   b. via the anterior superior alveolar artery
   c. via the nasopalatine artery
   d. via the sphenopalatine artery
   e. none of the above

51. The _____ gland's duct opens into the vestibule opposite the maxillary second molar.
   a. parotid
   b. submandibular
   c. sublingual
   d. buccal
   e. none of the above

52. Which of the following glands is mostly serous with some mucous acini?
   a. buccal
   b. sublingual
   c. parotid
   d. submandibular
   e. none of the above

53. The submandibular gland opens into the oral cavity
   a. opposite the maxillary second molar
   b. on the sublingual caruncle
   c. at the base of the labial frenum
   d. b and c
   e. none of the above

54. The serous glands of von Ebner are found
   a. in the cheek
   b. in the palate
   c. in the floor of the mouth
   d. in the tongue
   e. none of the above

55. The nerve supply to all salivary glands comes from the
   a. autonomic nervous system
   b. parasympathetic nervous system
   c. sympathetic nervous system
   d. voluntary nervous system
   e. a and b
   f. a and c

56. Which of the following major salivary glands has more than one duct?
   a. parotid
   b. submandibular
   c. sublingual
   d. both a and b above
   e. both b and c above

57. There are _____ pairs of cranial nerves.
   a. 5
   b. 7
   c. 9
   d. 12
   e. none of the above

58. Which of the following cranial nerves is involved with taste?
   a. glossopharyngeal
   b. vagus
   c. facial
   d. all of the above
   e. none of the above

59. The second part of the trigeminal nerve is known as the _____ division.
   a. mandibular
   b. ophthalmic
   c. pharyngeal
   d. maxillary
   e. none of the above

60. The nerve supply to the maxillary central incisors is the _____ nerve.
   a. greater palatine
   b. inferior alveolar
   c. posterior superior alveolar
   d. nasopalatine
   e. none of the above

61. The nerve supply to the mucosa of the lower lip is the _____ nerve.
   a. lingual
   b. anterior superior alveolar
   c. buccal
   d. mental
   e. none of the above

62. The nerve supply to the lingual gingiva of the maxillary central incisor is the
   a. anterior superior alveolar
   b. middle superior alveolar
   c. inferior alveolar
   d. lingual
   e. nasopalatine

63. Which of the following cranial nerves *does not* have parasympathetic fibers in its origin?
   a. III
   b. V
   c. VII
   d. IX
   e. X
   f. They *all* have parasympathetic fibers in their origin.

64. Which of the following clinical signs would you *not* find in stimulation of the sympathetic nervous system?
   a. increased heart rate
   b. increased respiration
   c. decreased blood supply to skin
   d. decreased blood supply to GI tract
   e. constriction of the pupil of the eye
   f. You would see *all* of the above signs.

65. Lymph nodes
   a. help return intercellular fluids to the bloodstream
   b. produce lymphocytes
   c. fight infection
   d. prevent spread of infection
   e. all of the above
   f. none of the above

66. A secondary node of involvement with infection of a maxillary premolar would be
   a. submental
   b. upper deep cervical
   c. submandibular
   d. lower deep cervical
   e. none of the above

67. The primary nodes of drainage for a maxillary central incisor are the
   a. submental nodes
   b. submandibular nodes
   c. retropharyngeal nodes
   d. upper deep cervical nodes
   e. none of the above

68. Fascial space infections in the region of the oral cavity could spread ultimately to the
   a. floor of the mouth
   b. side of the throat
   c. region behind the throat
   d. posterior chest region
   e. none of the above

69. Cancer of which of the following areas would have the best prognosis for a cure?
   a. posterolateral border of tongue
   b. maxillary sinus
   c. upper lip
   d. tip of tongue
   e. submandibular gland

70. Fascial space infection with swelling of the eye has most likely originated in the
   a. maxillary sinus
   b. orbital cavity
   c. maxillary incisor
   d. maxillary canine
   e. none of the above

Suggested Readings

Christensen JB, Telford IR: *Synopsis of gross anatomy,* ed 5, Hagerstown Md, 1988, JB Lippencott.

DuBrul E: *Sicher's oral anatomy,* ed 8, St Louis, 1988, Ishiyaku Euro.

Fehrenbach MJ, Herring SW: *Illustrated anatomy of the head and neck,* Philadelphia, 1996, WB Saunders.

Fried LA: *Anatomy of the head, neck, face and jaws,* ed 2, Philadelphia, 1980, Lea & Febiger.

Friedman SM: *Visual anatomy,* vol 1, Head and neck, Hagerstown Md, 1970, Harper & Row.

Gardner M: *Basic anatomy of the head and neck,* Baltimore, 1992, Williams & Wilkins.

Hiatt JL, Gartner LP: *Textbook of head and neck anatomy,* ed 2, Baltimore, 1987, Williams & Wilkins.

McClintic JR: *Human anatomy,* St Louis, 1983, Mosby.

McMinn RMH, Hutchings R, Logan B: *Color atlas of head and neck anatomy,* ed 2, St Louis, 1995, Mosby.

Paff GH: *Anatomy of the head and neck,* Philadelphia, 1973, WB Saunders.

Reed GM, Sheppard VF: *Basic structures of the head and neck,* Philadelphia, 1976, WB Saunders.

Seeley RR, Stephens TD, Tate PP: *Anatomy and physiology,* ed 3, St Louis, 1995, Mosby.

Short MJ: *Head, neck and dental anatomy,* ed 2, New York, 1994, Delmar.

Thibodeau G, Patton K: *Anatomy and physiology,* ed 2, St Louis, 1993, Mosby.

Wilson-Pauwels L et al: *Cranial nerves: anatomy and clinical comments,* St Louis, 1988, Mosby.

Wischnitzer S: *Outline of human anatomy,* Springfield, Ill, 1972, Charles C. Thomas.

UNIT IV

DENTAL
ANATOMY

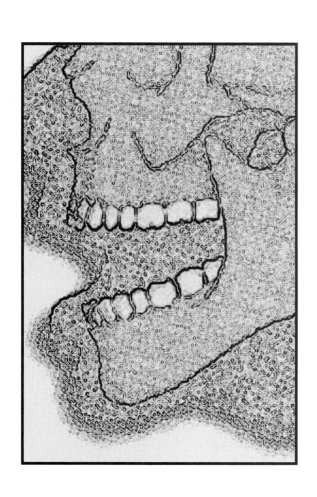

Chapter 21

The Tooth: Functions and Terms

OBJECTIVES
- To identify the different functions of the teeth
- To identify the different tissues that compose the teeth
- To differentiate between clinical and anatomic eruption
- To define single, bifurcated, and trifurcated roots
- To recognize how the functions of teeth determine their shape and size
- To understand the individual functions and therefore the individual differences that exist among incisors, canines, premolars, and molars
- To name and identify the location of the various tooth surfaces
- To name and identify the line angles of the teeth
- To name and identify the point angles of the teeth
- To define the terminology used in naming the landmarks of the teeth

FUNCTION OF TEETH

Teeth are very important in many functions of the body. They are essential for protecting the oral cavity, in acquiring and chewing food, and in aiding the digestive system in breaking down food. The teeth form a hard physical barrier that protects the oral cavity. This shield not only affords protection to the oral struc-tures, but the teeth themselves are formidable weapons. The group of mammals classified to the order *Carnivora* all have well-developed canines that they use as weapons to defend themselves and to attack and kill their prey. Lions and tigers are members of this order. The teeth also function in communication. They are necessary for proper speech, phonetics and even whistling. In many cultures their appearance can be a very positive sexual attraction. In dental anatomy the teeth are studied individually and collectively—their functions, anchorages, and relations to one another. Our study will therefore begin with a discussion of the individual tooth.

CROWN AND ROOT

Each tooth has a **crown** and **root** portion. The crown is covered with **enamel,** and the root portion is covered with **cementum.** The crown and root are joined at the **cementoenamel junction,** also called the **CEJ.** The line that demarcates it is called the **cervical line,** a line that is formed by the junction of the cementum of the root and the enamel of the crown (Fig. 21-1).

The crown portion of the tooth erupts through the **bone** and gum tissue. After eruption it will never again be covered with gum tissue. Only the cervical third of the crown in healthy young adults is partly covered by gingiva (gum tissue). The tooth continues to erupt from the bone and **gingival tissue** until all of the crown is exposed (Fig. 21-2).

There is a clinical difference between the amount of crown that could be erupted and the actual amount that is visible in the mouth. The **anatomic crown** is the whole crown of the tooth that is covered by enamel, whether erupted or not. The **clinical crown** is only that part seen above the gingiva. Any nonerupted area is not a part of the clinical crown of the tooth. Therefore, if all of the anatomic crown does not erupt, the part that is visible is considered the clinical crown, and the unerupted portion is part of the **clinical root** (Fig. 21-3). **Eruption** of a tooth is thus the moving of that tooth through its surrounding tissues so that the clinical crown gradually appears longer. The tooth may have a **single root** (see Fig. 21-1) or a **multiple root** with **bifurcation** or **trifurcation**—that is, division of the root portion into two or three segments

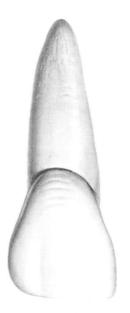

FIG. 21-1.   Maxillary right central incisor. The crown and root are separated by cementoenamel junction. (From Zeisz RC, Nuckolls J: *Dental anatomy,* St. Louis, 1949, Mosby.)

(Figs. 21-4 and 21-5). Each root has one **apex** or terminal end. The root is held in its position relative to the other teeth in the **dental arch** by being firmly anchored in the bony process of the jaw. The portion of the jaw that supports the teeth is called the **alveolar process.** The bony socket in which the tooth fits is called the **alveolus** (Fig. 21-6). Teeth in the upper part of the jaw are called **maxillary** teeth because they are anchored in the maxillary bone. In the lower jaw they are called **mandibular** teeth because they are anchored in the bone called the mandible.

TOOTH TISSUES

The four tooth tissues are enamel, **dentin,** cementum, and **pulp** (Fig. 21-7). The first three are **hard tissues;** the pulp is **soft tissue.**

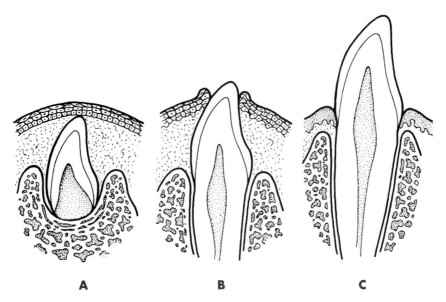

FIG. 21-2. **A,** Unerupted tooth. **B,** Beginning eruption. **C,** Young adult; eruption almost completed.

Enamel

Enamel forms the outer surface of the anatomic crown. It is thickest over the tip of the crown and becomes thinner until it ends at the cervical line. The color of enamel varies with its thickness and mineralization. The thicker the enamel, the whiter it appears. The thinner the enamel, the more it varies, from grayish white at the crown cusps' edges, to white in the middle of the tooth, and to yellow-white at the cervical line, where the thin enamel covering is translucent enough to show the yellow tint of the dentin underneath. The more mineralized the enamel, the more it lends itself to translucency. These two factors—the mineralization and the thickness of enamel—coupled with skin pigmentation, determine the color of the enamel.

Enamel is the most densely mineralized and hardest tissue in the human body. The chemical composition of enamel is 96% inorganic and 4% organic matter and water. This dense mineralization gives enamel the ability to resist the wear that the crown of a tooth is subjected to. The hard enamel does not wear very readily; rather, it wears down, grinds up, and crushes almost anything that a person subjects it to—nuts, seeds, ice cubes, even particles of bone, grit, sand, and leather.

Our ancestors wore the enamel off of their teeth. Their diet consisted of hard uncooked nuts, fruits, and grains. In addition, their food was unprocessed so that pieces of rock, sand, dirt, and grit were embedded in their food. Their lifestyle required chewing leather or bone to fabricate clothing. Often the life expectancy of our ancestors was directly related to whether or not they still possessed functional teeth. Those who were fortunate enough to have adequate enamel (durable, wear-resistant) were able to live longer and produce more offspring.

Present day humans rarely wear the enamel off of their teeth. Enamel is not only resistant to

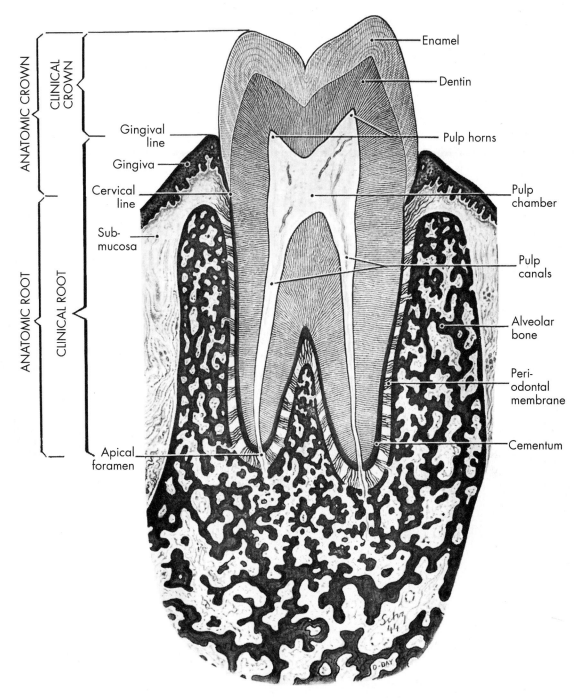

FIG. 21-3. Longitudinal section of a tooth. The clinical crown and root can change, but the anatomic crown-root ratio must always remain same. (From Zeisz RC, Nuckolls J: *Dental anatomy,* St. Louis, 1949, Mosby.)

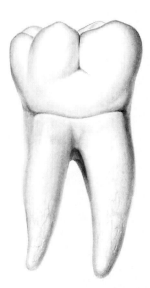

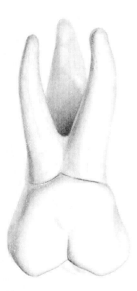

FIG. 21-4.   Bifurcated root. (From Zeisz RC, Nuck-olls J: *Dental anatomy,* St. Louis, 1949, Mosby.)

FIG. 21-5.   Trifurcated root. (From Zeisz RC, Nuck-olls J: *Dental anatomy,* St. Louis, 1949, Mosby.)

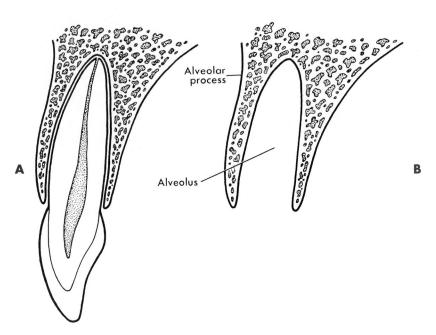

FIG. 21-6.   **A,** Tooth surrounded by a bony alveolus. **B,** Alveolus is the tooth socket in the alveolar process.

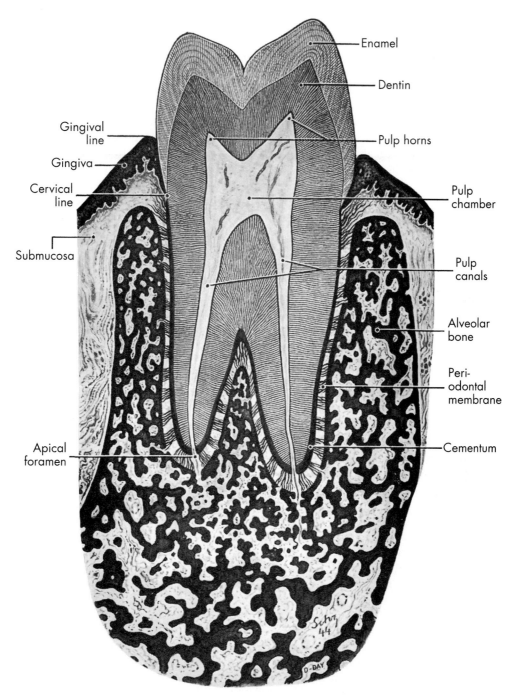

FIG. 21-7.   A pulp cavity is composed of pulp chambers, pulp horns, and root canals. (From Zeisz RC, Nuckolls J: *Dental anatomy*, St. Louis, 1949, Mosby.)

wear, but it is very durable and rather resistant to bacteria, mild acids, and tooth decay. The densely packed enamel is smooth, which gives the crown of the tooth a self-cleaning ability, making it difficult for food particles, bacteria, sticky carbohydrate material, and other debris to adhere to the surface of the tooth crown. This self-cleaning ability of enamel and its extreme hardness and resistance to wear make it a nearly perfect outer covering for the crown.

Dentin

Dentin forms the main portion or body of the tooth; it comprises the greatest bulk of the tooth because it forms the largest portion of the crown and root. Dentin is wrapped in an envelope of enamel, which covers the crown, and an envelope of cementum, which covers the root.

Dentin is a hard, dense, calcified tissue. It is softer than enamel but harder than cementum or bone. It is yellow in color and elastic in nature. Its chemical composition is 70% inorganic and 30% organic matter and water. Unlike enamel, dentin is capable of adding to itself. When it does this, the new dentin is called **secondary dentin.**

Secondary dentin is formed throughout the pulp chamber after the tooth erupts. In time, secondary dentin could completely fill the pulp chamber. **Reparative dentin** is the dentin that is laid down in response to caries or trauma.

Cementum

Cementum is a bonelike substance that covers the root, though the root is not covered with a perfect layer of cementum; there are voids exposing small patches of dentin. Its main function is to provide a medium for the attachment of the tooth to the alveolar bone. It is not as dense or as hard as enamel or dentin but is more dense than bone, to which it bears a physiologic resemblance. The chemical composition of cementum is 45% to 50% inorganic and 50% to 55% organic components. Cementum is quite thin at the cervical line but increases slightly in thickness at the apex of the root. The union of cementum and dentin is called the **dentinocemental junction.**

There are two types of cementum: **cellular cementum** and **acellular cementum.** Acellular cementum covers the entire anatomic root. Cellular cementum is confined to the apical third of the root and can reproduce itself, thereby compensating for the attrition (wear) that occurs on the crown of the tooth. Cellular cementum derives its name from the fact that the very cells that lie down and form the cementum eventually become trapped within newly formed cementum. The cells that produce cementum are called **cementoblasts.**

Cementum gives the tooth a mechanism of anchorage that protects and supports the tooth, yet it is self-adjusting and independent of the tooth's main nourishment system. The nutrition for cementum is derived from the outside of the tooth through blood vessels that come directly from the bone.

Pulp

Dental pulp is the nourishing, sensory, and dentin-reparative system of the tooth. It is composed of blood vessels, lymph vessels, connective tissue, nerve tissue, and special dentin-formation cells called **odontoblasts.**

The pulp is housed in the center of the tooth, with dentin surrounding the pulp tissue. The walls of the **pulp cavity** are lined with odontoblasts, the chief function of which is to lay down primary and secondary dentin. The odontoblasts form secondary dentin when the tooth is subjected to trauma from chemical, mechanical, or bacterial causes. Blood vessels bring in the nourishment necessary to activate and support the formation of secondary dentin. In addition, the blood vessels also supply the white blood cells necessary to fight bacterial invasion within the pulp. The lymph tissue filters the fluids within the tooth, and the nerve tissue is sensory in function and responds only to pain.

Anatomically the pulp is divided into two areas: the **pulp chamber** and the **pulp canals** or **root canals.** The pulp chamber is housed within the coronal portion of the tooth, and the pulp canals are located within the roots of the tooth. Together the pulp chamber and pulp canals are referred to as the pulp cavity; thus the pulp cavity runs the entire length of the interior of the tooth from the tip of the pulp chamber, the **pulp horns,** to the apex of the root canal (see Fig. 21-7).

TYPES OF TEETH

The functions of teeth vary, depending on their individual shape and size and their location in the jaws. The three basic food processing functions of the teeth are cutting, holding or grasping, and grinding.

Incisors

The **incisors** are designed to cut (incisor means "that which makes an incision, or cut"), and the biting edge is called an incisal edge (Fig. 21-8). The tongue side, or lingual surface, is shaped like a shovel to aid in guiding the food into the mouth (Fig. 21-9).

Canines

The **canines** are designed to function as holding or grasping teeth. The importance of these teeth can be seen in dogs, for example, whose genus, *Canis*, is named for these teeth. The dog uses the canines as a weapon or fighting tool. With them it pierces, holds its victim, and tears its victim's flesh.

In humans the canines also function to protect the jaw joint during side jaw movements. (See

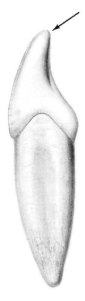

FIG. 21-8.   Mandibular central incisor. Notice the incisal edge *(arrow),* which incises or cuts food. (From Zeisz RC, Nuckolls J: *Dental anatomy,* St. Louis, 1949, Mosby.)

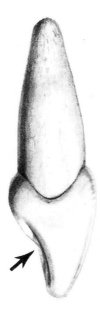

FIG. 21-9.   Arrow points to the shoveled-out lingual aspect of a maxillary right central incisor. (From Zeisz RC, Nuckolls J: *Dental anatomy,* St. Louis, 1949, Mosby.)

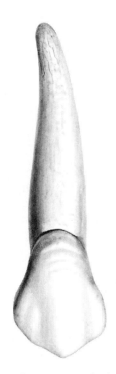

FIG. 21-10.   Maxillary canine. The bulk of the canine root affords resistance to displacement. (From Zeisz RC, Nuckolls J: *Dental anatomy,* St. Louis, 1949, Mosby.)

Chapters 25 and 28). The length and thickness of the canines afford lateral stress-bearing support during side-to-side jaw excursions. The canines are the longest teeth in human dentition. They are also some of the best anchored and most stable teeth because they have the longest roots (Fig. 21-10). Canine roots are shaped triangularly in **cross section.** This triangular root shape makes it possible for a canine to hold its place in the corner of the mouth. The shape resists anterior, posterior and lateral forces of displacement, as well as forces that would rotate or turn the tooth within its bony socket (Fig. 21-11).

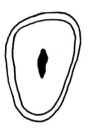

FIG. 21-11.   The triangular cross-sectional shape of the maxillary canine resists forces that would dislodge it.

Premolars

There are four maxillary and four mandibular **premolars.** Premolars are a cross between canines and molars. They are not as long as canines, and they usually have at least two **cusps** rather than one large ridge. Like canines, they aid in holding food, but they function to help grind rather than incise the food. Their pointed buccal cusps hold the food while the lingual cusps grind it, making their function similar to that of the molars.

Premolars are sometimes referred to as **bicuspids.** The term *bicuspid* is not accurate, however, because it implies only two cusps, and some premolars have three. Therefore, the term *premolar* is preferred (Fig. 21-12).

Molars

Molars are much larger than premolars, usually having four or more cusps. Also, molars are located more posteriorly than the premolars. The function of the 12 molars is to chew or grind up food. They do not incise food, and like premolars, they do not have incisal edges. Instead they have cusps, which are designed to interlock the upper and lower molars. There are four or five cusps on the occlusal surface of each molar, depending on its location and the occurrence of normal variations (Fig. 21-13). Maxillary (upper) and mandibular (lower) molars dif-

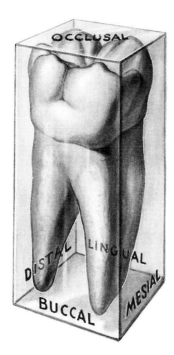

FIG. 21-15.   Surfaces of a mandibular right first molar. (From Zeisz RC, Nuckolls J: *Dental anatomy*, St. Louis, 1949, Mosby.)

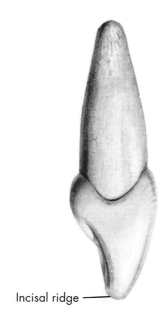

Incisal ridge ——————

FIG. 21-16.   Incisal ridge of the central incisor. Even though the incisal ridge is small, it is treated independently. (From Zeisz RC, Nuckolls J: *Dental anatomy*, St. Louis, 1949, Mosby.)

distal proximal surface faces away from the midline. The fifth surface of posterior teeth is called the **occlusal surface**—the biting surface of the tooth. It is also called the **occluding** or chewing surface. The occlusal surfaces of the lower posterior teeth hit against the occlusal surfaces of the upper teeth when the jaw closes (Figs. 21-14 and 21-15).

There is disagreement as to whether the anterior teeth have a fifth surface. They have a biting edge called an incisal ridge. Some authors contend that this **incisal ridge** is an incisal surface. Therefore any reference to the incisal surface is referring to the incisal ridge of an anterior tooth. After studying the sections on line and point angles (see below), it will make more sense to consider the anterior teeth as having five surfaces (Fig. 21-16).

DIVISION OF SURFACES

For the purpose of facilitating the location of various areas within a specific surface of a tooth, the surface is divided into thirds. The lingual surface of a tooth is divided into a **mesial**, a **middle**, and a **distal third**. The facial surfaces are divided in the same manner (Fig. 21-17). The proximal surfaces of a tooth are divided into a **facial**, a middle, and a **lingual third**.

The teeth can be divided into divisions perpendicular to these, so that any of the proximal,

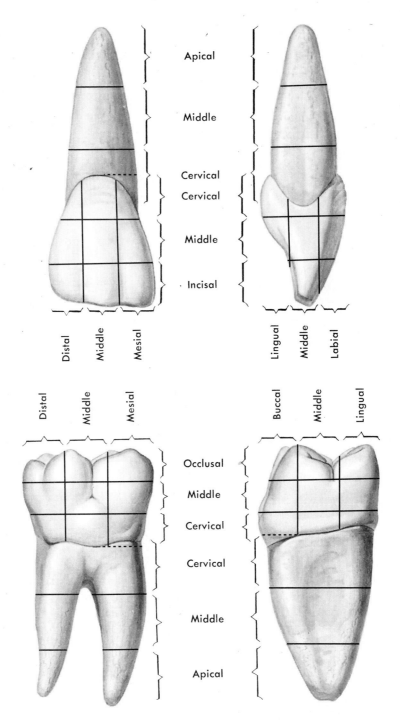

FIG. 21-17.   A maxillary right permanent central incisor and a mandibular right permanent first molar. (From Zeisz RC, Nuckolls J: *Dental anatomy,* St. Louis, 1949, Mosby.)

facial, or lingual surfaces can be further divided into an **incisal**, a middle, and a **cervical third**. On posterior teeth the incisal third is called the **occlusal third**.

LINE ANGLES

A **line angle** separates two surfaces of a tooth by forming the junction of the two surfaces. For instance, the junction of the buccal surface and the occlusal surface of a tooth is a line angle. Be-

cause the line angles are named according to the surfaces they join, the line angle that separates the buccal and the occlusal surfaces is called the buccoocclusal line angle (Figs. 21-18 and 21-19). Following are the various combinations.

Line Angles for Anterior Teeth	
Distolabial	Mesiolingual
Mesiolabial	Linguoincisal
Distolingual	Labioincisal
Line Angles for Posterior Teeth	
Distobuccal	Distoocclusal
Mesiobuccal	Mesioocclusal
Distolingual	Buccoocclusal
Mesiolingual	Linguoocclusal

POINT ANGLES

A **point angle** is the point at which three surfaces meet. For instance, the point at which the mesial, labial, and incisal surfaces join is called the mesiolabioincisal point angle (Figs. 21-20 and 21-21).

Point Angles for Anterior Teeth	
Mesiolabioincisal	Distolabioincisal
Mesiolinguoincisal	Distolinguoincisal
Point Angles for Posterior Teeth	
Mesiobuccoocclusal	Distobuccoocclusal
Mesiolinguoocclusal	Distolinguoocclusal

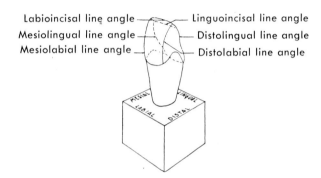

Labioincisal line angle — Linguoincisal line angle
Mesiolingual line angle — Distolingual line angle
Mesiolabial line angle — Distolabial line angle

FIG. 21-18.   Line angles for anterior teeth. (From Wheeler RC: *A textbook of dental anatomy and physiology,* Philadelphia, 1965, WB Saunders Co.)

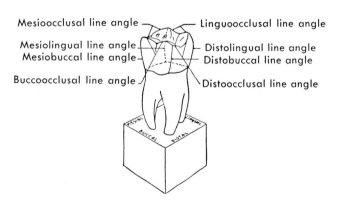

Mesioocclusal line angle — Linguoocclusal line angle
Mesiolingual line angle — Distolingual line angle
Mesiobuccal line angle — Distobuccal line angle
Buccoocclusal line angle — Distoocclusal line angle

FIG. 21-19.   Line angles for posterior teeth. (From Wheeler RC: *A textbook of dental anatomy and physiology,* Philadelphia, 1965, WB Saunders Co.)

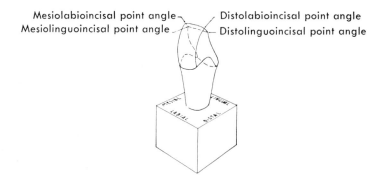

Mesiolabioincisal point angle   Distolabioincisal point angle
Mesiolinguoincisal point angle   Distolinguoincisal point angle

Fig. 21-20.   Point angles for anterior teeth. (From Wheeler RC: *A textbook of dental anatomy and physiology*, Philadelphia, 1965, WB Saunders Co.)

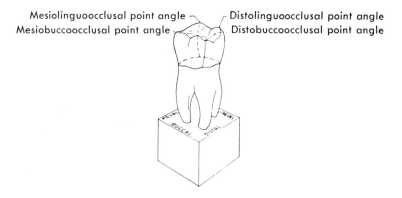

Mesiolinguoocclusal point angle   Distolinguoocclusal point angle
Mesiobuccoocclusal point angle   Distobuccoocclusal point angle

Fig. 21-21.   Point angles for posterior teeth. (From Wheeler RC: *A textbook of dental anatomy and physiology*, Philadelphia, 1965, WB Saunders Co.)

LANDMARKS

The student must know basic landmarks to be able to study individual teeth. When the crowns are formed, they develop from four or more growth centers called **lobes.** These lobes grow and eventually fuse, but a line remains on the erupted tooth where fusion of the lobes took place. These shallow grooves or lines that separate primary parts of the crown or root are called **developmental grooves** (Fig. 21-22).

Incisors, canines, and most premolars are de-veloped from three facial lobes and one lingual lobe. Second molars are developed from four lobes—two facial and two lingual. First molars are developed from five lobes; the maxillary has two facial and three lingual lobes, and the mandibular has two lingual and three facial lobes. In Fig. 21-22 the lines separating the lobes represent developmental grooves, and the lobes are numbered.

A **tubercle** is a small elevation of enamel on some portion of the crown of the tooth. It does

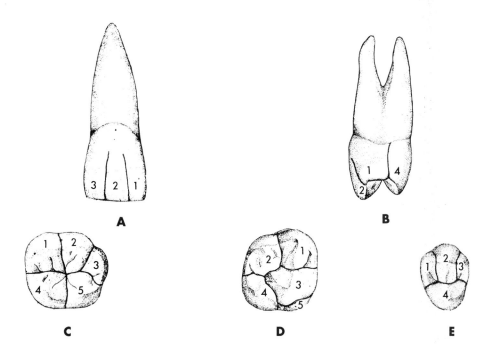

Fig. 21-22.   Lobes of teeth. **A,** Maxillary central incisor. **B,** Maxillary first premolar. **C,** Mandibular first molar. **D,** Maxillary first molar. **E,** Maxillary premolar. Lines separating lobes are developmental grooves. (From Wheeler RC: *A textbook of dental anatomy and physiology,* Philadelphia, 1965, WB Saunders Co.)

not always occur on the lingual surface of a tooth but can occur on an area such as the labial or occlusal surface (Fig. 21-23).

A **fossa** of a tooth is a depression or concavity, an area on the tooth that is indented, or concave. *Fossae* is the plural. The fossae are named for their location. For instance, a lingual fossa is on the lingual surface of a tooth.

On the anterior teeth there is a lingual fossa between the **marginal ridges** and incisal to the **cingulum** (cingula is the plural). These terms are further discussed in following sections in this chapter. When there is a pinpoint hole within the fossa or anywhere on the tooth, this depression is called a **pit.** Pits usually occur along the developmental grooves or in the fossae. On canines there are two lingual fossae; on premolars there

are triangular fossae on the occlusal surfaces, mesial or distal to the marginal ridges, and between cusps along the central developmental groove. Pits are named for their location on a tooth; thus a lingual pit occurs on the lingual surface of a tooth, and a buccal pit occurs on the buccal surface of a tooth.

A cusp is a mound on the crown portion of the tooth that makes up a major division of its occlusal or incisal surface. Cusps are found on premolars, molars, and canines. They are not, however, found on incisors. The difference between a tubercle, which is a smaller elevation on a tooth, and a cusp is that a cusp makes up a major or divisional part of the occlusal or incisal surface, and a tubercle does not.

A **ridge** is an elevated portion of a tooth that

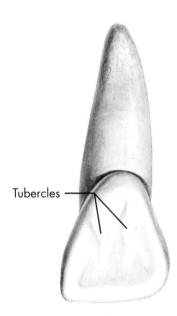

FIG. 21-23. Maxillary central incisor, lingual view. Tubercles of an anterior tooth extend from the cingulum onto the lingual fossa. (From Zeisz RC, Nuckolls J: *Dental anatomy,* St. Louis, 1949, Mosby.)

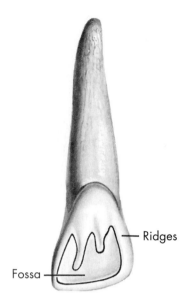

FIG. 21-25. Fossa and ridges of a tooth. The fossa is a concavity or depression, and the ridge is a convexity or bulge. (From Zeisz RC, Nuckolls J: *Dental anatomy,* St. Louis, 1949, Mosby.)

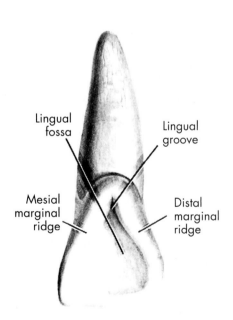

FIG. 21-24. Lingual view of the maxillary right central incisor. (From Zeisz RC, Nuckolls J: *Dental anatomy,* St. Louis, 1949, Mosby.)

runs in a line. Ridges are named for their location, such as the linguocervical ridge or the distal and mesial marginal ridges. All cusps have four ridges—buccal (or labial), lingual, mesial, and distal.

Marginal ridges are the rounded borders of enamel that form the mesial and distal shoulders of the occlusal surfaces of the posterior teeth and the mesial and distal shoulders of the lingual surface of the anterior teeth (Fig. 21-24).

A **concavity** is a carved-out section or area, like a cave. The opposite of concavity is **convexity**, a bulging out. The ridges of a tooth and a cusp tip are convex (Fig. 21-25).

Anterior Teeth

Anterior teeth show two developmental grooves on their labial surfaces. These two grooves separate the three lobes that form the labial surface (see Fig. 21-22, A). The fourth developmental lobe of anterior teeth occurs on the lin-

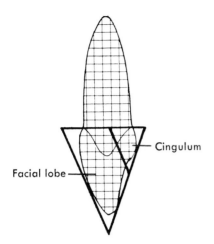

FIG. 21-26. The fourth developmental lobe or cingulum of an anterior tooth. The lingual fossa separates the cingulum from the three facial lobes. (From Wheeler RC: *A textbook of dental anatomy and physiology*, Philadelphia, 1965, WB Saunders Co.)

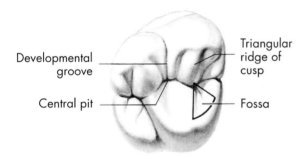

FIG. 21-27. Maxillary right second molar. (From Zeisz RC, Nuckolls J: *Dental anatomy*, St. Louis, 1949, Mosby.)

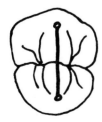

FIG. 21-28. Maxillary right first premolar. The transverse ridge is formed by the lingual ridge of the buccal cusp and the buccal ridge of the lingual cusp.

gual surface of the crown (Fig. 21-26). This fourth lobe is the cingulum, and it makes up the bulk of the cervical third of the lingual surface of an anterior tooth. The developmental line that separates this fourth lobe from the labial lobes is called the **lingual groove** or grooves (there may be more than one). The lingual fossa separates the lingual lobe from the other three lobes. A lingual developmental groove may not always be a single groove; rather, it may be several grooves interrupted by a tubercle (see Fig. 21-23).

Posterior Teeth

The most obvious landmarks on the posterior teeth are the cusps. The number will vary according to the tooth, and these are discussed under the individual teeth.

Aside from the marginal ridges on a posterior tooth, there are several additional types of ridges (Fig. 21-27). **Triangular ridges** are the main ridges on each cusp that run from the tip of the cusp to the central part of the occlusal surface. Thus the triangular ridge of the mesiobuccal cusp is the lingual ridge of the cusp that runs to the center of the occlusal surface, whereas the triangular ridge of the mesiolingual cusp is the buccal ridge that runs from the tip of the cusp to the center of the occlusal surface (see Fig. 21-27). A **transverse ridge** is the union of two triangular ridges, a buccal and a lingual, that cross the occlusal surface of a posterior tooth (Fig. 21-28).

Review Questions

1. What line separates the enamel from the cementum of the tooth?
2. How could a portion of the anatomic crown be a part of the clinical root?
3. How many roots are present in a trifurcated and in a bifurcated tooth?
4. Are maxillary teeth upper or lower jaw teeth?

5. Which tooth tissue composes the bulk of the tooth?
6. Which tooth tissue is the hardest?
7. Which tooth tissue is the softest?
8. Which tooth tissues have their own nourishment system?
9. Which tooth tissue is most like bone?
10. What is the main nourishment system of the tooth?
11. Name the different parts of the pulp cavity.
12. Is the pulp horn a part of the pulp chamber or the pulp canal?
13. What does the pulp tissue comprise?
14. A bifurcated tooth has how many roots?
15. What is the difference between the alveolus and the alveolar process?
16. Which is seen in the mouth first, the clinical or the anatomic crown?
17. What is the percentage of inorganic material in enamel? In dentin? In cementum?
18. Enamel is harder than dentin; dentin is harder than cementum. How does this correlate to the percentages of inorganic vs. organic materials present in these tissues?
19. What are the basic functions of the teeth? What determines which teeth have which functions?
20. What are the longest teeth in human dentition? Why are they considered the longest? How do the maxillary and mandibular compare?
21. Why is the term *bicuspid* inaccurate as compared with premolar?
22. What is the function of the molars, and how do the cusps perform this function?
23. How many premolars and how many molars are there in the permanent dentition?
24. How many surfaces are on a posterior tooth? Name them.
25. Which proximal surface is farther away from the midline, and which is closest to the midline?
26. If the anterior teeth do not have a fifth surface, what do they have that replaces the fifth surface?

27. What is a line angle? Name the six line angles for the anterior teeth and the eight for the posterior teeth.
28. What is a point angle?
29. The developmental grooves separate the lobes of a tooth. How many lobes does an anterior tooth have?
30. What separates the cingulum on an anterior tooth from the labial lobes?
31. A small elevation of enamel on some portion of the crown of a tooth is called a _____.
32. A small pinpoint depression that occurs along a developmental groove is a _____ _____.
33. Explain the difference between a tubercle and a cusp.
34. Which of the following items are convex and which are concave?
    a. Empty swimming pool
    b. Empty soup bowl
    c. Cave
    d. Ridge of a mountain
    e. Cusp tip
    f. Valley between two hills
    g. A marginal ridge
    h. Lingual fossa of an anterior tooth
35. Explain the difference between a developmental groove and a pit.
36. Identify the unlabeled surfaces of the mandibular lower right first molar that are missing in Fig. 21-29.
37. How many lobes or growth centers does it take to form the tooth in Fig. 21-30? Identify the two triangular ridges in Fig. 21-31.
38. Identify the two triangular ridges in Fig. 21-31.
39. A developmental elevated rounded mound of the crown that forms a major division of the occlusal surface is a:
    a. Lobe
    b. Tubercle
    c. Cusp
    d. Mamelon

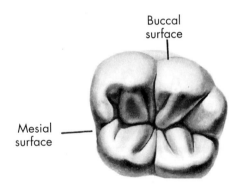

FIG. 21-29. (From Zeisz RC, Nuckolls J: *Dental anatomy*, St. Louis, 1949, Mosby.)

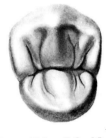

FIG. 21-31. (From Zeisz RC, Nuckolls J: *Dental anatomy*, St. Louis, 1949, Mosby.)

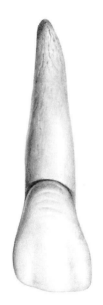

FIG. 21-30. (From Zeisz RC, Nuckolls J: *Dental anatomy*, St. Louis, 1949, Mosby.)

40. A developmental elevated projection on the incisal edge of a newly erupted incisor is a:
   a. Lobe
   b. Tubercle
   c. Cusp
   d. Mamelon

41. If a maxillary central incisor has an almost transparent incisal edge and a maxillary lateral incisor has a very white line covering its incisal edge, which incisor is more mineralized at its incisal edge?
   a. The central
   b. The lateral
   c. Not enough evidence to determine
   d. The white spot is a sign of a more mineralized and healthier incisal edge area.

42. How many roots does a trifurcated tooth have?

Turn to the sections in Chapter 5 concerning enamel composition, dentin composition, formation of regular dentin, and formation of secondary dentin and the section in Chapter 6 concerning cementum formation. These discussions contain much more detailed information about the material covered.

FUNDAMENTAL AND PREVENTIVE CURVATURES

Proximal Alignment of the Teeth and Protection of the Periodontium

OBJECTIVES

- To identify the successful characteristics of tooth shape and alignment in protecting the periodontium
- To understand that the teeth are shaped to align next to each other in order to preserve the dentition
- To identify the proximal contact areas
- To identify contact points

EVOLUTION OF FUNDAMENTAL AND PREVENTIVE CURVATURES AND PROXIMAL ALIGNMENT OF THE TEETH

Over millions of years of evolution the teeth have gradually developed a specific shape, with fundamental curvatures at certain areas on each tooth, representing successful adaptation toward the maintenance of the teeth within the dental arch. In other words, the curvatures aid the teeth in preventing disease, damage, bacterial invasion, and calculus buildup; dispersing excessive occlusal trauma and biting forces; and protecting the gingiva and **periodontium**. The periodontium comprises the supporting structures surrounding the teeth. If these tissues are damaged, then the vascularity, interdental gum tissue, gingiva, and finally the bone between and surrounding the teeth will be jeopardized, decreasing the life expectancy of the tooth within the dental arch.

Throughout evolution, the curvatures, by preserving the teeth, also increased the life expectancy and productivity of the possessor. As the life expectancy of the animal or person increased, so did the number of potential offspring. Thus through the process of evolution, and through successful traits outnumbering, outlasting, and outproducing the less successful traits, the teeth of modern humans possess certain successful characteristics of shape and **alignment** (their position in the jaw). Some of these successful adaptations and characteristics follow:

1. Specific location and size of proximal (mesial or distal) contact areas of various teeth
2. Size and location of interproximal spaces formed by the proximal contact surfaces
3. Location and effectiveness of the embrasures or spillways
4. Facial and lingual **contours** on the labial, buccal, and lingual surfaces of crowns
5. Amount of curvature of the cementoenamel junction on the mesial and distal surfaces of the various teeth
6. Self-cleaning qualities of the tooth; smoothness of the enamel; overall shape of the tooth to meet its function
7. Occlusal and incisal curvatures and contours

Proximal Contact Areas

The **proximal** (mesial or distal) **contact areas** of the teeth are the areas on the surfaces of the teeth where the proximal surfaces touch one another. The contact area between two teeth prevents food from packing between them. In a healthy mouth the contact surface formed is small enough to prevent a buildup of excessive amounts of bacteria, food, or proximal debris, but large enough to be an effective barrier and to prevent food from packing between the teeth. This affords protection to the underlying gum tissue between teeth. Finally, because the teeth do slightly touch, they offer support and anchorage to one another as well as resistance to displacement from traumatic forces.

Finally, we must remember that two adjacent teeth share the same interproximal bone. The same bone that supports the distal root portion of the first tooth also supports the mesial root portion of the second tooth. If something happens to cause the loss of this bone, it affects both teeth. Sometimes a periodontally involved tooth is removed to protect a neighboring tooth. However, this does not occur if the tooth is not adjacent to another tooth and does not jeopardize any other tooth by being retained.

The proximal contact areas are located on the mesial and distal surfaces of each tooth at the widest portion and at the greatest curvature. The **distal contact area** of one tooth touches the **mesial contact area** of the tooth posterior to it. For example, the distal contact area of the lower first premolar touches its neighbor, the lower second premolar.

Fig. 22-1 shows the contact areas of two premolars. The contact area on the distal surface

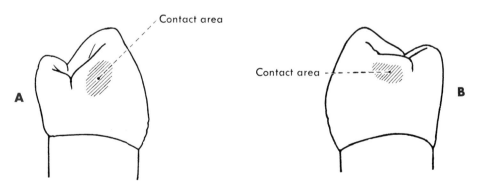

FIG. 22-1. Where the distal contact area *(shaded)* of the mandibular first premolar, **A,** touches the mesial contact area *(shaded)* of the second premolar, **B.** (From Zeisz RC, Nuckolls J: *Dental anatomy,* St. Louis, 1949, Mosby.)

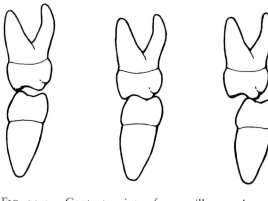

FIG. 22-2.   Contact points of a maxillary molar occluding with a mandibular molar in three different positions. A contact area is where two teeth in the same arch touch; a contact point is where a tooth in one arch touches a tooth in the opposite arch.

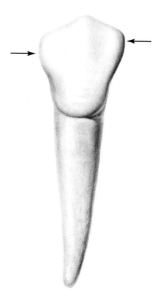

FIG. 22-3.   Buccal view of a lower first premolar. Contact areas *(arrows)*. (From Zeisz RC, Nuckolls J: *Dental anatomy,* St. Louis, 1949, Mosby.)

of the first premolar is called the distal contact area. What would the contact area on the mesial surface of the second premolar be called? The contact area is not just a point, but rather a flattened portion of the tooth where it actually touches the tooth next to it in the same dental arch.

A **contact point** differs from a contact area. A contact point is where the occlusal cusp of one tooth touches the occlusal portion of another tooth in the opposing arch (Fig. 22-2). The contact point of an upper tooth hits (occludes and makes contact with) the contact point of a lower tooth.

Looking at a buccal view of a tooth (Fig. 22-3), notice that the contact area occurs at the portion of the tooth that has the greatest curvature. In other words, the distal contact area occurs at the part of the distal portion of the tooth that bulges or curves out the most.

Even from an occlusal view it is apparent that, although the proximal contacts do not take up the entire surface, at least a considerable portion of the proximal surface does touch the adjacent tooth.

Interproximal Spaces

Interproximal spaces are triangular-shaped spaces between the teeth formed by the bone on one side and the proximal surfaces and their contact area on the other side (Fig. 22-4). The contact area forms the apex of the triangle, the proximal surfaces the sides, and the alveolar bone the base. These spaces are normally filled with gingival tissue called **papillary gingiva** or **interdental papilla.** By its presence the interdental papilla keeps food from collecting cervically to the contact areas between the teeth. The **interdental space** (space between teeth) provides a place for a bulk of bone, thus affording better anchorage and support. This space is wider cervically than occlusally in order to provide more access for the vascular support to nourish the interdental bone and papillary tissue. This

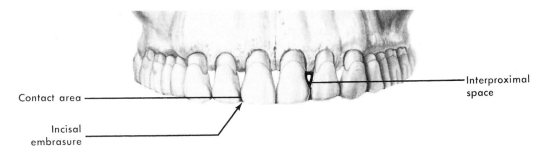

Contact area

Incisal embrasure

Interproximal space

FIG. 22-4.   Incisal embrasure *(arrow).* The area cervical to the contact area is a gingival embrasure, also called an interproximal space *(triangle).* (From Zeisz RC, Nuckolls J: *Dental anatomy,* St. Louis, 1949, Mosby.)

also affords a stronger bony base. When gingival recession occurs between the teeth, the interdental papilla and bone no longer fill the entire interproximal space; a void exists cervically to the contact area. This void is called a **cervical embrasure.** The more bone missing, the larger the interproximal space, because bone forms the base of the latter. The cervical embrasure could become larger because gum tissue receded while the bone level stayed the same. In this case the interproximal space would remain the same. Cervical embrasures occur frequently as a pathologic consequence of periodontal or orthodontic causes, and these embrasures offer a place in which bacteria, calculus, and food debris can accumulate (see Fig. 22-4).

Embrasures

Embrasures (spillways) are the spaces between the teeth that are occlusal to the contact areas (Fig. 22-5). They allow for the passage of food around the teeth so that food is not forced into the contact area between the teeth. These embrasures are named for their location in relation to the contact area. For instance, the space buccal to the contact area is the **buccal embrasure;** the **lingual embrasure** is lingual to the con-

tact area. The names of the embrasures are **facial** (buccal or labial), lingual, incisal, or **occlusal.** There is also a **gingival embrasure,** but only if the interproximal space is not occupied by any gingiva or bone. The gingival embrasure is gingival to the contact area and not usually present; it is the same as the cervical embrasure discussed in the last section. The embrasures have the following purposes:

1. They allow food to be shunted away from contact areas and thus keep food from being packed between the teeth.
2. They dissipate and reduce the forces of occlusal trauma brought to bear on the teeth, again by shunting food away from contact areas.
3. They are self-cleaning because of the rounded smooth surfaces that form the embrasures, allowing food to be swished away by saliva, ingested liquids, the cleaning action of other foods, and the friction of the tongue, cheeks, and lips.
4. They permit a slight amount of stimulation to the gingiva by frictional massage of food while at the same time protecting the gingiva from undue trauma. A poorly contoured embrasure leads to gingival irritation and breakdown.

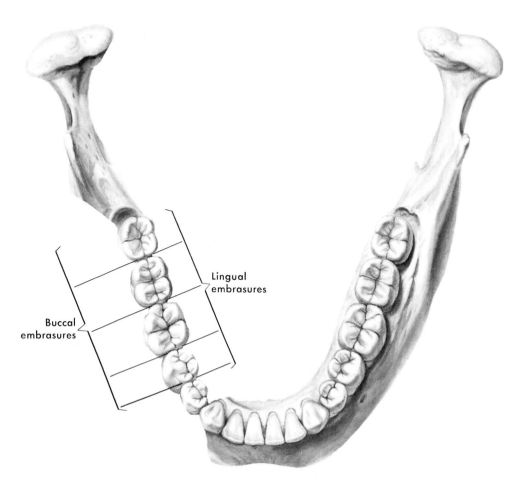

FIG. 22-5.   An occlusal view of proximal contact areas and embrasures. The width of the contact areas is not just a small point but an area of contact. Notice the position of the contact area with respect to the buccolingual dimensions of the tooth. (From Zeisz RC, Nuckolls J: *Dental anatomy,* St. Louis, 1949, Mosby.)

Location of the Contact Areas, Interproximal Spaces, and Embrasures

Facial view

The contact areas of the anterior teeth are located closer to the incisal surfaces of the teeth. The posterior teeth have their contact areas nearer to the middle third of the teeth. The more posterior the tooth, the more cervical is the location of its contact area. The one exception is the distal contact area of the maxillary canine, the location of which is in the center of the middle third of the tooth. This is more cervical than that of the first and second premolars, where the contact areas are just cervical to the junction of the occlusal and middle thirds of the tooth.

The more posterior teeth also have wider embrasures than more anterior teeth, at least in comparison with the occlusocervical dimensions of the tooth. The interproximal spaces of posterior teeth become shorter occlusocervically. Although the contact areas are at the same location, the teeth are shorter.

Occlusal view

The location of the contact areas and embrasures, as seen from the occlusal surface, shows that the contact areas of the anterior teeth are located in the center between the labial and lingual surfaces of the tooth. The posterior teeth have contact areas slightly buccal to the center of the teeth. Buccolingually the lingual embrasures are wider than the facial embrasures; the reason is that from their contact point outward, teeth are narrower on the lingual side than on the facial side (see Fig. 22-5).

Facial and Lingual Contours

Facial and **lingual contours** of the teeth also afford the correct amount of frictional massage to the gingiva by directing food off the teeth and against the gingiva at a proper angle (Fig. 22-6) (see the discussion on Periodontium on p. 273). Too much deflection of the food would leave some gingiva without the right amount of stimulation, whereas too little deflection would allow some food to be forced into the gingival crevice, the space that separates the tooth from the gingiva. Food packed into this crevice could cause gingival inflammation, periodontal disease, or tissue recession.

The correct degree of facial or lingual curvature allows for the proper deflection of food so that the right amount of tissue stimulation occurs and the gingival crevices are protected. In addition to these effects, the contour on the lingual surface should allow the tongue to rest against the tooth to promote the most efficient cleaning. Likewise, the facial height of contour allows for maximum cleaning of the lips and cheeks.

This contour varies in degree from tooth to tooth, but in general the location of the buccal

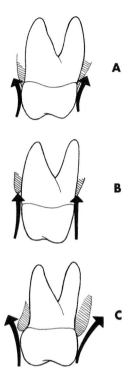

FIG. 22-6. The angle at which food is deflected from a tooth surface is determined by the buccal and lingual contours. **A,** Normal contour. **B,** Under contoured. **C,** Over contoured.

height of contour of anterior and posterior teeth will always be the same—at the cervical third of the tooth. The lingual height of contour of anterior teeth will also be at the cervical third of the tooth, but the **lingual crest of curvature** of posterior teeth will be at or near the middle third (Figs. 22-7 and 22-8). The crest of curvature refers to the widest part of the crown of the tooth; it is the same as the height of contour.

In young people most curvatures, buccal and lingual, lie beneath the gingiva. As the teeth erupt, the curvature becomes more clinically apparent. In the normal adult whose tooth eruption has been completed, the **gingival crest** is cervical to the buccal and labial contours of all

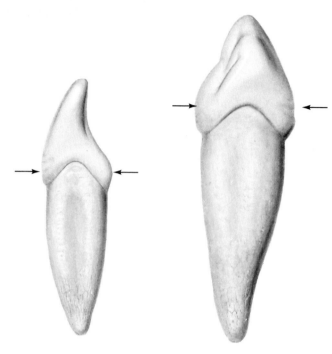

FIG. 22-7. Labial and lingual heights of curvature of mandibular and maxillary incisors and canines are located within the cervical thirds of teeth. Facial and lingual crests of curvature *(arrows)*. Also notice the curvature of the cervical lines (CEJ). (From Zeisz RC, Nuckolls J: *Dental anatomy,* St. Louis, 1949, Mosby.)

maxillary teeth and the lingual contour of anterior teeth. The **free gingiva** of the **cervical crest** covers the cervical enamel of the tooth. The normal amount of curvature found on most facial contours is approximately 0.5 millimeter (mm) and is somewhat less lingual on the anterior teeth.

On the lingual side of posterior teeth the crest of the gingiva is considerably more cervical than the lingual contour of the tooth. This is true because the height of contour on the lingual side of posterior teeth is located on the middle third of the crown. The amount of curvature on the lingual side of maxillary posterior teeth averages

approximately 0.5 mm, and on the mandibular posterior teeth, approximately 1 mm (see Figs. 22-7 and 22-8). The height of contour is the same as the crest of curvature and refers to the buccal or lingual width of a tooth. The contact areas refer to the mesial or distal crests of curvature of the tooth where it contacts adjacent teeth.

Curvature of the Cementoenamel Junction

As defined earlier, the cementoenamel junction (CEJ) is the line that marks the junction of the enamel and the cementum. It is also called the cervical line.

The curvature of the cervical lines (cementoenamel junction) on the mesial and distal surfaces of the teeth depends on the height of the contact area above the crown **cervix** and on the diameter of the crown labiolingually or buccolingually. The crowns of anterior teeth show greater curvature to the cervical line than do the posterior teeth. The anterior teeth are narrower labiolingually, and to afford more anchorage and bony support, nature may have allowed interdental bone between the teeth to protrude more incisally. The posterior teeth, which are wider buccolingually, have more bone support and therefore need not have this raised portion of bone between the teeth. Because of their cervicoincisal length, the anterior teeth need this added portion of bone for anchorage. The tooth crown is shaped on the mesial and distal surfaces to accommodate this needed bone. The enamel does not go so far gingivally on the mesial and distal surfaces as it could; instead, the cementum rises in an incisal direction in the middle of the tooth. This affords more cementum on which the bone can attach itself. The periodontal attachment follows the cervical line and connects the gingiva and the cementum. The periodontal ligament attaches the cementum to the bone.

The maxillary anterior teeth show the greatest amount of curvature of the cervical line. The more anterior the tooth, the greater the curvature. On the other hand, the mesial curvature of a tooth is greater than the distal curvature of the

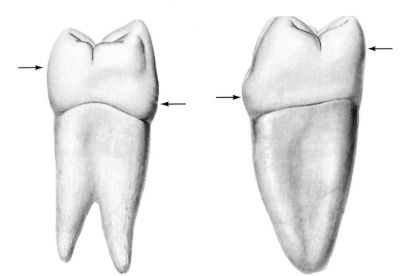

FIG. 22-8. The buccal height of curvature is at the cervical third, and the lingual height of curvature is at the middle third on the maxillary and mandibular premolars and molars. Buccal and lingual crests of curvature *(arrows)*. Notice the curvatures of the cervical lines (CEJ). (From Zeisz RC, Nuckolls J: *Dental anatomy,* St. Louis, 1949, Mosby.)

same tooth. The mandibular anterior teeth show less curvature than their maxillary counterparts do, generally less than 1 mm variation in cervical curvatures.

The posterior teeth in both arches show little variation. The mesial curvature of all posterior teeth usually averages about 1 mm, and the distal curvature is generally nonexistent or at least very slight, less than 0.5 mm. As a general rule, the curvature of the CEJ is usually about 1 mm less on the distal surface of the tooth than on the mesial surface. If a maxillary incisor has a 3.5 mm mesial curvature of the CEJ, the distal curvature may be 2.5 mm (Fig. 22-9).

Self-Cleaning Qualities of the Teeth

To a large extent the teeth are self-cleaning in that the crowns of the teeth are covered by a very smooth enamel. As mentioned previously, the smoothness of this enamel helps food and sticky substances slip off the crown of the tooth and allows the tooth to remain relatively free of bacteria, thus lessening decay and periodontal disease.

The shape of the crown also aids greatly in the prevention of periodontal disease by stimulating and cleaning the gingival tissue. It does this by deflecting the food onto the gingival tissue at a specific and proper angle. For instance, the shape of the incisors is like a shovel, and, accordingly, the incisor cuts its way through food and forces it toward the lingual surface onto the gingiva. In the case of the upper teeth, the food is directed toward the gingiva and onto the palate. Thus the shape of the incisor directs food off the incisor and onto the gingiva.

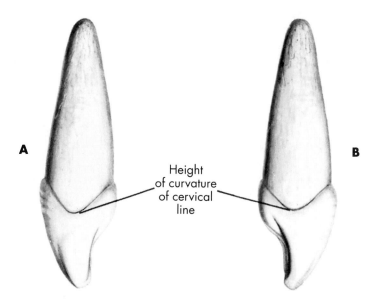

Height
of curvature
of cervical
line

FIG. 22-9.   The mesial curvature of the CEJ is greater than the distal curvature. **A,** Mesial view. **B,** Distal view. (From Zeisz RC, Nuckolls J: *Dental anatomy,* St. Louis, 1949, Mosby.)

The shapes of the teeth reflect their functions and their self-cleaning ability as well. As you know, the canine is a piercing tool. Like a spear it pierces through food. Because it is wedge shaped, it forces the food off the pointed canine cusp onto the cingulum and the gingiva. The premolars are shaped in such a way that food is deflected onto the occlusal surface of the premolar, where it is ground up by the cusps of the teeth in the opposing arch.

When food is introduced into the mouth, it is aided by the tongue and cheek in pushing the previously pulverized food back onto the surface of the molars. This process continues from molar to molar until the food reaches the back of the mouth and is swallowed. If there are deep pits and **fissures** on the occlusal surface of the tooth, some of the food debris will remain after eating. It would seem that deep pits, fissures, or holes in the enamel of the teeth would make cleaning difficult. Yet these pits and fissures do

provide a method of dissipating the extreme occlusal forces that result from the interdigitation of the cusps in the process of grinding up food. These little pits and fissures act as spillways on the occlusal surfaces of the teeth. Should these pits and fissures be too deep, nature has devised a way to eliminate them.

Primitive people, by eating natural raw foods, wore down some of the enamel of their teeth in the process of chewing, which resulted in the gradual obliteration of the pits and fissures. The wearing down of these pits and fissures could only be accomplished by the diet chosen. For over a million years humans chose to eat foods that were semi-raw or uncooked. In this form the food presented a certain amount of roughage in that it was hard and coarse and helped wear down the enamel. But the modern approach has found a way to avoid all this. Our diet of soft, overcooked, tacky, and sticky foods has resulted in an inability to wear down enamel; additionally, the stickiness of the food allows it to adhere to the tooth surface even when pits and fissures are not present. If our diet leaves a lot to be desired, it must also be said that our ingenuity does not—modern dentistry has found many more painless ways to obliterate the pits and fissures of teeth than through the abrasive action of eating. A pit can be polished out, making a tiny uncleanable hole into a small more cleanable fossa. This process is called an odontectomy or odontoplasty. A pit can also be filled in and covered with a sealant.

PERIODONTIUM

The periodontium is the supporting tissue adjacent to the teeth. It consists of the free gingiva, **attached gingiva,** and **alveolar mucosa,** as well as the cementum, periodontal ligament, and bone. These tissues are essential for the support and anchorage of the teeth. The curvatures and contact areas of the teeth must be shaped in such a way that they not only protect these tissues from excessive trauma but also keep them free of bacteria and offer frictional massage and stimulation.

The buccal and lingual contours of a tooth are shaped so that food is deflected off the tooth and onto the gingival tissue. The angle at which the food is deflected is specific (Fig. 22-10). The mechanical friction of the food must not place extreme pressure on the free gingiva because this part of the gingival apparatus cannot tolerate extreme trauma.

If the curvature is too extreme, the food will be deflected in such a way that the gingival tissue will not be stimulated and cleaned by the frictional action of the food that deflects off of it. In this situation bacteria will not be removed from the free gingival collar around the tooth, and the bacteria could then begin to destroy the gingival tissue. The tissue would become edematous, puffy, inflamed, and would bleed easily, eventually leading to the periodontal breakdown of the supporting structures.

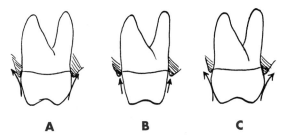

FIG. 22-10.   **A,** Normal curvatures as found on a maxillary molar. Arrows show the path of food as it is deflected over the curvatures onto the gingiva. **B,** A molar with little curvature and underdeveloped contours. The gingiva is likely to be stripped or pushed apically because of lack of protection and consequent overstimulation. **C,** A molar with excess curvature. The gingiva will be protected too much and will suffer from lack of proper stimulation. Food and bacteria may lodge under these curvatures, promoting pathological disturbance. (From Wheeler RC: *A textbook of dental anatomy and physiology,* Philadelphia, 1965, WB Saunders Co.)

When placing restorations or fillings, dentists must be careful not to over or under contour the restoration. However, while both over and under contouring of the buccal and lingual surfaces of teeth can cause periodontal disease, usually it is safer to under contour a restoration than to over contour it. Under contoured surfaces can occur thru the normal aging process where more and more root shows as an individual gets older.

The contact areas are equally essential to the health and maintenance of the periodontal tissue in the interproximal spaces. If **open contacts** are present the teeth do not touch each other at their contact areas, and food is allowed to pack between the teeth and remain there. The bacteria captured on and in the **gingival crevice** could then cause a periodontal breakdown of these tissues. If the contact area is so wide open, as in a diastema, that food can be forced into the interproximal space but not remain in this area because of the extremely large size of the space,

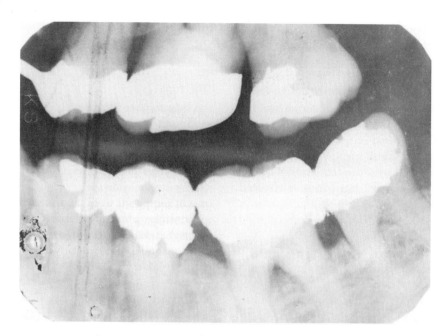

FIG. 22-11.   Large open contact between two upper molars and large overhanging restorations on bottom teeth.

then pathology can be prevented. The space must be large enough to ensure that bacteria and debris will be flushed out by the frictional massage of the food.

If the deflection of the food is at an extreme angle, a **recession** of the tissues away from the crown of the teeth could result. When gingival tissue recedes from the tooth, the root of the tooth becomes exposed. It is possible to have so much tissue stimulation or an improper angle of food deflection that the gum tissue recedes from the tooth.

When the missing part of a tooth is restored by some type of dental material, it is very important that the margins of the restoration be smooth and approximate the normal shape of the tooth as much as possible. If the margins are rough, they will allow bacteria to be retained around the restoration and thus cause gingival inflammation and decay. If the margin of the fill-ing or restoration is such that it extends far beyond the tooth, it will cause a condition known as **overhanging restoration,** a condition that allows for the buildup of plaque, bacteria, and food. Such a response would damage the gingival tissue (Fig. 22-11). Chapter 27 further explains the clinical implications of the material presented in this chapter.

Chapter 22 Review Questions

1. What normally fills the interproximal spaces between teeth? If this is missing, what do we call the void?

2. Name the embrasures and explain their function. Which embrasure is not always present and why?

3. Which teeth have the greater curvature of the cementoenamel junction, anterior or posterior? Mesial or distal?

4. What terms are synonymous with cementoenamel junction?

5. Does the diet a person chooses have any effect on gums and teeth?

6. What happens if a tooth is restored so that it has an overhanging restoration?

7. What happens if two adjacent teeth have open contact areas?

8. What is the difference between a contact area and a contact point?

9. Which of the following spaces in Fig. 22-12 will present the greatest potential for food impaction, periodontal disease, and caries:
   a. Interproximal space mesial to the upper first molar
   b. Interproximal space distal to the upper first molar
   c. Edentulous space mesial to the lower first molar

10. The buccal height of contour of anterior teeth is the _____ and of posterior teeth is the _____.
The lingual height of contour of anterior teeth is the _____ and of posterior teeth is the _____.
   a. cervical third of the tooth
   b. near middle of the tooth

11. The buccal crest of curvature is _____ the buccal height of contour.
   a. less than
   b. the same as
   c. lower than
   d. higher than

12. The normal amount of crest of curvature is _____.
   a. 1mm
   b. 0.5mm
   c. less than 0.5mm on the lingual of incisors
   d. at the cervical third except for mandibular posterior teeth
   e. b, c, and d

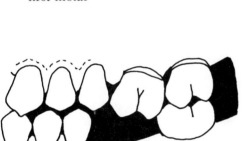

FIG. 22-12.

DENTITION

ARRANGEMENT OF TEETH

The general arrangement of teeth is referred to as the **dentition. Primary dentition** refers to the 20 **deciduous** teeth, often called baby teeth. **Secondary dentition** refers to the 32 permanent teeth (Figs. 23-1 and 23-2).

The dentition is divided into two **arches:** upper and lower. The teeth anchored within the upper jaw belong to the **maxillary arch.** The mandible is the bone that supports the lower arch of teeth, hence the name **mandibular arch.**

The mandibular and maxillary arches each compose one half of the dentition. In the permanent dentition of 32 teeth, each arch comprises 16 teeth. How many teeth are in an arch of the primary dentition? How many teeth compose the total primary dentition? Each arch is further divided into a right and a left half. Thus there are four **quadrants,** two in each arch. In the Palmer notation system, the quadrants are determined by the intersection of a vertical and a horizontal line. The maxillary quadrants are represented by numbers or letters above the horizontal line; the mandibular, below the line. The technical term for the dividing line between the right and left sides of the body is the **midsagittal plane.** In dentistry this is called the **midline,** or **median line,** of the face. The right and left quadrants are separated by this vertical line, which represents the midline of the skull when facing the patient. Thus each quadrant consists of one fourth of the dentition

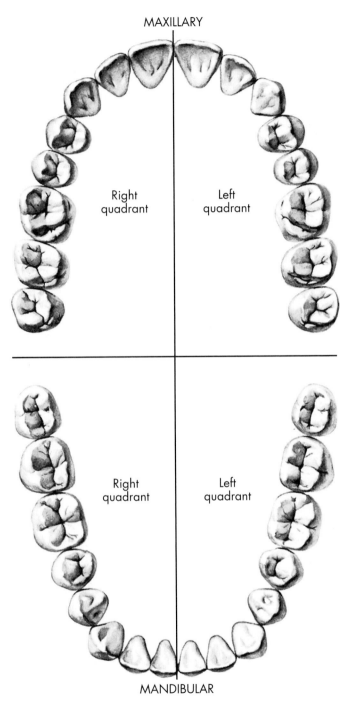

MAXILLARY

Right
quadrant

Left
quadrant

Right
quadrant

Left
quadrant

MANDIBULAR

Fig. 23-1. Permanent teeth or secondary dentition. Horizontal and vertical lines divide arches into quadrants. (From Massler M, Schour I: *Atlas of the mouth in health and disease,* ed 2, Chicago, 1975, American Dental Association.)

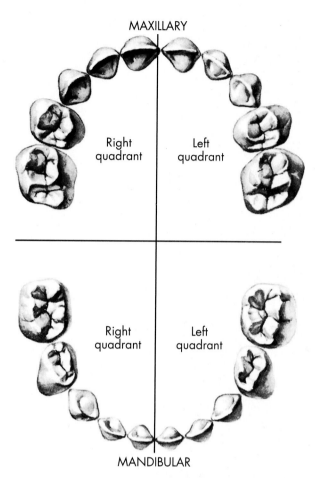

MAXILLARY

Right quadrant

Left quadrant

Right quadrant

Left quadrant

MANDIBULAR

FIG. 23-2. Deciduous teeth or primary dentition. (From Massler M, Schour I: *Atlas of the mouth in health and disease,* ed 2, Chicago, 1975, American Dental Association.)

and has a mirror image on the other side of the arch, as well as an opposing quadrant in the opposite arch.

Note that a permanent dentition quadrant has eight teeth—a central and a lateral incisor, a canine, a first and second premolar, and a first, second, and third molar. A deciduous (primary)

quadrant has five teeth—two incisors, a canine, and a first and second molar. There are no deciduous premolars.

The permanent teeth that replace or succeed the deciduous teeth are called **succedaneous** teeth. The permanent molars are called **nonsuccedaneous** teeth. They do not have predecessors, and they do not succeed or replace deciduous teeth. The permanent premolars replace the deciduous molars. How many teeth in the secondary dentition are nonsuccedaneous? How many are in each arch? How many are in each quadrant?

A **mixed dentition** refers to one that comprises some permanent teeth and some deciduous teeth. After a child's permanent teeth begin to erupt, there are several years of mixed dentition. Not all the deciduous teeth are replaced at one time. Some adults may also have a mixed dentition; this occurs when a deciduous tooth is retained even though the remainder of the teeth are permanent. If any combination of primary and secondary teeth are in the same dentition, then a mixed dentition is present.

If an adult has one retained primary tooth, with the rest being secondary teeth, what type of dentition does that person have? What would have to happen for that person to get a permanent dentition?

NAMING AND CODING TEETH

When identifying a specific tooth, list the dentition, arch, quadrant, and tooth name in that order. For example: permanent (dentition), mandibular (arch), right (quadrant), central incisor (tooth). Therefore, for example, we would refer to a "permanent mandibular right central incisor" rather than a "right mandibular permanent central incisor."

It is essential that each dental team be familiar with the various systems of naming and coding teeth. Although each office may use only one system, it is necessary that the personnel be familiar with all systems so that communication among dental offices is possible. Therefore the most popular systems will be discussed here.

Universal System

The **Universal system** uses the Arabic numerals 1 through 32 for permanent teeth and the letters A through T for the primary teeth. The number 1 is assigned to the most posterior molar on the upper right, the permanent maxillary right third molar. The highest number is given to the permanent mandibular right third molar (Fig. 23-3). Likewise, the letter *A* is given to the primary maxillary right second molar, and the letter *T* to the primary mandibular right second molar (Fig. 23-4).

What symbol would represent each of the following?
1. Secondary mandibular left first molar
2. Secondary maxillary right first premolar
3. Primary maxillary right first molar
4. Primary mandibular left central incisor
5. Permanent maxillary left first premolar
6. Deciduous mandibular right canine

What tooth is represented by each of the following symbols of the Universal system? 19, 5, B, O, 31, A, and I

Palmer Notation System

In the **Palmer notation system** each of the four quadrants is given its own prefix symbol or quadrant bracket. For instance, if the tooth is a maxillary tooth, the number or letter should be placed above the line of the bracket, thus indicating an upper tooth. Conversely, a mandibular tooth symbol should be placed below the line, indicating a lower tooth. Numbers or letters representing teeth from the right quadrant should be placed in a bracket with a line to their immediate right as we view it. This line indicates the midline or the midsagittal plane (refer to the diagram below). This system is a shorthand diagram of the teeth as if we were viewing the patient's teeth from the outside. The teeth in the right quadrant would have the midline bracket to the right of the numbers or letters, just as when looking at a patient—the midline is to the right of the teeth in the right quadrant.

The number or letter assigned to each tooth depends on its position relative to the midline. For example, the central incisors, the teeth closest to the midline, have the lowest number—the number 1 for permanent teeth and the letter *A* for deciduous teeth.

Study the diagram below and notice that there are 32 individual numbers, four of each number ranging from 1 to 8. In the Palmer notation system, the lowest number is closest to the midline. For instance, all central incisors, maxillary and mandibular, right or left, are given the number 1. All lateral incisors are given the number 2, all ca-

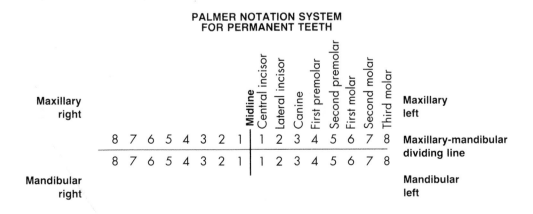

PALMER NOTATION SYSTEM
FOR PERMANENT TEETH

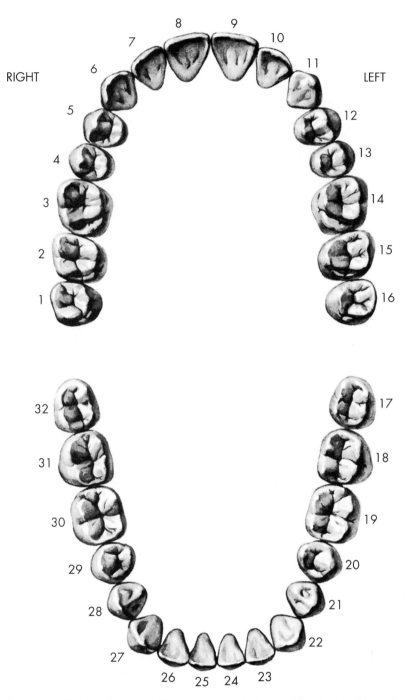

FIG. 23-3.   Universal system of permanent teeth. (From Massler M, Schour I: *Atlas of the mouth in health and disease,* ed 2, Chicago, 1975, American Dental Association.)

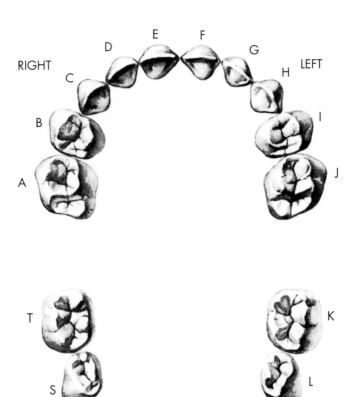

RIGHT   LEFT

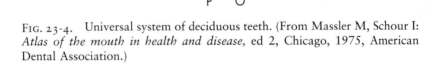

FIG. 23-4.   Universal system of deciduous teeth. (From Massler M, Schour I: *Atlas of the mouth in health and disease,* ed 2, Chicago, 1975, American Dental Association.)

nines the number 3, and the number 8 is assigned to the third molars. The farther from the midline, the higher the number assigned to the tooth. The number 6 is assigned to the first molars because it is the sixth tooth from the midline.

Each tooth is further identified as being maxillary or mandibular by its position above or below the horizontal maxillary–mandibular dividing line. In the diagram, notice that the number 1 appears at the four locations closest to the midline. Number 1 in all instances refers to a central incisor. By studying the midline bracket, we can identify whether the tooth belongs to a right or left quadrant. If the bracket is to the left of the letter or number, the tooth belongs to the left quadrant. The teeth are placed in relation to the midline as if one were looking at the patient, not looking from within the patient's mouth.

Study the following symbols:

$$\underline{\Big|\;\;1\;\;2\;\;4\;}$$
$$3\;\Big|$$

What can be determined from this diagram?

1. Three of the symbols (1, 2, and 4) are maxillary teeth because they are above the horizontal line.
2. One of the teeth (3) is a mandibular tooth. Why?
3. Numbers 1, 2, and 4 are in the maxillary left quadrant because the vertical line is to the immediate left of these numbers. This would also be the relationship of the vertical line to the teeth if one were looking *at* the patient.
4. Number 3 refers to a tooth in the mandibular right quadrant. Why?
5. Because number 1 refers to a central incisor, number 2 to a lateral incisor, and number 4 to the first premolar, these numbers refer to the maxillary left central and lateral incisors and the first premolar.

6. Because number 3 refers to a canine, number 3 in this diagram refers to the mandibular right canine.

If we wanted to represent only one tooth, such as the secondary maxillary left lateral incisor, the following symbol would be used:

All that we have done is eliminate some of the horizontal and vertical lines. The original symbol would have looked like this:

$$\underline{\Big|\;\;2}$$
$$\Big|$$

So far we have been using secondary (permanent) teeth in our examples of the Palmer notation system. Remember that the numbers 1 through 8 are used for permanent teeth and capital letters A through E for primary teeth. Refer to the diagram below for deciduous teeth.

PALMER NOTATION SYSTEM
FOR PRIMARY TEETH

					Central incisor	Lateral incisor	Canine	First molar	Second molar		
Maxillary right										Maxillary left	
	E	D	C	B	A	A	B	C	D	E	
Mandibular right	E	D	C	B	A	A	B	C	D	E	Mandibular left

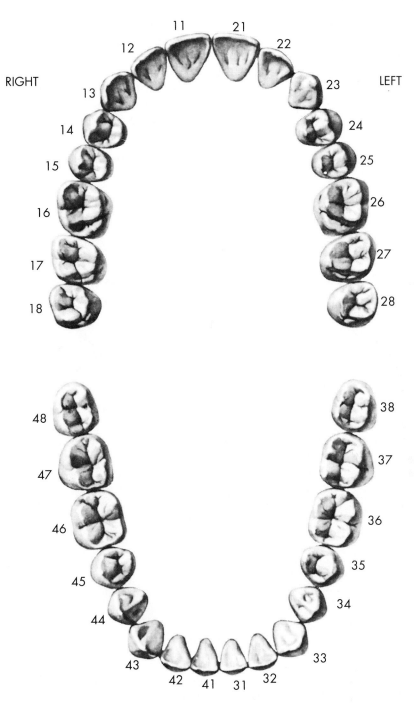

FIG. 23-5.   FDI system of permanent teeth. (From Massler M, Schour I: *Atlas of the mouth in health and disease,* ed 2, Chicago, 1975, American Dental Association.)

Which tooth is represented in each of the following?

What is the symbol for the primary mandibular right first molar?

FDI System

In the **FDI** (Federation Dentaire Internationale) **system** each tooth, deciduous or permanent, is given a two-digit number. No letters or duplicate numbers are used. It is similar to the

E ___

___ D

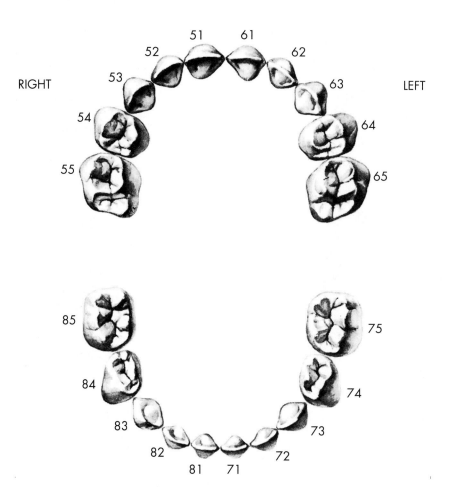

FIG. 23-6.   FDI system of deciduous teeth. (From Massler M, Schour I: *Atlas of the mouth in health and disease,* ed 2, Chicago, 1975, American Dental Association.)

Palmer notation system in that the second digit indicates the position of the tooth relative to the midline. The first digit indicates the quadrant and whether the tooth is permanent or deciduous. Looking at Fig. 23-5, notice that each tooth has its own specific two-digit number. The permanent maxillary right quadrant teeth are assigned numbers from 11 to 18, and the permanent maxillary left quadrant teeth, numbers 21 through 28. The permanent mandibular teeth are numbered 31 to 38 in the left quadrant and 41 to 48 in the right. Each quadrant is symbolized by a specific first digit, and all teeth in that quadrant have the same first digit. The second digit depends on the position the tooth occupies relative to the midline. The lowest number is given to the tooth closest to the midline.

Likewise, the deciduous teeth have their own first-digit number identifying each specific quadrant. Again, the second digit denotes the position the tooth occupies relative to the midline. See Fig. 23-6 for quadrant numbers.

Review Questions

1. Name two types of dentition and the number of teeth in each.
2. Name the different arches. How many teeth are present in a primary arch and how many in a secondary mandibular arch?
3. How many different quadrants are there?
4. Are any primary teeth succedaneous? If not, why not?
5. Name all the nonsuccedaneous permanent teeth.
6. Are secondary molars nonsuccedaneous?
7. A dentition composed of both primary and secondary teeth is called a _____ dentition.
8. How many dentitions are there?
9. Identify the following in the Universal system:
   a. Numbers 3, 5, 19, 28, 32
   b. Letters A, E, J, M, S
10. Give the correct Universal system symbol for the following:
   a. Primary maxillary left central
   b. Primary mandibular right first molar
   c. Primary maxillary right canine
   d. Permanent maxillary right second premolar
   e. Permanent mandibular right central incisor
11. Identify the following by dentition, arch, and quadrant:
   a. |8
   b. E|
   c. |1
   d. 6|
12. Translate the above four symbols of the Palmer system into the symbols of the Universal system.
13. Give the Palmer, Universal, and FDI symbols for the permanent mandibular right first molar.
14. Identify the following symbols. Which systems are they derived from, and which teeth do they represent?
   a. 8
   b. 8|
   c. E
   d. 1|
   e. 11
   f. 18

CHAPTER 24

DEVELOPMENT, FORM, AND ERUPTION

OBJECTIVES
- To understand how the tooth germs develop within the crypts
- To understand how the growth centers or lobes fuse and form a tooth
- To understand that this fusion can take a variety of forms, which result in different types of teeth—incisors, premolars, and molars
- To know how many lobes form each type of tooth and where the lobes are located
- To understand the eruption schedule of the deciduous and permanent teeth
- To understand some general rules about the eruption of teeth
- To understand the phenomena of mesial drift, root resorption, and exfoliation
- To understand the implications of the terms *impacted teeth, congenitally missing teeth, attrition, occlusal plane,* and *curve of Spee*
- To understand the periods of primary, mixed, and permanent dentition

DEVELOPMENT AND FORM

During the sixth week of fetal life (7 or 8 months before birth), tiny tooth buds, sometimes called **tooth germs,** begin to grow within the alveolar process of the fetus. Tooth germs are small clumps of cells that have the ability to form the tooth tissues (dentin, enamel, cementum, and pulp). Both the primary and secondary teeth develop from these tooth germs, which later are located within cavities of the alveolar process called **crypts.** (See Chapter 4 and Figs. 4-1 to 4-4.)

At this time the dentin and enamel begin to form, followed later in development by the cementum. The type of dentin formed at this early stage is called *primary dentin,* and it occurs before root completion. Secondary dentin is continually formed within the tooth by the same odontoblasts that form regular dentin. This process continues throughout one's entire lifetime. Secondary dentin differs from reparative dentin in that reparative dentin is laid down locally as protection for the pulp from irritation, caries, or trauma (see Chapter 5).

The earliest evidence of tooth formation occurs during the sixth week of embryonic life. At this time the dental lamina begins to form (see Chapter 4).

The primary teeth begin to calcify by about the fourth or fifth month of fetal life. The process of **calcification** is the hardening of the tooth tissues by the deposition of mineral salts within these tissues (Fig. 24-1). This process continues until about the third or fourth year after birth, when the deciduous roots become fully formed.

Soon after birth the permanent teeth begin to calcify and continue until about the twenty-fifth year, when the roots of the third molars become calcified. The last area of the tooth to become calcified is the apex of the root. (See Chapter 6.)

Developmental Lobes

Each tooth begins to develop from four or more growth centers. These centers grow out from the tooth germ and are known as **developmental lobes.** The lobes grow and develop within their bony crypt until they fuse. This fusion of the lobes is called **coalescence.** The junction that forms the union of these lobes is marked by lines on the tooth called **developmental grooves,** which can be seen on the tooth after it has erupted.

The number of developmental lobes necessary for the formation of a tooth depends on the particular tooth and how many cusps it has. For instance, all the anterior teeth develop from four lobes—three labial and one lingual. The three la-

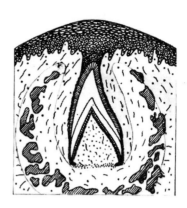

Fig. 24-1. Beginning of tooth calcification. The small hole in the bone in which a tooth bud germ forms is called a crypt; it later will become a tooth socket, which will house the root of the tooth. (From Massler M, Schour I: *Atlas of the mouth in health and disease,* ed 2, Chicago, 1975, American Dental Association.)

bial lobes form the labial surface of each tooth. The **mamelons,** which are evident after the eruption of incisor teeth, are the incisal ridges of these three labial developmental lobes, and they also are separated by developmental grooves (see Fig. 21-22).

In Fig. 24-2 notice how the three labial lobes fuse to form the entire labial surface. The only evidence that there ever were three separate lobes is at the incisal ridge, where the mamelons are distinct and separate, and on the labial surface of the tooth, where there are developmental lines or grooves. The three labial developmental lobes are called the *mesiofacial, centrofacial,* and *distofacial* lobes. The sole lingual lobe is called appropriately the *lingual lobe* and makes up the entire cingulum on the lingual surface of the tooth.

Lobes and Cusps

Premolars

The maxillary premolars are like the anterior teeth in that they have three facial lobes and one lingual lobe. However, unlike the anterior teeth,

MAMELONS

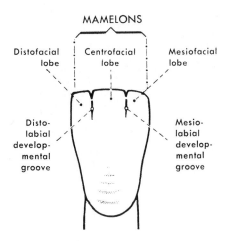

FIG. 24-2.   The incisal ridge of the three labial lobes is formed from mamelons. (From Zeisz RC, Nuckolls J: *Dental anatomy,* St Louis, 1949, Mosby.)

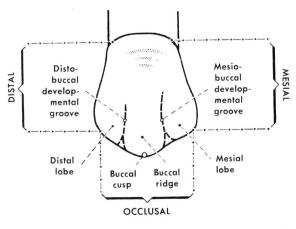

FIG. 24-4.   Buccal surface of a maxillary right second premolar. (From Zeisz RC, Nuckolls J: *Dental anatomy,* St Louis, 1949, Mosby.)

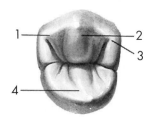

FIG. 24-3.   Four lobes of a maxillary second premolar. (See also Fig. 21-22, *B* and *E*.) (From Zeisz RC, Nuckolls J: *Dental anatomy,* St Louis, 1949, Mosby.)

the three facial lobes of maxillary premolars form one high buccal cusp instead of an incisal ridge, and the single lingual cusp forms a large lingual cusp rather than a cingulum. The names of the lobes are the same as those for the anterior teeth (Fig. 24-3).

The mandibular first premolar has the same number and arrangement of lobes as the maxillary premolars have; however, the lingual cusp of the mandibular first premolar is smaller than its maxillary counterpart. These teeth are termed

bicuspids because they have only two cusps, a buccal and a lingual. The mandibular second premolar varies; it may be a two-cusped or a three-cusped form. Because not all of these premolars have only two cusps, the term *premolar* is preferred.

The two-cusp variety of the mandibular second premolar is exactly the same in number and arrangement of lobes as the mandibular first premolar. The lingual cusp of this bicuspid is longer than that of the mandibular first premolar. The facial lobes and cusps of the three-cusp variety of the mandibular second premolar are exactly the same as on the first premolar, but the lingual lobes are quite different. First, there are two lobes, a mesiolingual and a distolingual lobe, instead of a single lobe, which results in two separate lingual cusps, with the mesiolingual cusp usually being larger than the distolingual cusp (Fig. 24-4). There is also a considerable difference in the number and location of the developmental grooves, with an additional groove located between the two lingual cusps. Further differences in anatomy are discussed in Chapter 32.

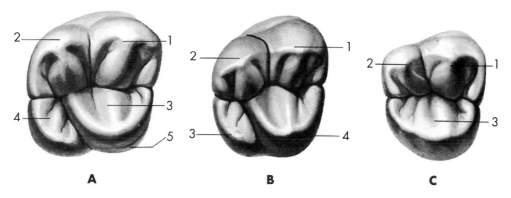

FIG. 24-5.   **A,** Maxillary first molar with five lobes. **B,** Maxillary second molar with four lobes. **C,** Maxillary third molar with three lobes. (From Zeisz RC, Nuckolls J: *Dental anatomy,* St Louis, 1949, Mosby.)

Molars

All molars have two facial and two lingual lobes, except the first molars, which usually have a fifth or minor lobe. For example, the maxillary first molar generally has five developing lobes: two major facial lobes (mesiobuccal and distobuccal), a mesiolingual lobe, one minor lobe (distolingual), and one **rudimentary lobe,** called the **lobe of Carabelli** or the **cusp of Carabelli.** Each of the four major and minor lobes develops into a cusp, which is named according to its lobe (e.g., the mesiobuccal lobe forms the mesiobuccal cusp). The lobe of Carabelli, which is located on the lingual surface of the mesiolingual cusp, develops into a tubercle (a small cusplike elevation).

The maxillary second molar often does not have a cusp of Carabelli; if it is present, it is much smaller in proportion to the other lobes. Second molars are much smaller than first molars in all cusp proportions as a rule, and the distolingual cusp, which is a minor cusp, is often even smaller in proportion. The minor cusp becomes smaller as the location becomes more posterior. Therefore it is not unusual for third molars to have only major cusps and no minor cusps. A maxillary third molar might have only three cusps, with little or no distolingual cusp. Additionally, the crown is usually smaller and the roots shorter than those of second or first molars (Figs. 24-5 and 24-6).

Special mention should be made about third molars in general. They are the most unpredictable of all the teeth. For instance, it is quite possible for mandibular third molars to be extremely well developed and better proportioned and larger than the first molars in the same mouth; however, they are more likely to be poorly formed and varying from three to eight cusps. They are likely to be deviated in form or missing entirely. Therefore, any general rule that applies to the regression of minor cusps or the size of teeth must be limited by the extreme variability of third molars.

ERUPTION

The first teeth to emerge into the oral cavity are the deciduous or primary teeth. Calcification of these teeth begins around the fourth month of fetal life. By the end of the sixth month, all the deciduous teeth have begun to develop. Normally no teeth are visible in the mouth at birth. Occasionally infants are born with erupted inci-

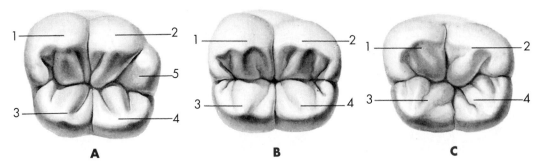

FIG. 24-6. **A,** Mandibular first molar with five cusps. **B,** Mandibular second molar with four cusps. **C,** Mandibular third molar. Each cusp is formed from one lobe. (From Zeisz RC, Nuckolls J: *Dental anatomy,* St Louis, 1949, Mosby.)

sor teeth, but these premature teeth are usually lost soon after birth. These teeth are not a part of the deciduous dentition.

The calcification process first forms the crown of the tooth, and root formation follows later. No two persons are exactly alike in calcification, crown and root formation, or eruption schedules. During enamel and dentin development, minerals are deposited in the forming tooth germs. However, any fever, metabolic dysfunction, childhood or nutritional disease, or physical illness or trauma can alter the formation of the teeth and even stop their formation or mineralization completely.

Although human dentition varies somewhat in all persons, certain approximations or averages are recognizable. Following is a list of deciduous teeth and approximate eruption times. It represents more recent data on eruption times than does Fig. 24-7.

Central incisors	6½ to 8 months
Lateral incisors	7 to 9 months
First molars	12 to 16 months
Canines	16 to 21 months
Second molars	21 to 30 months

The first general rule concerning eruption is that individual mandibular teeth usually precede the maxillary teeth in this process. The second rule is that the teeth in both jaws erupt in pairs, one on the right and one on the left. The third rule is that permanent teeth usually erupt slightly earlier in girls than in boys. There does not appear to be a sex difference in the eruption of deciduous teeth. Remember that these rules are not firm, and exceptions are numerous.

The first teeth to appear in the mouth are usually the deciduous mandibular central incisors. They generally erupt at the age of approximately 6½ to 7 months. Approximately a month later the maxillary central incisors can be seen. The deciduous mandibular lateral incisors emerge by about the seventh month, followed by the maxillary laterals about a month later.

To illustrate the variety that can exist, I have seen many instances in which the first two teeth to erupt were the maxillary central incisors. I have also seen a few instances in which all four mandibular incisors erupted before any of the maxillary incisors.

Next to erupt, at approximately 12 to 16 months of age, are the mandibular first deciduous molars, closely followed by the maxillary first deciduous molars. The deciduous canines erupt between 16 and 21 months of age, followed by the second molars between the twenty-first and thirtieth months. The deciduous second molars are often called the 2-year-old molars, and much of the cantankerous attitude of 2-year-olds is credited to the fact that the eruption of these large molars is painful.

All of the deciduous teeth are expected to have erupted by the time the child is 2½ years old. For the next 36 months as the child continues to grow, so too do the jaws, which support the teeth. The erupted teeth, however, do not become any larger. Consequently, by 5 years of age it is normal to have spaces and separations between the teeth, caused by the increased growth of the jaws.

Unfortunately, many people do not realize the importance of the deciduous teeth. They believe that because these teeth will be lost in the process of making way for the permanent teeth, they are unimportant and are left to suffer dental neglect. Terms such as *baby teeth* or *milk teeth* lend credence to this fallacy and should be discouraged.

With premature loss of deciduous teeth, normal jaw growth and development may not take place. The deciduous teeth must remain intact to retain the proper spacing for the permanent teeth that will replace them. So too must the deciduous dental arch help guide the first permanent molars into their normal position. These molars act as the foundation for the rest of the permanent dentition. To a large extent the proper position and location of the other permanent teeth are dependent on the first permanent molars being in their proper position (Fig. 24-7).

Normal growth and development of the jaws also depend on daily exercise. Premature loss of a deciduous tooth results in one side of the jaw developing differently from the other because the normal amount of exercise is not divided equally when one tooth is missing.

PERMANENT DENTITION

The first teeth of the permanent dentition to emerge into the oral cavity are usually the mandibular first molars, followed by the maxillary first molars within a few weeks. They emerge immediately distal to the deciduous second molars. Often they are called the 6-year molars because they erupt at approximately 6 years of age. Much larger than the deciduous molars, they cannot emerge into the oral cavity until sufficient jaw growth has occurred to allow space for them.

Along with the eruption of the permanent molars comes the phenomenon of **mesial drift.** Mesial drift is the tendency of the permanent molars to have an eruptive force toward the midline. This means that the permanent molars not only erupt occlusally to meet their antagonists in the opposite arch, but they also have an eruptive force that causes them to move mesially. This force is strong enough to move the permanent molars into any available space mesial to them. The phenomenon has two direct effects on the deciduous dentition: (1) the spaces between the deciduous teeth are closed as the first molar pushes the deciduous molars together; and (2) if a deciduous tooth is prematurely lost or if interproximal decay on the deciduous molar is not restored, the permanent first molar moves mesially into the available space. Because there is very little extra space left to allow room for the eruption of premolars and canines, the infringement of the permanent molar into this space may keep a premolar or canine from properly erupting.

The next permanent teeth to erupt are the central incisors—the mandibular at about 6 or 7 years of age and the maxillary at about 7 or 8 years. The permanent incisors take over the position that the deciduous incisors held. This is made possible because the deciduous incisors are exfoliated. **Exfoliation** is the process by which the roots of a baby tooth are resorbed and dissolved until so little root remains that the baby tooth falls out. As the permanent tooth erupts, osteoclastic cells destroy the root of the deciduous tooth. This phenomenon is called **resorption.** The pressure brought to bear on the deciduous root by the eruption of the permanent tooth triggers the body to activate certain bone-destroying

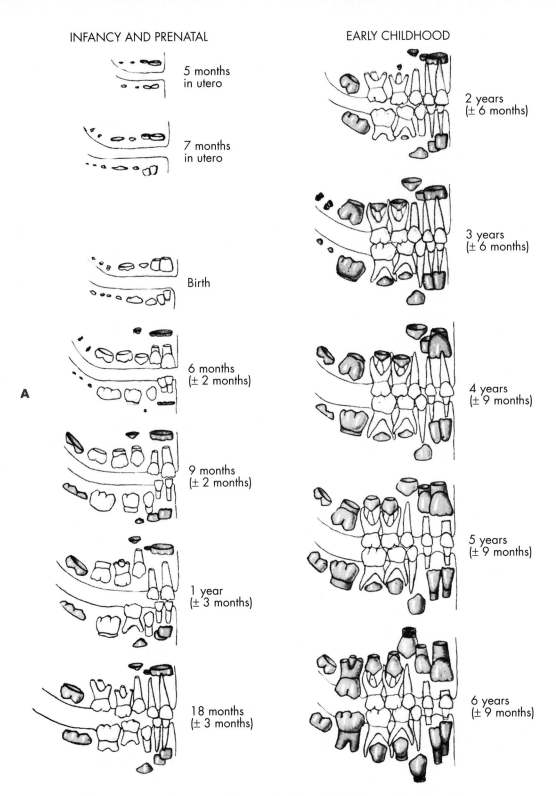

INFANCY AND PRENATAL

5 months
in utero

7 months
in utero

Birth

6 months
(± 2 months)

9 months
(± 2 months)

1 year
(± 3 months)

18 months
(± 3 months)

EARLY CHILDHOOD

2 years
(± 6 months)

3 years
(± 6 months)

4 years
(± 9 months)

5 years
(± 9 months)

6 years
(± 9 months)

A

FIG. 24-7. Development of human dentition. **A,** Deciduous dentition. (From Massler M, Schour I: *Atlas of the mouth in health and disease,* ed 2, Chicago, 1975, American Dental Association.)

Continued

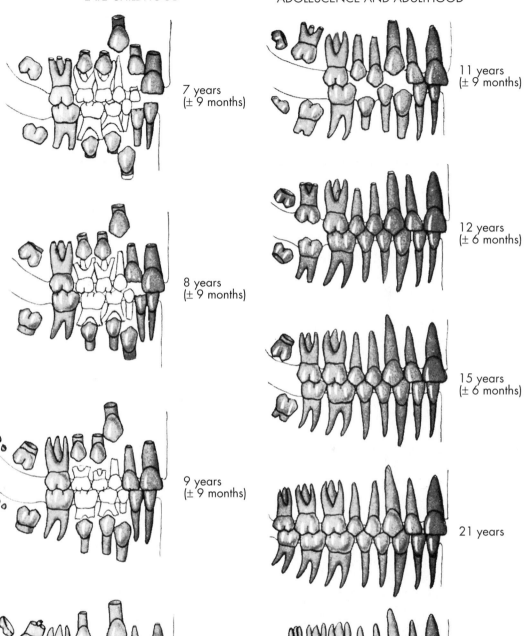

7 years
(± 9 months)

11 years
(± 9 months)

8 years
(± 9 months)

12 years
(± 6 months)

15 years
(± 6 months)

B

C

9 years
(± 9 months)

21 years

10 years
(± 9 months)

35 years

FIG. 24-7, CONT'D.   **B,** Mixed dentition, late childhood. **C,** Permanent dentition, adolescence and adulthood.

cells called **osteoclasts,** which destroy the roots of the deciduous teeth. As each deciduous root is destroyed, the tooth loses its anchorage, becomes loose, and finally exfoliates. During this process, the permanent tooth moves into the space that was occupied by the deciduous tooth.

It is not uncommon for the permanent incisors to erupt lingually to the deciduous incisors. Sometimes both central incisors are still in place, with the permanent central incisor located immediately lingual to the deciduous tooth. When the deciduous tooth is finally lost, pressure from the tongue forces the permanent tooth facially until it occupies its correct position in a balance between the lingual forces of the tongue and the facial forces of the lips.

The next teeth to erupt are the lateral incisors at 7 to 9 years of age, followed by the mandibular canines at 9 or 10 years. The maxillary canines do not erupt at this time. The developing incisors and canines are in a position lingual to the deciduous roots. Like the central incisors they can erupt lingual to their predecessors.

The mandibular canines are followed by the mandibular first premolars, but usually the maxillary first premolar erupts at about the same time or may even be earlier. The maxillary first premolar erupts at 10 to 11 years of age and the mandibular canines at 10 to 12 years.

The second premolars erupt at 10 to 12 years of age, with the maxillary premolars often preceding the eruption of the mandibular. This is the most common exception to the rule of mandibular teeth preceding the maxillary.

The maxillary canines then erupt at 11 or 12 years of age. It is very important that the deciduous teeth have maintained the proper amount of space for the canine to erupt. If the space is insufficient, the canine is forced to erupt facially toward the cheek or is unable to erupt at all. The latter situation occurs when the tooth is blocked out by the already erupted teeth and there is little available room.

At about the same time, 12 to 13 years of age, the mandibular second molars emerge, followed within months by their maxillary counterparts.

The permanent second molars are often called 12-year molars.

The third molars do not appear in the oral cavity until 17 years of age or later. There is much variation in the eruption of third molars, especially when one considers that third molars are the teeth most likely to be **impacted.** Impacted teeth are those that do not completely erupt but remain embedded in bone or soft tissue. Mandibular third molars are most often affected because the mandible has to grow enough to accommodate them. The maxillary third molars are the next most likely teeth to be impacted.

The third molars, maxillary and mandibular, are also the most common teeth to be congenitally missing. A **congenitally missing** tooth is one that never forms because a tooth bud was never produced from which it could form. This can be a hereditary trait.

The eruptive forces do not cease after the eruption of the third molars. Eruption continues because of **attrition,** the wearing away of the tooth through contact of its functioning surfaces.

As the teeth erupt and meet their antagonist in the opposite arch, they form what is known as the **occlusal plane.** Von Spee noted that the cusps and incisal ridges of the teeth tended to follow a curved line when the arches were observed from a point opposite the first molars. This line of occlusal surfaces is the occlusal plane. The curved alignment of the occlusal plane is named after von Spee and is called the **curve of Spee** (Fig. 24-8).

Following is an approximate breakdown of permanent tooth eruption:

Maxillary	
Central incisor	7 to 8 years
Lateral incisor	8 to 9 years
Canine	11 to 12 years
First premolar	10 to 11 years
Second premolar	10 to 12 years
First molar	6 to 7 years
Second molar	12 to 13 years
Third molar	17 to 22 years

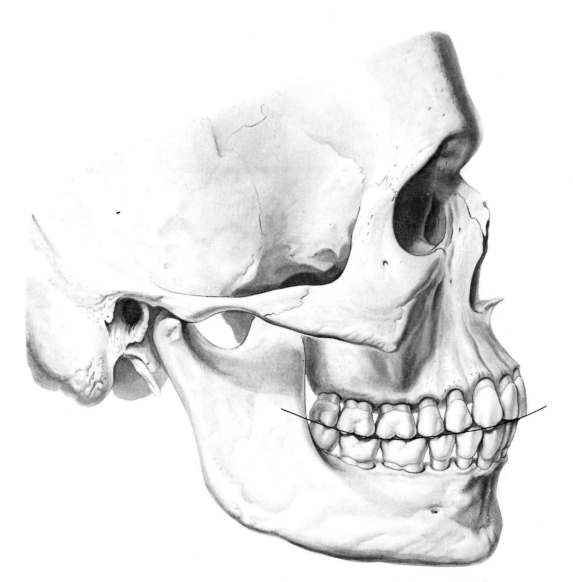

FIG. 24-8.   Occlusal plane (curve of Spee) rises to meet incisors and third molars. It dips down in area of first molars and second premolars. (From Zeisz RC, Nuckolls J: *Dental anatomy,* St Louis, 1949, Mosby.)

Mandibular	
Central incisor	6 to 7 years
Lateral incisor	7 to 8 years
Canine	9 to 10 years
First premolar	10 to 12 years
Second premolar	11 to 12 years
First molar	6 to 7 years
Second molar	12 to 13 years
Third molar	17 to 22 years

PERIODS OF DENTITION

The period of primary dentition begins with the eruption of the first deciduous tooth. This tooth, a central incisor, usually erupts 7 months after birth, but some erupt as early as 6 months or as late as 9 months after birth. The period of primary dentition lasts as long as only deciduous teeth are present. When the first permanent molar erupts, the period of primary dentition ends.

At about 6 years of age the period of **mixed dentition** begins. This period exists while both primary and secondary teeth are simultaneously present and ends when the last deciduous tooth is exfoliated and only permanent teeth remain.

The period of permanent dentition begins when the last primary tooth is lost and ends when the last permanent tooth is lost. This period usually begins at about 12 years of age and, it is hoped, does not ever end. If all of the permanent teeth are lost, no other period of dentition exists because there is no dentition. Such a condition is termed **edentulous,** meaning "no teeth."

Refer to Chapters 4 and 5 for a discussion of the formation of enamel, dentin, and pulp and to Chapter 34 for information concerning deciduous teeth.

Review Questions

1. Only primary teeth begin to develop in utero (during fetal life). T or F?
2. Which hard tissue of the tooth forms last?
   a. enamel
   b. dentin
   c. cementum
3. What does the term *coalescence* mean?
4. What do developmental grooves or lines separate?
5. From what lobe does the cingulum of an anterior tooth form?
6. What is a rudimentary lobe of the maxillary first molar called?
7. Which teeth erupt first, the deciduous first molars or the canines?
8. Which of the following statements are usually true about eruption?
   a. Girls' teeth erupt earlier than boys' teeth.
   b. Maxillary teeth erupt before their mandibular counterparts.
   c. Teeth in both jaws do not erupt in pairs.
   d. The eruption sequence varies little from person to person.
9. Name the first permanent tooth to erupt in the oral cavity.
10. If a child has spaces between the deciduous teeth at 5 years of age, these spaces will always remain, even after the permanent teeth have erupted. T or F?
11. Of the following, which is the only acceptable dental term?
    a. bicuspid
    b. premolar
    c. milk teeth
    d. baby teeth
12. Explain all of the various problems connected with premature loss of a deciduous molar.
13. With which teeth does the phenomenon of mesial drift occur, and what does it do?

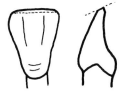

FIG. 24-9.

FIG. 24-10.

14. Which teeth are the most likely to be congenitally missing?
   a. central incisors
   b. lateral incisors
   c. third molars
   d. canines
15. Name the structures now worn off that used to be present on the incisal ridge of Fig. 24-9.
16. How many lobes are present in the mandibular premolar in Fig. 24-10? (Hint: It has three cusps.)
17. What periods of dentition might a 12-year-old boy be in? Give two possible reasons for each period of dentition.
18. When does the period of primary dentition end?
19. What deciduous teeth might an 11-year-old still have?
20. An orthodontist asks you to refer a patient back when the patient is out of mixed dentition. When would you send the patient to the orthodontist? What marks the end of the period of mixed dentition?

21. Permanent teeth show no evidence of development until the sixth month after birth. T or F?
22. Deciduous teeth begin to calcify as early as the fourth month of fetal life. T or F?
23. Deciduous teeth become fully formed somewhere around 3½ years after birth. T or F?
24. Permanent teeth continue to calcify until age 21 to 25. T or F?
25. A new drug has been developed. It is a wonderful drug but it has one very bad side effect. This side effect is that this drug can discolor teeth if taken during the period of tooth development.
   a. What age of patient should therefore avoid this drug to protect the permanent dentition?
   b. If this drug passes the placental barrier and affects the unborn fetal infant, then at what ages should it be avoided?

CHAPTER 25

OCCLUSION

OBJECTIVES
- To understand how the eruption schedule, growth, and ultimate alignment of the teeth are related
- To understand how muscle forces affect the alignment of the teeth
- To understand what the curve of Spee, the curve of Wilson, and the sphere of Monson are
- To understand in what way the teeth are aligned vertically—maxillary to mandibular
- To understand what centric occlusion is
- To understand the meaning of overjet, overbite, crossbite, and open bite, and to have some idea of how they occur
- To know and identify the three occlusal classifications
- To understand the relationship that exists between the teeth during lateral excursive movements

POSITION AND SEQUENCE OF ERUPTION

In the preceding chapter we studied the eruption patterns of teeth. The eruption schedule helps permanent teeth emerge in their proper position. The loss of certain deciduous teeth at the particular times allows the permanent teeth to move into key positions.

What about the deciduous teeth? What enables them to take their position for alignment? When we look at the deciduous teeth, they not only appear in a certain position that is normal for each tooth but also are arranged in a row, which is referred to as being in alignment.

Normally, the eruption schedule helps the deciduous teeth to take their proper position. For example, the central incisors come into position anterior to the lateral incisors because the centrals erupt before the lateral incisors. Facial development and growth encourages the teeth to erupt properly. The anterior teeth are not covered by as much bone, and therefore the tooth buds begin their formation earlier than those of the posterior teeth; the result is that most of the anterior teeth erupt before the posterior teeth. Some posterior teeth must actually wait until growth has occurred in the mandible because they are initially trapped under the **ramus of the mandible.** Thus the eruption pattern, facial development, and the sequence in which tooth buds begin forming all contribute to the eventual relationship of the teeth and jaws.

The development of **occlusion** begins with the eruption of the primary teeth (see Fig. 24-7, *A*). Usually the first teeth to erupt are the central incisors, with the mandibular teeth erupting slightly before the maxillary. The eruption of the lateral incisors, which occurs next, follows the same sequence.

At 16 months the primary molars erupt—an important event because the primary molars establish the vertical height of the primary occlusion. Primary molars also establish **intercuspation,** the mesial-distal and buccal-lingual relationships that determine how the upper teeth will touch, hit, and interlock with the lower teeth. The upper primary molars also help establish the anteroposterior (mesial-distal) relationship of the remaining deciduous teeth because their presence prompts the canines and second deciduous molars to erupt around them.

The primary dentition, which is usually complete by about 2½ years of age, erupts in a more upright position than secondary teeth replacements. The average overjet of primary teeth is 3.0 mm, and the average overbite is 2.5 mm. The primary occlusion has one of three possible anteroposterior molar relationships called steps or planes. The majority of children has a **mesial step** between the distal surfaces of the second primary molars (Fig. 25-1, *A*). The mandibular

molars are situated more mesially than their maxillary counterparts, thereby forming a mesial step. A smaller but still large group of children exhibits a **flush terminal plane,** with the distal surfaces of the deciduous second molars even with each other (Fig. 25-1, *B*). A still smaller minority has a **distal step** (Fig. 25-1, *C*). How would you describe a distal step in comparison with a mesial step or flush terminal plane? Note the large diastema or space in the mandibular arch between the canine and first molar.

As a child grows in height and weight, so too do the jaws. This growth of the mandible and maxilla results in horizontal and vertical growth of the dental arches. The teeth, however, remain the same size. Thus as the arches grow, spaces, called **diastemas,** form between the teeth. The largest spaces are often found mesial to the maxillary primary canines and distal to the mandibular canines. These spaces are called **primate spaces,** and although not always present, they are characteristic of all primates, including man (Fig. 25-2). As growth continues, diastemas also develop between the incisors.

DEVELOPMENT OF THE MESIAL STEP

The permanent molars erupt, and eventually touch the distal surfaces of the deciduous molars. As the permanent molars push up against the deciduous molars, they cause a chain reaction that pushes all of the spaces between the teeth closed. A mesial step occurs in the majority of individuals because closing the primary space allows room for the lower molars to move mesially.

A mesial step is further enhanced as the deciduous molars exfoliate and are replaced by the narrower permanent premolars. Extra space, called **leeway space,** is gained from this exchange of the second premolars. The earlier eruption cycle of the mandibular teeth allows them to capitalize on this exchange before the maxillary teeth, which further helps establish the mesial step (Fig. 25-3).

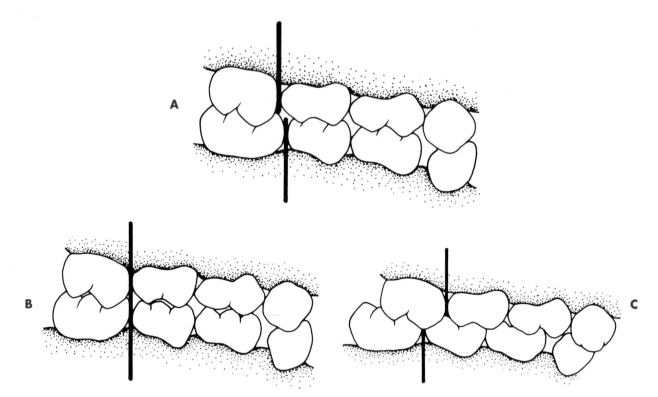

FIG. 25-1.   The relationships of the first permanent molars to each other are what determine step or plane. **A,** Mesial step. **B,** Flush terminal plane. **C,** Distal step.

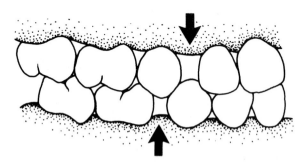

FIG. 25-2.   Primate spaces. These spaces occur in primary dentition. In the maxillary arch they are anterior to the canines. In the mandibular arch they are distal to the canines.

Finally the heads of the condyles of the mandible continue to grow later than the maxilla, allowing even further mesial mandibular advancement and ensuring in most instances a mesial step heading the patient toward a class I relationship. Further growth of the condyle head could push the patient into an extreme mesial step resulting in a class III relationship. A class II relationship could result if the mandible does not continue to grow or if the maxilla outgrows the mandible. It is possible for this type of relationship to occur on just one side while the other side maintains a class I relationship.

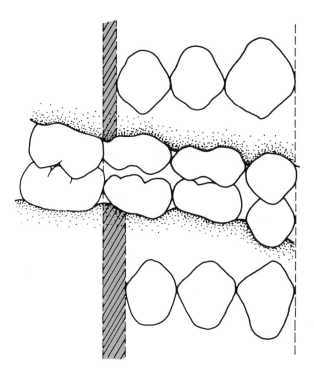

FIG. 25-3. Leeway space is extra space that deciduous canines and molars occupy to help save room for their permanent successors. These permanent teeth take up less space. The difference between the space deciduous teeth take up and that of their permanent replacements is called leeway space.

A deep bite could result if the condyle head is displaced distally in the glenoid fossa, if the posterior teeth do not erupt enough, if the muscles of mastication are so hyperactive that they prevent the eruption of the posterior teeth, or if the condyle grows at an angle that causes the jaw to develop in a less mesial direction.

The development of the occlusion is further influenced by hereditary factors such as congenitally missing teeth, impacted teeth, or the size and shape of muscle and bone. Controllable factors that also affect occlusal development include the premature loss of deciduous teeth, de-cayed teeth that were not restored, and harmful habits.

HORIZONTAL ALIGNMENT

After the teeth erupt into the oral cavity, the tongue acts as a huge internal force, pushing the teeth toward the lips and cheeks. Conversely, resistance from the muscles that form the cheeks and lips is the controlling factor that prevents the teeth from moving too far facially. The balance or relative equilibrium between the tongue and the facial muscles allows the teeth to be brought into proper alignment and to be maintained in their proper positions once they have erupted.

If this balance of forces is disturbed, a **malocclusion,** or an abnormal alignment of the teeth within the dental arches, can result. Abnormal forward thrusting of the tongue against the anterior teeth can cause such an imbalanced state (Fig. 25-4). Tongue thrusting causes the maxillary anterior teeth to **protrude** labially out of the mouth. This is especially true if there is an underdeveloped upper lip along with the tongue thrust.

An opposite situation can also occur if the lower lip is overdeveloped; the **retrusion** of the lower anterior teeth occurs. The patient is constantly tightening the lower lip against the lower anterior teeth. These lip muscles are so strong that the lower teeth will be pushed back into the mouth by this overdeveloped lower lip.

The lip, tongue, and cheek muscles and their relationship to one another are not the only factors that determine the alignment of the teeth. The intercuspation of the teeth helps prevent tooth deviations in a buccal or lingual direction. The maxillary posterior teeth have a buccal and a lingual cusp, and when the jaws are closed, the buccal cusps of the mandibular posterior teeth are interlocked between the buccal and lingual cusps of the maxillary teeth. This interlocking is similar to the interlocking of two gears.

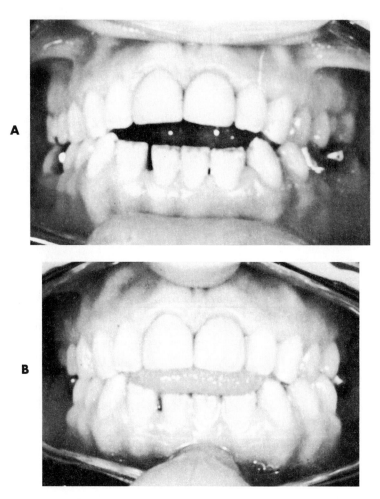

FIG. 25-4. Open bite resulting from tongue thrusting. A, Posterior teeth touch when jaws are closed, but space exists between anterior teeth. B, During swallowing, tongue closes space. (From Ross IF: *Occlusion: a concept for the clinician,* St Louis, 1970, Mosby.)

The alignment of previously erupted teeth in turn affects the alignment of successive teeth. Adequate space between teeth allows for complete and unhindered eruption of more teeth. If a tooth does not have room enough to erupt, it will deflect off the obstructing tooth and erupt out of alignment. It could also be blocked entirely by the obstruction and never erupt.

Other factors also influence the alignment of teeth. Mesial drift could account for the closure or loss of space necessary for tooth eruption. The size and shape of the jaws, the shape of the teeth, and the amount of lingual convergence of each tooth affect not only the alignment of the teeth but also the curvature of the dental arch and the spacing necessary for incoming teeth.

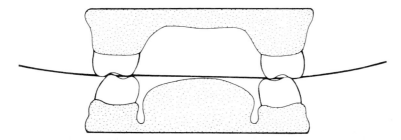

FIG. 25-5.   Curve of Wilson.

CURVE OF SPEE, CURVE OF WILSON, AND SPHERE OF MONSON

Usually the buccal cusp tips of posterior teeth, seen in alignment from a lateral view (see Fig. 24-8), conform to a fairly even curve in an anterior to posterior direction. This curve is known as the **curve of Spee.**

An occlusal curve exists for posterior teeth in a direction from right to left as seen from a posterior view (Fig. 25-5). This transverse occlusal curve is called the **curve of Wilson.**

The occlusal surfaces of the natural dentition are thought to be aligned in such a way that a spherical curve 8 inches in diameter could rest on the buccal cusp tips of the mandibular posterior teeth. The curves of Wilson and Spee, when studied simultaneously in three-dimensional alignment, demonstrate an illusion of the cusp tips of the mandibular posterior teeth resting on a sphere known as the **sphere of Monson** (Fig. 25-6). This theory has yet to be proved.

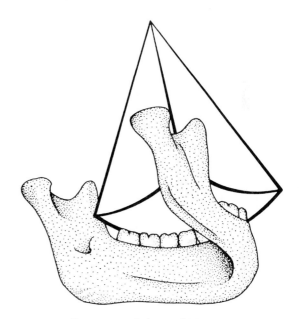

FIG. 25-6.   Sphere of Monson.

VERTICAL ALIGNMENT

We tend to think of the teeth as being vertically straight, but this is not true. The teeth are not positioned straight up and down in the mouth. As we have seen, the mandibular posterior teeth have a tendency to tip their crowns lingually and their roots laterally (Fig. 25-7). The maxillary posterior teeth tend to keep the crown straighter but with a slight buccal inclination, as well as a lingual inclination of the root (Fig. 25-8). From a lateral view, we can see that all the teeth, maxillary and mandibular, anterior and posterior, show a slight mesial inclination, with the possible exception of the maxillary third molar. Notice that the anterior teeth (Figs. 25-9 and 25-10) have a slight labial protrusion (a condition of being tipped forward), and from a frontal view their crowns seem to incline laterally. In other words, the anterior teeth tip out to

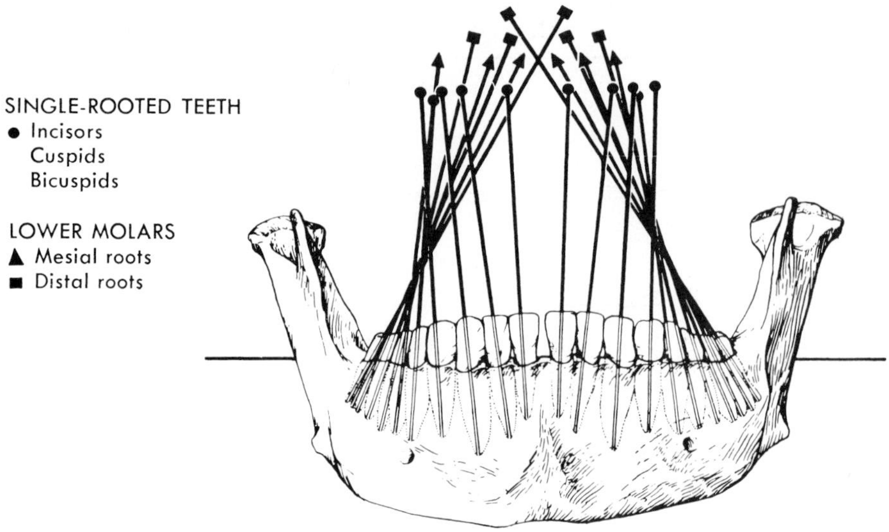

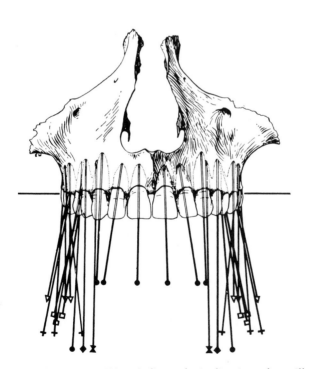

SINGLE-ROOTED TEETH
● Incisors
  Cuspids
  Bicuspids

LOWER MOLARS
▲ Mesial roots
■ Distal roots

FIG. 25-7.   Lines indicate the angle of inclination of teeth in relation to the mandible. (From Kraus BS, Jordon RE, Abrams L: *Dental anatomy and occlusion,* Baltimore, 1969, Williams & Wilkins Co.)

SINGLE-ROOTED TEETH
● Incisors
  Cuspids
  Upper second premolars

FIRST PREMOLAR
◆ Buccal roots
✗ Palatal roots

UPPER MOLARS
▽ Mesiobuccal roots
✛ Distobuccal roots
◻ Palatal roots

FIG. 25-8.   Lines indicate the inclination of maxillary teeth in relation to the maxillae. (From Kraus BS, Jordon RE, Abrams L: *Dental anatomy and occlusion,* Baltimore, 1969, Williams & Wilkins Co.)

SINGLE-ROOTED TEETH
- Incisors
  Cuspids
  Upper second premolars

FIRST PREMOLAR
- ◆ Buccal roots
- ✗ Palatal roots

UPPER MOLARS
- ▽ Mesiobuccal roots
- ✦ Distobuccal roots
- ◻ Palatal roots

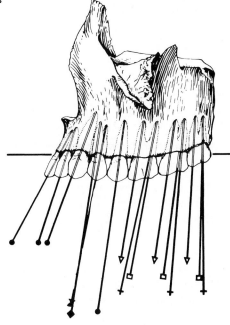

FIG. 25-9. A lateral view of the inclination of maxillary teeth. (From Kraus BS, Jordon RE, Abrams L: *Dental anatomy and occlusion*, Baltimore, 1969, Williams & Wilkins Co.)

SINGLE-ROOTED TEETH
- Incisors
  Cuspids
  Bicuspids

LOWER MOLARS
- ▲ Mesial roots
- ■ Distal roots

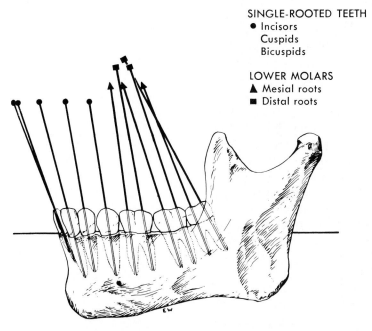

FIG. 25-10. A lateral view of the inclination of mandibular teeth. (From Kraus BS, Jordon RE, Abrams L: *Dental anatomy and occlusion*, Baltimore, 1969, Williams & Wilkins Co.)

the side and toward the front (see Figs. 25-7 and 25-8).

OCCLUSION

Occlusion is the term used to describe the relationship of the mandibular and maxillary teeth when the teeth are closed together or during excursive movements when the teeth are touching. When the jaws are completely closed together, there are two possible relationships. Either there is a relationship of the upper jaw to the lower jaw (centric relation) or a relationship of the upper teeth to the lower teeth (centric occlusion).

Centric Relation

Centric relation refers to the position of the mandible relative to the maxillae and is determined by the maximum contraction of the muscles of the jaw. This relationship of the mandible to the maxillae occurs during strong muscle contractions such as swallowing. It is the most stable and most posterior position that affords the strongest muscle contractions. It is a relationship of bone to bone brought about by allowing the muscles to contract in their most natural posture to their most comfortable and effective position. This posture does not have anything to do with the interdigitation of the teeth. Indeed, it may not be the position that allows the greatest intercuspation of the teeth.

Centric relation is defined as the most retruded relationship of the mandible to the maxillae when the condyles of the temporal mandibular joint are in their most upward, backward, and unstrained position in the glenoid fossae. It is a relationship also of the structural features of the temporal mandibular joint.

To experience centric relation, let your head tip as far back as possible and gently close your teeth together. Let your mandible go back as far as possible. You will notice this is different than your **habitual occlusion.** If you tip your head forward and close your teeth together as you

usually do, this is your centric occlusion. Is your mandible farther forward in your habitual centric occlusion or in your centric relation?

Centric Occlusion

Centric occlusion also refers to a position when the jaws are closed, but this position is de-

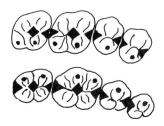

FIG. 25-11. Centric relation. Contacting marginal ridge areas are indicated by triangles, central fossae by diamonds, and occluding cusp tips by circles. The buccal cusp tips of the mandibular teeth contact the maxillary marginal ridges and the central fossae of the maxillary molars. The lingual cusp tips of the maxillary teeth contact the marginal ridges and central fossae of the mandibular molars.

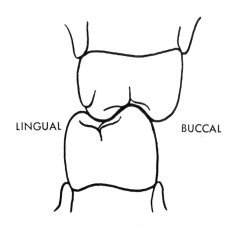

FIG. 25-12. Mesial view of the left first molars. In centric relation, teeth interconnect to their greatest potential. (From Ross IF: *Occlusion: a concept for the clinician,* St Louis, 1970, Mosby.)

termined by the way the teeth fit together. It is the jaw position that affords the greatest interdigitation of the teeth. It is related to tooth occlusion and not determined by muscle or bone. It is the habitual way that the teeth come together. Centric occlusion is sometimes called **acquired centric occlusion,** habitual occlusion, **convenience occlusion,** or **intercuspal position (ICP).** This is the way your teeth fit together out of habit without planning or forethought. With the jaws closed, the occlusal surfaces of the maxillary teeth touch the occlusal surfaces of the mandibular teeth. The lingual cusps of the maxillary premolars and molars rest in the deepest parts of the occlusal sulci of the mandibular premolars and molars, and the buccal cusps of the mandibular premolars and molars rest in the deepest parts of the sulci of the maxillary premolars and molars (Figs. 25-11 and 25-12).

When the jaws are closed in centric occlusion, the cusps of the maxillary teeth overlap the cusps of the mandibular teeth so that the maxillary teeth are facial to the mandibular teeth. Although the cusps of the maxillary teeth do not directly touch the cusps of the mandibular teeth on closure of the jaw, it is possible for the cusps to come into contact when the mandible slides from side to side. Notice that the maxillary cusps are located facial to the mandibular cusps.

The amount of facial horizontal overlap of the maxillary teeth is called an **overjet.** Notice in Fig. 25-13 that the maxillary incisors are facial to the mandibular incisors. Line A represents the amount of horizontal overlap, or overjet.

In Fig. 25-14 notice that the maxillary incisors also vertically overlap the mandibular incisors. Line A indicates the amount of vertical overlap or **overbite.** Overbite is the extension of the incisal edges of the maxillary anterior teeth below the incisal edges of the mandibular anterior teeth in a vertical direction (Fig. 25-15).

If one or more teeth in the mandibular arch are located facial to their maxillary counterparts,

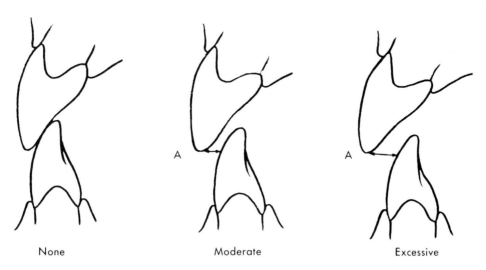

None   Moderate   Excessive

FIG. 25-13. Moderate and slight overbite. Line *A* indicates the difference in overbite; the amount of overjet is same in both examples. (From Ross IF: *Occlusion: a concept for the clinician,* St Louis, 1970, Mosby.)

Moderate   Slight

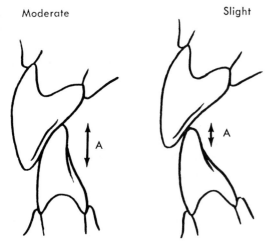

FIG. 25-14.   Overjet.

a condition known as **crossbite** occurs. Fig.25-16 illustrates a mandibular right first molar in cross-bite. Notice that the buccal cusp of the mandibular molar is located facial to the buccal cusp of the maxillary molar. A crossbite condition can exist between any number of teeth. It can be caused by a loss of space in the deciduous arch such that the maxillary second premolar, which is one of the last teeth to replace a deciduous tooth, might be blocked out to the lingual side of the other maxillary teeth. Then, if the lower premolar erupted normally, a maxillary crossbite of the second premolar could occur. A crossbite of all the mandibular teeth can occur if there is a disease that causes the patient's mandible but not the maxillae to continue growing. Such a condition is **acromegaly.** In this disease, growth hormone causes the mandible to grow faster than the maxilla. As a result, the mandib-

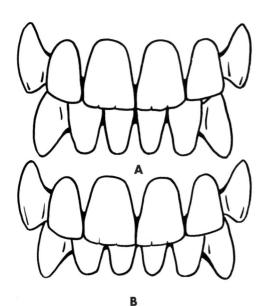

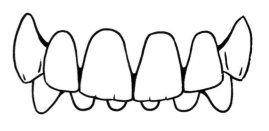

FIG. 25-15.   **A,** Slight overbite. **B,** Moderate overbite. **C,** Excessive overbite. (From Ross IF: *Occlusion: a concept for the clinician,* St Louis, 1970, Mosby.)

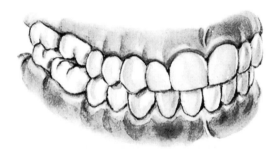

FIG. 25-16.   Posterior crossbite of right first molars. (From Massler M, Schour I: *Atlas of the mouth in health and disease,* ed 2, Chicago, 1975, American Dental Association.)

ular teeth are eventually positioned in crossbite with the maxillary teeth.

An even more common cause of crossbite can also occur if the maxillae bones do not grow in proportion to the mandible. When this happens the maxillary teeth are bilaterally in crossbite or edge to edge with the mandibular teeth. In most of these situations the patient forces their teeth to one side in order to close completely together as in centric occlusion. The other side displays full crossbite of most or all of the posterior teeth on that side. The midline of the anterior teeth is off, and the maxillary and mandibular midlines do not line up because the patient is forcing the mandible to one side to get a more functional bite.

OPEN BITE

When the teeth are in centric occlusion, the maxillary and mandibular teeth should touch each other. The occlusal surfaces of the posterior teeth should touch, and the anterior teeth should touch in such a way that the incisal edges of the mandibular anterior teeth almost or just barely touch the lingual surfaces of the maxillary anterior teeth. If the anterior teeth do not touch but are widely separated when in centric occlusion, the condition known as **open bite** exists. An open bite exists when the anterior teeth of the maxillary

arch do not overlap the mandibular teeth in a vertical direction. Such a condition can be caused by either a thumb-sucking or a tongue-thrusting habit. In either situation a powerful force is exerted against the anterior teeth when the jaws close. In thumb-sucking the patient's thumb or fingers rest between the maxillary and mandibular anterior teeth, thereby preventing the teeth from touching each other. Thus a force is exerted that pushes the anterior teeth back into the bone and prevents them from erupting. The outcome is a wide separation of the anterior teeth when the jaws close (see Fig. 25-4).

A tongue-thrusting habit places the tongue between the anterior teeth every time the patient swallows. The act of swallowing requires the jaws to come together and the lips to close, which seals off air spaces and results in a negative pressure. If the patient has poor tongue placement or if open spaces exist between the front teeth, the following sequence occurs. First the patient places the tongue against these open spaces or against the anterior teeth. When the patient swallows, closing the jaws, the tongue pushes against the anterior teeth. The result is a protrusion of the maxillary anterior teeth, with the pressure preventing the teeth from erupting normally. In the normally developed swallowing pattern this situation is prevented because the tongue is placed against the roof of the mouth, not against the teeth. When the tongue thrusts during jaw closure, it exerts pressure on the palate rather than on the teeth.

OCCLUSAL CLASSIFICATION

There are two basic classifications of occlusion. The first is based on the relationship of the bone of the maxilla to the bone of the mandible. This system, because it is related to the bones, is referred to as the **skeletal classification.** The second system is based on the relationship of the teeth of the mandible to the teeth of the maxilla. It is called the **dental classification** because it is concerned with the teeth.

A   **B**

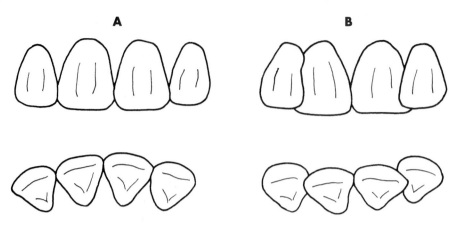

FIG. 25-17.   **A,** Class II, division I—maxillary incisors are in good alignment. **B,** Class II, division II—maxillary central incisors are retruded lingually behind the lateral incisors.

The skeletal classification is divided into three classes of relationship (Figs. 25-17 and 25-18).

Class I—The maxilla and mandible are in normal relationship to each other.

Class II—The mandible is retruded and thus retrognathic. The mandible has a distal relationship with the maxilla.

Class III—The mandible is protruded and thus prognathic. The mandible has a mesial relationship with the maxilla.

The dental classification is based on the relationship of the teeth. Usually the canines or the first permanent molars are used in dental classifications.

Angle's classification system is the most popular dental classification system in use today. His system is based primarily on the relationship of the permanent first molars to each other and to a lesser degree on the relationship of the permanent canines to each other. In centric occlusion there are three relationships that can exist between the first molars. In the normal relationship the maxillary first molar is slightly posterior to the mandibular first molar. The mesiobuccal cusp of the maxillary first molar is directly in line with the buccal groove of the mandibular first molar. Such a relationship is called a **class I occlusal relationship** or a **neutroclusion** (Fig. 25-19 (also see Fig. 25-18, *A*)).

A **class II occlusal relationship** or a **distoclusion** exists when the maxillary first molar is even with or anterior to the mandibular first molar. In this relationship the buccal groove of the mandibular first molar is posterior to the mesiobuccal cusp of the maxillary first molar (Fig. 25-20). Could such a relationship be present if the maxillary teeth protruded or if the mandibular teeth retruded?

There are two separate class II divisions. Class II, division I occurs when the permanent first molars are in class II and the permanent maxillary central incisors are in their normal, slightly protruded position (see Figs. 25-17, *A,* 25-18, *B,* 25-19, and 25-20). Class II, division II occurs when the permanent first molars are in class II relationship and the permanent maxillary central incisors are retruded and inclined lingually (see Figs. 25-17, *B,* 25-18, *C,* 25-19, and 25-20).

A class II, division II relationship frequently occurs when the following scenario is present:

1. Deep overbite
2. Crowded maxillary anteriors

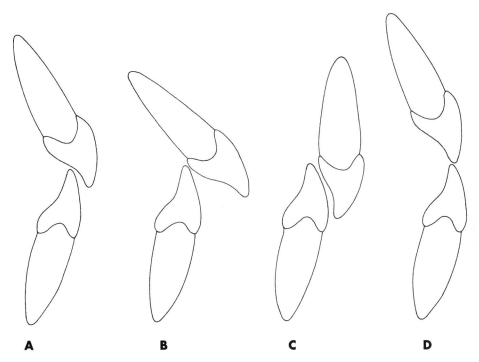

FIG. 25-18. Types of malocclusion. **A,** Class I. **B,** Class II, division I, severe overjet, deep overbite. **C,** Class II, division II, deep overbite, no overjet. **D,** Class III, edge-to-edge maxillary central even to or lingual to lower central.

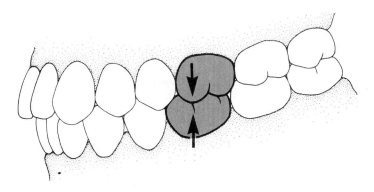

FIG. 25-19. Class I occlusal relationship.

3. Normal overjet

4. Excessive masseter muscle development

A **class III occlusal relationship** or a **mesiocclusion** exists when the buccal groove of the mandibular first molar is more anterior than normal to the mesiobuccal cusp of the maxillary first molar (Fig. 25-21) (also see Fig. 25-18, *D*). This relationship would be present if the maxillary teeth retruded or if the mandibular teeth protruded.

It is possible for both sides of the mandible to be in different classes.

The canines can be used in a dental classification system as follows:

Class I—The distal surface of the mandibular canine is within one premolar's width of the mesial surface of the maxillary canine.

Class II—The distal surface of the mandibular canine is distal to the mesial surface of the maxillary canine by a width of at least one premolar.

Class III—The distal surface of the mandibular canine is mesial to the mesial surface of

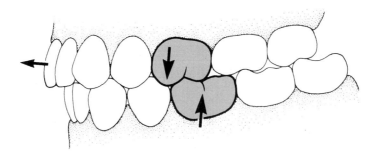

FIG. 25-20.   Class II, division I occlusal relationship.

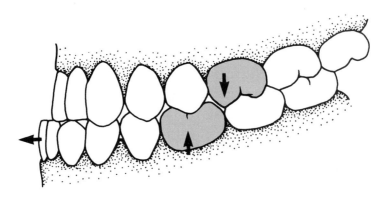

FIG. 25-21.   Class III occlusal relationship.

a maxillary canine by at least a width of one premolar.

Another form of dental classification involves the incisor relationships (see Fig. 25-18).

Class I—The mandibular incisors occlude with or lie directly below the middle of the lingual surfaces of the maxillary incisors (see Fig. 25-17).

Class II—The incisal margins of the mandibular incisors lie behind the middle part of the lingual surfaces of the maxillary incisors. Division I means that the maxillary centrals (and possibly laterals) are protruded labially. Division II means that the maxillary centrals only have their incisal edges tipped more lingually and the maxillary centrals may be retruded lingually to the laterals (see Fig. 25-18, *B* and *C*).

Class III—The incisal margins of the mandibular incisors lie in front of the middle of the lingual surface of the maxillary incisors (see Fig. 25-18, *D*).

LATERAL MANDIBULAR GLIDE (LATERAL EXCURSION)

In **lateral excursion** the mandible moves toward the right or left side. The side to which the mandible moves is referred to as the **working side,** and the other side is referred to as the **nonworking side** when no teeth are contacting on this side. When working with artificial teeth as in denture construction, this nonworking side is referred to as the **balancing side.** When making dentures it is important to have both sides continue to contact and touch even in side movements. This keeps the denture balanced and avoids tipping. Natural teeth do not need to balance, and therefore the nonworking side may or may not be in contact (Fig. 25-22). When teeth are contacting on the nonworking side, it is called the balancing side.

A working-side contact exists when the mandible is moved to one side, with buccal cusps of the maxillary and mandibular teeth touching each other and the lingual cusps directly over each other on the same side to which the mandible moved. If you slide your lower jaw to the right, the working side is on the right.

A balancing side contact occurs on the opposite side that the jaw moves toward. If you move the lower jaw to the right, a balancing side contact would exist if you still hit on the left posterior side.

In lateral mandibular glide, only a few pairs of interlocking cusps make occlusal contact. The canines carry the bulk of the contact. This is referred to as a **canine rise** because the mandibular canine opens the bite by gliding down the lingual surface of the maxillary canine. In lateral excursion the last two teeth to touch, in an almost cusp tip-to-cusp tip arrangement, should be the canines. If the lateral glide is to the right, the last two teeth to touch should be the right canines.

It is common to have the premolars occluding as well as the canines in lateral excursion. When the premolars also occlude during lateral excursion it is called **group function.** The canines should still be the dominant occluding teeth; the premolars only assist through part of the lateral slide.

In natural dentition the cusps on the nonworking side rarely touch at all. In fact, having balancing side interferences during lateral excursion can have detrimental effects on the temporomandibular jaw joint. The reverse is true in artificial dentition where light balancing contact

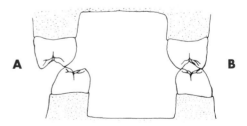

FIG. 25-22. Lateral excursion. **A,** Balancing side. **B,** Working side.

is needed to prevent the denture from dislodging. Dividing the forces equally in artificial teeth helps prevent the dentures from tipping or displacing during lateral movement of the jaw. Heavy balancing side interferences are still to be avoided. Most dentures do tip slightly during side excursions and this seems to dissipate the lateral forces enough to prevent the jaw joint problems seen in natural dentition.

PROTRUSION

Protrusion is when the mandible moves forward from centric occlusion. In protrusion the only teeth that should touch are the anterior teeth. The mandibular anterior four incisors should glide across the maxillary four incisors as the mandible moves forward. No other teeth except possibly the canines may touch, and then only slightly. No posterior teeth should touch in a mandibular protrusive movement (see Fig. 25-21).

PREMATURE CONTACT

When the jaw closes, all of the posterior teeth should come into contact at the same time. If one tooth hits ever so slightly more than the others, it becomes an interference and bears more force than the others. It is called a **premature contact.** The anterior incisors may also hit but not harder than the posteriors. If the anteriors do hit in centric occlusion, it is called **anterior coupling.**

A premature contact will cause the jaw to deflect before allowing the rest of the teeth to occlude. If the path of the lower jaw movement deflects from its true course, the temporomandibular jaw joint must be put into a stretched or abnormal position, which can cause the following results.

1. The temporomandibular joint undergoes abnormal stress, causing damage to the ligaments or to the muscles of the joint. Often the jaw joint affected is the one from the opposite side of the mouth that has the premature contact.

2. The muscles that act as **antagonists** to the muscles of mastication become tired, sore, and tender if one set of muscles is forced to be overexerted because of a premature contact. Eventually that set of muscles exhibits symptoms of overutilization.

3. The tooth that is hitting prematurely becomes sensitive to percussion and tender during chewing. It may become mobile, and x-ray examination may reveal a widening of the periodontal ligament.

4. The responsible tooth may become cracked or broken. Even under the normal stress of occlusion, when all of the teeth are hitting at the same time, the occluding cusps undergo a contact pressure of 300 pounds per square inch. In premature contact the force extended to the offending cusp could be thousands of pounds per square inch.

FUNDAMENTALS OF IDEAL OCCLUSION IN PERMANENT DENTITION

Ideal occlusion is the result of the maxillary bones and the mandibular bone in proper harmony with each other. The condyles of the mandible are in their most favorable location within the glenoid fossae. At the same time the muscles of the face and jaws must be in balance with each other and with the above-mentioned bones. Finally, the occlusion of the teeth and how they interlock is most stable when all of the above-mentioned bones, muscles, and joints are synchronized to be in balance and harmony with one another. Is ideal occlusion a matter of luck, wishful thinking, or a dream? No, it actually happens. The function of the bones, muscles, and joints helps guide and balance the other structures until a harmony of forces results in a balanced occlusion, not by accident but rather by the design, function, and symmetry of these structures as they interrelate. When these all occur in a well-balanced, harmonious environment, a well-balanced, harmonious occlusion results.

E. H. Angle found that the most ideal occlusion is a class I occlusion. The class I molar relationship exists when the mesiobuccal cusps of the first permanent molar fall within the groove between the mesiobuccal and middle buccal cusps of the lower first molar. A class I canine relationship exists when the distal surface of the mandibular canine is within one premolar's width of the mesial surface of the maxillary canine. The lower canine should then be positioned in the embrasure located between the upper canine and the upper lateral incisor.

In the ideal occlusion the occlusal plane is almost flat with a slight curve of Spee, which deepens with age. The teeth have good, tight proximal contacts with no spaces between teeth. There are no rotated teeth, and the upper and lower arches are symmetrical and well formed. All of the crowns of the teeth are tipped slightly mesially, with the exception of the upper third molar. The maxillary third molar is almost straight up and down with a slight distal inclination. The crown inclination labiolingually and buccolingually is such that the incisors flair labially and the rest of the teeth flair lingually. Finally, the maxillary first molar is tipped mesially so that it touches the mandibular first and second molars. This is called a **stolarized molar,** and in the ideal occlusion the distal marginal ridge of the permanent maxillary first molar touches the mesial marginal ridge of the permanent mandibular second molar as well as the middle of the mandibular first molar (Fig. 25-23).

Because all humans are different, only a few experience ideal occlusion. However, it is easier to discover malocclusions when one is familiar with the ideal. It is also helpful to study the skeletons of our ancestors to discover how our occlusion developed. In the 1930s Dr. P.R. Begg studied more than 800 Australian aboriginal skulls. He noted that while some class II and class III malocclusions occurred, there were proportionately fewer in Australian aboriginal

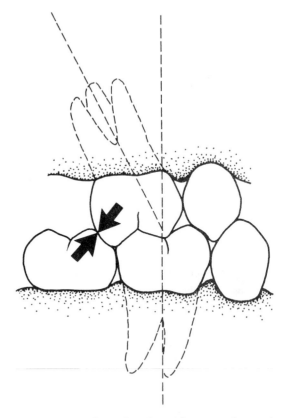

Fig. 25-23. Stolarized molars. The upper first molar is tipped forward so its distal marginal ridge touches the mesial marginal ridge of the lower second molar and the middle of the mandibular first molar. To do this the upper molar must have a mesial tip that allows its distal marginal ridge to come further occlusally than its mesial marginal ridge.

skulls than in modern humans, and he postulated that this occurred for two reasons: first, there were far fewer malocclusions because of overcrowding or excess tooth size; and second, some of the more severe anomalies were so detrimental to Stone Age man that their incidence was kept relatively low by natural selection, which limited survival rates.

Begg noted that Stone Age people had extensive attrition of their teeth. He concluded that the diet of primitive aborigines was abrasive enough to wear down not only the occluding surfaces but the interproximal surfaces of the teeth as well. There was an average of 1 mm of wear on the proximal surfaces of each tooth, which accumulated to 7.5 mm of wear per arch. Through mesial drift the posterior teeth took advantage of this wear and closed the arch length, and the extra space provided by interproximal wear allowed the third molars additional arch space to erupt.

Begg surmised that there seemed to be an adaptive mechanism that allowed the mandible to move anteriorly. As the incisors were worn down, the mandible moved forward to maintain an edge-to-edge bite. This enabled the posterior teeth to occlude with the jaw in an anterior position with no overjet or overbite. The occlusal cusps were worn flat so the jaw could have full occlusion in class I or in protrusive movement.

This occlusal wear shortened the crown length, but the teeth erupted to compensate for the loss of vertical height. The supraeruptive forces of the teeth compensated for this occlusal wear just as mesial drift took advantage of the opportunity to close the spaces left from interproximal wear. The dentition of primitive people had extreme occlusal wear, which led to the shortening of the anatomic crowns and the preservation of the vertical bite via supraeruption.

The vast majority of Stone Age skulls studied by Begg had class I occlusions, with only 12% having class II, division I occlusions; 1% having class II, division II occlusions; and only 3% having class III occlusions. According to Begg, "Class II, division II and class III malocclusions are far more serious afflictions physically for Stone Age man than they are for civilized man. This is because of the harm that these two forms of malocclusion do to Stone Age man by interfering with his proper masticatory function and by producing severe dental disease."

In Stone Age people the deep incisor overbite of class II, division II malocclusion interfered with lateral movement of the lower teeth and jaw. This was a less effective form of mastication of food and required more effort and time. In addition, the incisors would undergo severe attrition faster because the maxillary incisors were inclined lingually, which caused the incisors to abscess when the pulps were exposed. The resulting bacterial infections could have adversely affected survival rates (Fig. 25-24). The extreme early wear of the incisors in class III could have also resulted in lower survival rates for the same reason (Fig. 25-25).

According to Begg then, the survival of our ancestors was affected by the class of dental occlusion they possessed. More class I occlusions were successfully passed on through genetics. This was the result of attrition rather than jaw placement, temporomandibular joint structure, or muscle-to-bone relationships.

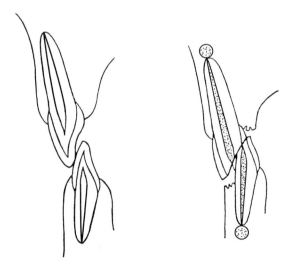

FIG. 25-24. Incisal wear, such as that seen in Stone Age human's attritional class II, division II malocclusion, may cause exposure and death of the tooth pulp. (From Begg PR, Kesling PC: *Begg orthodontic theory and technique,* Philadelphia, 1977, WB Saunders.)

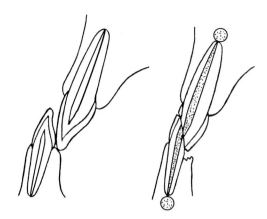

FIG. 25-25. Incisal wear, such as that seen in Stone Age human's attritional class III malocclusion, may cause pulp exposure. (From Begg PR, Kesling PC: *Begg orthodontic theory and technique*, Philadelphia, 1977, WB Saunders.)

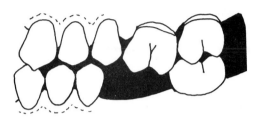

FIG. 25-26. Premature occlusal contact of the maxillary first molar. To avoid premature occlusal contact, the mandible moves backward during closing.

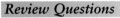

Review Questions

1. What affects the alignment of the teeth?
2. Which muscle forces affect the alignment of the teeth?
3. What is the difference between the curve of Spee and the curve of Wilson?
4. Define the following terms:
    a. open bite
    b. overbite
    c. overjet
    d. centric occlusion
    e. working side
    f. balancing side
5. Which occlusal classification has the distal surface of the mandibular canine distal to the mesial surface of the maxillary canine by a width of at least one premolar?
6. Which occlusal classification is Fig. 25-26?
7. What is meant by mesial step?

8. If an occlusion with a mesial step proceeds without problems, which of the following will most likely result?
    a. class I
    b. class II
    c. class III
    d. distal step
9. Which factors influence occlusion?
    a. heredity
    b. unrestored deciduous decayed molars
    c. impacted deciduous teeth
    d. congenitally missing teeth
    e. growth of the condyles
    f. eruption sequence of teeth
    g. leeway space
    h. primate space
10. Outline the elements of the ideal occlusion.
11. Outline some of the differentiating features of the occlusion of primitive people.
12. What marks the beginning of the development of occlusion?
13. What determines the height of the primary occlusion?
14. Define or explain the term *intercuspation*.
15. Which molar relationship is more common in children: the flush terminal plane or the distal step?

CHAPTER 26

DENTAL ANOMALIES

OBJECTIVES
- To define dental anomaly
- To discuss intrinsic factors
- To discuss extrinsic factors
- To discuss the difference between hereditary and congenital factors
- To define the various anomalies listed in this chapter

A N ANOMALY is defined as something that is noticeably different or that deviates from the ordinary or normal. Dental anomalies are deviations of dental tissue origin and therefore are derived from the dental tissues enamel, dentin, or cementum. Anomalies can be extreme variations or just slight deviations. They can be caused by a multitude of things or by just one small variation in the environment.

Some abnormalities result from **intrinsic** factors, such as heredity, metabolic dysfunction, or mutations; other causes are more **extrinsic,** such as physical or chemical trauma, biologic agents, nutritional deficiencies, stress, habits, or environmental conditions. In many instances anomalies result from a combination of intrinsic and extrinsic factors.

If a condition occurs because of an individual's genetic makeup, the condition is termed **hereditary.** If the condition occurs at or before birth, it is termed **congenital.** A congenital condition is sometimes the result of heredity, and sometimes a hereditary condition does not become evident until years after birth. If a condition exhibits some evidence of an in-herited tendency but such evidence is incon-clusive, it is often referred to as a **familial tendency.** If a condition results during the formation and development of a dental structure, it is referred to as a *developmental anomaly.*

CLASSIFICATION OF DENTAL ANOMALIES

Anomalies resulting in a variation in the size of teeth are called **macrodontia,** which is when teeth are too large, (Fig. 26-1) and **microdontia,** which is when teeth are too small (Fig. 26-2).

Anomalies resulting in a variation in the number of teeth are **hyperdontia** (multiple or extra teeth) (Fig. 26-3) and **anodontia** (too few teeth) (Fig. 26-4). Total anodontia exists if no teeth are present at all, and partial anodontia, if less than the normal number of teeth are present. True anodontia is the congenital absence of teeth. It may involve the permanent dentition, the primary dentition, or both. If the primary teeth are congenitally missing, their permanent replacements will also be absent.

The most commonly missing permanent teeth are the third molars, and the maxillary thirds are absent more often than the mandibular. The next most likely teeth to be missing are the permanent maxillary lateral incisors. Between 1% and 2% of the population are missing at least one permanent maxillary lateral incisor. The third most frequently missing tooth is the permanent mandibular second premolar. About 1% of the population are affected. The least likely permanent teeth to be missing are the canines.

Hyperdontia is not an uncommon anomaly. It has been reported that from 0.1% to 3.6% of individuals from various populations have too many teeth. These extra teeth are referred to as **supernumeraries.** Supernumerary teeth are most commonly located in the midline and molar regions of the maxillae, followed by the premolar region of the mandible, whereas other sites are only rarely involved. Maxillary supernumerary teeth outnumber mandibular nine to one.

Supernumerary teeth arising in the midline of the maxillae are termed **mesiodens** (Fig. 26-5), and are the most common supernumeraries. The maxillary distomolars are the next most com-

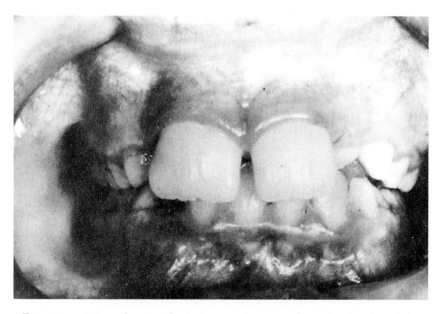

FIG. 26-1.   Macrodontia. The incisor teeth are too large for the size of the oral cavity.

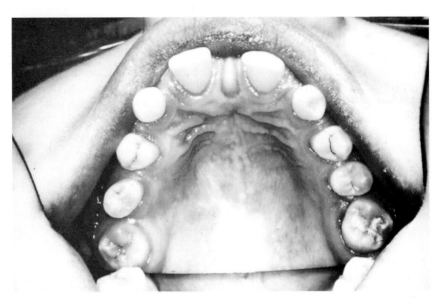

FIG. 26-2. Microdontia. Although some lateral incisors are missing, the teeth are too small for the size of the oral cavity.

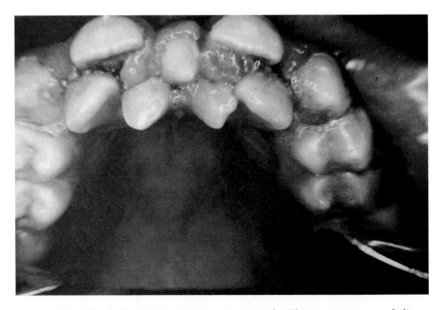

FIG. 26-3. Hyperdontia or supernumerary teeth. There are extra teeth lingual to the regular dentition.

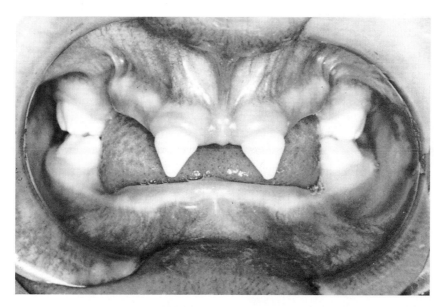

FIG. 26-4.   Anodontia. This particular case illustrates partial anodontia. There is a large number of missing teeth.

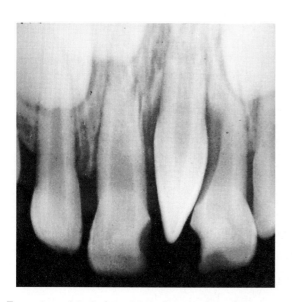

FIG. 26-5.   Mesiodens. Note the peg-shaped supernumerary tooth between maxillary incisors.

mon supernumerary teeth. These **distomolars** are also called fourth molars and are located distal to the maxillary third molars. Mandibular distomolars do occur but not nearly as often as in the maxilla. A supernumerary tooth situated buccally or lingually to a molar is called a **paramolar;** they are usually small and rudimentary. The next most likely location for supernumeraries is the premolar area of the mandible. Only 10% of all supernumeraries occur in the mandible.

If a supernumerary resembles a regular tooth, it is termed *supplemental;* if it is cone shaped, it is called **conical;** and if it is very small, it is called **tubercle.**

Supernumerary teeth are much more common in the permanent than in the primary dentition.

ANOMALIES IN SHAPE

Odontoma

An **odontoma** (Fig. 26-6) is a tumorous anomaly of calcified dental tissues. There are two types of odontoma: complex, which consists

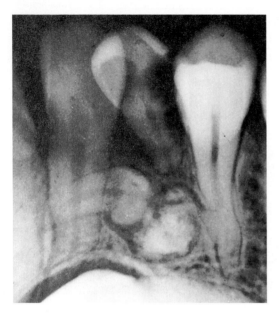

FIG. 26-6.   Odontoma. The two odd-shaped, calcified structures in the middle of the field are odontomas.

of a single mass of dentin, cementum, and enamel in a large blob or unspecified shape; and compound, which consists of several small masses that more or less resemble rudimentary teeth. Although compound odontomas may sometimes resemble multiple mesoderms because they resemble small supplemental teeth, they are smaller.

Dens in Dente

Dens in dente (Fig. 26-7) is a developmental variation thought to occur when the outer surface of the tooth crown invaginates or turns itself inward before mineralization. The term, *dens in dente* means "tooth within a tooth." An x-ray image of a dens in dente shows what appears to be a tooth actually within a tooth (see Fig. 26-7, *A*). This invagination allows communication between the oral cavity and the inner enamel-lined cavity, which could be considered

an extremely deep pit. Permanent maxillary lateral incisors are the teeth most frequently affected by dens in dente.

Dilaceration

A dilacerated tooth (Fig. 26-8) is a tooth that has a sharp bend or curve in the root or crown. It appears as though the tooth suddenly bent under pressure. The term *dilaceration* should only be used to describe teeth with very sharp bends.

Dwarfed Roots

A condition in which the roots of the teeth are extremely short in comparison with their crowns is called dwarfed roots (Fig. 26-9).

Gemination

Gemination (Fig. 26-10) is an anomaly that arises when a tooth attempts to divide itself or partially twin itself by splitting its tooth germ. It therefore is a developmental anomaly. Gemination could result in twin teeth. In most cases, however, geminated teeth are only partially split. Usually the geminated teeth have a single root and a common pulp canal. A tooth split into two crowns with one root would be termed a *bifid tooth* or *bifurcated crown*.

One form of gemination called twinning occurs when a single tooth germ splits, forming two nearly identical teeth but remaining fused as one, usually with a single root and a single pulp ca-nal. This is more commonly seen in the anterior area and occurs more frequently in primary dentition than in permanent dentition.

Fusion

Fusion (Fig. 26-11) occurs when two adjacent tooth germs unite. The two teeth may be united along a part of or the entire length of the tooth. They may be joined by their crowns or their roots. The fusion of the teeth must be made at the dentin. If the teeth are only connected by their cementum, then it is not fusion but concrescence that has occurred. For fusion to exist, two

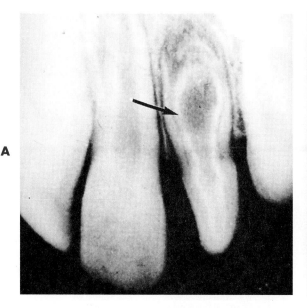

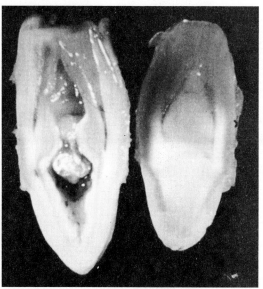

FIG. 26-7.   **A,** Radiograph of dens in dente. There is enamel growing within the tooth *(arrow),* or "tooth in tooth." **B,** A dens in dente has been extracted and sectioned in half, showing the enamel growing within the tooth.

teeth must be joined; therefore there is one less tooth than the normal complement.

Concresence

Concrescence (Fig. 26-12) is a type of fusion that occurs after the roots have formed. It is thought to occur sometimes as a result of trauma. It involves two approximating roots contacting and fusing by a deposition of cementum. It can occur before or after eruption.

Hypercementosis

Hypercementosis (Fig. 26-13) is the deposition of excessive amounts of secondary cementum. This usually occurs at the apex of the tooth and often along the entire length of the root.

Cementoma

Cementoma (Fig. 26-14) is a form of hypercementosis that is also associated with localized destruction of the bone.

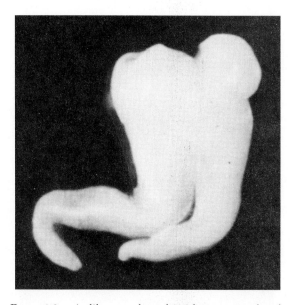

FIG. 26-8.   A dilacerated tooth with numerous bends in the root. This anomaly makes tooth extraction very difficult.

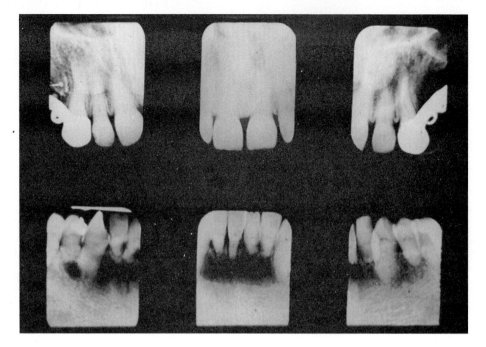

FIG. 26-9. Dwarfed roots. Most of the tooth roots in this patient have never fully developed.

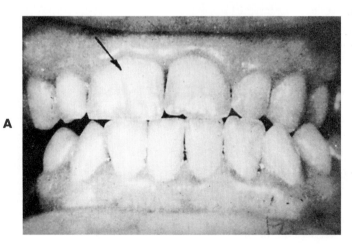

A

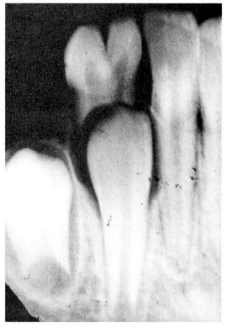

B

FIG. 26-10. **A,** Gemination. There is a groove in the central incisor *(arrow)* where two teeth have begun development. **B,** This radiograph shows how two teeth have grown from one tooth. This anomaly is much more obvious than that illustrated in *A*.

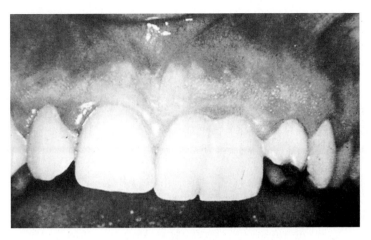

FIG. 26-11. Fusion. The central and lateral incisors have fused in their development. They are fused at both the enamel and dentin.

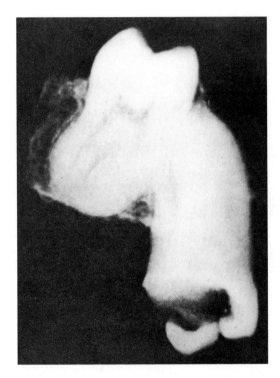

FIG. 26-12. Concrescence. Two teeth grew separately but then fused at their cemental surfaces and were joined together.

Enamel Pearls

Enamel pearls (Fig. 26-15) are small masses of excess enamel on the surface of the teeth located apically to the cementoenamel junction (CEJ). They are frequently found at the bifurcation or trifurcation area and are formed by a small misplaced group of ameloblasts.

Hutchinson's Incisors

Hutchinson's incisors (Fig. 26-16) are notched incisors, sometimes called *screwdriver shaped*, that are formed as a result of prenatal syphilis. The notched incisors are characteristic of congenital syphilis, as are **mulberry molars**—irregular-shaped molars with poorly formed cusps.

Enamel Dysplasia

Enamel dysplasia includes two types of abnormal enamel development: **enamel hypoplasia** and **enamel hypocalcification.** Enamel hypoplasia, which is caused by any condition that inhibits enamel formation, may leave small pits or grooves at different levels in the crown (Fig. 26-17). They are formed by a local disturbance

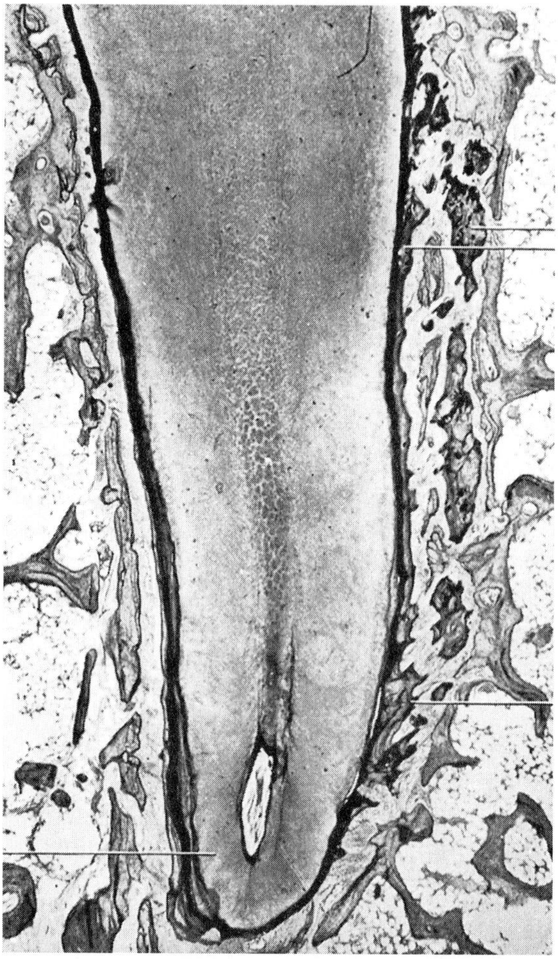

FIG. 26-13. Hypercementosis. Note the localized area of hypercementosis, which may be referred to as *hyperplastic cementum*. (From Bhaskar SN: *Orban's oral histology and embryology,* ed 10, St Louis, 1986, Mosby.)

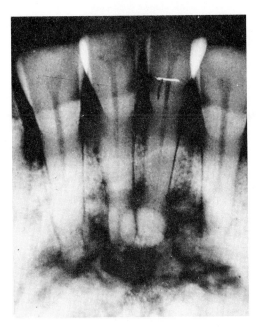

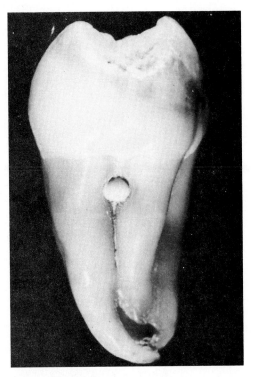

FIG. 26-14. Cementoma. Note the thickened radiopaque area of cementum at the apexes of the central incisors with localized bone destruction around them.

FIG. 26-15. Enamel pearl. There is a small ball of enamel in the bifurcation of this molar. It always is found in bifurcations or trifurcations of teeth.

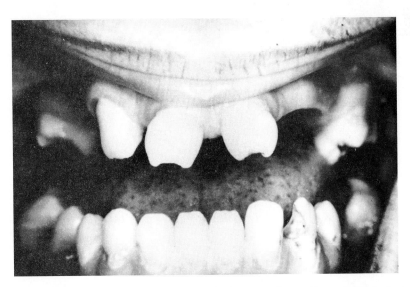

FIG. 26-16. Hutchinson's incisors with the typical notching of the incisal edges of the incisors as a result of congenital syphilis.

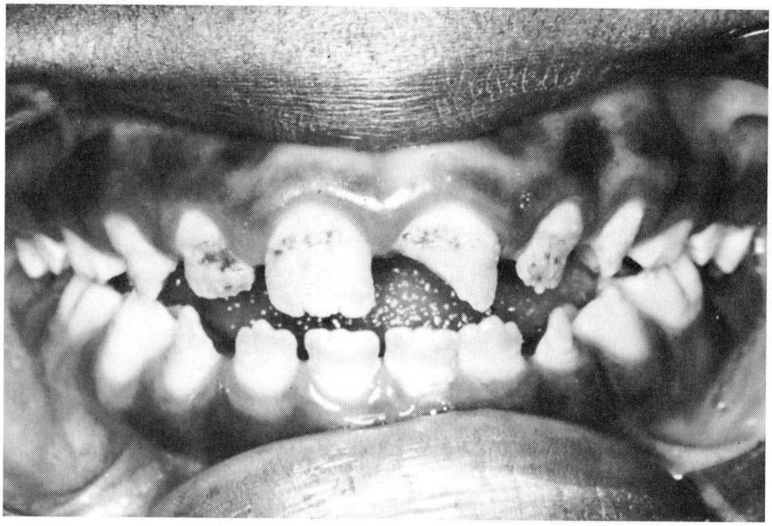

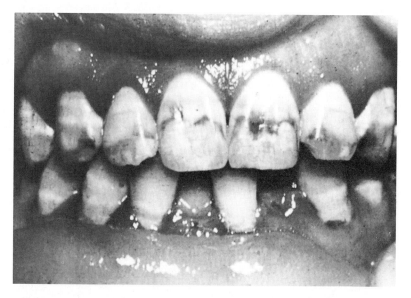

FIG. 26-17.   Enamel hypoplasia. There is pitting on the surfaces of the maxillary central and lateral incisors where the enamel is thin.

FIG. 26-18.   Enamel fluorosis is discoloration of the teeth from too much fluoride. This usually results from drinking natural well water with high fluoride content.

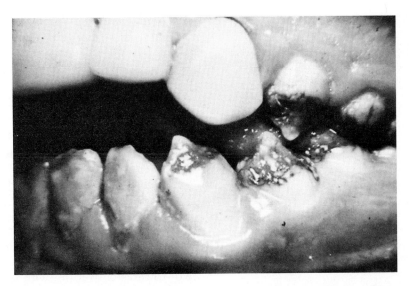

FIG. 26-19. Amelogenesis imperfecta. The enamel is soft and chips off easily. Note the chipped and misshapen areas.

in the enamel formation. Such situations can be caused by inflammation, fever, systemic disease, and even heredity. Enamel hypocalcification is caused by a condition that inhibits the calcification of enamel.

Enamel fluorosis

One of the most common forms of enamel hypocalcification is **enamel fluorosis** (Fig. 26-18), a discoloration of enamel caused by an excessive amount of fluoride in the tooth structure. This can occur naturally from well water with excess amounts of fluoride or accidentally by a child's taking vitamins with fluoride, fluoride mouthwashes, or fluoride supplements either in excess or in combination with fluoridated water. The enamel discoloration can range from small white flecks to large opaque areas to brownish spots, sometimes with pits. In severe cases, large areas of the crown are a brownish color. These discolored areas are called **mottled enamel.**

See Fig. 24-7 to see at what age a developmental anomaly could occur to a maxillary permanent central incisor.

Amelogenesis imperfecta

Amelogenesis imperfecta (Fig. 26-19) is another developmental anomaly related to hypocalcification, but one that is hereditary rather than acquired. In the typical form of amelogenesis imperfecta the enamel of the permanent and deciduous teeth is affected. Sometimes, however, only the permanent teeth are affected. The enamel, when present, is very thin, is stained various shades of yellow and brown, and easily fractures away.

Turner's tooth

Turner's tooth (Fig. 26-20) is a hypocalcification of a single tooth, usually a maxillary incisor. The condition occurs if a developing permanent tooth is affected by a local infection or trauma. Something, bacteria or trauma, disturbs the ameloblastic layer, which results in a hypoplasia of the enamel.

Dentinogenesis Imperfecta

Dentinogenesis imperfecta (Fig. 26-21) is a hereditary dentinal developmental abnormality.

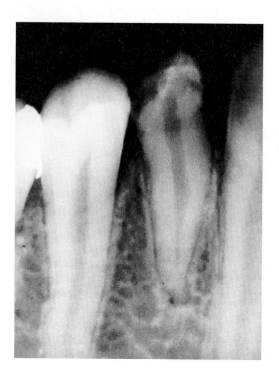

FIG. 26-20.   Turner's tooth. Note the lack of calcification of the crown of this tooth. The tooth was affected while the crown was forming but was not affected later when the root was forming.

The dentin is colored gray, brown, or yellow, but the tooth exhibits an unusual translucent hue. The most striking feature of this condition is that the pulp chambers and root canals are completely filled in with dentin. This total obliteration of the pulp tissue occurs because the dentinal tissue continues to form dentin until all of the root canal and pulp chambers are completely filled.

Tetracycline Staining

Another dentinal developmental condition is **tetracycline staining** (Fig. 26-22). This condition occurs when an expectant mother or a young child whose tooth crowns are still developing takes the antibiotic tetracycline. The teeth of the developing fetus or the young child discolor, ranging from yellow to brown or grayish blue.

ABNORMAL CROWN SHAPES

The maxillary third molars followed by the mandibular third molars are the most likely of the teeth to show variety and abnormalities in the size, number, and shape of the cusps. They can range from a single peg-shaped crown to a multicusped large or small variation of the first or second molar.

The most common malformed anterior tooth is the maxillary lateral incisor, which is peg shaped in more than 1% of the population.

Mandibular second premolars vary from a two- to three-cusp form, with several variations of each.

Accessory cusps or tubercles can occur on any tooth, but are most commonly found on maxillary molars.

ABNORMAL ROOT FORMATION

The maxillary second premolars very frequently have two bifurcated roots, although more often only one. The maxillary first premolars usually do have two roots, although in 40% of cases they have one. It is not uncommon for the mandibular second premolars or canines to have accessory roots, a second root sometimes bifurcated only at the apical third. In all of the above, if two roots are present, one will be buccal and one lingual.

Mandibular canines and premolars are the single-rooted teeth most likely to be affected by accessory roots. Third molars are the most likely multirooted teeth to possess accessory roots.

A severe bend or distortion in the tooth root and crown of more than 40 degrees is termed a dilaceration, most often seen in mandibular third molars. A sharp curvature or twist of a tooth root only is called **flexion.**

The condition of concrescense as mentioned before occurs when two adjacent teeth are fused

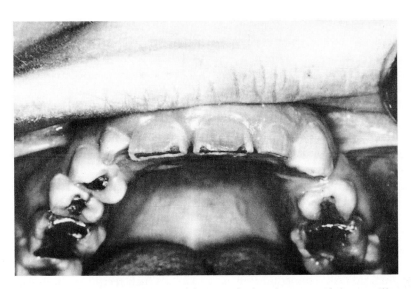

FIG. 26-21.   Dentinogenesis imperfecta with discoloration of the maxillary anterior teeth. Enamel frequently chips away because the poorly developed dentin beneath it does not support it.

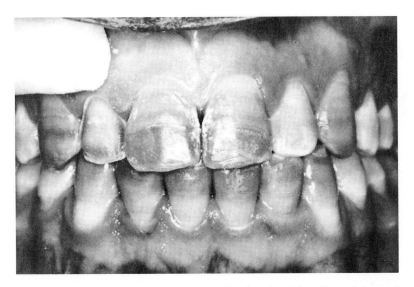

FIG. 26-22.   Tetracycline staining. Note the discolored banding of the teeth. This individual was taking tetracycline for an extended period of time, and most of the teeth were affected.

together at their roots through cementum only. This is different from fusion because these teeth were originally separate and became joined after eruption. Concrescense is most frequently seen in the maxillary molar region.

Maxillary teeth with normal sized crowns and abnormally short roots are not uncommon. These roots are termed *dwarfed roots*. This condition can occur in mandibular incisors as well (see Fig. 26-9).

Excessive cementum formation around the apical third of a root after a tooth has erupted is termed *hypercementosis*. It first appears on x-ray films as a radiolucent dark area that is sometimes mistaken for a periapical abcess. Later this area appears opaque on x-ray film as it becomes more mineralized. This condition is not pathologic.

Review Questions

1. What is an anomaly?
2. Name some extrinsic and intrinsic factors that may cause anomalies.
3. What is the difference between hereditary and congenital factors?
4. What is the difference between hyperdontia and anodontia?
5. What is an odontoma?
6. What is the difference between gemination and fusion?
7. What is the cause of Hutchinson's incisors and mulberry molars?
8. What is the difference between amelogenesis imperfecta and dentinogenesis imperfecta?
9. What is tetracycline staining, and when does it occur?
10. What is mottled enamel?
11. What is familial tendency?
12. Which teeth are the most likely to be congenitally missing?
13. In which arch do supernumerary teeth occur with more frequency?
14. Of the following, which affect only the root of the tooth?
    a. Flexion
    b. Dilaceration
    c. Dwarfed roots
    d. Cementoma
    e. Hypercementosis
    f. All but b
    g. All but a

CHAPTER 27

SUPPORTING STRUCTURES

The Periodontium

OBJECTIVES
- To understand the relationships within the gingival unit, a supporting structure of the teeth
- To understand the terminology of the gingival unit and to identify its various parts
- To understand how the gingival unit functions
- To understand how the attachment apparatus is related to the gingival unit
- To understand the relationship of cementum, periodontal ligament, and alveolar bone
- To understand how the fibers of the periodontal ligament function in tooth movement and shock absorption

THE PERIODONTIUM consists of those tissues that support the teeth. It is divided into a **gingival unit** and an **attachment unit** or **attachment apparatus:**

I. Gingival unit
  A. Gingiva
    1. Free gingiva
    2. Attached gingiva
  B. Alveolar mucosa
II. Attachment unit
  A. Cementum
  B. Alveolar bone
  C. Periodontal ligament

GINGIVAL UNIT

The gingiva is made up of free and attached gingiva (Fig. 27-1). Composed of very dense mucosa called **masticatory mucosa,** it has a thick **epithelial** covering and **keratinized cells.** The underlying **mucosa** is composed of dense collagen fibers (Table 27-1 on page 334). This type of masticatory mucosa is also found on the hard palate. Masticatory mucosa is well designed to withstand the trauma to which it is subjected in grinding food.

The rest of the mouth is lined with a different type of mucosa called **lining mucosa.** This type makes up the alveolar mucosa. It is thin and

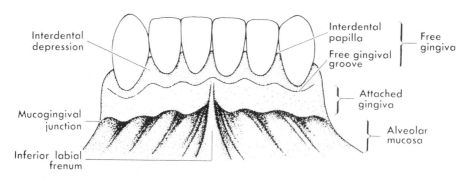

FIG. 27-1. Anatomy of a normal gingival unit of a periodontium.

TABLE 27-1.	Characteristics of Gingiva and Alveolar Mucosa	
Tissue characteristics	Free and attached gingiva	Alveolar mucosa
Type of mucosa	Masticatory	Lining
Tone	Tightly bound	Movable and elastic
Epithelium	Thick epithelial layer	Thin epithelial layer
	Keratinized	Nonkeratinized
	Rete peg formation	No rete peg formation
Texture	Stippled surface (like an orange peel)	Smooth
Color	Light pink	Red to bright red
Fiber	Collagenous fibers	Collagenous fibers and elastic fibers

freely movable and tears or injures easily. The epithelium covering this lining mucosa is thin and nonkeratinized. Its mucosa is composed of loose connective tissue and muscle fibers.

Free Gingiva

Free gingiva is the gum tissue that extends from the gingival margin to the base of the gingival sulcus. The attached gingiva extends from the base of this sulcus to the mucogingival junction. Alveolar mucosa is found apical to the mucogingival junction and is contiguous with the rest of the mucous membrane of the cheeks and lips and the floor of the mouth. Free gingiva is usually light pink in color and averages between 0.5 to 2 mm in depth.

The free gingival margin around a fully erupted tooth is located next to the enamel about 0.5 to 2 mm coronal to the cemento-enamel junction (CEJ). It forms a collar, which is separated from the tooth by the gingival sulcus. This gingival sulcus is the space between the free gingiva and the tooth. The bottom of the sulcus is influenced by the curvature of the cervical line of the tooth. A healthy gingival sulcus will rarely exceed 2.5 mm in depth.

The gingival papilla is the free gingiva located in the triangular interdental spaces. The apex in the anterior teeth is rather sharp but is more blunt in the posterior teeth. The shape of gingival papilla is greatly affected by the location of the contact area of the adjacent teeth, by the shape of the interproximal surfaces of the adjacent teeth, and by the CEJ of the adjacent teeth. Inflammation of the gingival papilla is easily recognized because the area takes on a redder color than normal and exhibits a puffy appearance with some blunting of its apex.

The inner portion of the gingival sulcus is lined with nonkeratinized epithelium; the outer portion is the free gingiva, which is covered with keratinized epithelium. The attached gingiva begins at the base of the gingival sulcus. A gingival groove often occurs on the outside of the free gingiva and corresponds to the base of the sulcus. This groove is not always present but is to be considered a normal part of the anatomy when present. The attached gingiva extends apically from the base of the sulcus and is attached to the bone and the cementum by a dense network of collagenous fibers. It often has a stippled texture, resembling the dimpled surface of an orange. Stippling becomes evident before the teeth erupt and becomes even more so in adult gingiva. The attached gingiva is highly keratinized and is covered by **stratified squamous epithelium** in which **rete peg formation** is evident. The dimpling effect is caused by the rete peg formation, which is simply the irregular binding of the epithelium to the bone by collagen fibers. This causes depressions or dimples where the epithelium is pulled tight to the bone. The color of the gingiva varies from light to dark pink and may contain pigment, correlating to the skin pigmentation of the person. The darker a person's skin color is, the more likely the gingiva will be darker and contain **melanin.**

Attached Gingiva

The gingiva is connected to the tooth by a meshwork of collagenous fibers. These fibers are formed by **fibroblasts,** which are the principal cells of connective tissue. All fibers embedded in the cementum are known as **Sharpey's fibers;** they extend from the cementum to the papillary area of the gingiva. These fibers pass out from the cementum in small bundles (Fig. 27-2, *A*). Some of the fibers *(A)* curve toward the mucosa of the free gingiva and interlace with one another. Other fibers *(B)* pass directly across from the cementum to the gingiva. Still further apically, other fibers *(C)* pass from the cementum over the alveolar crest and turn apically between the outer periosteum of the alveolar process and the outer epithelial covering of the attached gingiva.

On the proximal side (Fig. 27-2, *B*), the connective tissue fibers arise from a higher level on the cementum because of the curvature of the CEJ on the interproximal surfaces of the teeth. This curvature allows more room for the cementum to attach to the gingiva. Attachment is made possible by groups of connective tissue fibers. The most occlusal group travels to the papillary layer of the epithelium of the interdental papilla. The next layer of fibers passes occlusally into the interproximal gingiva. The next layer of fibers, the transseptal *(TS)* group, travels completely across the interproximal space and attaches to the adjacent tooth. These transseptal fiber bundles bind one tooth to another. Additionally, circular bands of connective tissue fibers surround the teeth, tying them together (Fig. 27-3).

The function of these gingival fibers is to keep the gingiva closely attached to the tooth surface. These fibers prevent the free gingiva from being peeled away from the tooth and keep the attached gingiva firmly attached. They also prevent the apical migration of the epithelial attachment and resist gingival recession.

The blood supply of the gingival tissue comes from the **supraperiosteal** vessels. These in turn originate from the lingual, mental, buccal, infraorbital, and palatine arteries. The gingiva is quite rich in capillary vascularity, and the alveolar mucosa is equally **vascular** but more red. Its deep color is attributed to numerous shallow blood vessels.

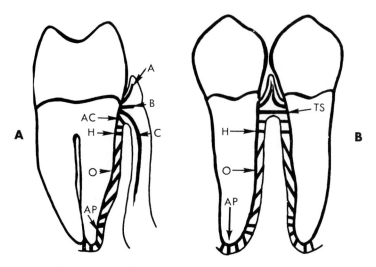

FIG. 27-2. The principal fiber groups of a gingival unit and an attachment unit. **A,** Gingival fibers: groups *A*, *B*, and *C* are seen in buccolingual sketch. **B,** Transseptal fibers *(TS)* are seen in the mesiodistal sketch. Periodontal ligament fibers include: alveolar crest fibers *(AC)*, horizontal fibers *(H)*, oblique fibers *(O)*, and apical fibers *(AP)*. (From Kraus BS, Jordon RE, Abrams L: *Dental anatomy and occlusion,* Baltimore, 1969, Williams & Wilkins Co.)

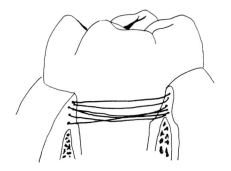

FIG. 27-3.   Circular fibers of a gingival unit.

Alveolar Mucosa

The alveolar mucosa joins the attached gingiva at the mucogingival junction and is continuous with the rest of the tissues of the **vestibule.** This tissue is thin and soft and rather loosely attached to the underlying bone. Alveolar mucosa is composed of lining mucosa, and its **submucosa** contains loose connective tissue and fat. The epithelium is smooth, thin, and nonkeratinized.

ATTACHMENT UNIT

The attachment unit comprises the cementum, the periodontal ligament, and the alveolar bone. Cementum is hard, bonelike tissue covering the roots of the teeth. The **periodontal ligament** is the tissue that surrounds the roots of the teeth and connects them to alveolar bone. The alveolar bone is the thin covering of compact bone that surrounds the teeth; when viewed radiographically, it is called the **lamina dura** (Figs. 27-4 and 27-5). The function of the attachment apparatus is not only supportive, but also nutritive, formative, and sensory. The supportive function is to maintain the support for the tooth in the bone and to prevent its movement. The

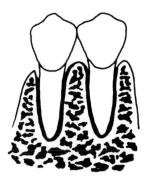

FIG. 27-4.   This sketch of a radiograph shows that the periodontal ligament separates the lamina dura from the tooth. Notice the width of the periodontal ligament and the direction of the bone trabeculae. The black space around the root of the teeth is the periodontal ligament.

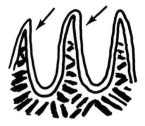

FIG. 27-5.   An overview of Fig. 27-4, depicting the lamina dura *(arrows)* and the direction of the bone trabeculae.

nutritive and sensory functions are fulfilled by the blood vessels and nerves. The nerves act as indicators of pressure or pain around the tooth. The formative function is to replace cementum, periodontal ligament, and alveolar bone, and is accomplished by specialized cells called **cementoblasts,** fibroblasts, and osteoblasts. In addition to these functions, the periodontal ligament acts as a suspensory mechanism that keeps the root and bone from abrading each other. The periodontal ligament also acts as a hammock of live tissue whose fibers cushion the impact between

tooth and bone upon the exertion of pressure. The fibers themselves become taut, thus dissipating the pressure and at the same time allowing the nerves associated with these fibers a method of measuring and equating the amount of pressure.

Cementum

Cementum can be cellular or acellular. Both types are formed by cementoblasts, but in the cellular type, the cementoblasts become embedded in the cementum. The acellular type is free of embedded cementoblasts and is clear and without structure.

Acellular cementum always covers the cervical third of the root and sometimes extends over almost all of the root except the apical portion. Cellular cementum covers the apical portion of the root and sometimes may form over acellular cementum. Cellular cementum is like bone in character and in the way it can be resorbed and added to. Like bone, cementum grows by the **apposition** (addition) of new layers, one on another. Changes in function and pressure influence the growth activity of cementum.

Both cellular and acellular cementum have collagen fibers embedded within them. These fibers, known as Sharpey's fibers, are the embedded ends of connective tissue fibers of the periodontal membrane. Some are embedded in cementum and some in bone.

Alveolar Bone

The type of bone that lines the sockets in which the roots of teeth are held is called *alveolar bone proper.* The socket in which the tooth rests is called an *alveolus.* These alveoli are a part of the alveolar process that surrounds and supports the teeth in the maxilla and mandible. Alveolar bone proper is thin and compact, with many small openings through which blood vessels, nerves, and lymphatic vessels pass. The alveolar bone that forms the alveolus around a tooth's bony socket contains Sharpey's fibers. What other hard tissue has Sharpey's fibers? Sharpey's fibers are part of what membrane?

Bone tissue is continually undergoing change. The architectural arrangement of the **trabeculae** is directly related to the demands of function. Even bone apposition and resorption are related to the functional demands placed on the bone. Compared with cementum, bone is an extremely active tissue. Very slow apposition of cementum occurs, whereas the alveolar bone undergoes changes readily. Under normal conditions bone is constantly in flux, undergoing tissue growth (apposition) and resorption in a finely coordinated way. Bone may be laid down on one end and resorbed on the other. The extreme difference between bone and cementum in their ability to undergo remodeling poses a significant problem. The two tissues are tied together by the periodontal ligament, which must make adjustments for the variation in their abilities.

Bone, like cementum, consists of an **organic matrix** and **inorganic matter**. The organic matrix comprises collagen and intercellular substance; the inorganic matter comprises **apatite crystals** of calcium, phosphate, and carbonates.

Alveolar bone is deposited next to the periodontal ligament and is supported by a more compact bone. The bone forming the alveoli is dependent on the functional demands of the tooth. If a tooth undergoes long-standing loss of function, as when the antagonists in the opposite arch are lost, the alveolar bone undergoes changes. If the teeth are subjected to **occlusal stress,** the supporting bone will be composed of thicker and more numerous trabeculae. The bone itself undergoes resorption when pressure is exerted on it and opposition when tension is placed on it. Sharpey's fibers, embedded in the bone at one end and in the cementum at the other, are capable of expressing such tension. The term **bundle bone** applies when numerous layers of bone are added to the socket wall. Bundle bone forms the immediate attachment of the periodontal ligament.

Periodontal Ligament

The fibers of the periodontal ligament attach to the alveolar bone and to the cementum. They are arranged in the following five groups:

1. **Alveolar crest group**—fibers extending from the cervical area of the tooth to the alveolar crest
2. **Horizontal group**—fibers running horizontally from the tooth to the alveolar bone
3. **Oblique group**—fibers running obliquely from the cementum to the bone
4. **Apical group**—fibers radiating apically from the tooth to the bone (see Fig. 27-2)
5. **Interradicular group**—periodontal fibers between roots of multirooted teeth

This arrangement of fibers provides a hammock of tissue bundles that support the tooth within the bone. They not only tie the tooth to the bone but also prevent it from being pushed into the bone. They insulate the tooth and bone, thereby minimizing the trauma of being pushed together. This shock absorption function is also helped by the roots of the teeth and by fluids within the periodontal ligament. The shapes and sizes of the roots of the teeth help dissipate occlusal stresses in both a lateral and apical direction. In multirooted teeth the forces can be distributed between the roots of the same tooth. Additionally, the fluids within the periodontal ligament act as a hydraulic pressure system on the walls of the alveolus.

Because the fibers are constantly subjected to a variety of pressures exerted on the tooth, the periodontal ligament is constantly undergoing functional change. The main portion of the periodontal ligament is composed of bundles of white collagenous connective tissue fibers. These fibers extend from and are embedded in the cementum of the tooth and the alveolar bone and are bundled together like the many strands of a rope.

In addition to the collagen fibers, the periodontal ligament contains fibroblasts, one of the cellular elements of the periodontal ligament. They are found in alignment with the collagen fibers, arranged in groups. The periodontal ligament also contains small blood and lymph vessels and nerves. Loose connective tissue surrounds these vessels and nerves.

The tooth itself is actually suspended by this periodontal ligament in such a way that it is allowed some degree of movement within the bony cavity. For instance, if pressure is exerted on the mesial surface, the periodontal fibers on the distal surface are compressed and allow more space between the tooth and the bone. This ability of the periodontal ligament to expand allows the tooth to tip, rotate, or be compressed within the bony cavity. Even total bodily movement is possible because of the periodontal ligament. An example of this is the constant abrading of neighboring teeth, not only occlusally but also interproximally. This causes wear on the contact areas and occlusal surfaces. Two forces that are active within the mouth allow for movement of the tooth. The first is mesial drift, which allows the tooth to move forward within the oral cavity, thus closing the spaces lost from interproximal wear. The second is an active eruption force of the tooth, which causes the tooth to migrate occlusally until it occludes with an antagonist. Both forces can be activated fairly rapidly because of the periodontal ligament's ability to tense and compress and the bone's ability to change the shape and size of the socket.

CLINICAL CONSIDERATIONS

There are several clinical situations that should be discussed. The first of these concerns how a tooth can move within a bony alveolus. Such movement is accomplished by several mechanisms already discussed.

For a tooth to move through bone, a force of some type must be acting on it. This force causes pressure on the root, periodontal ligament, and bone. It compresses the periodontal ligament and the alveolar bone on one side of the root. If this force continues for a long enough time, a biomechanical system of osteoclastic cells (bone-destroying cells) is initiated. The osteoclasts destroy bone to make room for the compressed tissues. If the pressure is extreme, the osteoclastic cells may even resorb portions of the root of the tooth.

On the other side of this same tooth root, the periodontal ligament is pulled taut. This results in a pulling force on the alveolar bone on that side of the socket. This constant tension causes an opposite biomechanical system. Osteoblastic cells (bone-forming cells) start laying down bone. These osteoblasts produce bone in response to tension, which aids in relieving the tension on the periodontal ligament. The net effect is that the tooth moves away from the force by remodeling bone. On one side bone is destroyed, and on the other side bone is formed.

The following are some of the forces that exert pressure on the teeth:

1. Active eruption—tooth eruption into the oral cavity, and eruption to compensate for occlusal **abrasion**
2. Mesial drift—the mesial movement of molars to compensate for proximal abrasion
3. Masticatory occlusal forces—tooth occlusion during chewing
4. Orthodontic corrective forces—a dentist or orthodontist's placing pressure-causing appliances on the teeth to correct malocclusion
5. Traumatic occlusal forces—teeth being subjected to premature contact during occlusion

The first four of these forces can tip, rotate, or move the tooth because of the bone-remodeling system just mentioned. These forces must be relatively constant for the bone-remodeling mechanisms to be activated.

The last of these forces, occlusal trauma, is not a consistent, constant force. It is usually intermittent and consequently does not result in tooth movement as much as tooth mobility. Although some osteoclastic activity occurs, it may be the result of constant pressure from inflam-

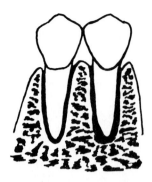

FIG. 27-6.   The tooth on right shows widening of the periodontal ligament, indicating tooth mobility.

mation caused by trauma more than the external force of the occlusion. In general the periodontal ligament is tensed and torn, the space between the cementum and the lamina dura is enlarged and widened, the lamina dura is compressed, and the tooth becomes loose and mobile within the socket (Fig. 27-6).

Review Questions

1. Which of the following are true of attached gingiva?
    a. The tissue is soft and movable.
    b. The epithelial layer is thick and keratinized.
    c. The tissue can have a stippled texture.
    d. The tissue is fixed and firmly attached to the bone and cementum.
2. Which is most true of cementum?
    a. Sharpey's fibers are embedded in it.
    b. It is always smooth.
    c. Acellular cementum covers the apical end of the tooth.
    d. It is resorbed as easily as bone.

3. Which is true of Sharpey's fibers?
    a. They can embed in bone only.
    b. They can embed in cementum only.
    c. They can embed in either bone or cementum.
    d. The same fiber could embed in bone at one end and in cementum at the other.
4. When the tooth is subjected to occlusal stress, it relieves this stress by which of the following mechanisms?
    a. The periodontal ligament tenses.
    b. The fluids in the periodontal ligament absorb some force.
    c. The walls of the alveolus spread the force out and divide it over a wider area.
5. Define the following by researching the index and glossary:
    a. rete peg formation
    b. stratified squamous epithelium
6. Which statements are true about fibers A, B, and C in Fig. 27-7?
    a. They are called Sharpey's fibers.
    b. They attach only the free gingiva to the cementum.
    c. They are called transseptal fibers.
    d. They are embedded in the cementum.
7. Draw and label the periodontal ligament fibers in Fig. 27-8 (a mandibular first molar).
8. The free gingiva extends from the gingival margins to the base of the gingival sulcus. T or F?
9. The attached gingiva extends from the gingival sulcus to the interdental space. T or F?
10. The gingival sulcus is the space between the tooth and the mucogingival fold. T or F?
11. The gingival papilla is located in the interdental space. T or F?
12. The alveolar bone when seen on the x-ray is called lamina dura. T or F?

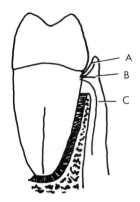

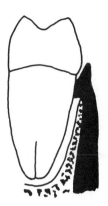

FIG. 27-7.   Mesial view of a permanent mandibular left first molar.

FIG. 27-8.   Mesial view of a permanent mandibular left molar.

CLINICAL
CONSIDERATIONS

WHEN STUDYING clinical considerations of an existing dental condition, there are two alternatives: either the circumstances are preventive in nature, enhancing the ability of the oral tissues to protect themselves, or they are potentially pathologic. It is important to recognize the difference. It is bad enough not to recognize a potentially pathologic situation, but it is worse to be the cause of it because of ignorance in therapeutic treatment. It is for this reason that a study of preventive clinical situations is important.

PREVENTIVE CLINICAL CONSIDERATIONS

Preventive clinical considerations include tooth form, shape, and arrangement that aid in the prevention of dental problems such as decay, occlusal trauma, and periodontal disease.

Decay and Periodontal Disease

Remember that the teeth are encased in a hard, smooth outer covering, the enamel, which offers protection from the accumulation of bacteria and debris (plaque). The smoothness of the enamel makes the adherence of plaque more difficult. This self-cleaning ability of the enamel therefore helps resist decay because decay is caused by bacterially produced acids that etch away the tooth surface. If the bacteria cannot accumulate and adhere to the tooth surface, decay cannot occur. Likewise, some prevention of periodontal disease is attributable to the very smoothness of this enamel because bacteria that destroy gum and bone tissue are also prevented from accumulating on the tooth.

It is important to remember, however, that not all periodontal disease is caused by bacteria. If the tooth has rough pits, grooves, or fissures, these areas will allow debris to accumulate and provide a breeding ground for bacteria. The same is true if the tooth has rough margins on its restorations or if interproximally the tooth has an overhanging restoration—that is, a restoration that does not stay within the confines of the tooth form but protrudes into the gingival tissue. Bacteria can adhere around the margins of the excess material and lead to disease within the gum and tooth tissues. Restoration of any tooth must follow the normal anatomy of that tooth. A restoration must be polished smooth so that the tooth can resume normal function, and the jaw its normal anatomy. Dental personnel provide a valuable service in preventive dentistry by polishing dental restorations. It is much more comfortable for patients to undergo the polishing of their restorations than their replacement (Fig. 28-1).

Likewise, tooth sealants can be placed in the grooves and pits on the occlusal of the molars.

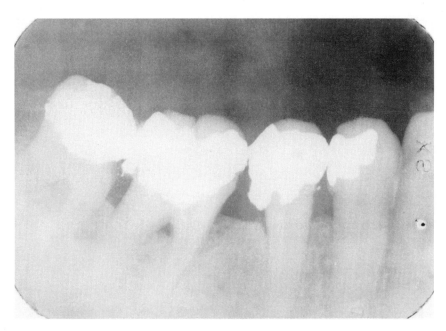

FIG. 28-1. Radiograph showing periodontal disease caused by bacteria, which are harbored by overextended restoration.

This is to prevent decay from forming in these hard to clean areas.

Rough surfaces on the roots of teeth and extra projections of cementum and calculus can also lead to decay and to the breakdown of periodontal tissues. It therefore becomes extremely important for dental professionals not only to remove calculus and stain from the roots of the teeth but also to smooth any rough areas on the root that may be formed from irregularities in the cementum or defects within the root formation.

This regular root cleaning, which can prevent disease by destroying any plaque-trapping areas that could harbor bacteria, is sometimes called **root planing.** The dental professional must always remember how thin the envelope of cementum is that wraps around the root. A painful situation occurs when bare dentin is exposed because the cementum is stripped away from part of the root of a tooth.

Trauma

The hardness of enamel helps prevent occlusal wear or attrition, but this same hardness allows the full impact of trauma to be transferred from tooth to bone. If a tooth prematurely contacts another, only the two teeth will bear the initial brunt of forces when the jaws are closed. A more ideal situation is to have all the teeth hit equally upon closure of the jaw, without any teeth hitting prematurely. This allows for the forces exerted to be dissipated over all the teeth. Should one tooth hit with a greater force than the rest of the teeth, it will be traumatized by this excess force. Such a situation is known as **occlusal trauma** and results in disease of the periodontal tissue, cracking of the enamel of the tooth, and possible fracture of the tooth (Fig. 28-2).

Occlusal trauma can also occur during eating. It is necessary to have spillways between the teeth to allow for the dissipation of forces. This dissipation of occlusal forces occurs because the

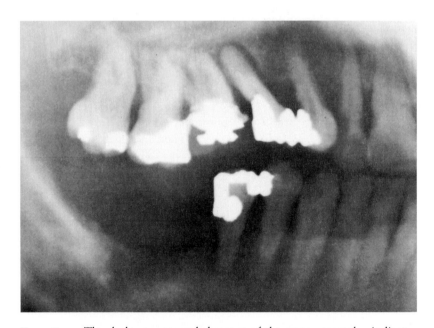

FIG. 28-2.   The dark area around the root of the upper premolar indicates bone loss caused by occlusal trauma.

spillways allow the food to escape from between the teeth.

Contours of Teeth

The contours of the teeth, buccally and lingually, determine the angle at which food is deflected off the teeth and onto the gingiva. If the buccal or lingual contours are underdeveloped (undercontoured), food and debris are pushed into the gingival crevice. If the buccal and lingual contours are overdeveloped (overcontoured), the food and debris pass off the tooth and onto the gingiva at a poor angle. This results in gingival inflammation because the gum tissue is denied proper frictional massage (see Fig. 22-6.)

An excess of contour, such as more than 1 mm of lingual contour on mandibular molars, creates an oral hygiene problem. If the tooth contour presents extreme undercuts, the natural cleaning action of the tongue and friction of the food and cheeks become ineffective. Special oral hygiene devices and instructions must be given to the patient.

THERAPEUTIC CONSIDERATIONS

Maintaining Form in Restorations

Because it is very important in the restoration of teeth to reconstruct a tooth in its anatomic form, it is important to know the anatomic shape of each individual tooth. We also need to know contact areas and buccal and lingual contours. For instance, an overhanging restoration

or an open interproximal contact is undesirable in restoring a tooth in the interproximal area. Measures should be taken to keep the filling material from impinging on the tissue. To prevent such overflow, a metal band is placed around the tooth and wedged into position (Fig. 28-3). This matrix band retains the material being packed against the tooth, and the wedge forces the inside of the matrix band against the tooth so that no excess filling material can overflow into the gingiva. The wedge also forces the teeth apart so that a tight interproximal contact can be made. There should be no rough margins or excesses on the marginal line of the filling and the tooth; they should be as smooth as possible, with the tooth restored to its proper form and function.

Deep pits and fissures that occur naturally should not be recreated in the teeth to be restored. The deep pits and grooves only become plaque traps. The buccal and lingual contours, however, should be restored in the best possible manner so that the gingiva is carefully protected.

The pulp tissue of the tooth should also be protected during a tooth restoration. Any trauma to the pulp tissue of a tooth creates serious complications. For example, if one were to hit his or her finger with a hammer, an inflammatory process would ensue. The finger would immediately be painful, and soon blood would rush to the injured area. The finger would swell, and heat from the increased vascularity would be felt. The same factors exist for inflammation within the pulp cavity. If trauma occurs, the pul-

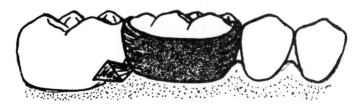

FIG. 28-3.   A matrix band wedged interproximally with a wooden wedge to prevent an overhanging restoration.

pal tissues become inflamed, caused by an increase in the blood flow to that area. Unlike the finger, however, pulpal tissue cannot swell; it is encased in hard tooth structures. The pulp cavity walls are formed from dentin (Fig. 28-4), which makes it virtually impossible for the pulpal tissue to expand. As the pressure from the increased vascularity builds up within the pulp cavity walls, the veins within the pulp tissue begin to close. Because arteries have thicker walls than the veins, and because they are less affected by pressure, they maintain the blood supply; however, the veins, with thinner walls, collapse. Because the only opening into the pulp cavity is the small **apical foramen** at the root apex, very little internal pressure closes this opening. As soon as the apical foramen is obstructed, blood flow is stopped and the tooth literally chokes itself off from fresh oxygenated blood. The result is that the tooth's pulpal tissues die from lack of oxygen (see Fig. 28-4).

Maintaining Proper Bite in Restorations

The dentist and auxiliary should check a patient's bite after a restoration is in place by having the patient bite on articulating (ink) paper. This is done to ensure that no part of the restoration is hitting prematurely, which would result in occlusal trauma to the tooth and eventual fracture of the restoration or even the tooth itself. Even if the tooth hits with just slightly more contact than the rest of the teeth, the result is extreme trauma. First, the tooth, by hitting prematurely, becomes sore because it is carrying more than its share of the burden of occlusal stress. Second, the soreness of the tooth leads to inflammation of the periodontal and other supporting tissues. Third, with inflammation, edema occurs; pressure and swelling within the tissues push the tooth out of its bony socket in an attempt to relieve some of these stresses. Fourth, the tooth now extends farther from the bony socket than it did before it was inflamed and hits the opposing teeth sooner and harder. Thus the tooth undergoes even more severe occlusal trauma, resulting in more inflammation, swelling, and pain. The tooth is forced to extend even farther from the bony socket to relieve this new pressure from the inflammation and edema. If untreated, the cycle could be irreversible. Therefore the dentist must make sure that any new dental restorations fit properly according to the patient's bite.

Pain

When diagnosing dental pain, it is important to remember that the nerve centers within the tooth are not the only nerve centers capable of eliciting pain around the tooth. If a tooth is severely damaged such that the nerve of the tooth has degenerated or even been obliterated, the tooth could still cause pain. Even an endodontically treated tooth, whose pulp cavity has been completely **debrided** of all traces of nerve tissue

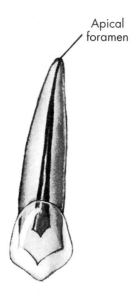

Apical foramen

FIG. 28-4.   The pulp tissue of a tooth is encased by hard dentin. The only pathway for blood's vital support is through the apical foramen. (From Massler M, Schour I: *Atlas of the mouth in health and disease,* ed 2, Chicago, 1975, American Dental Association.)

and filled with root canal filling material, can respond to pain if the tooth is touched. The reason is that the nerve tissues in the periodontal ligament and surrounding bone tissue are still alive. If trauma or infection from any source, such as periapical involvement or periodontal abscess, are present, the nerves in the supporting structures around the tooth will respond to the pain. The nerve within the pulp cavity can give only a response to pain, whereas nerves within the periodontal tissue can give either a pain response or a pressure response. A patient who reports feeling pain from within a tooth may be experiencing pain from the periodontal tissues or surrounding bone. A careful clinical examination is therefore absolutely necessary, because false and referred pains are common.

A common form of pain occurs when the gum recedes and the root of the tooth is exposed. The cementum leaves bare areas of dentin uncovered, and the dentin elicits pain whenever air, sweets, hot, or cold come into contact with it. Dentin can become nature's warning system of gum disease.

Tooth Migration

If a tooth is fractured so that it no longer hit its antagonist in the opposite arch, within 24 hours the tooth would begin to erupt to meet this antagonist. This is called **tooth migration.** The same thing would happen if a dentist cut a tooth for a crown preparation and the occlusal surface were cut away; the tooth would no longer hit its antagonist and would erupt to try to meet the antagonist. If an impression had been taken of the tooth preparation at that time so that the crown could be made, then when the crown was ready 2 weeks later, the tooth would have moved. The crown then might not fit. To avoid this problem, a well-placed temporary restoration is made to fit the crown preparation. This temporary must not only replace the interproximal areas (to prevent mesial drift), but must also restore the cut preparation to a functional occlusion to prevent the tooth from erupting to meet its antagonist.

If a tooth were removed and not replaced, the tooth in the opposite arch might **supraerupt** (erupt past the occlusal plane in an attempt to meet its antagonist), which would destroy the effectiveness of the contact areas between this tooth and its neighboring teeth. With the contact areas changed, food impaction could occur. In the opposite arch mesial drift would begin to cause any teeth immediately posterior to the extraction site to move in a mesial direction. This would usually cause the posterior teeth to become mesially tipped as well. In Fig. 28-5 notice what has happened to the interproximal spaces and contact areas. All of this resulted because a tooth was removed and not replaced.

INTERRELATION OF THE DENTAL STRUCTURES

Let us look at the dental tissue collapse initiated by the loss of a single tooth, a mandibular first molar (see Fig. 28-5). The maxillary first molar supraerupts to meet its missing mandibular antagonist. Notice the relocation of the mesial and distal contact areas of the maxillary first molar. This causes food impaction between the maxillary teeth interproximally. Plaque adheres to these poor contact areas, which results in decay. Food debris and plaque also cause gingival irritation and periodontal breakdown. Finally, premature occlusal contact occurs in centric occlusion because the distal area of the maxillary first molar prematurely hits the mesial area of the mandibular second molar. When the mandible goes into protrusive movement, the distal area of the maxillary first molar hits the mesial area of the mandibular second molar. (In protrusive movement only the anterior teeth should occlude; the posterior teeth disengage.)

This occlusal trauma results in mobility of the affected teeth and finally migration and tipping of these teeth. The mandibular second premolar migrates and tips distally and results in an open contact between the mandibular premolars. This open contact can cause a periodontal pocket

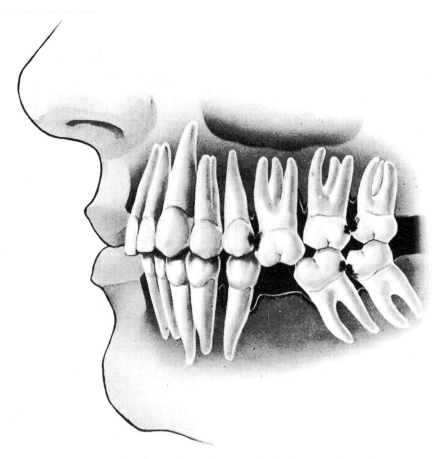

FIG. 28-5. Dental tissues collapse because of a failure to replace the missing mandibular first molar. (From Massler M, Schour I: *Atlas of the mouth in health and disease,* ed 2, Chicago, 1975, American Dental Association.)

with loss of the lamina dura and formation of infraosseous periodontal pockets.

The teeth are not the only structures traumatized. The temporomandibular joint and especially the lateral pterygoid muscles suffer from trauma caused by premature occlusal contacts.

The combination of occlusal trauma and mesial drift cause the mandibular second molar to move mesially and tip gingivally. This in turn causes a poor contact area between the distal mandibular second molar and the mandibular third molar, which results in a periodontal

pocket between these two molars. This malpositioned contact area allows the bacteria to build up initiate dental decay of the interproximal surfaces of these two molars. The mesial drift of the mandibular third molar causes the second molar to move into the decay area on the second molars, causing a poor occlusal relationship between the two third molars.

All of this helps to illustrate the importance of good preventive dentistry and the interrelationships that exist within the oral cavity. All of the dental structures interrelate in a biomechanical system. Each mechanism protects and supports the others in some way. The breakdown of any one of these systems destroys the circle of mutual protection. If the contour of teeth is destroyed, sooner or later the gingiva and bone tissue are destroyed. If the occlusal relationship is destroyed, there is damage to the bone, teeth, gums, and temporomandibular joint. Even the muscles responsible for movement of the jaw become traumatized and spasmodic. When an occlusal prematurity exists, the patient subconsciously tries to avoid this occlusal discrepancy. To do this, the patient overexerts the lateral pterygoid muscle. This muscle becomes overworked, trying to protrude the jaw to avoid the premature contact. This is only one example among numerous possibilities.

The best dentistry is preventive dentistry. Preventive dentistry maintains the oral structures in their most mutually protective harmony. It intercepts disease at the earliest possible time so that the most natural, self-protective, functional, and preventive balances can be restored and maintained by these tissues. The clinical considerations are endless, but here it is intended that the student of dental anatomy merely have an example of how to apply the basic principles of dental anatomy to the clinical experience. Never cease to be alert and observant. Your reward will be the comfort of patients, pride in your work, and the progress of the dental profession.

Review Questions

1. If a dentist restores a tooth in such a way that it is the first tooth to touch its antagonist when the patient closes his mouth, which of the following clinical problems could result?
   a. Inflammation of the nerve of the tooth
   b. Occlusal trauma
   c. Tooth mobility
   d. Tooth migration
   e. Pain
   f. Nerve involvement
   g. Fracture of the restoration or the tooth
   h. Inflammation of the supporting structures of the tooth
   i. All of the above

2. If a dentist cuts a crown preparation but does not place a temporary restoration properly, which of the following could occur?
   a. Gingival inflammation of the supporting structures because of bacterial build-up around the margins of the temporary restoration
   b. Occlusal trauma to the tooth and temporary restoration
   c. Tooth migration to avoid occlusal trauma
   d. Supraeruption of the tooth to meet its antagonist
   e. Pain caused by trauma, inflammation, or bacterial involvement
   f. Sensitivity to hot or cold fluids
   g. Tipping or mesial drifting of the tooth

3. What could happen to the nerve of a tooth if the tooth became inflamed because of occlusal traumatization?

4. Name all of the possible pathologic situations present in Fig. 28-6.

5. You find an overhanging restoration on an x-ray. It does not show any bone loss radiographically. You use an explorer to examine the gingival area next to the overhang in the patient's mouth. What findings would you consider healthy?

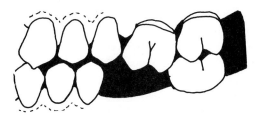

FIG. 28-6.

a. The presence of a 4-mm pocket
b. The depth of the gingival sulcus exceeding 3 mm
c. The presence of pus and blood upon probing the area
d. No bleeding upon probing the sulcus a depth of 2.5 mm (pink and firm papillary gingiva)

6. What can be done to prevent dental disease (caries and periodontal disease)?
   a. Polishing restorations
   b. Sealants
   c. Smoothing off or replacing overhanging restorations
   d. Grinding down teeth that are hitting prematurely
   e. All of the above

7. Which of the following will illicit a pain response in an area of gum recession?
   a. Cold
   b. Swells
   c. Air
   d. Heat
   e. All of these
   f. None of these

8. A healthy gingival sulcus rarely exceeds:
   a. 3 mm
   b. 3.5 mm
   c. 4 mm
   d. 2.5 mm

CHAPTER 29

TOOTH IDENTIFICATION

IT IS rare to find a full set of teeth in which every tooth met all the anatomic criteria of what a perfect tooth should be; there is too much variation among individual teeth. When studying tooth identification, it is important to remember the extreme amounts of variation possible. The individual tooth you are trying to identify may meet most of the criteria of a maxillary central incisor, may be missing certain criteria for a maxillary central incisor, and may even meet some of the criteria of a maxillary canine or lateral incisor, yet it may still be a maxillary central incisor. Only after compiling all of the characteristics of the tooth in question and categorizing these characteristics, that one can identify the individual tooth—and then only after it becomes apparent that the tooth meets more characteristics of one type of tooth than another.

Following is a description of general characteristics of each of the teeth by their respective groupings: incisors, canines, premolars, and molars.* In identifying teeth it is necessary to be able to differentiate among the left and right teeth in any particular group.

---

*The term *facial* has been used synonymously with *labial* and *buccal*. In general, the terms *labial* and *buccal* will be used because they are most commonly accepted; however, *facial* will also be used. *Facial* can be substituted for *labial* and *buccal* and vice versa.

GENERAL RULES OF TOOTH IDENTIFICATION

1. The curvature of the cementoenamel junction (CEJ) is usually about 1 mm less on the distal surface of the tooth than on the mesial.
2. Tooth roots do not always curve; however, if they do curve, they usually curve distally, especially at the apex of the root. It is not uncommon, however, for the root to curve toward mesially.
3. The distal incisal edges of anterior teeth are more rounded than the mesial incisal edges.
4. Mandibular anterior teeth tend to wear on their labial incisal edges, whereas maxillary teeth wear on their lingual incisal edges. Unless a person has a class III occlusion, the maxillary teeth are facial to the mandibular teeth.
5. Permanent molars are generally smaller in height and have fewer cusps the more posteriorly they are positioned. For example, permanent first molar usually has five cusps and is larger than a second or third molar. A mandibular first molar has a distal cusp on its facial surface, and a maxillary first molar has a cusp of Carabelli. The second and third molars are less likely to have these cusps; however, when they do, cusps are less well developed and are more like tubercles than cusps.
6. Permanent molars tend to have more **secondary** and **tertiary anatomy** the more posteriorly they are positioned. Secondary anatomy consists of extra grooves and pits in addition to

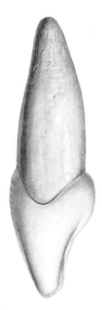

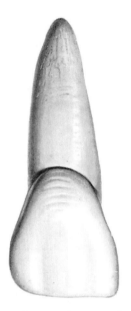

Fig. 29-1. Maxillary right central incisor, mesial view. (From Zeisz RC, Nuckolls J: *Dental anatomy*, St Louis, 1949, Mosby.)

Fig. 29-2. Maxillary right central incisor, labial view. (From Zeisz RC, Nuckolls J: *Dental anatomy*, St Louis, 1949, Mosby.)

the main primary developmental anatomy. These grooves and pits are more shallow than the primary anatomy and are more likely to be found on second and third molars. Tertiary anatomy refers to the extremely shallow and even more numerous grooves, pits and lines that third molars often have, giving them a more wrinkled appearance than first or second molars.

7. The roots of molars tend to be shorter and closer together the more posteriorly the molars are positioned, and the roots are often fused into one. First molars have the widest and longest roots of all molars.

8. There is more variation of anatomy the more posteriorly the molars are positioned. Third molars are more wrinkled and unpredictable in shape than second or first molars; they could have six cusps or one single conical

cusp. They are also more likely to be congenitally missing than other molars.

INCISORS

1. Incisal two thirds appear flattened on labial and lingual sides (Fig. 29-1)
2. Incisal "biting" edge, not a cusp (Fig. 29-2)

Maxillary

1. Crown wider mesiodistally than faciolingually (Figs. 29-3 and 29-4)
2. Root has triangular cross section, being broader on facial side

Central

1. Greater crown-to-root ratio than lateral incisors (crown larger, root about same as or smaller than lateral incisors) (Figs. 29-5 and 29-6)

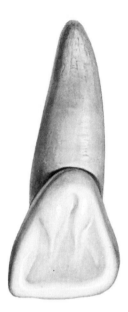

FIG. 29-3. Maxillary right central incisor, lingual view. (From Zeisz RC, Nuckolls J: *Dental anatomy,* St Louis, 1949, Mosby.)

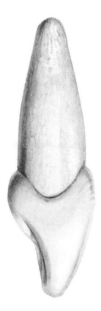

FIG. 29-4. Maxillary right central incisor, distal view. (From Zeisz RC, Nuckolls J: *Dental anatomy,* St Louis, 1949, Mosby.)

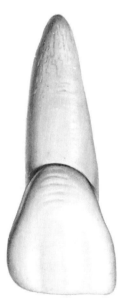

FIG. 29-5. Maxillary right central incisor, labial view. (From Zeisz RC, Nuckolls J: *Dental anatomy,* St Louis, 1949, Mosby.)

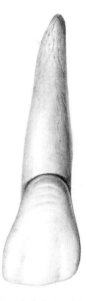

FIG. 29-6. Maxillary left lateral incisor, labial view. (From Zeisz RC, Nuckolls J: *Dental anatomy,* St Louis, 1949, Mosby.)

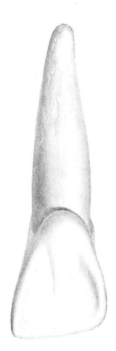

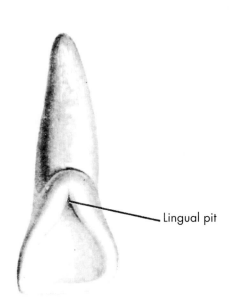

FIG. 29-7. Maxillary right lateral incisor, lingual view. (From Zeisz RC, Nuckolls J: *Dental anatomy*, St Louis, 1949, Mosby.)

FIG. 29-8. Maxillary right lateral incisor, lingual view. (From Zeisz RC, Nuckolls J: *Dental anatomy*, St Louis, 1949, Mosby.)

2. Mesioincisal angle relatively sharp (90-degree angle), with contact area in incisal third
3. Broad, smooth lingual fossa with well-developed cingulum

Lateral
1. Lesser crown-to-root ratio than central incisors (crown smaller, root about same as or larger than central incisors)
2. Mesioincisal angle rounded, with contact area at junction of middle and incisal thirds
3. Small cingulum, often with a lingual pit (Figs. 29-7 and 29-8)

Right-left
1. Mesioincisal angles more square than distoincisal angles (Fig. 29-9)

2. Crest of cervical line more often displaced toward distal from labial or lingual view
3. Mesiocervical line curves more incisally than distocervical line (Figs. 29-10)

Mandibular
1. Smaller than maxillary central or lateral incisor (Figs. 29-11 and 29-12)
2. Crown wider faciolingually than mesio-distally
3. Root with oval cross section
4. Incisal edge wears on labial surface (Fig. 29-13); incisal edge angled toward the lingual side

Central
1. Incisal view—incisal edge perpendicular to faciolingual axis of tooth

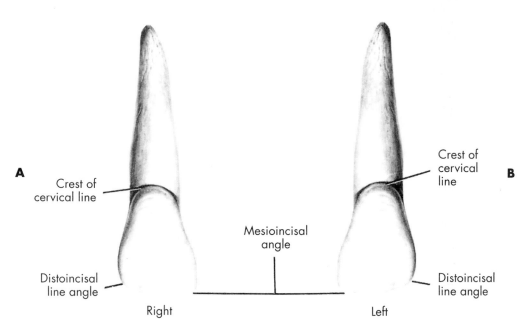

FIG. 29-9.   **A,** Maxillary right lateral incisor. **B,** Maxillary left lateral incisor. (From Zeisz RC, Nuckolls J: *Dental anatomy,* St Louis, 1949, Mosby.)

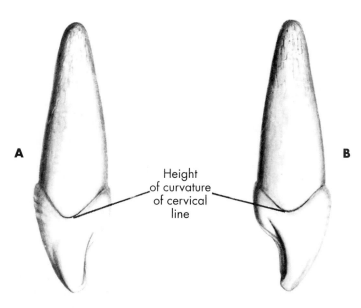

FIG. 29-10.   **A,** Maxillary right lateral incisor, mesial view. **B,** Maxillary right lateral incisor, distal view. (From Zeisz RC, Nuckolls J: *Dental anatomy,* St Louis, 1949, Mosby.)

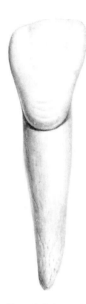

FIG. 29-11.   Maxillary left lateral incisor is shown inverted for comparison. (From Zeisz RC, Nuckolls J: *Dental anatomy,* St Louis, 1949, Mosby.)

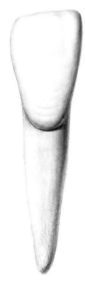

FIG. 29-12.   Mandibular right lateral incisor. (From Zeisz RC, Nuckolls J: *Dental anatomy,* St Louis, 1949, Mosby.)

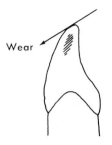

FIG. 29-13.   Mandibular right lateral incisor, mesial view.

FIG. 29-14.   Mandibular right central incisor, incisal view. (From Zeisz RC, Nuckolls J: *Dental anatomy,* St Louis, 1949, Mosby.)

FIG. 29-15.   Mandibular right lateral incisor, incisal view. (From Zeisz RC, Nuckolls J: *Dental anatomy,* St Louis, 1949, Mosby.)

2. Mesial and distal lobes appear identical (Fig. 29-14)

Right-left

1. Cervical line curves more incisally on mesial than on distal surface
2. Height of curvature of cervical line on mesial greater than on distal surface
3. Root tip may have slight distal curve
4. Incisal edge worn wider on distal surface

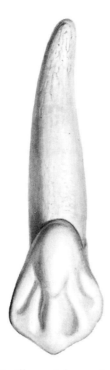

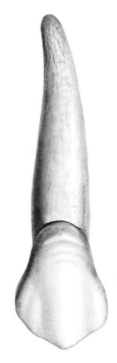

FIG. 29-16. Maxillary right canine, lingual view. (From Zeisz RC, Nuckolls J: *Dental anatomy*, St Louis, 1949, Mosby.)

FIG. 29-17. Maxillary right canine, labial view. (From Zeisz RC, Nuckolls J: *Dental anatomy*, St Louis, 1949, Mosby.)

Lateral
1. Incisal view—distoincisal edge angled toward lingual side
2. Distal lobe appears larger than mesial lobe (Fig. 29-15)

Right-left
1. Cervical line curves more incisally on mesial than on distal surface
2. Incisal view—distal half of incisal edge rotated toward lingual side
3. Incisal edge worn wider and longer on distal surface

CANINES

1. Single conical cusp with well-developed mesiofacial lobe

2. Lingual cusp ridge from cusp tip to lingual fossa

Maxillary

1. Lingual surface has well-developed marginal ridges, cingulum, and fossa (Fig. 29-16)
2. Larger and bulkier crown than incisors and lower canines; more distal convexity (Fig. 29-17)
3. Cusp tip directly midcenter over root

Right-left
1. Cervical line curves more incisally on mesial than on distal surface (Figs. 29-18 and 29-19)
2. Incisal view—distofacial lobe elongated or pulled out

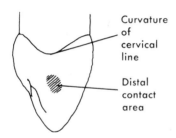

FIG. 29-18.   Maxillary right canine, distal view.

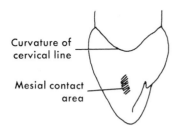

FIG. 29-19.   Maxillary right canine, mesial view.

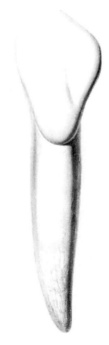

FIG. 29-20.   Mandibular right canine, lingual view. (From Zeisz RC, Nuckolls J: *Dental anatomy,* St Louis, 1949, Mosby.)

3. Facial view—distal surface rounded and contact area located more cervically

Mandibular

1. Lingual surface almost smooth with poorly developed ridges, cingulum, and fossa (Fig. 29-20)
2. Narrower mesiodistal width than maxillary
3. More wear on facial (labial) surface (Fig. 29-21) when compared with maxillary canine

PREMOLARS

1. At least two cusps, one a single facial cusp, with one or two lingual cusps

Maxillary

1. Two major cusps, one buccal and one lingual, approximately equal in size

2. Distinctly wider faciolingually than mesiodistally
3. Proximal view—facial and lingual cusps nearly same height and both located over root trunk (Fig. 29-22)

First premolar

1. Facial cusp slightly longer than lingual cusp (Fig. 29-23)
2. Frequently has two roots, buccal and lingual
3. Occlusal surface has well-developed central groove, with little supplemental grooving
4. Mesial surface has depression above contact area starting below cervical line and usually extending onto root

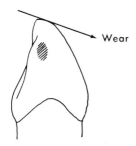

FIG. 29-21. Mandibular right canine, mesial view. (From Zeisz RC, Nuckolls J: *Dental anatomy,* St Louis, 1949, Mosby.)

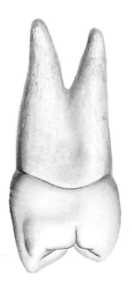

FIG. 29-23. Maxillary right first premolar, mesial view. (From Zeisz RC, Nuckolls J: *Dental anatomy,* St Louis, 1949, Mosby.)

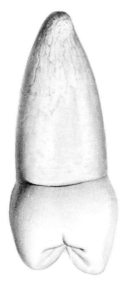

FIG. 29-22. Maxillary right second premolar, distal view. (From Zeisz RC, Nuckolls J: *Dental anatomy,* St Louis, 1949, Mosby.)

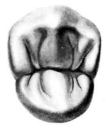

FIG. 29-24. Maxillary right first premolar, occlusal view. (From Zeisz RC, Nuckolls J: *Dental anatomy,* St Louis, 1949, Mosby.)

Right-left
1. Mesial marginal groove
2. Cervical line on mesial curves more occlusally than on distal surface
3. Occlusal view—mesiofacial cusp ridge forms 90-degree angle with mesial marginal ridge; distofacial cusp ridge forms rounded angle with distal marginal ridge (Fig. 29-24)

Second premolar
1. Facial and lingual cusps nearly same height (Fig. 29-25)
2. Usually single rooted
3. Short central groove, with frequent and numerous supplemental grooves

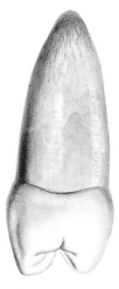

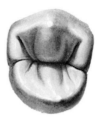

FIG. 29-26.   Maxillary right second premolar, occlusal view. (From Zeisz RC, Nuckolls J: *Dental anatomy*, St Louis, 1949, Mosby.)

FIG. 29-25.   Maxillary right second premolar, mesial view. (From Zeisz RC, Nuckolls J: *Dental anatomy*, St Louis, 1949, Mosby.)

4. No depression on mesial or distal crown surfaces

Right-left

1. Lingual cusp displaced slightly toward mesial side (Fig. 29-26)

Mandibular

1. Prominent facial cusp with one or two much smaller lingual cusps
2. Nearly equal faciolingual and mesiodistal widths
3. Proximal view—facial cusp much larger; facial cusp tip at or near midaxis of root; lingual cusp(s) extend lingually past lingual border of root (Fig. 29-27)

First premolar

1. Proximal view—occlusal surface tilted strongly toward lingual side (Fig. 29-28)
2. Occlusal view—oval outline with strong transverse ridge and no central pit (Fig. 29-29)

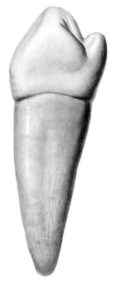

FIG. 29-27.   Mandibular right first premolar, mesial view. (From Zeisz RC, Nuckolls J: *Dental anatomy*, St Louis, 1949, Mosby.)

Right-left

1. Cervical line on mesial surface curves more occlusally than on distal surface
2. Frequently a depression or groove where mesial marginal ridge joins lingual cusp ridge (Fig. 29-30)
3. Distal marginal ridge more prominent

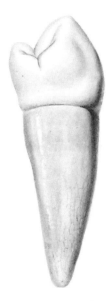

FIG. 29-28.   Mandibular right first premolar, proximal view. (From Zeisz RC, Nuckolls J: *Dental anatomy*, St Louis, 1949, Mosby.)

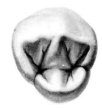

FIG. 29-29.   Mandibular right first premolar, occlusal view. (From Zeisz RC, Nuckolls J: *Dental anatomy*, St Louis, 1949, Mosby.)

Second premolar
1. Occlusal view—pentagonal outline, with a central pit and no transverse ridge (Fig. 29-31)
2. Proximal view—occlusal surface less lingually tilted (Fig. 29-32)
3. May have two lingual cusps

Right-left
1. Proximal view—more of occlusal surface

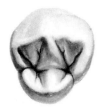

FIG. 29-30.   Mandibular left first premolar, occlusal view. (From Zeisz RC, Nuckolls J: *Dental anatomy*, St Louis, 1949, Mosby.)

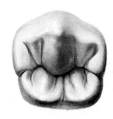

FIG. 29-31.   Mandibular right second premolar, occlusal view. (From Zeisz RC, Nuckolls J: *Dental anatomy*, St Louis, 1949, Mosby.)

visible from distal than from mesial because of distal inclination of crown axis to root axis

MOLARS
1. Three to five cusps, with at least two facial

Maxillary
1. Crowns wider faciolingually than mesiodistally
2. Three roots: two on facial and one on lingual side

First molar
1. Occlusal view—strong **oblique ridge** less likely to be crossed by a groove (Fig. 29-33)
2. Three roots widely separated
3. Frequently has a fifth cusp (Carabelli's) on mesiolingual cusp (Fig. 29-34)

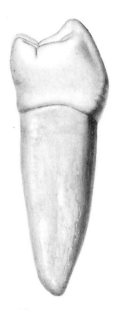

FIG. 29-32.   Mandibular right second premolar, distal view. (From Zeisz RC, Nuckolls J: *Dental anatomy,* St Louis, 1949, Mosby.)

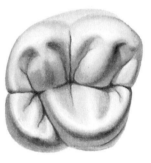

FIG. 29-33.   Maxillary right first molar, occlusal view. (From Zeisz RC, Nuckolls J: *Dental anatomy,* St Louis, 1949, Mosby.)

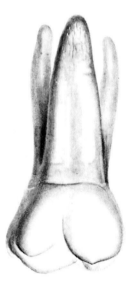

FIG. 29-34.   Maxillary right first molar, lingual view. (From Zeisz RC, Nuckolls J: *Dental anatomy,* St Louis, 1949, Mosby.)

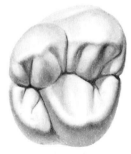

FIG. 29-35.   Maxillary right second molar, occlusal view. (From Zeisz RC, Nuckolls J: *Dental anatomy,* St Louis, 1949, Mosby.)

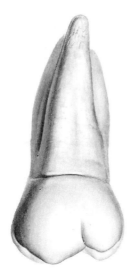

FIG. 29-36. Maxillary right second molar, lingual view. (From Zeisz RC, Nuckolls J: *Dental anatomy*, St Louis, 1949, Mosby.)

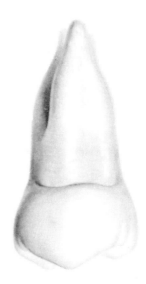

FIG. 29-37. Maxillary right third molar, lingual view. (From Zeisz RC, Nuckolls J: *Dental anatomy*, St Louis, 1949, Mosby.)

Right-left
1. Mesiolingual cusp always much larger than distolingual cusp

Second molar
1. Occlusal view—smaller oblique ridge usually interrupted by a groove (Fig. 29-35)
2. Roots closer together (Fig. 29-36)
3. No fifth cusp
4. Distolingual cusp smaller than on first molar

Right-left
1. Mesiolingual cusp always much larger than distolingual cusp

Third molar
1. Distolingual cusp progressively smaller or missing entirely (Fig. 29-37)
2. Roots either fused or very close together and much shorter
3. No oblique ridge (Fig. 29-38)

Right-left
1. Distofacial cusp much shorter than other molars
2. Roots curved distally

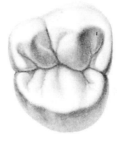

FIG. 29-38. Maxillary right third molar, occlusal view. (From Zeisz RC, Nuckolls J: *Dental anatomy*, St Louis, 1949, Mosby.)

Mandibular
1. Crowns wider mesiodistally than faciolingually
2. Two roots: one mesial and one distal

First molar
1. Three facial cusps and two facial grooves (Fig. 29-39)

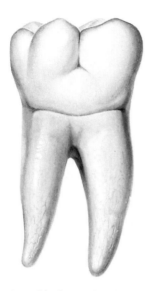

FIG. 29-39. Mandibular right first molar, buccal view. (From Zeisz RC, Nuckolls J: *Dental anatomy*, St Louis, 1949, Mosby.)

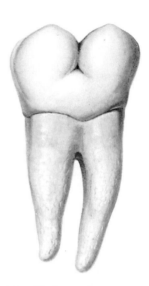

FIG. 29-41. Mandibular right second molar, buccal view. (From Zeisz RC, Nuckolls J: *Dental anatomy*, St Louis, 1949, Mosby.)

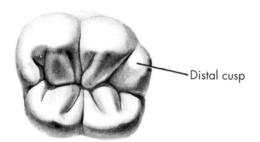

—Distal cusp

FIG. 29-40. Mandibular right first molar, occlusal view. (From Zeisz RC, Nuckolls J: *Dental anatomy*, St Louis, 1949, Mosby.)

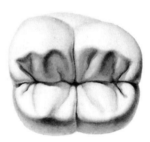

FIG. 29-42. Mandibular right second molar, occlusal view. (From Zeisz RC, Nuckolls J: *Dental anatomy*, St Louis, 1949, Mosby.)

2. Roots widely separated and relatively vertical

Right-left

1. Distal cusp is smallest facial cusp (Fig. 29-40)

Second molar

1. Only two facial cusps and one facial groove (Fig. 29-41)
2. Occlusal groove well defined but travels straight mesial to distal and forms a cross (+) with facial and lingual grooves (Fig. 29-42)

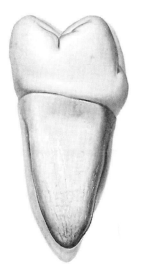

FIG. 29-43. Mandibular right second molar, distal view. (From Zeisz RC, Nuckolls J: *Dental anatomy,* St Louis, 1949, Mosby.)

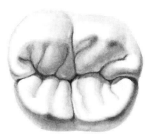

FIG. 29-44. Mandibular right third molar, occlusal view. (From Zeisz RC, Nuckolls J: *Dental anatomy,* St Louis, 1949, Mosby.)

3. Roots close together
Right-left
1. Buccal height of contour in cervical third; lingual height of contour in middle third (Fig. 29-43)
Third molar
1. Secondary and tertiary anatomy (Fig. 29-44)
2. Short roots, often fused and curved distally

Right-left
1. Crown tapers distally; wider faciolingually on mesial than on distal surface (also true of mandibular first and second molars)

Review Questions

1. Which anterior incisors are much wider mesiodistally than faciolingually?
2. Which incisors, centrals or laterals, have the greater crown-to-root ratio?
3. Which incisors are nearly identical?
4. In general, does the cervical line curve more incisally on the mesial or the distal surface?
5. Which has more developed lingual marginal ridges, the maxillary or mandible?
6. On incisors, which incisal line angle is more rounded, mesial or distal?
7. Which incisor has its incisal edge worn on the labial side, maxillary or mandibular?
8. Which mandibular incisor is longer?
9. Which canine has more distal convexity?
10. Which is more concave, the inside or the outside of a football helmet?
11. On canines, which surface is least convex, mesial or distal?
12. Which premolars are most likely to have two roots?
13. Which premolar is most likely to have three cusps?
14. Which premolar is most likely to have a well-defined mesial marginal groove?
15. Which molars, first or second, are most likely to have five cusps?
16. Name the smallest of the five cusps of a mandibular first molar.
17. The fifth cusp of a maxillary first molar is located on what other cusp?

18. The roots are closer together on a first or second molar?

19. The roots are longest on a first or second molar?

20. Which molar is most likely to have three buccal cusps?

21. If two teeth look identical, such as two mandibular incisors, the one that shows greater curvature of the cementoenamel junction (CEJ) is more likely the:
   a. Central
   b. Lateral
   c. Neither

22. If the root of the tooth described in question 21 has a curve of the root at its apex, this curve more likely points:
   a. Mesially
   b. Distally
   c. Neither

23. If this same tooth has a rounded incisal ridge on the same side toward which the root curves, this rounded edge is more likely to be the:
   a. Mesial incisal ridge
   b. Distal incisal ridge

CHAPTER 30

INCISORS

OBJECTIVES
- To identify the particular anatomic features of incisor teeth
- To compare maxillary central incisors with maxillary lateral incisors
- To compare maxillary incisors with their mandibular incisor counterparts
- To identify an extracted incisor
- To recognize the normal and the deviated anatomic forms of incisor teeth

THERE ARE eight permanent incisors, four maxillary (upper) and four mandibular (lower). The maxillary incisors consist of two central and two lateral incisors, as do the four mandibular incisors (Fig. 30-1).

The most prominent teeth in the mouth are the maxillary incisors. The maxillary central incisors are larger than the lateral incisors, but these teeth complement each other in form and function. The central incisors erupt in the seventh or eighth year, and the lateral incisors a year or so later.

MAXILLARY INCISORS

Central Incisors

Evidence of calcification	3 months
Eruption	7-8 years
Root completed	10 years

A maxillary central incisor (Fig. 30-2) is the widest mesiodistally of any of the anterior teeth. Its labial appearance is less rounded than that of a maxillary lateral incisor or canine. The crown usually looks symmetrical and normally formed, having a nearly straight incisal edge, a mesial side with a straight outline, and the distal side more curved. The mesioincisal angle is relatively sharp, and the distoincisal angle is much more rounded.

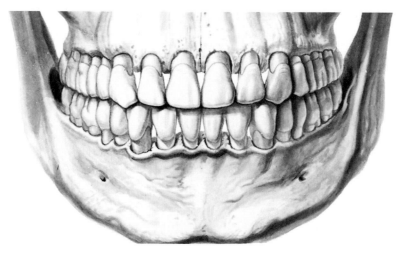

FIG. 30-1.   Anterior view of the lower portion of an adult skull. (From Zeisz RC, Nuckolls J: *Dental anatomy,* St Louis, 1949, Mosby.)

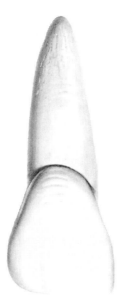

FIG. 30-2.   Maxillary right central incisor. (From Zeisz RC, Nuckolls J: *Dental anatomy,* St Louis, 1949, Mosby.)

Maxillary central incisors usually develop normally. Two anomalies that sometimes occur are a short root or an unusually long crown. A third is gemination where the tooth shows evidence of attempting to divide itself.

Labial aspect (Fig. 30-3; see also Fig. 30-8, *A*)

The labial surface of the crown of the maxillary central incisor is slightly convex, bulging out from the cervical portion of the crown. The enamel surface is very smooth. When the tooth first erupts, mamelons can be seen on the incisal ridge. These mamelons are rounded portions of the incisal ridge of newly erupted teeth. Each mamelon forms the incisal ridge portion of one of the labial primary lobes. Developmental lines on the labial face divide the surface into three parts, each developmental line separating a primary lobe.

From this facial view, the distal outline of the crown is more rounded or convex than the mesial outline, the height of curvature being higher toward the cervical line. The cervical line crests slightly distal to the center of the tooth.

The incisal outline is usually regular and straight across the incisal ridge after the tooth

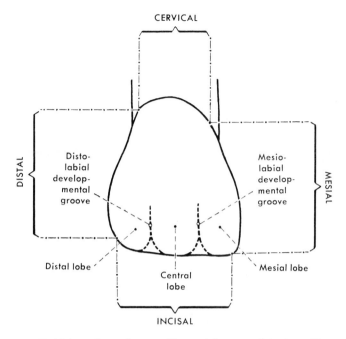

CERVICAL

DISTAL

Disto-
labial
develop-
mental
groove

Mesio-
labial
develop-
mental
groove

MESIAL

Distal lobe

Central
lobe

Mesial lobe

INCISAL

FIG. 30-3.   Labial surface of a maxillary right central incisor. (From Zeisz RC, Nuckolls J: *Dental anatomy*, St Louis, 1949, Mosby.)

has been in function long enough to wear down the mamelons. When an incisor first erupts, the incisal portion of the crown is rounded and the mamelons are quite distinct. This ridge portion is then called the *incisal ridge*. However, normal use eventually wears down the rounded ridge into a flat edge, and therefore the term **incisal edge** is more appropriate than ridge.

The root of a central incisor from the labial aspect is cone shaped and has a blunt apex in most instances. The root is usually 2 to 3 mm longer than the crown, though the root-to-crown ratio varies considerably.

Lingual aspect (Fig. 30-4; see also Fig. 30-8, *B*)

The lingual outline of a maxillary central incisor is the reverse of that found on the labial aspect. The labial surface of the crown is smooth, whereas the lingual surface is bordered by rounded convexities and a concavity. The outline

of the cervical line is similar, but immediately below the cervical line is a smooth convexity called the *cingulum*.

Mesially and distally confluent with the cingulum is a shallow concavity called the *lingual fossa*. The marginal and incisal ridges, which are rounded convexities, border the lingual fossa. Usually there are developmental grooves extending from the cingulum into the lingual fossa.

The crown and root taper lingually; the lingual portion of the root is narrower than the labial portion.

Mesial aspect (Fig. 30-5; see also Fig. 30-8, *D*)

The crown of a maxillary central incisor is triangular, with the base of the triangle at the cervix and the apex at the incisal ridge. The incisal ridge of the crown is centered over the middle of the root. This alignment is characteristic of maxillary central and lateral incisors.

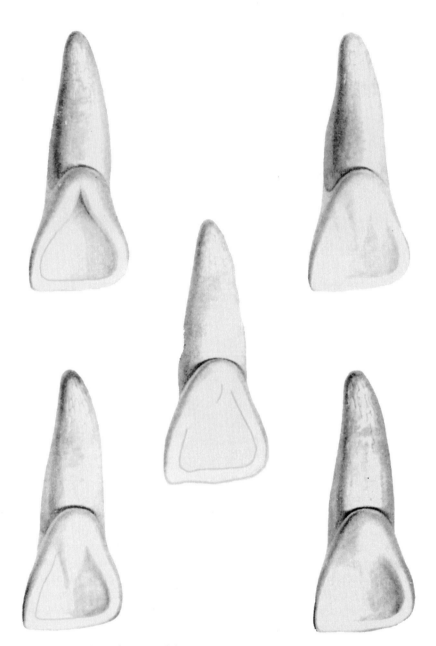

FIG. 30-4.   Lingual views of five permanent maxillary right central incisors.
(From Zeisz RC, Nuckolls J: *Dental anatomy*, St Louis, 1949, Mosby.)

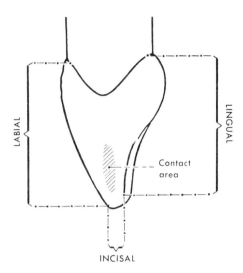

FIG. 30-5. Mesial surface of a maxillary right central incisor. (From Zeisz RC, Nuckolls J: *Dental anatomy*, St Louis, 1949, Mosby.)

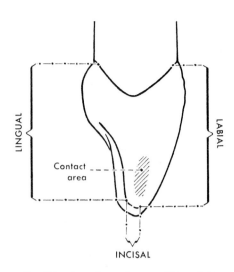

FIG. 30-6. Distal surface of a maxillary right central incisor. (From Zeisz RC, Nuckolls J: *Dental anatomy*, St Louis, 1949, Mosby.)

The labial outline of the crown from the crest of curvature to the incisal edge is slightly convex, with the height of curvature about one third of the way down from the cervical line. The cervical curvature is greater on the mesial surface of these teeth than on any surface of any other teeth in the mouth.

Distal aspect (Fig. 30-6; see also Fig. 30-8, *E*)

There is a little difference between the distal and mesial outlines of maxillary central incisors. The cervical line indicating the cementoenamel junction (CEJ) is less curved on the distal surface than on the mesial. It is generally true that if there is a difference in the curvatures of the mesial and distal cervical lines of the same tooth, the mesial curvature will be greater. For example, if mesial curvature is 2.5 mm, the distal might be 1.5 mm.

Incisal aspect (Fig. 30-7; see also Fig. 30-8, *C*)

The incisal ridge tends to slope lingually as a result of the lower incisors coming more frequently into contact with the lingual edge than

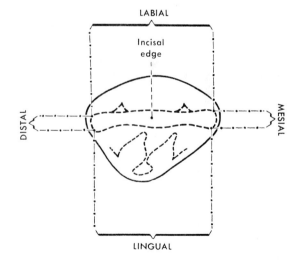

FIG. 30-7. Incisal edge of a maxillary right central incisor. (From Zeisz RC, Nuckolls J: *Dental anatomy*, St Louis, 1949, Mosby.)

with the facial edge of the maxillary incisor. From an incisal view, the crown shows a triangular shape, with its apex on the lingual surface. (See Fig. 30-8 for all of the views of a maxillary right central incisor.)

Lateral Incisors

Evidence of calcification	1 year
Eruption	8-9 years
Root completed	11 years

Maxillary lateral incisors complement the central incisors in function and resemble each other in form. Lateral incisors are small in all dimensions except root length. The features—curvatures, concavities, and convexities—of the lateral incisors are more prominent and show more distinction and contrast than those of the central incisors. These teeth differ from the central incisors in that their individual development varies considerably. Maxillary lateral incisors vary in form more than any other teeth in the mouth except the third molars. If the variation is too great, it is considered a developmental anomaly. A common situation is to find maxillary lateral incisors that have a nondescript, pointed form; such teeth are called **peg-shaped lateral incisors.** In some persons the lateral incisors are missing entirely. Maxillary lateral incisors are more likely to be congenitally missing than any other teeth except the third molars. One type of malformed maxillary lateral incisor displays a large, pointed tubercle as part of the cingulum; some have deep developmental grooves that extend down the root lingually with a deep fold in the cingulum. Other maxillary lateral incisors show twisted roots or distorted crowns.

Labial aspect

Although the labial aspect (Fig. 30-9, A) of a maxillary lateral incisor may appear to resemble that of a central incisor, it usually has more curvature, with a rounded incisal ridge and rounded angles mesially and distally. The distal outline is always more rounded and the height of contour more cervical than the mesial outline.

The labial surface of the crown is more convex than that of a central incisor, and as a rule, the root length is greater in proportion to the crown length than that of a central incisor. The root is often about one and one half times the length of the crown.

Lingual aspect

The lingual view (Fig. 30-9, B) of a lateral incisor shows more contrast than the same view of a central incisor. Mesial and distal marginal ridges are pronounced and the cingulum is usually prominent, with a tendency toward deep developmental grooves within the lingual fossa where it joins the cingulum. The linguoincisal ridge is better developed, and the lingual fossa is more concave and circumscribed than that of the central incisor.

Mesial aspect

The mesial aspect (Fig. 30-9, D) of a maxillary lateral incisor is similar to that of a small central incisor, except that the root appears longer.

Distal aspect

The distal aspect (Fig. 30-9, E) of the maxillary lateral incisor is the same as the mesial aspect except for less curvature of the cervical line.

Incisal aspect

The incisal aspect (Fig. 30-9, C) of these teeth sometimes resembles that of the central incisors or a small canine. The cingulum and the incisal ridge, however, may be large; the labiolingual dimension may be greater than usual in comparison with the mesiodistal dimension. If these variations are present, the teeth show a strong resemblance to the canines.

All maxillary lateral incisors exhibit more convexity labially and lingually from the incisal aspect than do the maxillary central incisors.

Root

The maxillary central incisor usually has a straight, thick, cylindrically shaped root. The maxillary lateral incisor has a narrower root mesiodistally; the root is as long as that of the central incisor but appears thinner. The apical por-

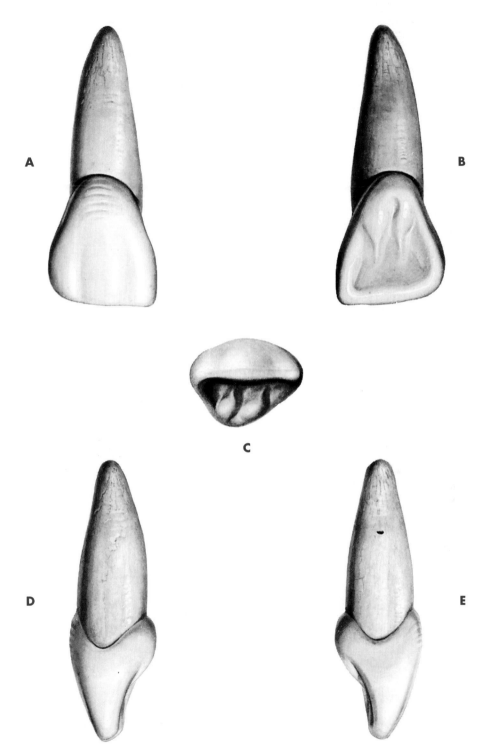

FIG. 30-8.   A maxillary right central incisor. **A,** Labial view. **B,** Lingual view.
C, Incisal view. **D,** Mesial view. **E,** Distal view. (From Zeisz RC, Nuckolls J:
Dental anatomy, St Louis, 1949, Mosby.)

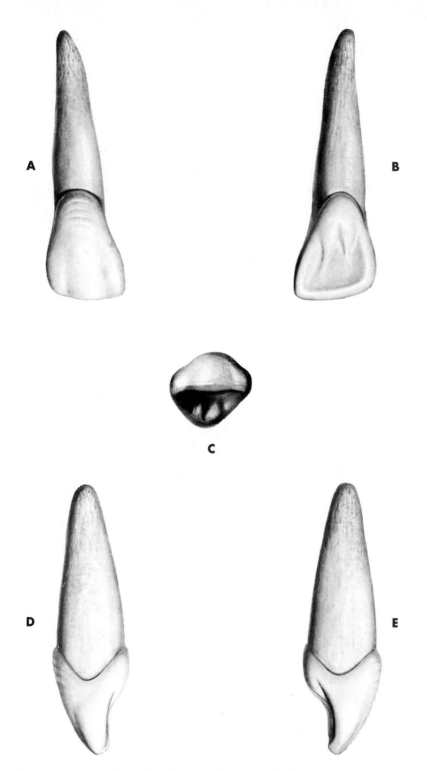

F𝐈𝐆. 30-9.   A maxillary right lateral incisor. **A,** Labial view. **B,** Lingual view.
C, Incisal view. **D,** Mesial view. **E,** Distal view. (From Zeisz RC, Nuckolls J:
Dental anatomy, St Louis, 1949, Mosby.)

tion of the lateral incisor's root often curves distally and ends in a sharp apex rather than in a blunt, straight apex as in the central incisor.

Neither maxillary central nor lateral roots shows evidence of division, bifurcation, indentation, or a proximal groove.

Pulp Cavity

The pulp cavity varies in size with the age of the tooth. When the tooth first erupts, the pulp cavity is very large and the root is incompletely formed, so the canal becomes funnel shaped in the region of the apical foramen. As the tooth develops completely, the entire pulp cavity to the apex of the root becomes smaller, and the dentin becomes thicker in both the crown and the root. The apical foramen is then very small. This process continues throughout the life of the tooth. It

is not unusual to find in very elderly persons that the entire pulp cavity has become calcified and there is solid dentin filling the entire root canal. This variation in the size of the pulp cavity with aging is common to all of the permanent teeth.

The pulp cavity of the maxillary central incisor (Fig. 30-10) mirrors the configuration of the tooth. There is only one root canal, which is rather large. The pulp chamber lies in the coronal portion of the tooth and presents three sharp elongations: the mesial, distal, and central pulp horns. The central pulp horn is usually shorter and more rounded than the other two.

The pulp cavity of the maxillary lateral incisor is quite simple, comprising only a pulp chamber and a single pulp canal. The chamber is similar to that of the maxillary central incisor but usually does not have three sharp pulp horns.

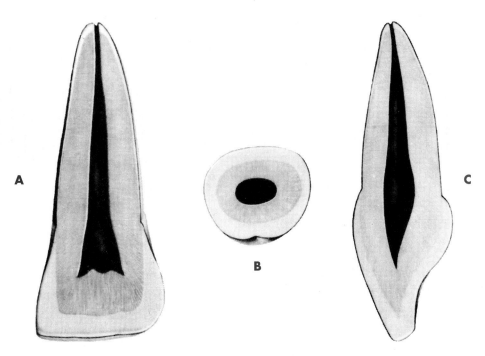

FIG. 30-10.   The pulp cavity of a maxillary right central incisor. **A,** Distomesial section, lingual view. **B,** Cross section, incisal view. **C,** Linguolabial section, mesial view. (From Zeisz RC, Nuckolls J: *Dental anatomy,* St Louis, 1949, Mosby.)

More often the pulp chamber ends incisally as one rounded form or two less sharp pulp horns, a mesial and distal (Fig. 30-11).

Pertinent Data

Maxillary central incisors

	Right	Left
Universal Code	8	9
International Code	11	21
Palmer notation	1⏌	⎳1
Number of roots	1	
Number of pulp horns	3	
Number of developmental lobes	4	

Location of proximal contact areas
Mesial: incisal third
Distal: junction of incisal and middle thirds

Height of contour
Facial: cervical third, 0.5 mm
Lingual: cervical third, 0.5 mm

Identifying characteristics. These incisors are the largest and most prominent incisors. The distoincisal angle is more rounded than the mesioincisal angle. The lingual surface has a prominent cingulum, broad lingual fossa, and distinct marginal ridges. The pulp cavity is one large single chamber and root canal.

Maxillary lateral incisors

	Right	Left
Universal Code	7	10
International Code	12	22
Palmer notation	2⏌	⎳2
Number of roots	1	
Number of pulp horns	1 to 3	
Number of developmental lobes	4	

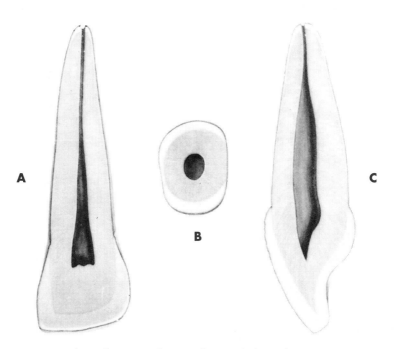

FIG. 30-11. The pulp cavity of a maxillary right lateral incisor. **A,** Distomesial section, lingual view. **B,** Cross section, incisal view. **C,** Linguolabial section, mesial view. (From Zeisz RC, Nuckolls J: *Dental anatomy,* St Louis, 1949, Mosby.)

Location of proximal contact areas
Mesial: junction of incisal and middle thirds
Distal: middle third
Height of contour
Facial: cervical third, 0.5 mm
Lingual: cervical third, 0.5 mm

Identifying characteristics. The lingual anatomic features are similar to those of the central incisors but are more highly developed and have more prominent marginal ridges and deeper lingual fossae. Lateral incisors are more likely to have a lingual pit. The cingulum may be smaller or even almost absent. The labial surface resembles that of a central incisor but is more convex. The crown-to-root ratio is less than in a central incisor because the crown is usually smaller, whereas the root is almost as long. In all other ways the lateral incisors appear as smaller, more rounded versions of the central incisors.

MANDIBULAR INCISORS

Central Incisors

Evidence of calcification	3 months
Eruption	6-7 years
Root completed	9 years

The smallest teeth in the mouth are the mandibular central incisors. How does this differ from the maxillary teeth? Which are larger, the maxillary central or lateral incisors?

A mandibular central incisor occludes only with one opposing tooth, a maxillary central incisor (see Fig. 30-1).

Similar to other anterior teeth, a mandibular central incisor is derived from four lobes, three labial and one lingual. When mandibular incisors erupt, mamelons can be seen on the incisal ridges.

Of all the teeth, mandibular central incisors are the most difficult to identify as either right or left. They are bilaterally symmetrical and very difficult to differentiate. The following features will not always be obvious but if present may support a good guess.

1. The distoincisal angle is just slightly greater than the mesioincisal.
2. The distofacial line angle is more rounded than the mesiofacial (Fig. 30-12).
3. The cervical line crests slightly toward the distal side (Fig. 30-13).
4. A straight line drawn between the endpoints of the distofacial line angle *(y)* compared with a straight line drawn between the endpoints of the mesiofacial line angle *(x)* is shorter (Fig. 30-14).

Labial aspect

The labial aspect (Fig. 30-15) exhibits a very smooth facial surface. The gingivoincisal outline is almost straight up and down. On both the mesial and distal surfaces the height of contour is at the incisal third.

Lingual aspect

The lingual view (Fig. 30-16) presents a cingulum much smaller than that of the maxillary

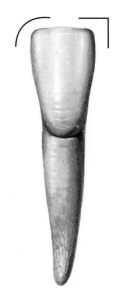

FIG. 30-12.   The distofacial line angle of a mandibular right central incisor is more convex than the mesiofacial line angle. (From Zeisz RC, Nuckolls J: *Dental anatomy,* St Louis, 1949, Mosby.)

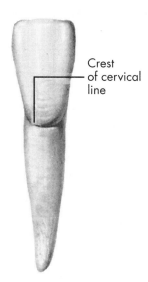

Crest
of cervical
line

FIG. 30-13.   The cervical line of a mandibular right central incisor has its crest slightly toward the distal surface. (From Zeisz RC, Nuckolls J: *Dental anatomy*, St Louis, 1949, Mosby.)

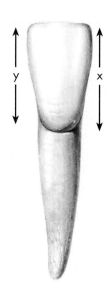

y   *x*

FIG. 30-14.   Line *x* is longer than line *y*. (From Zeisz RC, Nuckolls J: *Dental anatomy*, St Louis, 1949, Mosby.)

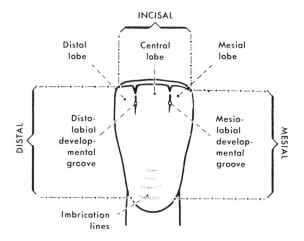

FIG. 30-15.   The labial surface of a mandibular right central incisor. (From Zeisz RC, Nuckolls J: *Dental anatomy*, St Louis, 1949, Mosby.)

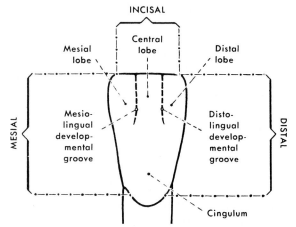

FIG. 30-16.   The lingual surface of a mandibular right central incisor. Notice that there are no pits or tubercles. (From Zeisz RC, Nuckolls J: *Dental anatomy*, St Louis, 1949, Mosby.)

anteriors. There are no tubercle extensions or lingual pits, and the fossa is very shallow.

Mesial and distal aspects

The proximal views (Fig. 30-17) reveal that the incisal edge tends toward the lingual half of the tooth and slants labially from this edge.

The height of contour at the cervical third is about 0.5 mm on the labial and lingual surfaces.

Is the cervical curvature greater mesially or distally? There is not always a difference between the amount of cervical curvature on the mesial and distal sides, but if there is a difference, the mesial side will show more curvature.

Incisal aspect

The incisal view (Fig. 30-18) shows wear on the incisal ridge. Notice that incisal wear occurs toward the facial aspect. In what way do the maxillary central incisors wear? When the upper teeth touch the lower teeth, the lower incisors touch the lingual surface of the upper incisors. Therefore the upper incisors wear down the lingual part of their incisal ridges, and the lower incisors wear down the labial portion of their incisal ridges. (Fig. 30-19 shows all of the views of a mandibular right central incisor.)

Lateral Incisors

Evidence of calcification	4 months
Eruption	7-8 years
Root completed	10 years

The mandibular lateral incisors appear to have nearly the same form as the mandibular central incisors. Indeed, it is very difficult to tell them apart. In general, the following principles help differentiate between the mandibular lateral and the mandibular central incisors in the same mouth. Mandibular lateral incisors are bigger, wider, and longer than the mandibular centrals; they are wider mesiodistally and longer gingivoincisally. This situation is different from that of the maxillary incisors. The laterals are wider because their distal development lobe is larger than the distal lobe of mandibular centrals. Lateral incisors have more prominent anatomic fea-

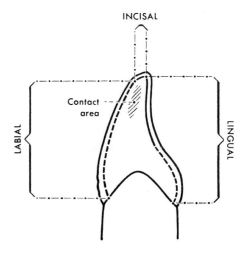

FIG. 30-17.   The mesial surface of a mandibular right central incisor. (From Zeisz RC, Nuckolls J: *Dental anatomy,* St Louis, 1949, Mosby.)

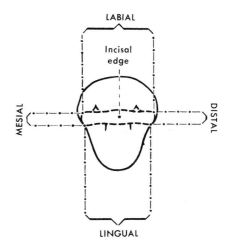

FIG. 30-18.   The incisal surface of a mandibular right central incisor. (From Zeisz RC, Nuckolls J: *Dental anatomy,* St Louis, 1949, Mosby.)

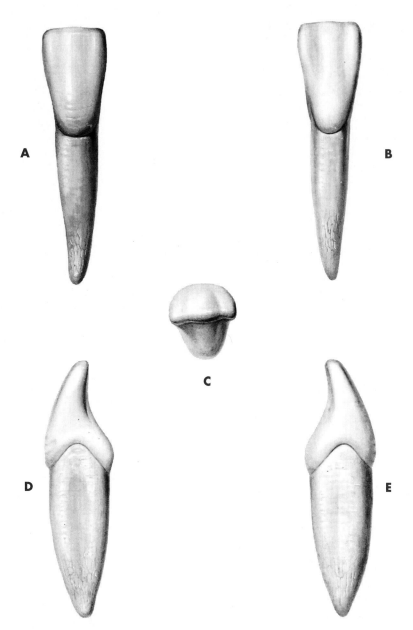

FIG. 30-19.   A mandibular right central incisor. **A,** Labial view. **B,** Lingual view. **C,** Incisal view. **D,** Mesial view. **E,** Distal view. (From Zeisz RC, Nuckolls J: *Dental anatomy*, St Louis, 1949, Mosby.)

tures on the lingual aspect than do the central incisors. In mandibular teeth the difference is not so extreme as in the maxillary; however, the lateral incisors are still slightly more convex and concave than their counterparts, the central incisors, in the same mouth.

The laterals have greater facial curvature than the central incisors have. The endpoints of the mesiofacial line angle are farther apart than those of the distofacial line angle (Fig. 30-20).

Labial aspect

The labial view (Fig. 30-21) shows a more rounded appearance mesially and distally. The developmental grooves on the labial surface are all deeper on the lateral incisors as compared with the central incisors. The height of contour at the contact areas is at the incisal third on the mesial and distal aspects. The distal contact area is slightly more gingival than mesial. This is generally true of all teeth.

Lingual aspect

When compared with the lingual view of the central incisors, the lingual view of the lateral incisors (Fig. 30-22) shows more prominent features. The ridges are more developed, the fossa appears, and enamel tubercles often extend into the fossa. A lingual pit is also more often, but still rarely, present.

There is much more deviation in the form of a lateral incisor. All features are usually more prominent if present.

Mesial and distal aspects

The proximal views (Fig. 30-23) reveal that the height of contour on the labial and lingual surfaces is at the gingival third. Notice that a lateral incisor is thicker than a central incisor at the linguoincisal ridge.

A lateral incisor is narrower labiolingually, thus making an already thicker linguoincisal ridge appear much thicker in comparison. Once again the cervical curvature is greater on the mesial than on the distal side.

Incisal aspect

The incisal view (Fig. 30-24) depicts a rounded general appearance for the lateral inci-

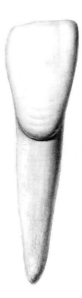

FIG. 30-20.   The distal lobe of a mandibular right lateral incisor is larger than the distal lobe of a central incisor. (From Zeisz RC, Nuckolls J: *Dental anatomy,* St Louis, 1949, Mosby.)

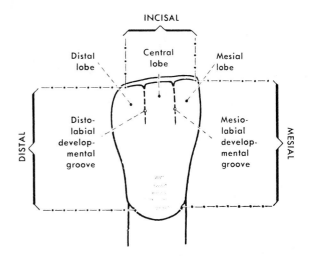

FIG. 30-21.   The labial surface of a mandibular right lateral incisor. (From Zeisz RC, Nuckolls J: *Dental anatomy,* St Louis, 1949, Mosby.)

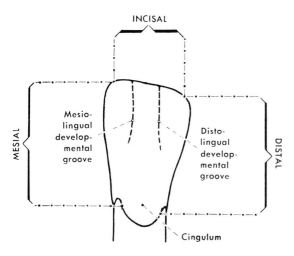

FIG. 30-22.   The lingual surface of a mandibular right lateral incisor. (From Zeisz RC, Nuckolls J: *Dental anatomy,* St Louis, 1949, Mosby.)

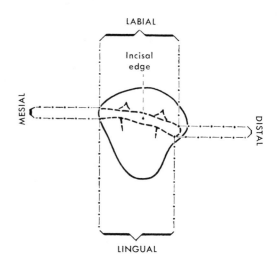

FIG. 30-24.   The incisal surface of a mandibular right lateral incisor. (From Zeisz RC, Nuckolls J: *Dental anatomy,* St Louis, 1949, Mosby.)

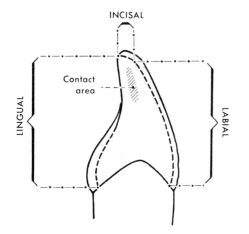

FIG. 30-23.   The distal surface of a mandibular right lateral incisor. (From Zeisz RC, Nuckolls J: *Dental anatomy,* St Louis, 1949, Mosby.)

sors, and the developmental grooves appear deeper.

The lateral incisors appear to be rotated on their root axis because the distal developmental lobe of the mandibular lateral incisors is larger and located more lingually than its mesial lobe. The reason for this extra bulk and lingual location is that the laterals have to curve distally to fit into the mandibular arch. Remember that the mandibular arch curves more than the maxillary because it has to fit inside the maxillary arch.

Root

The root of a mandibular incisor is usually straight. The root of the lateral incisor is slightly wider, thicker, and longer than that of the central incisor. The apex of the lateral incisor's root may point labially or distally. Proximal grooves are commonly found on the root surface, giving the appearance of a double root (Fig. 30-25).

Pulp Cavity

The pulp cavities of the mandibular central and lateral incisors are simple. They usually have three pulp horns and a single root canal.

The root canals of all four mandibular incisors are similar to their maxillary counterparts. They are straight and narrow and present very

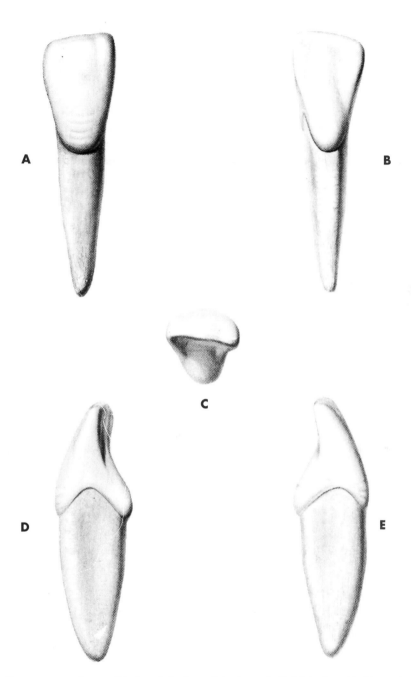

FIG. 30-25.   A mandibular right lateral incisor. **A**, Labial view. **B**, Lingual view. **C**, Incisal view. **D**, Mesial view. **E**, Distal view. (From Zeisz RC, Nuckolls J: *Dental anatomy*, St Louis, 1949, Mosby.)

little variation. The mandibular lateral pulp canal is larger and may show more variation than the central. It is a rare occurrence for either to have two root canals (Fig. 30-26).

Pertinent Data

Mandibular central incisors

	Right	Left
Universal Code	25	24
International Code	41	31
Palmer notation	1⌐	⌐1
Number of roots	1	
Number of pulp horns	3	
Number of developmental lobes	4	

Location of proximal contact areas
Mesial: incisal third
Distal: incisal third
Height of contour
Facial: cervical third, less than 0.5 mm
Lingual: cervical third, less than 0.5 mm
Identifying characteristics. The distoincisal and mesioincisal angles are nearly identical. The lingual surface is shallow, with no prominent features. The crown is wider faciolingually than mesiodistally. The root is oval shaped in cross section. The incisal edge shows wear on the facioincisal edge. From a proximal view the incisal edge appears to be tilted toward the lingual side.

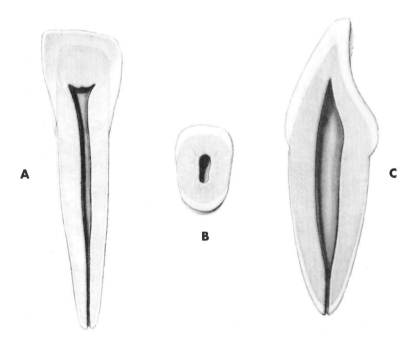

FIG. 30-26. The pulp cavity of a mandibular right lateral incisor. The pulp cavity of a mandibular central is nearly identical to the lateral but smaller. **A,** Mesiodistal section, lingual view. **B,** Cross section, incisal view. **C,** Labiolingual section, mesial view. (From Zeisz RC, Nuckolls J: *Dental anatomy,* St Louis, 1949, Mosby.)

Mandibular lateral incisors

	Right	Left
Universal Code	26	23
International Code	42	32
Palmer notation	2⏋	⌐2
Number of roots	1	
Number of pulp horns	3	
Number of developmental lobes	4	

Location of proximal contact areas
Mesial: incisal third
Distal: incisal third
Height of contour
Facial: cervical third, less than 0.5 mm
Lingual: cervical third, less than 0.5 mm
Identifying characteristics. The crown is similar to that of the mandibular central incisors. The distal lobe is more highly developed than the mesial. The distal incisal ridge angles toward the lingual as if rotating on the root axis. The crown and the root are slightly larger than those of the central incisors.

Review Questions

1. A permanent maxillary central incisor, as compared with a maxillary lateral incisor in a proximal view, is:
   a. thicker at the incisal edge.
   b. identical at the incisal edge.
   c. thinner at the incisal edge.
   d. similar but smaller overall.
2. Which of the following is not characteristic of the maxillary central incisors?
   a. distal line angle that is shorter in the facial view than in the mesial view
   b. rounded distoincisal angle
   c. mesial line angle that is nearly straight
   d. rounded mesioincisal line angle

3. With normal wear, the incisal edge of the maxillary incisors:
   a. slopes up toward the facial side.
   b. flattens.
   c. slopes up toward the lingual side.
   d. becomes more rounded.
4. The mesiofacial line angle of the maxillary central incisors differs from the distal in that it is:
   a. less rounded.
   b. longer.
   c. sharper.
   d. all of the above.
5. In contrast to the maxillary lateral incisors, the maxillary central incisors usually have how many pulp horns?
   a. 1 or 2
   b. 2 or 3
   c. 3
   d. 4
6. Which of the following anatomic features of the mandibular incisors provides evidence of the four developmental lobes of these teeth?
   a. mamelons and faint developmental lines at eruption
   b. lingual pit, marginal ridges, and incisal edge
   c. mamelons, faint developmental lines at eruption, and cingulum
   d. incisal edge and lingual concavity
7. The proximal contact area on the distal surface of a mandibular lateral incisor is located incisocervically:
   a. in the incisal third.
   b. at the junction of the incisal and middle thirds.
   c. just cervical to the junction of the incisal and middle thirds.
   d. in the middle third.
8. The structure of the mandibular lateral incisors, when compared with the mandibular centrals, is:
   a. identical but larger.
   b. almost identical but smaller.

c. almost identical but larger.

d. the same.

9. The mesiodistal crown width of the maxillary lateral incisors, when compared with the central incisors, is:

a. greater.

b. smaller.

c. about equal.

d. sometimes smaller but more often greater.

10. The distofacial line angle of maxillary lateral incisors, when compared with the maxillary central incisors, is:

a. the same.

b. more rounded.

c. less rounded.

d. very straight.

11. Which is the more acute incisal angle on the maxillary central incisors?

a. facial

b. mesial

c. distal

d. lingual

12. In contrast to a mandibular incisor, a maxillary incisor can be identified by which of these?

a. its rotated incisal edge

b. central location of its cingulum

c. prominent longitudinal grooves on the root

d. prominent lingual features of the crown

13. Where does the height of contour of the facial and lingual surfaces of the anterior teeth occur?

a. mesial third

b. incisal third

c. middle third

d. cervical third

14. Which anterior teeth have the most prominent and widest crowns (mesiodistally) in the permanent dentition?

a. maxillary canines

b. mandibular lateral incisors

c. mandibular canines

d. maxillary central incisors

15. A more prominent cingulum is found on which tooth?

a. maxillary central

b. mandibular central

c. mandibular lateral

d. maxillary lateral

16. The curvature of the cementoenamel junction of maxillary centrals is:

a. higher on the mesial than any other tooth distal or mesial.

b. higher on the distal than the mesial.

c. highest toward the mesial on the facial surface.

d. the same as the cervical line and crests more toward the mesial on the facial surface.

17. Which incisor is more likely to be congenitally missing:

a. maxillary central

b. mandibular central

c. mandibular lateral

d. maxillary lateral

18. Which incisor can have less than 3 pulp horns?

a. maxillary central

b. mandibular central

c. mandibular lateral

d. maxillary lateral

19. Which incisor occludes with only one tooth?

a. maxillary central

b. mandibular central

c. mandibular lateral

d. maxillary lateral

20. Which incisor is the smallest in crown and root?

a. maxillary central

b. mandibular central

c. mandibular lateral

d. maxillary lateral

CHAPTER 31

CANINES

OBJECTIVES

- To understand the function of a canine tooth in relation to its shape
- To understand the calcification and root completion schedules in relation to the eruption dates of the canines
- To recognize the resemblance of the canines to the other anterior teeth
- To understand how the canines are different from the other anterior teeth, as well as how they are similar to some posterior teeth
- To recognize and identify the anatomic structure and landmarks of the canine teeth
- To compare maxillary and mandibular canines and identify each

THE FOUR maxillary and mandibular permanent canines, one on each side of each jaw, are the longest teeth in the mouth. Located at the corners of the mouth, they are well anchored in the bone by their extremely long roots. Their location requires extra anchorage, which is furnished by the length and the shape of their roots as well as a special projection of bone called the **canine eminence.** The term *canine* brings to mind the fanglike teeth of dogs, which are members of the animal family *Canidae*.

In function the canines act as holding and tearing tools and assist both the incisors and premolars. In addition, their V shape at the corner of the mouth allows for dissipation of pressures that can force the premolars to protrude out of the mouth or the incisors farther into the mouth. The self-cleaning qualities of the canines, their smooth, pointed shape, the thickness of their crowns, and their strong anchorage make the canines the most stable teeth in the mouth.

Maxillary Canines

Evidence of calcification	4 months
Enamel completed	6-7 years
Eruption	11-12 years
Root completed	13-15 years

A maxillary canine (Fig. 31-1) resembles an incisor in its composition of four developmental lobes, three facial and one lingual. The three facial lobes resemble the facial lobes of the incisors except that the middle facial lobe extends farther incisally when the tooth is viewed from the labial or lingual aspect. This middle lobe extension results in the formation of a single cusp. The cusp tip is formed by the junction of four ridges. One of the ridges extends along the middle lobe of the tooth on its most facial part; another extends along the lingual part. The other two ridges run from the mesioincisal and distoincisal corners. All four ridges converge to form the cusp tip.

The lingual lobe of a canine is much larger and thicker than the lingual lobe of an incisor, which results in the canine being much wider labiolingually than a maxillary incisor is. The cingulum of a maxillary canine also shows greater development in that it is larger and bulkier than the cingulum on any of the other anterior teeth.

Labial aspect (Figs. 31-2; see also Fig. 31-1, A)

The crown and root of a maxillary canine are narrower mesiodistally than those of a maxillary central incisor. The cervicoincisal length of the crown is much larger on a maxillary canine than on any other anterior tooth, except the maxillary central incisor and the mandibular canine. Although these teeth usually have longer crowns than a maxillary canine has, the roots of the maxillary canines are longer and thus make them the longest teeth in the mouth.

Mesially the outline of the crown is straighter than laterally with a slight convexity at the contact area. The center of the mesial contact area is approximately at the junction of the middle and incisal thirds of the crown.

Distally the outline of the crown is rounded in appearance because the distal contact area is usually at the center of the middle third of the crown. This position makes the distal convexity appear larger and more uniform. How does this differ from the location of the mesial contact area? Which contact area is located more incisally, the mesial or the distal?

The labial surface of the crown is smooth. The developmental lines are two shallow depressions dividing the three labial lobes. The middle lobe is much larger and has greater development than the other lobes, resulting in a ridge on the labial surface of the crown. This ridge ends incisally at the cusp tip, which is centered in the middle of the tooth (from the facial view).

The cervical line crests slightly mesial to the center of the tooth.

The root of a maxillary canine is slender in comparison with the crown and is conical in shape with a blunt root apex. It is not unusual for the root to turn sharply to the distal or mesial side in the apical third. A general rule is that most roots, if they do have an apical curvature, will point toward the distal side. Although this rule applies to almost all single-rooted teeth, there are exceptions. If an apical curvature is not present, the root itself will have a tendency to point more often toward the distal than to the mesial side.

Lingual aspect (Figs. 31-3; also see Fig. 31-1, B)

The root of a maxillary canine tapers toward the lingual surface. The lingual sides of both the crown and root are narrower than the labial sides.

Compared with the facial line, the cervical line shows a more even curvature, and the crest is straighter and centered over the middle of the tooth.

The most obvious structure on the lingual surface of a maxillary canine is the well-developed cingulum. It is huge in comparison with those of all the other anterior teeth.

Confluent to the cingulum and running from the cusp tip is a well-developed lingual ridge. This ridge runs from the cusp tip on the lingual side to the cingulum. Unlike other anterior teeth that have a lingual fossa, this area on a maxillary

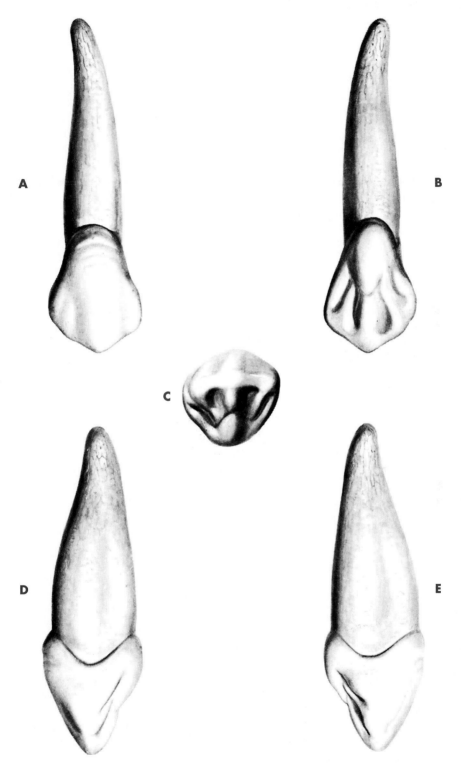

FIG. 31-1.   A maxillary right canine. **A,** Labial view. **B,** Lingual view. **C,** Incisal view. **D,** Mesial view. **E,** Distal view. (From Zeisz RC, Nuckolls J: *Dental anatomy,* St Louis, 1949, Mosby.)

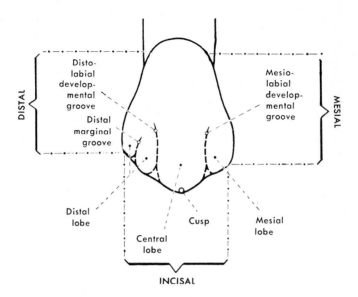

FIG. 31-2.   The labial surface of a maxillary right canine. (From Zeisz RC, Nuckolls J: *Dental anatomy,* St Louis, 1949, Mosby.)

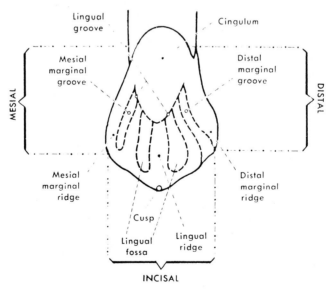

FIG. 31-3.   The lingual surface of a maxillary right canine. (From Zeisz RC, Nuckolls J: *Dental anatomy,* St Louis, 1949, Mosby.)

canine is occupied by a lingual ridge, which divides the lingual side of the three facial lobes, creating two separate lingual fossae, one on the mesial and one on the distal side of the lingual ridge. These fossae are bordered by a mesial and a distal marginal ridge, respectively. When present, these fossae are called the mesial and distal lingual fossae. The borders of the lingual fossae are the incisal ridge, the lingual ridge, and the mesial or distal marginal ridge.

Sometimes the lingual surface of a canine crown is so smooth that no concavities or fossae are present. Usually the cingulum and marginal ridges are less developed in these instances, with little evidence of developmental grooves.

The lingual side of the root is narrower than the labial side. A cross-sectional view of the root appears triangular, with the lingual portion more tapered than the labial.

Mesial aspect

The functional form of a maxillary canine is evident on the mesial view (Fig. 31-4; see also Fig. 31-1, D). The wedge-shaped outline of the crown shows the canine to have greater labiolin-

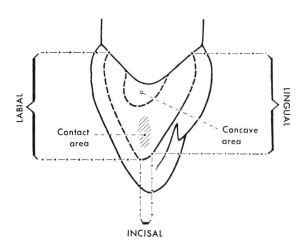

FIG. 31-4. The mesial surface of a maxillary right canine. (From Zeisz RC, Nuckolls J: *Dental anatomy*, St Louis, 1949, Mosby.)

gual bulk than any other anterior tooth. The greatest measurement labiolingually is at the cervical third. This is because of the huge cingulum of the lingual side and the more convex labial outline of the canine. The entire labial surface is more convex from the cervical line to the cusp tip than any other maxillary anterior tooth. The cervical line curves toward the cusp an average of 2.5 mm.

The root of a canine is broad labiolingually and is usually extremely long. The end of the root apex is blunt and may often curve to the lingual or distal lingual side. The mesial surface of the root shows much labiolingual development, with a shallow developmental depression extending from the cervical line halfway to the apex of the root. This developmental depression appears to almost divide the single root into two roots. In extremely well-developed roots it helps anchor a canine in the bone and prevents root rotation.

The mesial surface of a canine crown is entirely convex throughout except for a small area between the contact area and the cervical line, which may be flat.

Distal aspect

The distal aspect (Fig. 31-5; see also Fig. 31-1, E) of a maxillary canine shows the same form and outline as the mesial view does. However, the cervical line shows less curvature toward the cusp tip. The distal marginal ridge is more developed and heavier in outline than the mesial marginal ridge. Although both the mesial and the distal surfaces show a slightly flat or concave area above the contact area, the distal surface displays much more concavity. The root surface on the distal aspect may show a more pronounced developmental depression than that on the mesial aspect.

Incisal aspect

An incisal view (Fig. 31-6; see also Fig. 31-1, C) of a maxillary canine shows that the tooth is not only wide mesiodistally but also has the thickest labiolingual measurement of any anterior tooth. Although these two measurements

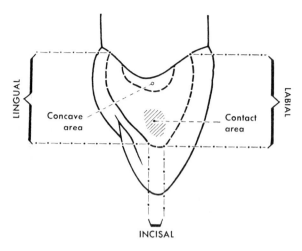

FIG. 31-5.   The distal surface of a maxillary right canine. (From Zeisz RC, Nuckolls J: *Dental anatomy*, St Louis, 1949, Mosby.)

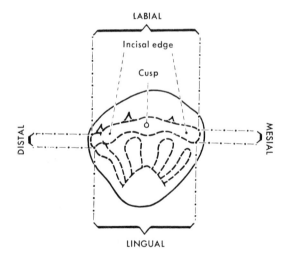

FIG. 31-6.   The incisal edge of a maxillary right canine. (From Zeisz RC, Nuckolls J: *Dental anatomy*, St Louis, 1949, Mosby.)

are about equal, the crown is usually larger in a labiolingual direction. The cusp tip is labial to the center of the crown labiolingually and mesial to the center mesiodistally.

The distal aspect of the crown appears thinner than the mesial. Indeed, it seems to stretch out to make contact with the first premolars.

Root

The root of the upper canine is usually the longest of any tooth in the mouth. It is very strong and firmly embedded in the maxilla. In a cross-sectional view the root appears to taper from the labial toward the lingual areas. From a proximal view a longitudinal groove may be seen. The apical portion will often point distally but seldom mesially.

Pulp cavity

The pulp cavity of the maxillary canine (Fig. 31-7) consists of a large pulp chamber and a single root canal. The pulp chamber has one single pulp horn, which extends toward the tip of the cusp. The root canal is usually straight but can be tortuous when the root is curved.

Pertinent Data

Maxillary canines

	Right	Left
Universal Code	6	11
International Code	13	23
Palmer notation	3⌋	⌊3
Number of roots	1	
Number of pulp horns	1	
Number of cusps	1	
Number of developmental lobes	4	

Location of proximal contact areas
Mesial: Junction of incisal and middle thirds
Distal: Middle third
Height of contour
Facial: Cervical third, 0.5 mm
Lingual: Cervical third, 0.5 mm
Identifying characteristics. The maxillary canines are the longest teeth in the mouth. They have a single cusp with mesial and distal ridges forming an incisal edge. The cingulum is promi-

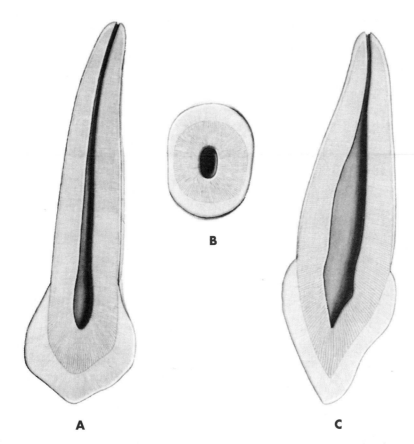

FIG. 31-7.   The pulp cavity of a maxillary right canine. **A,** Distomesial section, lingual view. **B,** Cross section, incisal view. **C,** Linguolabial section, mesial view. (From Zeisz RC, Nuckolls J: *Dental anatomy,* St Louis, 1949, Mosby.)

nent, and a prominent facial ridge is off-center toward the mesial side. The mesiofacial lobe forms the facial ridge of the cusp, and the centrofacial lobe forms the lingual ridge of the cusp. This lingual ridge divides the mesial and distal fossae. The distofacial ridge is longer and more rounded than the mesiofacial ridge.

Mandibular Canines

Evidence of calcification	4 months
Enamel completed	7 years
Eruption	9-10 years
Root completed	13 years

The mandibular canines resemble the maxillary canines in that they have the same wedge-shaped outline, long crown and root, and well-developed cingulum. They differ from the maxillary canines, however, in the following ways.

1. A mandibular canine crown is narrower mesiodistally by about 0.5 mm.
2. A mandibular canine crown length is as long as that of a maxillary canine and sometimes longer.
3. The root may be as long as that of a maxillary canine but more often is shorter.

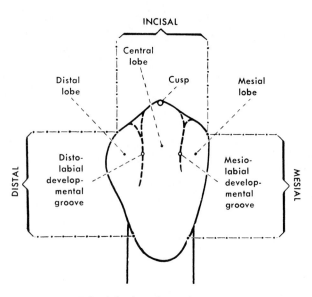

FIG. 31-8.   The labial surface of a mandibular right canine. (From Zeisz RC, Nuckolls J: *Dental anatomy,* St Louis, 1949, Mosby.)

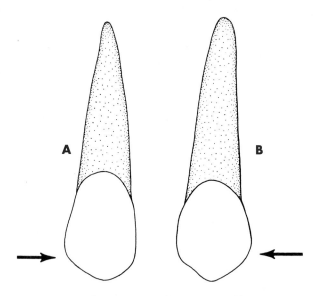

FIG. 31-9.   Comparison of, **A**, a mandibular, and, **B**, a maxillary left canine.

4. The labiolingual measurement of the crown and the root is usually a fraction of a millimeter less than for a maxillary canine. How then does the total length of a mandibular tooth—crown and root—compare with the other teeth?

5. The lingual surface of a mandibular canine is smoother, the cingulum is less developed, and the marginal ridges are less prominent than those of a maxillary canine. The lingual surface of a mandibular canine resembles the lingual surface of the other mandibular anterior teeth.

6. The cusp tip of a mandibular canine is not as well developed as that of a maxillary canine, and the cusp ridges are thinner labiolingually.

7. The cusp tip of a mandibular canine may be centered more lingually than a maxillary canine cusp tip.

8. An anomaly of a mandibular canine is bifurcated roots, where a mandibular canine has two roots, one buccal and one lingual. Usually only the apical third of the root is bifurcated.

Labial aspect

From the labial view (Fig. 31-8), a mandibular canine shows a straighter mesial outline than does a maxillary canine. The distal outline resembles that of a maxillary canine, which means that the mesial outline of a mandibular canine is less convex than is its distal outline. Which surface, mesial or distal, shows the greater convexity on a maxillary canine? Is it the same for a mandibular canine?

The distal contact area is more incisal on a mandibular canine than the same contact area on its maxillary counterpart and is located somewhat cervical to the junction of its incisal and middle thirds (Fig. 31-9). Where is the distal contact on a maxillary canine? The mesial contact area of a mandibular canine is nearer the mesioincisal point angle than is its maxillary counterpart, at the incisal third of the tooth. Where is the mesial contact area of a maxillary canine?

Facially the cervical line of a mandibular canine is more symmetrically contoured than the cervical line of a maxillary canine. The cervical line of a maxillary canine is less uniform, cresting slightly mesial to the midline of the tooth.

Lingual aspect

The lingual surface (Fig. 31-10) of the crown of a mandibular canine is flatter than that of a maxillary canine. Lingual features are less prominent—the cingulum is relatively smooth, the marginal ridges are less distinct, and the lingual fossae and ridge are less pronounced.

The lingual surface of a mandibular canine resembles the other mandibular anterior teeth but has a larger cingulum and a pronounced lingual ridge. The cingulum is larger and more developed than those on the other mandibular anterior teeth. Compared with a maxillary canine, a mandibular canine's cingulum tapers more lingually and is less developed.

The lingual ridge of a mandibular canine is less distinct than the same ridge on a maxillary canine except toward the cusp tip where it is raised. There are no lingual pits on the mandibular canines.

A mandibular canine resembles the other mandibular teeth from a lingual view in that the marginal ridges and lingual fossae are flatter than those of maxillary teeth. In fact, the lingual surfaces of all the mandibular teeth are smoother and more hollowed than those of their maxillary counterparts.

Mesial aspect

A mandibular canine resembles its maxillary counterpart from a mesial view (Fig. 31-11; see also Fig. 31-14, *D*), having the same wedge shape and pointed cusp. It differs from a maxillary canine in that it has a less developed cingulum and thinner marginal ridges. The cusp tip of a mandibular canine is more lingually inclined, whereas the cusp tip of a maxillary is centered slightly labially. As the canines become abraded with wear, this discrepancy in the centering of a canine cusp tip becomes more apparent. The reason for the lingual incline of the mandibular

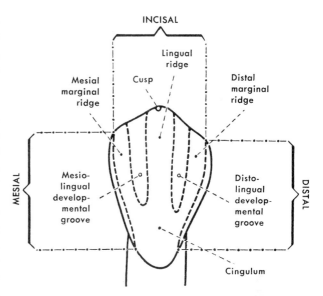

FIG. 31-10. The lingual surface of a mandibular right canine. (From Zeisz RC, Nuckolls J: *Dental anatomy*, St Louis, 1949, Mosby.)

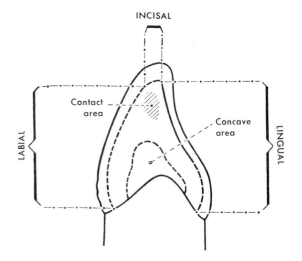

FIG. 31-11. The mesial surface of a mandibular right canine. (From Zeisz RC, Nuckolls J: *Dental anatomy*, St Louis, 1949, Mosby.)

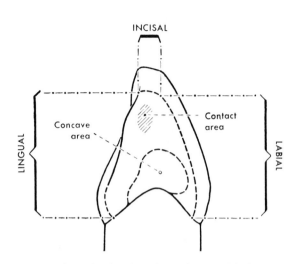

FIG. 31-12.   The distal surface of a mandibular right canine. (From Zeisz RC, Nuckolls J: *Dental anatomy,* St Louis, 1949, Mosby.)

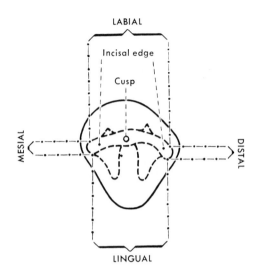

FIG. 31-13.   The incisal edge of a mandibular right canine. (From Zeisz RC, Nuckolls J: *Dental anatomy,* St Louis, 1949, Mosby.)

canine is apparent given the position of a mandibular canine in relation to its maxillary counterpart when the two are touching.

The cervical line curves more toward the incisal portion than does the cervical line on a maxillary canine.

The roots of the mandibular and maxillary canines are similar except that a mandibular canine's root may be more pointed at the apex. The developmental depression on the root of a mandibular canine is more pronounced, and sometimes the root is bifurcated.

Distal aspect

The distal aspect (Fig. 31-12; see also Fig. 31-14, *E*) of a mandibular canine resembles a maxillary canine except for those features mentioned in the discussion of the mesial aspects.

Incisal aspect

From an incisal view (Fig. 31-13; see also Fig. 31-14, *C*) the incisal edge of a mandibular canine slants toward the lingual side with the distal incisal ridge slanting more lingually than the me-

sial side. The cusp tip is located more lingually on a mandibular canine than on a maxillary canine. In all other ways the mandibular canines resemble the maxillary canines. (Fig. 31-14 shows all views of a mandibular right canine.)

Root

The root of the mandibular canine is the longest mandibular root, and of all the tooth roots it is second only to the root of the maxillary canine; it is wide labiolingually and narrow mesiodistally. Some specimens show a bifurcated root in the apical third. It is the anterior tooth root most likely to be bifurcated. When the root is bifurcated, one branch is labial and the other lingual. The single-rooted form is much more common, and if deep longitudinal grooves are present on the proximal surfaces of the root, then there is a tendency for two root canals to form even if these join together at the apex. Bifurcated or not, the mandibular canine root is flatter than the maxillary canine root on the distal or mesial surface.

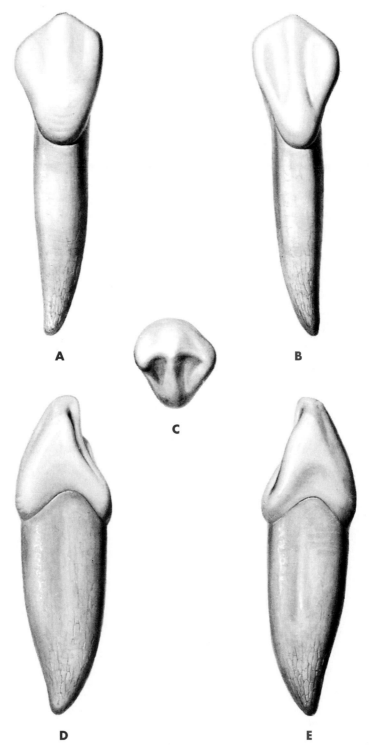

FIG. 31-14.   A mandibular right canine. **A,** Labial view. **B,** Lingual view. **C,** Incisal view. **D,** Mesial view. **E,** Distal view. (From Zeisz RC, Nuckolls J: *Dental anatomy,* St Louis, 1949, Mosby.)

Pulp cavity

The pulp cavity of the mandibular canine resembles that of the maxillary canine in that they both have a large pulp chamber and usually a single root canal. There is also only one pulp horn present.

The major difference between the two teeth is that the mandibular canine may have two separate root canals. When this happens, one canal is to the labial side and the other is to the lingual side. The canals may join at the apex or have separate apical foramina. When the root is bifurcated, there are almost always two canals, each with its own apical foramen (Fig. 31-15).

Pertinent Data

Mandibular canines

	Right	Left
Universal Code	27	22
International Code	43	33
Palmer notation	3⌐	⌐3
Number of roots	1 or 2	
Number of pulp horns	1	
Number of cusps	1	
Number of developmental lobes	4	

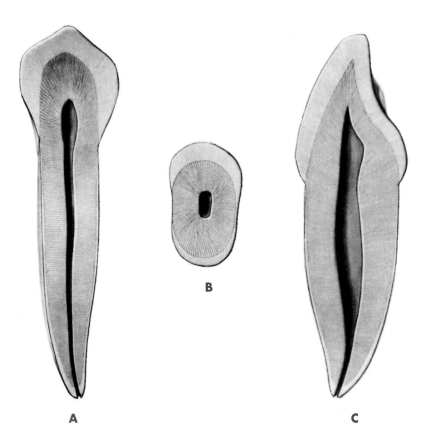

A   **B**   **C**

FIG. 31-15. The pulp cavity of a mandibular right canine. **A,** Mesiodistal section, lingual view. **B,** Cross section, incisal view. **C,** Labiolingual section, mesial view. (From Zeisz RC, Nuckolls J: *Dental anatomy,* St Louis, 1949, Mosby.)

Location of proximal contact areas
Mesial: Incisal third
Distal: Just cervical to the junction of incisal and middle thirds
Height of contour
Facial: Cervical third, less than 0.5 mm
Lingual: Cervical third, less than 0.5 mm
Identifying characteristics. The crown is similar to that of the maxillary canine but narrower and smoother. It has less prominent lingual features. From a proximal view, the cusp tip is inclined lingually. From an incisal view, the distal end of the incisal edge is rotated lingually. They have the longest roots in the mandibular arch, with longitudinal grooves on the root.

Review Questions

1. A maxillary canine can be distinguished from a mandibular canine by which of the following characteristics?
   a. A mandibular canine has a less prominent cingulum.
   b. The mesial side of a mandibular canine crown and root is relatively straight.
   c. The incisal edge of a mandibular canine is located lingual to the center of the tooth.
   d. All of the above.
2. Which of the following is characteristic of the root of a mandibular canine?
   a. It is longer than the root of a maxillary canine.
   b. The root is never bifurcated.

c. It is flattened or slightly concave on the mesial and distal surfaces.
   d. All of the above.
3. Generally, on the lingual surface of a maxillary canine there is (are):
   a. one fossa.
   b. two fossae.
   c. three fossae.
   d. four fossae.
4. Compared with other anterior teeth, a mandibular canine is the most likely to have:
   a. longitudinal grooves.
   b. a root that is narrow mesiodistally.
   c. two root canals.
   d. any or all the above.
5. A mandibular canine root sometimes bifurcates into a:
   a. mesiofacial and distolingual root.
   b. facial and lingual root.
   c. mesial and distal root.
   d. none of the above; the mandibular canine root does not bifurcate.
6. Canine teeth exhibit:
   a. a facial ridge.
   b. a lingual ridge.
   c. a mesial marginal ridge.
   d. all of the above.
7. The bony projection that is a part of the support for canines is called a _____ ____ _____.
8. Facially the cervical line crests slightly mesial to the center of the tooth. T or F?
9. The contact area of a canine is located more toward the junction of the mesial and middle third on the distal surface. T or F?
10. The mesial contact areas are located more cervically than the distal contact areas. T or F?

CHAPTER 32

PREMOLARS

OBJECTIVES
- To identify an extracted premolar as maxillary or mandibular, first or second, right or left
- To recognize and name the pertinent dental anatomic form of each tooth—cusps, ridges, developmental grooves, triangular grooves, pits, and developmental depressions
- To make comparisons between maxillary and mandibular premolars
- To discuss the major differences and similarities between the maxillary first and second premolars
- To describe briefly the various occlusal forms possible for a mandibular second premolar
- To compare the mandibular first premolars with the mandibular second premolars (development, shape, and diversities of anatomic form)
- To understand how development occurs through the formation and fusion of the lobes
- To understand how the form of a tooth relates to its ultimate function

THE PREMOLARS succeed the deciduous molars. There are eight premolar teeth—two in each quadrant. How many maxillary and how many mandibular premolars are there? The term *premolar* implies that these are the teeth that will be located immediately anterior to the permanent molars. In the study of human dentition the term *bicuspid* is often used in place of *premolar*. This is inaccurate because *bicuspid* presupposes that a tooth has only two cusps. In human dentition, however, mandibular premolars show variation from one to three in the number of cusps. Thus the use of the term *bicuspid* is discouraged in favor of the term *premolar*.

The maxillary first and second premolars, as well as the mandibular first premolars, are developed from four lobes just like the anterior teeth. The mandibular second premolars usually develop from five lobes—three buccal and two lingual.

The buccal cusp of a premolar is developed from three labial lobes, as in the anterior teeth. The primary difference in development is that the lingual cusp, which is extremely well formed, develops from the single lingual lobe. In anterior teeth the lingual lobe forms the cingulum of the incisors and canines. In premolars this single lingual lobe forms an extremely well-developed lingual cusp.

In the case of the three-cusp form (the mandibular second premolar) there are two lingual lobes, each of which forms a separate small lingual cusp. There is also a two-cusp form of the mandibular second premolar, which develops from just four lobes. How many lingual lobes would it have? The lingual cusps of the mandibular premolars are small and **afunctional** when compared with the larger lingual cusps of the maxillary premolars.

The premolar crowns and roots are shorter than those of the canines.

MAXILLARY PREMOLARS

First Premolars

Evidence of calcification	1½ years
Enamel completed	5-6 years
Eruption	10-11 years
Root completed	12-13 years

Maxillary first premolars (Fig. 32-1) have two cusps, a buccal and a lingual. The buccal cusp is usually 1 mm or more longer than the lingual cusp. These teeth are also the only premolars that normally have two roots, a buccal and a lingual, though occasionally there is only a single root.

Most maxillary first premolars have two roots and two pulp canals. Even when only one root is present, two pulp canals can usually be found. It

is not uncommon for maxillary second premolars to also have two roots; however, there is usually only one.

Facial (buccal) aspect (Fig. 32-2; see also Fig. 32-1, *A*)

A maxillary first premolar is similar in appearance to a maxillary canine. However, the crown is shorter and narrower mesiodistally, and unlike a canine, the mesial and distal contact areas are at about the same level. The mesial and distal marginal ridges are also sharper than those of a canine.

The tip of the facial cusp is located distally to the midline and separates the occlusal border into a long, straight mesial ridge and a short, convex distal ridge. The mesial ridge may even have a slight indentation at the junction of the mesial and middle lobes. From the contact areas cervically, the distal border is straight, whereas the mesial border is more concave. Two developmental lines on the facial surface mark the coalescence of the developmental lobes. The facial surface of the crown is convex, and an extremely well-developed middle facial lobe is present.

Lingual aspect

From the lingual view (Fig. 32-3; see also Fig. 32-1, *B*), the crown converges toward the lingual cusp, which is shorter than the facial cusp. The tip of the lingual cusp is located slightly toward the mesial side of the midline.

Mesial aspect

On the mesial surface (Fig. 32-4; see also Fig. 32-1, *C*) of the crown, a groove extends from the mesial marginal ridge cervically. This groove is called the **mesial marginal groove**. It crosses the mesial marginal ridge and runs from the occlusal third to the middle third of the crown, lingual to the contact area. The mesial surface can also be identified by a **mesial developmental depression** located cervically to the mesial contact area. The concavity continues cervically from above the contact area across the cervical line, where it joins a deep **developmental depression** between the roots. The mesial marginal groove is not

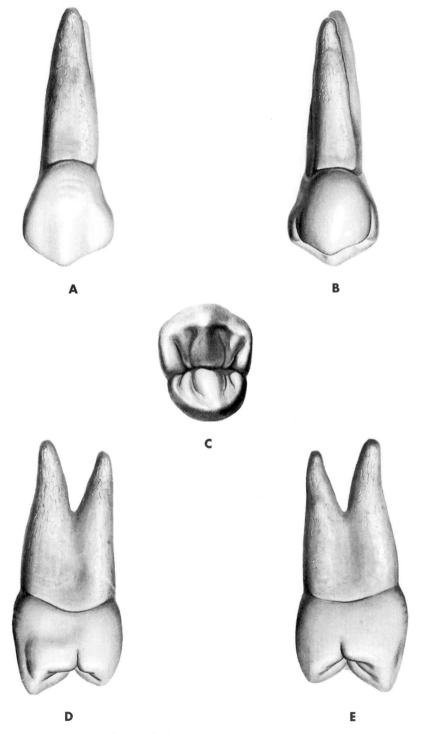

FIG. 32-1. A maxillary right first premolar. **A,** Buccal view. **B,** Lingual view. **C,** Occlusal view. **D,** Mesial view. **E,** Distal view. (From Zeisz RC, Nuckolls J: *Dental anatomy,* St Louis, 1949, Mosby.)

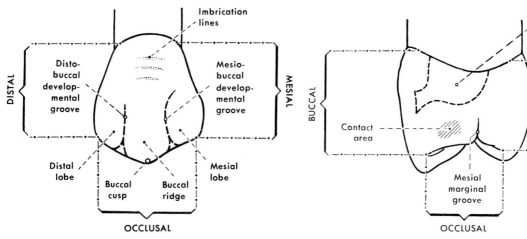

FIG. 32-2. The buccal surface of a maxillary right first premolar. (From Zeisz RC, Nuckolls J: *Dental anatomy,* St Louis, 1949, Mosby.)

FIG. 32-4. The mesial surface of a maxillary right first premolar. (From Zeisz RC, Nuckolls J: *Dental anatomy,* St Louis, 1949, Mosby.)

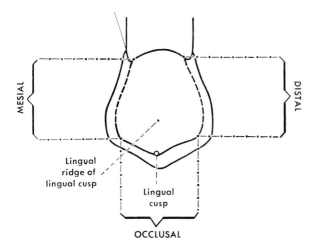

FIG. 32-3. The lingual surface of a maxillary right first premolar. (From Zeisz RC, Nuckolls J: *Dental anatomy,* St Louis, 1949, Mosby.)

always present, but the mesial developmental depression usually is.

The facial outline is convex with the crest of contour located within the cervical third of the crown. The lingual outline is also convex with its crest of contour located within the middle third of the crown. The curvature of the cervical line is greater on the mesial surface than on the distal surface.

Distal aspect

From the distal view (Fig. 32-5; see also Fig. 32-1, *E*) a maxillary first premolar is similar to the mesial view, except there is usually no groove crossing the distal marginal ridge and no developmental depression is present. Some specimens show a distinct distal **marginal groove,** but the mesial marginal groove is deeper and more obvious. The cervical line is less curved on the distal surface than on the mesial surface. The crown also appears more rounded and smooth. Both the buccal and lingual cusp tips are centered over the root. This is also true from the mesial view. All maxillary premolars have their cusp tips centered over their root.

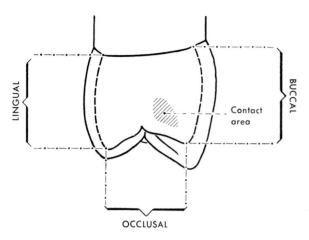

FIG. 32-5.   The distal surface of a maxillary right first premolar. (From Zeisz RC, Nuckolls J: *Dental anatomy*, St Louis, 1949, Mosby.)

Occlusal aspect

The occlusal surface (Fig. 32-6; see also Fig. 32-1, *C*) shows two well-developed cusps. The lingual cusp is more pointed than the facial cusp, but the facial cusp is much larger and longer than the lingual. Each cusp has four ridges emanating from it, and each ridge is named according to its location—facial, lingual, distal, and mesial.

On the facial cusp, the facial ridge descends from the cusp tip cervically onto the facial surface. The mesial and distal ridges descend from the cusp tip to their respective point angles. They are called the mesial and distal cusp ridges.

The lingual cusp ridge extends from the cusp tip lingually to the central area of the occlusal surface. Any ridge that runs from the cusp tip to

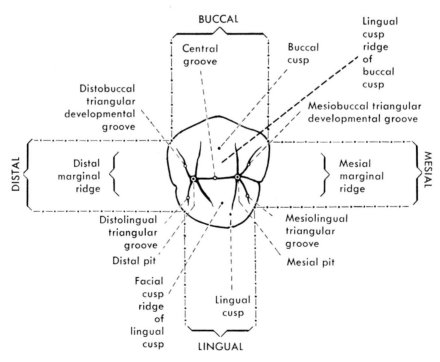

FIG. 32-6.   The occlusal surface of a maxillary right first premolar. (From Zeisz RC, Nuckolls J: *Dental anatomy*, St Louis, 1949, Mosby.)

the central groove of the occlusal surface is called a triangular ridge. Examples are the lingual cusp ridge of the buccal cusp and the buccal cusp ridge of the lingual cusp, which runs from the cusp tip of the lingual cusp to the central groove (Fig. 32-7).

The lingual cusp has four ridges, like its counterpart the buccal cusp. The lingual cusp ridge of the lingual cusp extends onto the lingual surface. The mesial and distal cusp ridges extend from the cusp tip to their respective point angles and fuse into the mesial and distal marginal ridges.

When two triangular ridges join, after traversing the tooth buccolingually, they form a transverse ridge. Thus a transverse ridge exists on the occlusal surface of a maxillary first premolar. It is formed by the union of the two triangular ridges—the lingual cusp ridge of the buccal cusp and the facial cusp ridge of the lingual cusp. In Fig. 32-7, notice the transverse ridge formed by the two joining triangular ridges.

From the occlusal aspect, close observation reveals that the crown is wider on the buccal surface than on the lingual surface. Notice also that the buccolingual dimension of the crown is much greater than the mesiodistal dimension.

The primary anatomic features comprise the major structures, grooves, and pits that are pertinent to the teeth. They must occur regularly with uniformity in shape and size.

Thus primary grooves are sharp, deep, and V shaped. They occur consistently and mark the junction of major anatomic boundaries. All developmental grooves are primary grooves because they occur routinely and are of major importance to anatomic development. Developmental grooves mark the union of what structures?

Secondary grooves are of lesser importance. They differ from primary grooves in that they usually are shallower and more irregular in shape, giving the tooth a more wrinkled appearance. They are not always present.

As a general rule, first premolars and first molars will have fewer secondary anatomic features. Second premolars and second molars will have more secondary grooves and pits. Third molars will have even more secondary anatomic grooves, pits, and fissures. Therefore the third molars will appear more wrinkled because of the more numerous and shallow anatomic features.

There are few secondary grooves on the occlusal surface of a maxillary first premolar. In most instances the surface is relatively smooth. A well-defined **central developmental groove** divides the tooth buccolingually. A **mesial marginal developmental groove** extends from the central developmental groove, across the mesial marginal ridge, and onto the mesial surface of the tooth.

Two developmental grooves connect to the central groove just inside the mesial and distal marginal ridges. These grooves are the **mesio-**

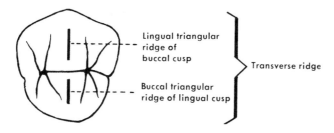

FIG. 32-7.   The occlusal surface of a maxillary right first premolar. (From Zeisz RC, Nuckolls J: *Dental anatomy*, St Louis, 1949, Mosby.)

buccal developmental groove and the **distobuccal developmental groove.** Each can connect at opposite ends of the central developmental groove, at which point they usually end in a deep depression in the occlusal surface called the *mesial* and *distal developmental pits*.

The triangular depression that harbors the mesiobuccal developmental groove is called the *mesial triangular fossa*. Likewise, the depression in which the distobuccal developmental groove lies is called the distal triangular fossa. The terms *mesiobuccal developmental groove* and *mesiobuccal triangular groove* are synonymous.

Root

The root of a maxillary first premolar may be either single or bifurcated. The bifurcated root form is far more common, but even in the single root form two root canals are usually present.

The number of pulp horns corresponds to the number of cusps—in this case, two.

On the bifurcated root form there is one buccal (facial) and one **palatal** (lingual) **root.** The buccal root is larger and longer than the palatal root (see Fig. 32-1, *D* and *E*).

On the single-rooted form, grooves are usually present lengthwise in the middle of the root, giving the appearance of a root trying to divide itself. The mesial root surface will have a more highly developed root groove.

Pulp cavity

The pulp cavity (Fig. 32-8) of the maxillary first premolar has two pulp horns, one for each cusp, and two root canals, one for each root. Sometimes there is only one undivided root. When this occurs, there are still usually two root canals, although they often combine to form one

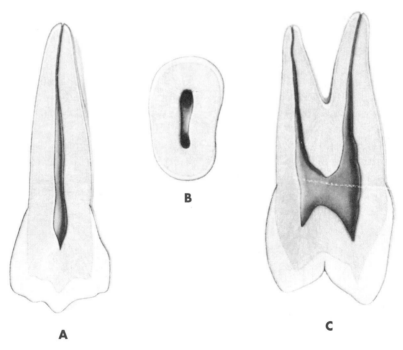

FIG. 32-8. The pulp cavity of a maxillary right first premolar. **A,** Mesiodistal section, buccal view. **B,** Cross section, occlusal view. **C,** Buccolingual section, distal view. (From Zeisz RC, Nuckolls J: *Dental anatomy,* St Louis, 1949, Mosby.)

apical foramen. In some specimens with only one root there may be only one single root canal.

General characteristics

The maxillary first premolars exemplify some characteristics that are common to all posterior teeth when compared with anterior teeth.

1. The posterior teeth have a greater faciolingual measurement in relation to their mesiodistal measurements.
2. The mesial and distal contact areas are broader and closer to the same level on the tooth.
3. The mesial and distal curvature of the cervical line is less.
4. The crown measurements cervicoocclusally are less, giving the appearance of shorter crown length.

Second Premolars

Evidence of calcification	2 years
Enamel completed	6-7 years
Eruption	10-12 years
Root completed	12-14 years

Maxillary second premolars (Fig. 32-9) resemble the maxillary first premolars in both form and function. The crown, however, has a less angular and more rounded appearance. The second premolars also vary from the first in that they usually have only one root. How many roots do the maxillary first premolars have?

Second premolars vary individually more than first premolars. A maxillary second premolar may have a crown that is noticeably smaller cervicoocclusally and mesiodistally. On the other hand, it may be larger in those dimensions and usually is.

Generally the root of a second premolar is longer than that of a first premolar. Although a second premolar usually has only one root, it is not unusual to find these premolars with two roots.

Facial (buccal) aspect

From the buccal view (Fig. 32-10; see also Fig. 32-9, *A*), it is evident that the buccal cusp of a second premolar is not as long as that of a first premolar, and it appears less pointed. Also, a second premolar has the same general markings as the first, but they are not as well defined.

Lingual aspect

Little variation can be seen from the lingual view (Fig. 32-11; see also Fig. 32-9, *B*) except that the lingual cusp is almost the same length as the buccal cusp.

Mesial aspect

The mesial view (Fig. 32-12; see also Fig. 32-9, *D*) shows the difference in cusp length between the maxillary first and second premolars. The buccal cusp of a second premolar is shorter than the buccal cusp of a first premolar, and the lingual cusp is almost as long; thus the buccal and lingual cusps are nearly the same length.

There is no deep developmental groove crossing the mesial marginal ridge, just as there is no deep developmental depression on the mesial surface of the crown; instead, the crown surface is convex. A shallow developmental groove bisects the single root form, giving the appearance of two roots fused into one.

Distal aspect

The distal view (see Fig. 32-9, *E*) shows that the features of the first and second premolars are the same, except that the buccal and lingual cusps of a second premolar are more even in length.

Occlusal aspect

The occlusal outline (Fig. 32-13; see also Fig. 32-9, *C*) is more rounded than that of a first premolar, and the second premolar is ovoid rather than hexagonal.

There appears to be more distance between the cusp tips buccolingually than on the first premolar, and the lingual cusp is almost as wide as the buccal. Is this true of a first premolar?

The groove pattern is less distinct than in the first premolar, and the grooves are shorter, shallower, and more irregular. The central developmental groove is also shorter and more irregular, with numerous supplemental grooves radiating from it, giving the occlusal surface a more wrinkled appearance.

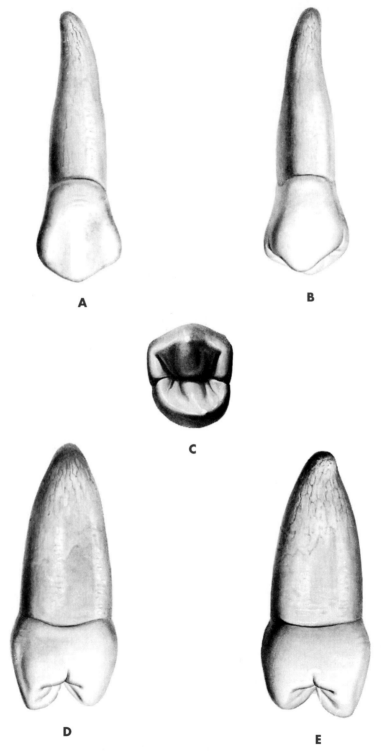

Fig. 32-9. A maxillary right second premolar. **A,** Buccal view. **B,** Lingual view. **C,** Occlusal view. **D,** Mesial view. **E,** Distal view. (From Zeisz RC, Nuckolls J: *Dental anatomy,* St Louis, 1949, Mosby.)

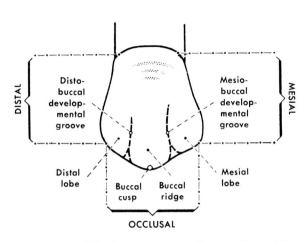

FIG. 32-10.   The buccal surface of a maxillary right second premolar. (From Zeisz RC, Nuckolls J: *Dental anatomy,* St Louis, 1949, Mosby.)

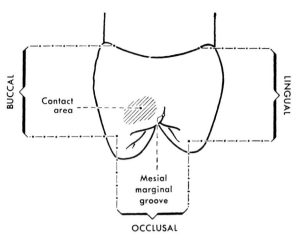

FIG. 32-12.   The mesial surface of a maxillary right second premolar. *Note:* Although mesial and distal marginal grooves are present in all maxillary second premolar drawings, the actual grooves are shallower than the mesial marginal groove of a maxillary first premolar. (From Zeisz RC, Nuckolls J: *Dental anatomy,* St Louis, 1949, Mosby.)

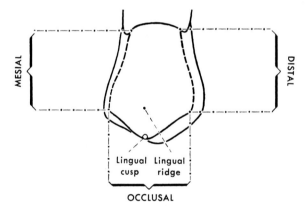

FIG. 32-11.   The lingual surface of a maxillary right second premolar. (From Zeisz RC, Nuckolls J: *Dental anatomy,* St Louis, 1949, Mosby.)

least a portion of the root. A bifurcated root similar to that of a first premolar is common; this form has two root canals.

Pulp cavity

The pulp cavity (Fig. 32-14) of the maxillary second premolar has two pulp horns and a single root canal. The single-rooted form is more common; it is also more common to have one root canal. If two canals are present, they usually join to form one single apical foramen, although it is not rare to find two apical foramina. In the bifurcated root there are two canals and two apical foramina.

Pertinent Data

Maxillary first premolars

	Right	Left
Universal Code	5	12
International Code	14	24
Palmer notation	4⌋	⌊4
Number of roots	2	

Root

The root of a maxillary second premolar is usually single with a longitudinal groove on the mesial and distal surfaces. This groove gives the appearance of a single root dividing into two, buccally and lingually. Usually there is only one root canal, but often a divided canal occurs in at

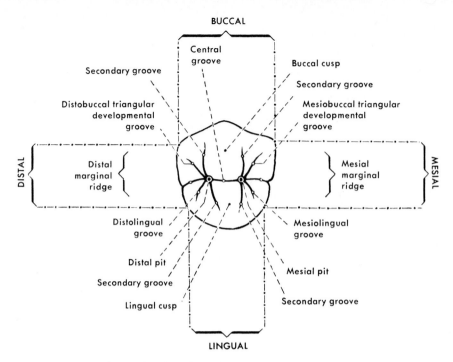

FIG. 32-13. The occlusal surface of a maxillary right second premolar. (From Zeisz RC, Nuckolls J: *Dental anatomy,* St Louis, 1949, Mosby.)

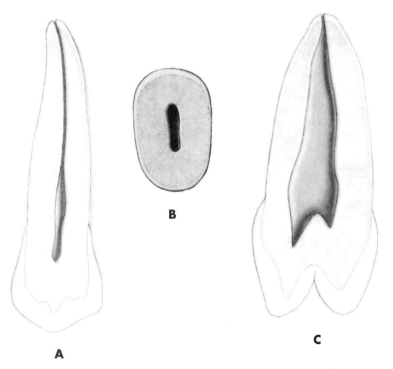

A

B

C

FIG. 32-14. The pulp cavity of a right maxillary second premolar. **A,** Mesiodistal section, buccal view. **B,** Cross section, occlusal view. **C,** Linguobuccal section, mesial view. (From Zeisz RC, Nuckolls J: *Dental anatomy,* St Louis, 1949, Mosby.)

Number of pulp horns	2
Number of cusps	2
Number of developmental lobes	4

Location of proximal contact areas.
Mesial and distal: Just cervical to the junction of occlusal and middle thirds
Height of contour.
Facial: Cervical third, 0.5 mm
Lingual: Middle third, 0.5 mm
Identifying characteristics. Maxillary first premolars have bifurcated roots, and a longitudinal groove is present on each root. The mesial surface shows a developmental fossa. The mesial marginal groove crosses the mesial marginal ridge and extends onto the mesial surface. The facial cusp is wider and longer than the lingual cusp. The mesial ridge of the facial cusp may have a slight concavity.

Maxillary Second Premolars

	Right	Left
Universal Code	4	13
International Code	15	25
Palmer notation	5⌋	⌊5
Number of roots	1	
Number of pulp horns	2	
Number of cusps	2	
Number of developmental lobes	4	

Location of proximal contact areas.
Mesial and distal: Just cervical to the junction of occlusal and middle thirds
Height of contour.
Facial: Cervical third, 0.5 mm
Lingual: Middle third, 0.5 mm
Identifying characteristics. Maxillary second premolars usually have a single root. About 40% have two root canals. The buccal and lingual cusps are nearly equal in length. The buccal cusp is shorter than that of a first premolar. The entire crown, especially the occlusal outline, is less angular and more rounded than that of a maxillary first premolar. The occlusal surface has more supplemental grooves. The occlusal developmental grooves are shorter, shallower, and more irregular.

Maxillary First Premolars Compared With Maxillary Second Premolars

The following features are more true for a maxillary first premolar than for a maxillary second premolar:

1. It usually has two roots.
2. It usually has two root canals, even if it has only one root.
3. It has a mesial developmental fossa.
4. Its mesial marginal ridge is crossed by a mesial marginal developmental groove.
5. The lingual and buccal cusps are not nearly the same height—the buccal is longer.
6. The occlusal outline is less rounded in the first premolars.
7. The facial contour is more angular.
8. The occlusal grooves are not as short, shallow, or irregular as those of the second premolars.
9. It has fewer secondary anatomic features and fewer supplemental grooves.
10. It has a shorter buccal cusp.

MANDIBULAR PREMOLARS

First Premolars

Evidence of calcification	2 years
Enamel completed	5-6 years
Eruption	10-12 years
Root completed	12-13 years

The mandibular first premolars (Fig. 32-15) have many of the characteristics of the mandibular canines. Like the canines, they have a dominant facial cusp, which is the only part that occludes with the maxillary teeth.

As a rule, the mandibular first premolars are always smaller than the mandibular second premolars. In most cases this is not true of the maxillary premolars.

The mandibular first premolars develop from

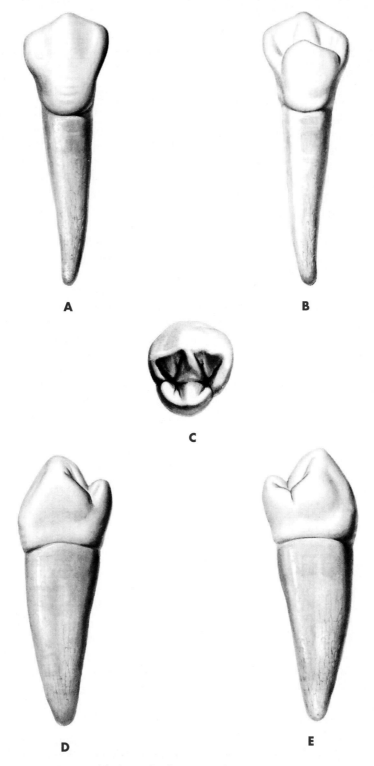

FIG. 32-15. A mandibular right first premolar. **A,** Buccal view. **B,** Lingual view. **C,** Occlusal view. **D,** Mesial view. **E,** Distal view. (From Zeisz RC, Nuckolls J: *Dental anatomy,* St Louis, 1949, Mosby.)

four lobes, just as the maxillary first and second premolars do. The three facial lobes form the large buccal cusp, and the single lingual lobe forms into a lingual cusp. This lingual cusp is much smaller than the lingual cusp of the maxillary premolars. It is so small in height and width that it does not occlude with any of the maxillary teeth. It is for this reason that the lingual cusp of the mandibular first premolars is considered afunctional. As in the case of the maxillary premolars, each cusp has its own pulp horn. How many pulp horns would the mandibular first premolars have?

Facial (buccal) aspect

A mandibular first premolar resembles a mandibular canine from the facial view (Fig. 32-16; see also Fig. 32-15, A). This premolar has nearly the same buccolingual measurement as a canine, and like the canine it has a sharp buccal cusp. The middle buccal lobe is well developed. The mesial cusp ridge is shorter than the distal cusp ridge, but the contact areas are almost at the same level mesially and distally. They are located slightly occlusal to the midpoint of the tooth cervicoincisally. In what third of the tooth are the contact areas located?

A mandibular premolar is more convex than a maxillary premolar at the cervical and middle thirds.

The root of this tooth is usually 3 mm or more shorter than that of a mandibular canine.

Developmental depressions are often seen between the three lobes. However, developmental lines are usually not present.

Lingual aspect (Fig. 32-17; see also Fig. 32-15, B)

The crown and root of a mandibular first premolar taper lingually. Like a canine, a first premolar is broader mesiodistally on the buccal cusp portion of the tooth than on the part developed from the lingual lobe. The lingual cusp is small in comparison to the buccal cusp.

The occlusal surface slopes toward the lingual side in a cervical direction. On each side of the triangular ridge, mesial and distal occlusal pits can be seen within the fossae.

The most striking and characteristic identifying feature of this tooth is the mesiolingual developmental groove, which separates the mesial marginal ridge from the lingual cusp.

Mesial aspect

From the mesial view (Fig. 32-18; see also Fig.

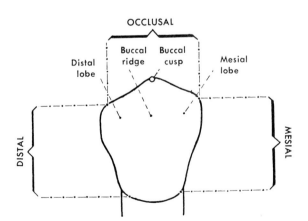

FIG. 32-16. The buccal surface of a mandibular right first premolar. (From Zeisz RC, Nuckolls J: *Dental anatomy,* St Louis, 1949, Mosby.)

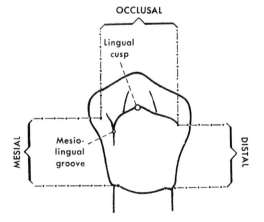

FIG. 32-17. The lingual surface of a mandibular right first premolar. (From Zeisz RC, Nuckolls J: *Dental anatomy,* St Louis, 1949, Mosby.)

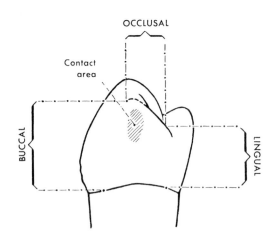

FIG. 32-18.   The mesial surface of a mandibular right first premolar. (From Zeisz RC, Nuckolls J: *Dental anatomy,* St Louis, 1949, Mosby.)

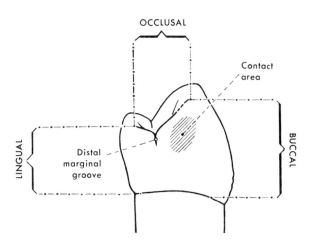

FIG. 32-19.   The distal surface of a mandibular right first premolar. (From Zeisz RC, Nuckolls J: *Dental anatomy,* St Louis, 1949, Mosby.)

32-15, *D*), the buccal cusp overshadows the smaller lingual cusp. The tip of the buccal cusp is centered directly over the root, and the tip of the lingual cusp is centered lingually to the root. How does this differ from the maxillary premolars?

The buccal crest of curvature is located in the cervical third of the crown, the lingual crest near the middle third.

The mesiolingual developmental groove can be seen between the mesiobuccal and the lingual lobes.

Distal aspect

The distal view (Fig. 32-19; see also Fig. 32-15, *E*) resembles the mesial except for the following characteristics:

1. There is no mesiolingual developmental groove.
2. The distal marginal ridge is much more developed than the mesial ridge, and its continuity is unbroken by any deep developmental lines.
3. The curvature of the cervical line is less than the 1 mm usually found on the mesial.
4. The distal contact area is broader than the

mesial, though it is centered in the same relationship to the crown.

5. The root exhibits more convexity distally than mesially and rarely shows a developmental groove.
6. A shallow developmental depression, less prominent than on the mesial, is often found.

Occlusal aspect

The occlusal aspect (Fig. 32-20; see also Fig. 32-15, *C*) displays considerable individual variation. Much more variation exists on either mandibular first or second premolars than on their maxillary counterparts.

The crown converges sharply toward the lingual side, the marginal ridges are well developed, and the lingual cusp is small.

The buccal cusp shows a heavy facial triangular ridge and a smaller lingual triangular ridge. Two depressions, the mesial and distal fossae, are visible, one on each side of the lingual triangular ridge of the buccal cusp.

The mandibular first premolars are the only premolars that may have a transverse ridge that does not cross an occlusal developmental groove. The mesial developmental groove extends from

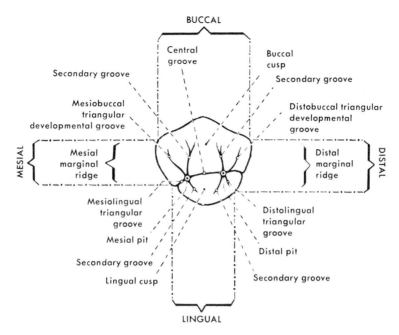

FIG. 32-20.   The occlusal surface of a mandibular right first premolar. A central groove is not always present. (From Zeisz RC, Nuckolls J: *Dental anatomy*, St Louis, 1949, Mosby.)

the mesial fossa lingually, between the mesial marginal ridge and the lingual cusp, and onto the lingual surface. Either fossa may contain a pit. What would the name of these pits be, should they occur? Does a mandibular first premolar always have a central developmental groove?

Root

A mandibular first premolar is normally single rooted. The mesial and distal surfaces are usually slightly convex. If a longitudinal groove is present, then the mesial and distal surfaces may be concave. Occasionally, there may be two roots, a buccal and a lingual. A deep longitudinal groove will separate the roots on the proximal sides in such cases.

Pulp Cavity

The pulp cavity of the mandibular first premolar comprises two pulp horns, a pulp chamber, and a single root canal. The buccal pulp horn is dominant, and the lingual pulp horn is small and insignificant. Each pulp horn is located within a cusp (Fig. 32-21).

Second Premolars

Evidence of calcification	2½ years
Enamel completed	6-7 years
Eruption	11-12 years
Root completed	13-14 years

A mandibular second premolar (Fig. 32-22) is always larger than a mandibular first premolar. From a labial view, the crown resembles a first premolar in its general shape and in the fact that the contact areas, mesially and distally, are near the same level. The buccal cusp is shorter, however, and the root is longer.

The lingual cusps of a second premolar are much more developed, and both marginal ridges

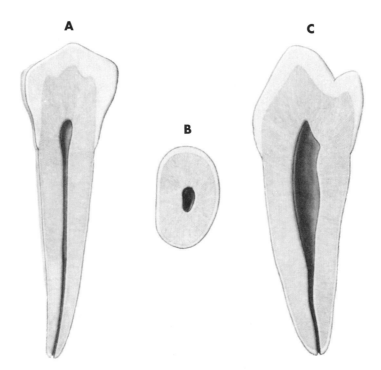

FIG. 32-21.   The pulp cavity of a mandibular right first premolar. **A,** Mesiodistal section, buccal view. **B,** Cross section, occlusal view. **C,** Buccolingual section, mesial view. (From Zeisz RC, Nuckolls J: *Dental anatomy,* St Louis, 1949, Mosby.)

are higher. This produces a more efficient occlusion with its maxillary antagonist. Therefore a mandibular second premolar functions more like a molar than a canine. How does this differ from a mandibular first premolar?

There are two common forms of this tooth, the three-cusp and the two-cusp type, with one pulp horn in each cusp. The three-cusp form has how many lingual pulp horns? How many pulp horns does the two-cusp form have?

The three-cusp form resembles the mandibular molars in the following ways:

1. It has two lingual cusps formed from two separate developmental lobes.
2. It has two lingual pulp canals.
3. It has afunctional lingual cusps.

4. It has higher mesial and distal marginal ridges.
5. The marginal ridges function in occlusion, offering more efficient contact and intercuspation of the teeth, despite the fact that lingual cusps are afunctional.

The single root of a second premolar is larger and longer than that of the first. It is sometimes bifurcated, but this is rare.

Facial (buccal) aspect

From the buccal view (Fig. 32-23; see also Fig. 32-22, *A*) a mandibular second premolar appears to have a shorter buccal cusp than that of a first premolar. Also, the mesiobuccal and distobuccal cusp ridges are more rounded. The mesial and distal contact areas are broad, and

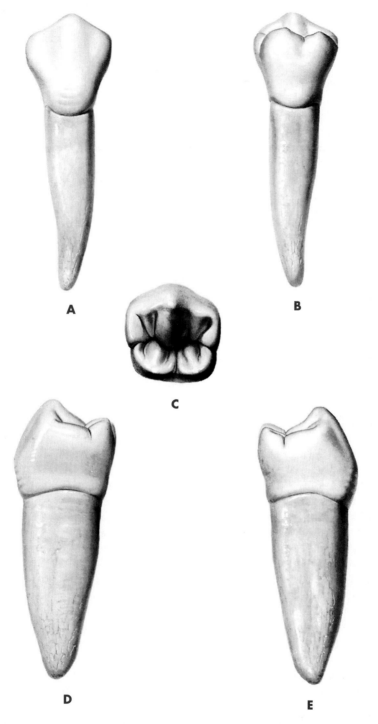

Fig. 32-22. A mandibular right second premolar. **A,** Buccal view. **B,** Lingual
view. **C,** Occlusal view. **D,** Mesial view. **E,** Distal view.

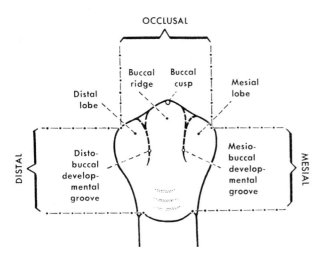

FIG. 32-23.   The buccal surface of a mandibular right second premolar. (From Zeisz RC, Nuckolls J: *Dental anatomy*, St Louis, 1949, Mosby.)

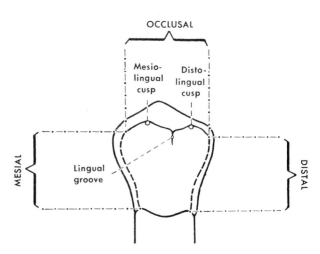

FIG. 32-24.   The lingual surface of a mandibular right second premolar. (From Zeisz RC, Nuckolls J: *Dental anatomy*, St Louis, 1949, Mosby.)

they are located just cervical to the junction of the middle cervical third of the crown.

The root is wider mesiodistally and slightly longer, with a more blunt apex.

Lingual aspect

The lingual view (Fig. 32-24; see also Fig. 32-22, *B*) of a second premolar shows much variation because there are two different cusp forms. In general, however, the following statements are true of a mandibular second premolar as compared with the first premolar.

1. The lingual lobes are developed to a greater degree. At least one lingual cusp will be longer than a lingual cusp of a first premolar.
2. In the three-cusp form there is a **mesiolingual** and a **distolingual cusp.** The mesiolingual cusp is usually the wider and longer of the two cusps, which are divided by a lingual groove.
3. In the two-cusp form the single lingual lobe is higher than on a mandibular first premolar. There is no groove on the lingual lobe, as in the three-cusp form, but a developmental depression can be seen distolingually where the

lingual cusp ridge joins the distal marginal ridge.

4. The lingual surface of the root is wider than that of a first premolar. Thus the convergence of the root toward the lingual side is less. This is true even though the root is wider buccally, because the root is much wider lingually than on a first premolar, resulting in less convergence toward the lingual side.

The lingual portion of the crown and root is slightly convex.

Mesial aspect (Fig. 32-25; see also Fig. 32-22, *D*)

A second premolar differs mesially from a first premolar in the following ways:

1. The buccal cusp is shorter, and its tip is located more to the buccal side.
2. The crown and root are wider buccolingually.
3. The lingual lobe shows more development.
4. The marginal ridge is at a right angle to the long axis of the tooth.
5. There is no mesiolingual developmental groove.

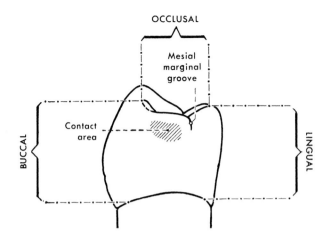

FIG. 32-25.   The mesial surface of a mandibular right second premolar. (From Zeisz RC, Nuckolls J: *Dental anatomy,* St Louis, 1949, Mosby.)

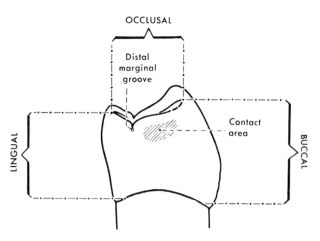

FIG. 32-26.   The distal surface of a mandibular right second premolar. (From Zeisz RC, Nuckolls J: *Dental anatomy,* St Louis, 1949, Mosby.)

6. The root is longer, and the apex is more blunt.

Distal aspect

From the distal view (Fig. 32-26; see also Fig. 32-22, *E*) more of the occlusal surface can be seen because the distal marginal ridge is at a lower level than the mesial marginal ridge.

As a general rule, the crowns of all posterior teeth, maxillary or mandibular, are tipped distally to the long axis of the root. Thus, if a specimen is held vertically, more of the occlusal surface of a posterior tooth can be seen from the distal aspect. Another general rule is that more roots of posterior teeth will tip toward the distal side. In other words, the apex of the root will curve distally.

Occlusal aspect (Fig. 32-27; see also Fig. 32-22, *C*)

In both the two- and three-cusp forms the buccal cusp is similar. In the three-cusp form the buccal cusp is the largest, the mesiolingual cusp the next largest, and the distolingual cusp the smallest.

Each of the three cusps has a well-developed triangular ridge separated by deep developmental grooves. These grooves form a wide pattern

on the occlusal surface. The three developmental grooves are the mesial, the distal, and the lingual grooves. Three pits may be present—a central, a mesial, and a distal. Of the three, the central pit is the most likely to be present. Mesial and distal **triangular fossae** are also present.

Supplemental grooves are more commonly found on a second premolar than on a first, and the developmental grooves are usually not so deep.

In the two-cusp type, as compared with the three-cusp type, the following observations can be noted:

1. The occlusal outline of the crown is more rounded.
2. The lingual surface of the crown is more convex and tapers toward lingually.
3. There is no lingual developmental groove.
4. There is only one well-developed lingual cusp on the two-cusp form, and it is located directly opposite the buccal cusp in a lingual direction.
5. There is usually no central pit; a mesial or distal pit is much more likely.

In the three-cusp type, the groove pattern is

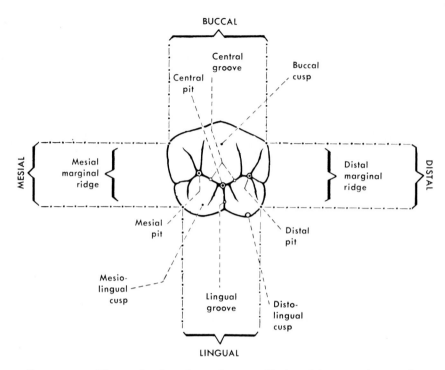

FIG. 32-27.   The occlusal surface of a mandibular right second premolar (three-cusp variety). (From Zeisz RC, Nuckolls J: *Dental anatomy,* St Louis, 1949, Mosby.)

commonly called a Y-groove pattern. In the two-cusp type, the groove pattern can be either a U- (sometimes called C-) or H-groove pattern (Figs. 32-28 through 32-30) depending on whether the central developmental groove is straight mesio-distally or curves buccally at its ends. The central groove of the two-cusp form terminates in mesial and distal fossae. If lingual triangular grooves radiate from these fossae, the H-groove pattern is present.

The Y-groove pattern as seen in the three-cusp form is by far the most dominant form, occurring with much more frequency than the two-cusp forms. Of the less prevalent two-cusp forms, the H-groove pattern is more common than the U-groove pattern.

According to Julian Woelfel, in his text *Den-*

tal Anatomy: Its Relevance to Dentistry, 43% of lower second premolars have two cusps, 54.2% have three cusps, and 2.8% have four cusps. His sample comprised 1532 specimens.

As a general rule, second premolars and second molars have shallower developmental grooves than first premolars and first molars. They also have more secondary grooves. In general, the more posterior the tooth, the more wrinkled it appears.

Root

The root of the mandibular second premolar is similar to that of the first premolar. It is longer and wider buccolingually. There is no tendency for it to bifurcate as the mandibular first premolar sometimes does (see Fig. 32-22).

The distal surface of the root of both premo-

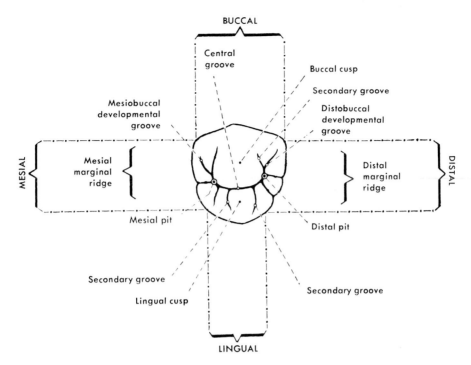

Fig. 32-28. Occlusal surface, U type (two-cusp variety). (From Zeisz RC, Nuckolls J: *Dental anatomy,* St Louis, 1949, Mosby.)

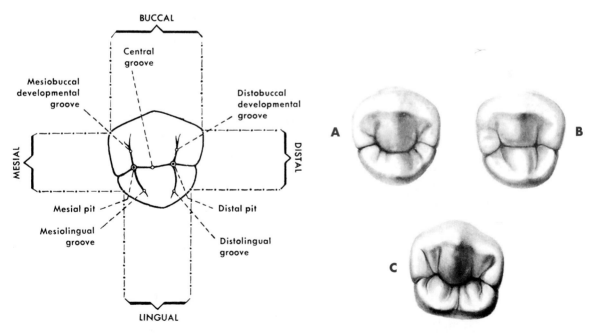

Fig. 32-29. Occlusal surface, H type (two-cusp variety). (From Zeisz RC, Nuckolls J: *Dental anatomy,* St Louis, 1949, Mosby.)

Fig. 32-30. Occlusal views. A, U type. B, H type. C, Y type. (From Zeisz RC, Nuckolls J: *Dental anatomy,* St Louis, 1949, Mosby.)

lars, first and second, is more likely to have a longitudinal depression in the middle third. The mesial surface is far less likely to have such a longitudinal depression. This is just the reverse of the maxillary premolars.

Pulp cavity

The pulp cavity (Fig. 32-31) of the mandibular second premolar shows two pointed pulp horns, three in the three-cusp variety. The pulp horns are more pointed than in the mandibular first premolar. A single root canal is present, with even less tendency to have divided root canals than in the first premolar.

Pertinent Data

Mandibular first premolars

	Right	Left
Universal Code	28	21
International Code	44	34
Palmer notation	4⌐	⌐4
Number of roots	1	
Number of pulp horns	1 or 2	
Number of cusps	2	
Number of developmental lobes	4	

Location of proximal contact areas.

Mesial and distal: Just cervical to junction of occlusal and middle thirds

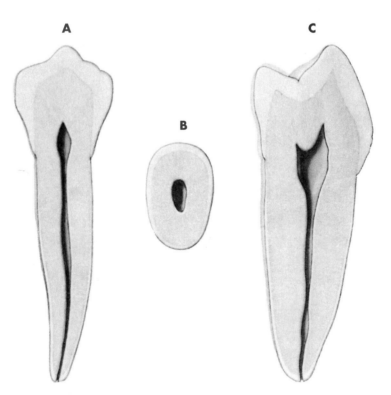

A

B

C

FIG. 32-31.   The pulp cavity of a mandibular right second premolar. **A**, Mesiodistal section, buccal view. **B**, Cross section, occlusal view. **C**, Buccolingual section, mesial view. (From Zeisz RC, Nuckolls J: *Dental anatomy*, St Louis, 1949, Mosby.)

Height of contour.
Facial: Cervical third, 0.5 mm
Lingual: Middle third, 1 mm

Identifying characteristics. Mandibular first premolars have two cusps, one large buccal cusp and one small lingual cusp. The buccal cusp is centered directly over the root. The lingual cusp is centered lingual to the root and is afunctional and nonoccluding. The occlusal surface slopes sharply lingual in a cervical direction. The mesiobuccal cusp ridge is shorter than the distobuccal cusp ridge. It has a mesiolingual developmental groove and one root.

Mandibular second premolars

	Right	Left
Universal Code	29	20
International Code	45	35
Palmer notation	5⌐	⌐5
Number of roots	1	
Number of pulp horns	2 or 3	
Number of cusps	2 or 3	
Number of developmental lobes	4 or 5	

Location of proximal contact areas.
Mesial and distal: Just cervical to junction of occlusal and middle thirds

Height of contour.
Facial: Cervical third, 0.5 mm
Lingual: Middle third, 1 mm

Identifying characteristics. Mandibular second premolars have two or three cusps. The buccal cusp is very large. If two lingual cusps are present, the mesiolingual is the larger. Although the lingual cusps are larger than on the first premolar, they are afunctional and do not occlude with the maxillary teeth. A second premolar has more secondary anatomic features and more variation than any other tooth except a third molar. The two-cusp form has a U- or H-groove pattern. A mesiolingual groove is rare and is poorly developed if present. The three-cusp form has a lingual developmental groove between the two lingual cusps. The single root is longer and larger than that of a first premolar.

Review Questions

1. In which of the following is a maxillary second premolar different from a maxillary first premolar?
   a. number of developmental lobes
   b. size of cusps and number of roots
   c. existence of a central groove
   d. location of proximal contacts
2. Which of the following best describes the functional cusp(s) of a mandibular first premolar?
   a. both facial and lingual
   b. facial
   c. lingual
   d. neither facial nor lingual
3. Which tooth in the human dentition is most likely to be derived from five developmental lobes?
   a. maxillary right first premolar
   b. maxillary right second premolar
   c. mandibular left first premolar
   d. mandibular right second premolar
4. In comparing the mandibular and maxillary first premolars,
   a. the facial cusp of a mandibular premolar is more lingually located.
   b. the lingual cusp is more facially located.
   c. the occlusal surface of a mandibular first premolar is relatively large.
   d. the occlusal outline is wider mesiodistally in the lingual portion of the mandibular first premolar.
5. A maxillary first premolar may be identified by:
   a. a noticeable mesial concavity in the cervical area.
   b. rounded cusps of nearly equal height.
   c. long supplemental grooves.
   d. a single root canal.
6. Which of the following best describes the location of the proximal contacts of a maxillary second premolar?
   a. just cervical to the junction of the occlusal and middle thirds

b. just occlusal to the junction of the cervical and middle thirds
c. just cervical to the junction of the cervical and middle thirds
d. just occlusal to the junction of the occlusal and middle thirds

7. The mandibular first and second premolars are distinguished with respect to:
a. the usual number of cusps.
b. the average number of root canals in 100 specimens.
c. the incisocervical location of proximal contacts.
d. the number of developmental lobes forming the facial portion.

8. Usually the most striking identifying characteristic of a mandibular first premolar is which of the following grooves?
a. central
b. mesiolingual
c. faciolingual
d. mesial

9. Which of the following groove patterns is the most dominant form of mandibular second premolars?
a. the Y-groove pattern
b. the C-groove pattern
c. the H-groove pattern
d. the U-groove pattern

10. When the triangular ridge of the buccal cusp joins the triangular ridge of the lingual cusp, it is known as a:
a. triangular ridge.
b. marginal ridge.
c. transverse ridge.
d. occlusal ridge.

11. One permanent premolar has the most pronounced cervical concavity of any of the premolars, which requires special consideration when a matrix band is adapted. The premolar and the proximal surface where the concavity is located is the:
a. distal surface of a mandibular second premolar.

b. mesial surface of a maxillary first premolar.
c. distal surface of a maxillary second premolar.
d. mesial surface of a maxillary second premolar.

12. Which of the permanent premolars often has fewer pulp horns than the other premolars?
a. maxillary first premolar
b. maxillary second premolar
c. mandibular first premolar
d. mandibular second premolar

13. A cusp has how many ridges?
a. 2
b. 3
c. 4
d. 5

14. If you examined an extracted premolar tooth and found a single root, a symmetrical rounded effect of the crown in all aspects, and many secondary grooves arising from the central groove, you could assume it to be a:
a. maxillary first premolar.
b. maxillary second premolar.
c. mandibular first premolar.
d. mandibular second premolar.

15. A premolar with a root that is most commonly bifurcated is a:
a. maxillary first premolar.
b. mandibular first premolar.
c. maxillary second premolar.
d. mandibular second premolar.

16. Which of the following is true concerning longitudinal grooves?
a. They are often present on the mesial and distal sides of maxillary second premolars.
b. They are more common on the distal side of mandibular premolars than the mesial side.
c. They are usually present on maxillary premolars.
d. All of the above.

17. Posterior teeth are wider buccolingually than anterior teeth. T or F?

18. Lower premolars have buccal afunctional cusps. T or F?

19. Posterior teeth are higher cervicoocclusally. T or F?

20. Mesial and distal contact areas of premolars are broader than contact areas of anterior teeth. T or F?

MOLARS

OBJECTIVES

- To understand the lobe formations of the crowns of molars
- To compare the formations of first, second, and third molars
- To understand the anchorage of the roots as a resistance to forces of displacement
- To describe the details of the various molars
- To make comparisons among the various molars: maxillary and mandibular, as well as first, second, and third molars
- To identify each molar

THE TWELVE permanent molars are the largest and strongest teeth in the mouth by virtue of their crown bulk size and their root anchorage in bone (Fig. 33-1). Their primary function is to grind or crush food.

The permanent molars erupt long after all the deciduous teeth have already erupted. The first permanent molars erupt distal to the primary second molars. In humans usually the first permanent teeth to erupt are the first molars. It is only after these molars have erupted that the permanent incisors begin replacing the deciduous incisors.

The following chart shows the approximate eruption time for molars. Bear in mind that there is much individual variation. Which teeth usually erupt first, the mandibular or the maxillary?

Eruption Times of Molars			
	Eruption	Enamel completion	Root completion
First molar	6-7 years	4 years	9-10 years
Second molar	11-13 years	7-8 years	14-16 years
Third molar	17-22 years	12-16 years	18-25 years

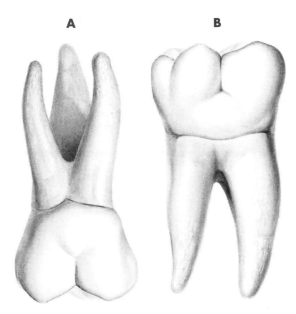

FIG. 33-1.   **A,** Maxillary first molar. **B,** Mandibular first molar. (From Zeisz RC, Nuckolls J: *Dental anatomy,* St Louis, 1949, Mosby.)

 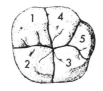

FIG. 33-2.   Lobes of molars. (From Wheeler RC: *A textbook of dental anatomy and physiology,* Philadelphia, 1965, WB Saunders Co.)

Whose teeth usually erupt first, boys' or girls'? (Refer to Chapter 24.)

The molars are nonsuccedaneous teeth—that is, they do not replace any primary teeth. They are referred to as **accessional,** or nonsuccedane-

ous, as opposed to succedaneous teeth, which do replace deciduous teeth.

Generally, the first molars are formed from five lobes, but some second and third molars may have only four lobes. The lobes in Fig. 33-2 are numbered in the order of their size, number 1 being the largest.

In general each cusp of a molar is formed from its own lobe. For instance, a maxillary first molar forms from five lobes, three of which form major cusps. These major cusps are large and well developed, characteristic of, and usually present on all maxillary molars—first, second, and third. The fourth lobe on a maxillary first molar forms a minor cusp. A minor cusp has smaller proportions and less development. It is less functional than the major cusps and is not always present on second and third molars. The maxillary first molars have a fifth lobe, which develops into a supplementary cusp. A supplementary cusp is completely afunctional and is not usually present on either the second or third molars. First molars are the most highly developed and largest of the molars and are more likely to have minor and supplementary cusps in addition to their major cusp.

The maxillary molars have only three major cusps, one minor cusp, and sometimes one supplementary cusp. The mandibular molars usually have four major cusps and sometimes one minor cusp. (See Figs. 24-4 and 24-5.)

The minor cusps of the maxillary teeth are the distolingual cusps; those on the mandibular teeth are the distal cusps. The supplementary cusp occurs only on a maxillary first molar. However, it may not be present at all.

In review, the most developed of the molars are the first molars, whether maxillary or mandibular. The second molars usually have no supplementary cusps, and the minor cusps are even more minor in relation to the major cusps. Third molars may not develop minor cusps at all. A maxillary third molar may have only three major cusps, or a mandibular third molar may have four major cusps.

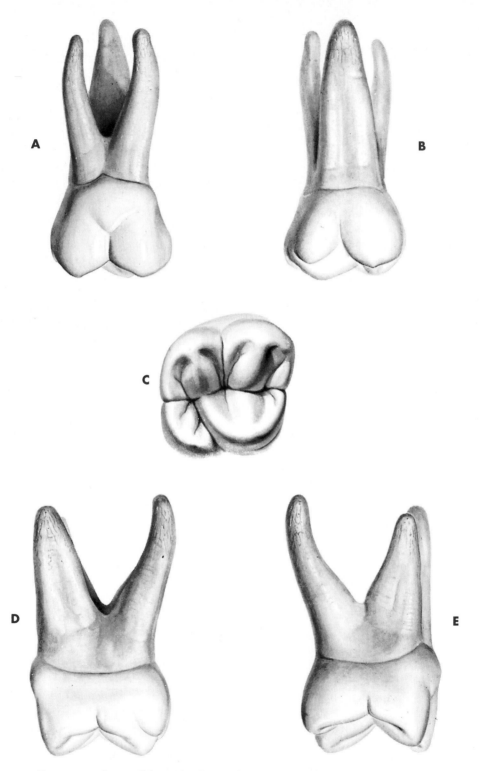

FIG. 33-3. A maxillary right first molar. **A,** Buccal view. **B,** Lingual view. **C,** Occlusal view. **D,** Mesial view. **E,** Distal view. (From Zeisz RC, Nuckolls J: *Dental anatomy,* St Louis, 1949, Mosby.)

MAXILLARY MOLARS

First Molars

Evidence of calcification	Birth
Enamel completed	4 years
Eruption	6-7 years
Root completed	9-10 years

The maxillary first molars (Fig. 33-3) are normally the largest teeth in the maxillary arch. There are three molars on each side—the first, second, and third maxillary molars. Each has three well-developed major cusps and one minor cusp, all of which are functional. The fifth or supplemental cusp, which is afunctional, is called the cusp or tubercle of Carabelli. This fifth cusp is usually found on all maxillary first molars.

The crown of a first molar is broad mesiodistally and buccolingually and just slightly wider buccolingually than mesiodistally. Of the four functional cusps, two are found on the buccal and two on the lingual side.

Facial (buccal) aspect

From the buccal view (Fig. 33-4; see also Fig. 33-3, A) four cusps can usually be seen—mesio-buccal, distobuccal, mesiolingual, and distolingual. The two lingual cusps are not located directly behind the buccal cusps but are distal and lingual to them. Although the mesiobuccal cusp is broader than the distobuccal cusp, the latter is usually sharper and longer. The mesiobuccal cusp forms an obtuse angle (more than 90 degrees), where its mesial slope meets its distal slope at the cusp tip. The distobuccal cusp usually forms a less obtuse angle where the mesial slope meets the distal slope.

The buccal developmental groove divides the two buccal cusps. This groove runs in a line parallel to the long axis of the tooth, terminating halfway from its point of origin to the cervical line of the crown. Although not very deep at any point, at its terminal end it splits into a buccal pit with two small grooves radiating from it.

The cervical line is irregular and curved, generally toward the occlusal side at the mesial and distal ends.

The mesial outline is straight from the cervical line to the mesial contact area. Below the contact area it curves distally until it reaches the mesio-

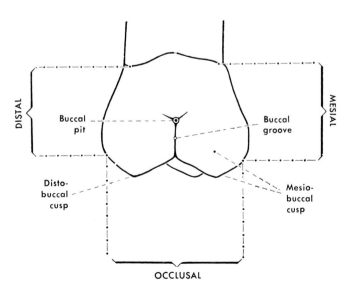

FIG. 33-4. The buccal surface of a maxillary right first molar. (From Zeisz RC, Nuckolls J: *Dental anatomy,* St Louis, 1949, Mosby.)

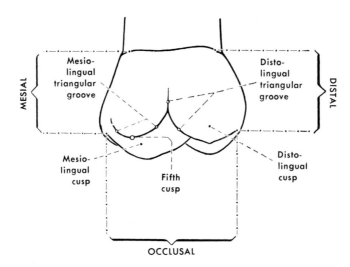

Fig. 33-5.   The lingual surface of a maxillary right first molar. (From Zeisz RC, Nuckolls J: *Dental anatomy*, St Louis, 1949, Mosby.)

buccal cusp tip. The height of curvature is just cervical to the junction of the middle and occlusal thirds.

Distally the outline of the crown is convex, and the contact area is in the center of the middle third.

Lingual aspect

The lingual cusps alone can be seen from the lingual aspect (Fig. 33-5; see also Fig. 33-3, *B*). The mesiolingual cusp is much longer and larger than either of the buccal cusps. Wider mesiodistally and buccolingually, the mesiofacial cusp is the next largest, although it is not as long as the distofacial cusp. The distolingual cusp is the smallest and the shortest of the functional cusps. Of course, the cusp of Carabelli is the shortest and smallest of all five cusps, but it is afunctional. In fact, the cusp of Carabelli is not a cusp at all but rather a tubercle. A **fifth-cusp developmental groove,** called the **mesiolingual groove,** separates the cusp of Carabelli from the mesiolingual cusp.

The outline of the crown is as straight mesially as it is buccally. The distal outline is more convex because of the roundness of the distolingual cusp. The **lingual developmental groove** extends from the center of the lingual surface occlusally, between the two lingual cusps, where it curves sharply to the distal side and becomes the **distal oblique groove.** These two grooves (lingual and distal oblique grooves) are sometimes considered to be one and are then referred to as the **distolingual developmental groove.**

The distolingual cusp of a maxillary first molar is functional even though it is small. On a first molar the distolingual cusp occupies approximately 40% of the lingual surface and the mesiolingual cusp occupies the other 60%. The distolingual cusp is progressively smaller on the maxillary second and third molars.

All three roots can be seen from the lingual aspect. On the average, the roots are about twice as long as the crown. The lingual root is usually longer than either of the two buccal roots, which are the same length.

Mesial aspect

The mesial aspect (Fig. 33-6; see also Fig. 33-3, *D*) of a maxillary first molar usually shows a clear profile of the cusp of Carabelli. The lingual crest

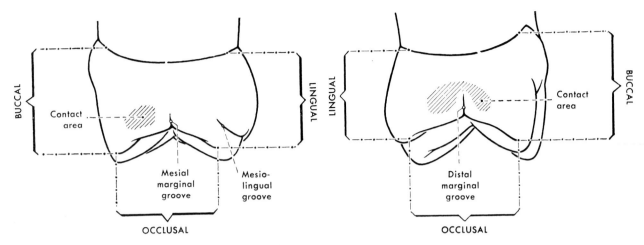

FIG. 33-6. The mesial surface of a maxillary right first molar. (From Zeisz RC, Nuckolls J: *Dental anatomy*, St Louis, 1949, Mosby.)

FIG. 33-7. The distal surface of a maxillary right first molar. (From Zeisz RC, Nuckolls J: *Dental anatomy*, St Louis, 1949, Mosby.)

of curvature is at the center of the middle third of the crown, the buccal crest at the cervical third. The cervical line is slightly convex mesially.

Distal aspect (Fig. 33-7; see also Fig. 33-3, *E*)

The crown has the tendency to taper distally. The buccolingual measurement of the crown on the mesial side is greater than the same measurement distally. The distal cervical line is usually straighter and less curved than that on the mesial side. Although the distal surface of the crown is convex and smooth, there is a slight concavity on the distal surface of the root trunk from the cervical line to the distobuccal root.

The distal marginal ridge is shorter and less prominent than the mesial marginal ridge, and more of the occlusal surface in general can be seen from the distal view.

The distobuccal root is the narrowest of all three roots.

Occlusal aspect

A maxillary first molar has a rhomboidal occlusal outline (Fig. 33-8; see also Fig. 33-3, *C*). The molar crown is wider mesially than distally; it is also wider lingually than buccally. This is the

only tooth that is wider lingually than buccally. Is the occlusal outline of a maxillary first molar more like a square or more like a square that has been squashed sideways? What is the difference between a rhomboidal and a square form?

Other anatomic structures

There are two major fossae and two minor fossae on maxillary first molars. The major fossae are the **central fossa**, which is mesial to the oblique ridge, and the distal fossa, which is distal to the oblique ridge. The minor fossae are the mesial fossa and the distal triangular fossa, both of which are located on the inside of their respective marginal ridges.

The **central developmental pit** lies in the central fossa. The **buccal developmental groove** radiates from this pit buccally between the two buccal cusps. The central developmental groove lies in a mesial direction, originating in the central developmental pit and terminating at the mesial triangular fossa. Here it is joined by the mesiofacial and mesiolingual triangular grooves, which appear as branches of the **central groove**. The mesial marginal groove, a

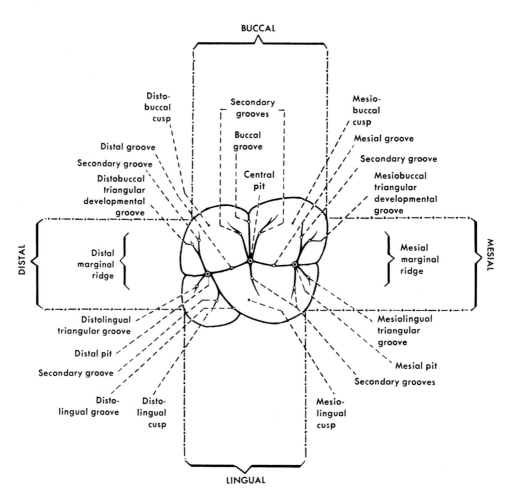

Fig. 33-8.   The occlusal surface of a maxillary right first molar. (From Zeisz RC, Nuckolls J: *Dental anatomy,* St Louis, 1949, Mosby.)

branch of the central groove, lies between these two triangular grooves and may cross the mesial marginal ridge of the crown. The **mesial pit** is found in the mesial triangular fossa.

Sometimes another developmental groove radiates from the central pit in a distal direction. If it crosses the oblique ridge, joining the central and distal fossae, it is called the **transverse groove of the oblique ridge** or the distal part of the central developmental groove.

The **oblique ridge** is a transverse ridge and is unique to maxillary molars. A transverse ridge is formed by two triangular ridges joining together and crossing the surface of a posterior tooth diagonally rather than straight across buccolingually. In this case the triangular ridge of the mesiolingual cusp joins the triangular ridge of the distobuccal cusp. This cannot happen unless the ridges cross the tooth transversely, as opposed to buccolingually. Therefore the oblique ridge runs from the tip of the mesiolingual cusp to the tip of the distobuccal cusp.

The distal fossa of a maxillary first molar runs parallel with and distal to the oblique ridge. This fossa is long and narrow rather than circular. In this fossa lies the distal oblique groove from which it takes its shape.

The **distal pit** is found in the distal fossa.

The distal triangular fossa is mesial to the distal marginal ridge. The distal oblique groove terminates in the distal triangular fossa, where the distal oblique groove gives off three branches, the distofacial triangular groove, the distolingual triangular groove, and the **distal marginal groove.**

The primary grooves of the maxillary first molars are as follows:

1. Facial groove
2. Central groove (two parts—mesial and distal)
3. Distolingual groove (two parts—lingual and distal oblique grooves)
4. Mesiolingual groove (cusp of Carabelli groove)
5. Mesial marginal groove
6. Distal marginal groove
7. Mesiofacial triangular groove
8. Mesiolingual triangular groove
9. Distolingual triangular groove
10. Distofacial triangular groove

As a point of clarification, it should be mentioned that triangular grooves are primary grooves that separate a marginal ridge from the triangular ridge of a cusp. These triangular grooves end in a triangular fossa. In studying the central groove, notice that the triangular groove is a continuation of the central groove. As the central groove goes toward the marginal ridge, it separates into two or three branches. The two outer Y-shaped branches curve between the marginal ridge and the triangular ridges of the buccal and lingual cusps. The part of the groove that lies between the cusp ridge and the marginal ridge is the triangular groove. The two triangular grooves are bisected by a third groove, which lies between them. This groove connects with the marginal ridge and is called the marginal groove.

Second Molars

Evidence of calcification	3 years
Enamel completed	7-8 years
Eruption	11-13 years
Root completed	14-16 years

A maxillary second molar (Fig. 33-9) supplements a first molar's function. Generally speaking, the differences that occur between the first and second molars are even more accentuated between the first and third molars. In other words, certain characteristics in form and development occur in a first molar that occur to a lesser degree in a second molar and possibly not at all in a third molar. What are these characteristics? Following is a list of several traits that may occur, but in general they have a tendency to be more accentuated in a second molar and most accentuated in a third molar.

1. The maxillary molar crowns are shorter occlusocervically and narrower mesiodistal-

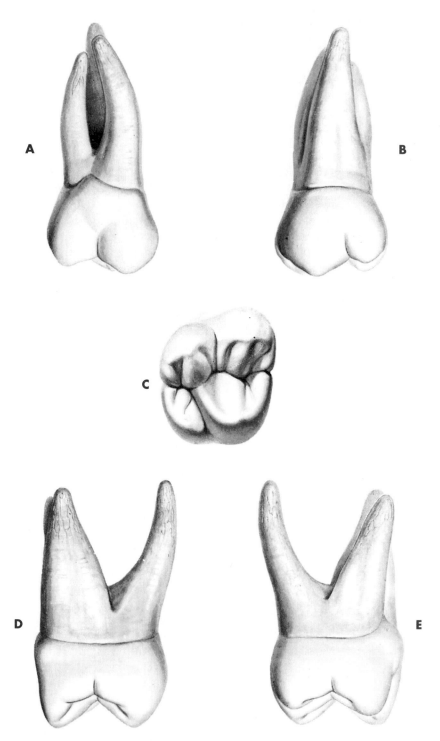

FIG. 33-9.   A maxillary right second molar. **A,** Buccal view. **B,** Lingual view.
C, Occlusal view. **D,** Mesial view. **E,** Distal view. (From Zeisz RC, Nuckolls J:
Dental anatomy, St Louis, 1949, Mosby.)

ly in the second molars than in the first molars. The third molars continue to be smaller in all crown proportions, including buccolingually.

2. The molar crowns show more **supplemental (secondary) grooves** and pits on the second molars than on the first. The third molars show even more supplemental grooves, as well as **accidental (tertiary) grooves** and pits.

3. The oblique ridge is less prominent on the second molars and in some instances disappears almost entirely on the third molars.

4. The fifth lobe, or cusp of Carabelli, usually disappears on the second molars and occurs infrequently on the third molars.

5. The distolingual cusp is less developed on the maxillary second molars and disappears almost entirely on most maxillary third molars.

6. The occlusal outline of the second molars is less rhomboidal and more heart shaped. A third molar is even more heart shaped in occlusal outline.

7. The roots of the second molars have a ten-

dency to lie closer together and may even be fused.

8. The mesiobuccal roots of the second and third molars have a greater tendency to curve distally in their apical third. The distobuccal root of a maxillary second molar is straighter than that of a maxillary first molar, with little or no mesial curvature. The third molar's distobuccal root has a tendency to curve distally in its apical third.

9. The roots of the second molars are almost as long and sometimes even longer than those of the first molars. The roots of the third molars are almost always smaller than those of either the first or second molars.

10. The second molars show more variety of form than the first molars, not only in the crown but also in root development. The third molars show unlimited variety in crown and root formations and are often congenitally missing.

Facial (buccal) aspect (Fig. 33-10; see also Fig. 33-9, *A*)

The crown of a maxillary second molar is shorter cervicoocclusally and narrower mesiodis-

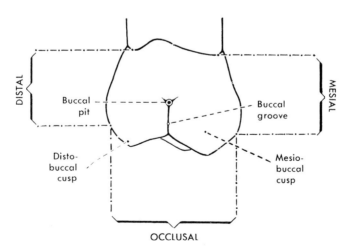

FIG. 33-10.   The buccal surface of a maxillary right second molar. (From Zeisz RC, Nuckolls J: *Dental anatomy,* St Louis, 1949, Mosby.)

tally than that of a maxillary first molar. The distobuccal cusp also is smaller.

The buccal roots are about the same length as each other and are closer together. The distobuccal root is straighter up and down than that of the maxillary first molar, and it has no mesial curvature. The mesiobuccal root has a greater curvature distally at its apical third.

Lingual aspect

The lingual view (Fig. 33-11; see also Fig. 33-9, B) of a maxillary second molar shows no fifth cusp (cusp of Carabelli). The distolingual cusp is smaller than that of the first molars.

Mesial aspect

The mesial view (Fig. 33-12; see also Fig. 33-9, D) shows the second molar crown to be shorter than the first molar, but its buccolingual measurement is about the same as that of a maxillary first molar. The roots are closer together.

Distal aspect

The distobuccal cusp is smaller than the mesiobuccal cusp, thus more of the mesiobuccal cusp can be seen from the distal view (Fig. 33-13; see also Fig. 33-9, E).

Occlusal aspect

The occlusal outline (Fig. 33-14; see also Fig. 33-9, C) of the crown of a maxillary second molar is less rhomboidal than that of a maxillary first molar. The increase in size of the mesiolingual cusp and the absence of the cusp of Carabelli makes this possible. Also the distolingual cusp is smaller.

The mesiodistal diameter of the crown is smaller, but the buccolingual diameter is about the same as that of a maxillary first molar.

The mesiobuccal and mesiolingual cusps are just as developed as in a first molar. The distobuccal cusp is just barely smaller, and the distolingual cusp is noticeably smaller.

More supplemental grooves and pits are present on a maxillary second molar than on a maxillary first molar.

Third Molars

Evidence of calcification	7 years
Enamel completed	12-16 years
Eruption	17-22 years
Root completed	18-25 years

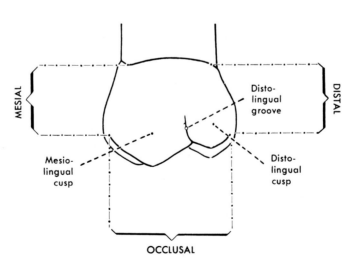

FIG. 33-11. The lingual surface of a maxillary right second molar. (From Zeisz RC, Nuckolls J: *Dental anatomy,* St Louis, 1949, Mosby.)

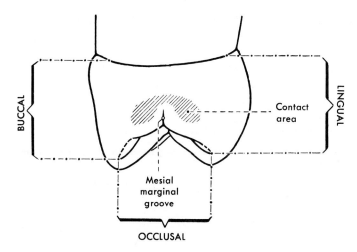

FIG. 33-12.   The mesial surface of a maxillary right second molar. (From Zeisz RC, Nuckolls J: *Dental anatomy,* St Louis, 1949, Mosby.)

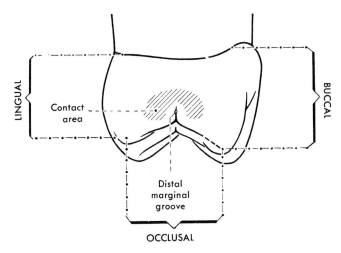

FIG. 33-13.   The distal surface of a maxillary right second molar. (From Zeisz RC, Nuckolls J: *Dental anatomy,* St Louis, 1949, Mosby.)

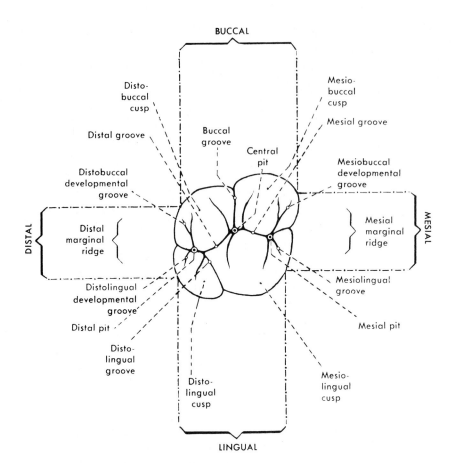

BUCCAL

Disto-buccal cusp

Distal groove

Buccal groove

Central pit

Mesio-buccal cusp

Mesial groove

Distobuccal developmental groove

Mesiobuccal developmental groove

DISTAL

Distal marginal ridge

MESIAL

Mesial marginal ridge

Distolingual developmental groove

Mesiolingual groove

Distal pit

Disto-lingual groove

Mesial pit

Disto-lingual cusp

Mesio-lingual cusp

LINGUAL

Fig. 33-14.   An occlusal view of a maxillary second molar. (From Zeisz RC, Nuckolls J: *Dental anatomy,* St Louis, 1949, Mosby.)

A maxillary third molar varies more than any other maxillary tooth in size, shape, and relative position to the other teeth. Rarely is it as well developed as a maxillary second molar. It often appears as a developmental anomaly or does not form at all. What term is descriptive of the latter situation?

The crown of a third molar is shorter than that of a second molar, and the roots tend to fuse into one fused root.

The occlusal outline of a maxillary third mo-

lar is heart shaped. The distolingual cusp is poorly developed or even absent (Fig. 33-15).

There is a tendency of third molars to become impacted. If a tooth does not erupt because it is obstructed by bone or another tooth, or if it is prevented from eruption because of the angle at which it is situated within the bone, it is said to be impacted. Third molars, maxillary or mandibular, have a greater tendency to be impacted than any other teeth. The impaction of third molars is to a large extent caused by an underdevel-

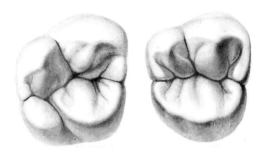

FIG. 33-15. Occlusal surfaces of maxillary right third molars. (From Zeisz RC, Nuckolls J: *Dental anatomy,* St Louis, 1949, Mosby.)

oped jaw and hence insufficient space to accommodate them. Thus they are blocked out and prevented from erupting.

Our ancestors' need for third molars was critical. The eruption of the third molars helped push together the remaining teeth, especially necessary if a portion of a tooth or a whole tooth was lost through attrition or accident.

As civilization advanced, survival became less dependent on keeping one's teeth. More and more persons survived without third molars. Today the congenital absence of third molars presents no problem whatsoever. Congenitally missing third molars are a modern genetic trend in humans, which is becoming more dominant. More and more persons will never have one or more third molars formed, and they will suffer no consequences because of it.

Roots

Maxillary molars are **trifurcated** and have three roots—mesiobuccal, distobuccal, and lingual—connected to a single **root trunk** (Figs. 33-16 and 33-17). These trifurcated roots give maxillary molars sturdy anchorage against forces that would tend to displace them. The lin-

gual root is the longest, and the distobuccal is the shortest.

All three roots are usually visible from the buccal view (see Fig. 33-16). The two buccal roots incline distally, with the mesiobuccal root starting to curve at its middle third. The distal root is usually straighter and tends to curve mesially at its middle third.

A deep developmental groove runs buccally between the bifurcation and the cervical line. The point of bifurcation of the two buccal roots is located about 4 mm apical to the cervical line. The point of bifurcation for deciduous molars is much less. Deciduous molars have a shorter root trunk than permanent molars do. The buccal roots of deciduous molars flare apart rather than curve toward each other.

The following are several characteristics of maxillary molar roots:

1. The roots become shorter the more posterior the maxillary molar is. The maxillary first molar has the longest roots, and the third molar the shortest.
2. The roots become less divided the more posterior the maxillary molar is. The roots of the maxillary first molar are much more divided than those of the second or third molar. The third molar often has fused roots.
3. The roots become more varied in shape, size, and direction of curvature the more posterior the maxillary molar is.

Pulp Cavity

The pulp cavity of a maxillary molar (Figs. 33-18 and 33-19) consists of a pulp chamber and three main pulp canals, one for each root. The lingual root canal is by far the largest, the distobuccal is the smallest, and the mesiobuccal is slightly larger than the distobuccal.

There is a tendency for the maxillary first molar to have four root canals, with two canals in the mesiobuccal root. In the fused-root form there may be only one large root with one root

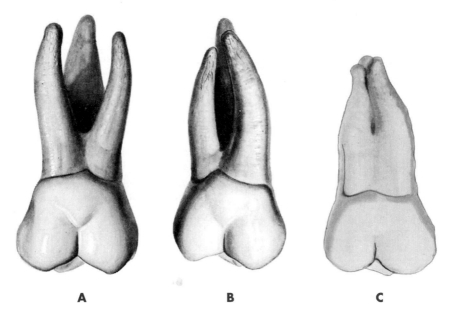

FIG. 33-16. A buccal view of maxillary right molars. **A,** First molar. **B,** Second molar. **C,** Third molar. Notice how the roots tend to be closer together when the molars are farther distally. Third molar roots are often fused. (From Zeisz RC, Nuckolls J: *Dental anatomy*, St Louis, 1949, Mosby.)

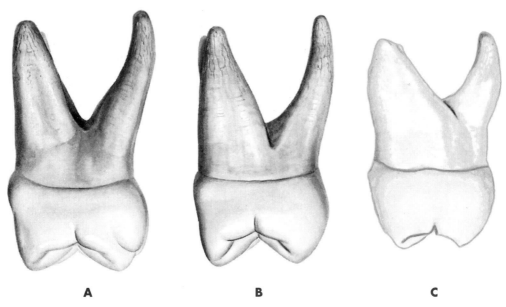

FIG. 33-17. A mesial view of maxillary right molars. **A,** First molar. **B,** Second molar. **C,** Third molar. The first molar has the longest roots, and the third molar has the shortest. (From Zeisz RC, Nuckolls J: *Dental anatomy*, St Louis, 1949, Mosby.)

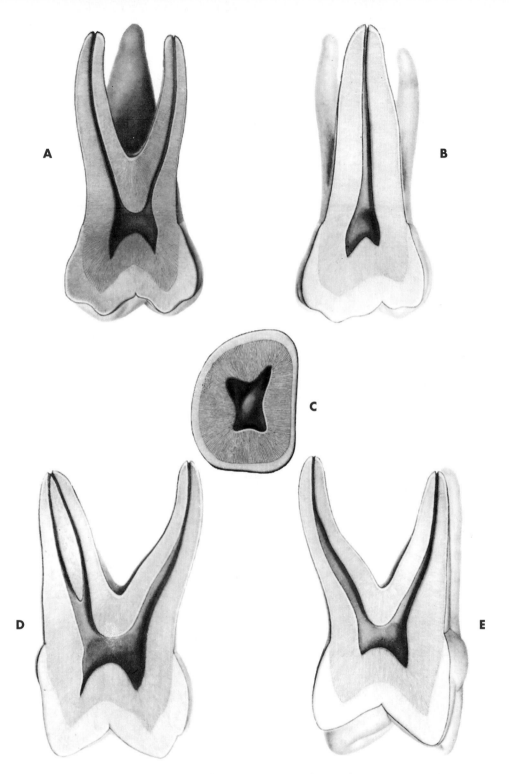

FIG. 33-18. The pulp cavity of a maxillary right first molar. **A,** Mesiodistal section, buccal view. **B,** Distomesial section, lingual view. **C,** Cross section, occlusal view. **D,** Linguobuccal section, mesial view. **E,** Buccolingual section, distal view. Notice that the mesiobuccal root has two root canals within one root. (From Zeisz RC, Nuckolls J: *Dental anatomy,* St Louis, 1949, Mosby.)

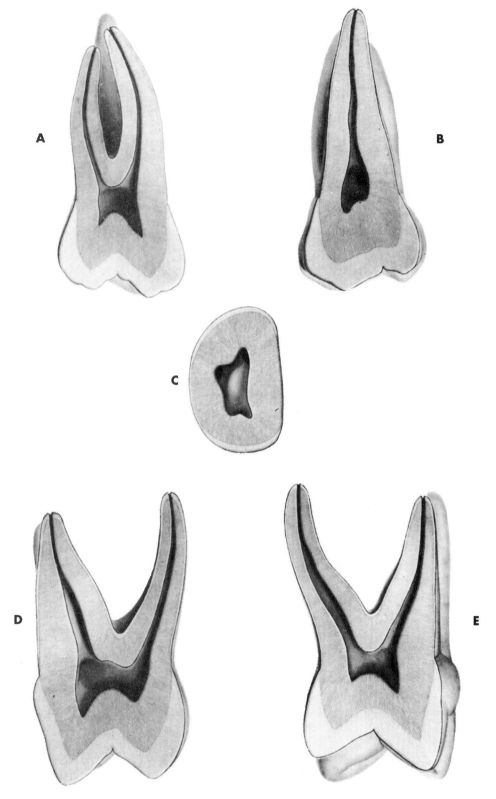

Fig. 33-19. For legend see opposite page.

Fig. 33-19.   The pulp cavity of a maxillary right second molar. **A,** Mesiodistal section, buccal view. **B,** Distomesial section, lingual view. **C,** Cross section, occlusal view. **D,** Linguobuccal section, mesial view. **E,** Buccolingual section, distal view. Notice that the mesiobuccal root has two root canals within one root. (From Zeisz RC, Nuckolls J: *Dental anatomy,* St Louis, 1949, Mosby.)

canal. If there are four roots, as in some maxillary third molars, there may be four root canals, one for each root.

There usually is one pulp horn for each cusp. The maxillary molars would then have four pulp horns—mesiobuccal, distobuccal, mesiolingual, and distolingual.

Pertinent Data

Maxillary first molars

	Right	Left
Universal Code	3	14
International Code	16	26
Palmer notation	6 ⌋	⌊ 6
Number of roots	3	
Number of pulp horns	4	
Number of cusps	4	
		5 (including cusp of Carabelli)
Number of developmental lobes	5	

Location of proximal contact areas.
Mesial: Middle third
Distal: Middle third
Height of contour.
Facial: Cervical third, 0.5 mm
Lingual: Middle third, 0.5 mm
Identifying characteristics. A cusp of Carabelli may be present. The occlusal outline is square or rhomboidal rather than triangular. The distolingual cusp is well developed. There is a prominent oblique ridge and distolingual grooves. The crown is nearly as wide mesiodistally as buccolingually. The three roots are widely separated.

Maxillary second molars

	Right	Left
Universal Code	2	15
International Code	17	27
Palmer notation	7 ⌋	⌊ 7
Number of roots	3	
Number of pulp horns	4	
Number of cusps	4	
Number of developmental lobes	4	

Location of proximal contact areas.
Mesial: Middle third
Distal: Middle third
Height of contour.
Facial: Cervical third, 0.5 mm
Lingual: Middle third, 0.5 mm
Identifying characteristics. These teeth are similar to maxillary first molars except that the fifth cusp is usually absent and the distolingual cusp is not as developed. The oblique ridge is less prominent. The crown is shorter occlusocervically and narrower mesiodistally. It is just as wide buccolingually. The occlusal outline of the crown is rhomboidal to heart shaped. The three roots are less separated.

Maxillary third molars

	Right	Left
Universal Code	1	16
International Code	18	28
Palmer notation	8 ⌋	⌊ 8
Number of roots	1 to 4	
Number of pulp horns	1 to 4	
Number of cusps	3 to 5	
Number of developmental lobes	4	

Comparison Chart of Maxillary Molars

Aspect	First molar	Second molar	Third molar
Buccal	Widest of the three mesiodistally	Intermediate in width mesiodistally	Smallest in width
	Buccal cusps equal in height	Distobuccal cusps slightly shorter than mesiobuccal	Distobuccal cusps much shorter than mesiobuccal
	Distobuccal root apex curves mesially	Distobuccal root straight	All roots show pronounced distal inclination
Lingual	Distolingual cusp well formed	Distolingual cusps smaller in width and height	Distolingual cusp usually missing
Mesial	Mesial marginal ridge tubercles numerous and pronounced	Mesial marginal ridge tubercles less numerous and less pronounced	Mesial marginal ridge tubercles absent
Occlusal	Crown outline square to rhomboidal	Rhomboidal form more pronounced in crown outline	Triangular or heart-shaped crown outline
	Oblique ridge smaller	Oblique ridge often absent	
Roots	Wide apart	Closer together	Usually fused

Location of proximal contact areas.
Mesial: Middle third
Distal: None
Height of contour.
Facial: Cervical third, 0.5 mm
Lingual: Middle third, 0.5 mm
Identifying characteristics. These teeth vary more in form than any others. They usually do not have a distolingual cusp. The occlusal outline is heart shaped with three cusps. The roots, usually three, have a tendency to be very close together or to fuse with an extreme distal inclination.

Review Questions

PART A

1. Which cusp of a maxillary first molar has the widest mesiodistal measurement?
2. Which two cusps join to form the oblique ridge?

3. Which of the five cusps of a maxillary first molar is the least developed?
4. Which of the four functional cusps is least developed?
5. On which cusp is the tubercle of Carabelli located?
6. Which cusps surround the central fossa?
7. Are the terms *mesiolingual groove* and *developmental groove of the cusp of Carabelli* synonymous?
8. Are the terms *distolingual groove* and *distal oblique groove* synonymous?
9. Are the terms *mesiolingual triangular groove* and *mesiolingual groove* synonymous?
10. If a mesial pit is present on a maxillary first molar, in which fossa is it located? Where is the distal pit found?
    a. central fossa
    b. distal fossa
    c. mesial triangular fossa
    d. distal triangular fossa
11. Which of the following is more likely to be present only on maxillary first molars?
    a. oblique ridge
    b. distolingual cusp

c. cusp of Carabelli

d. distobuccal root with its apex curved slightly mesially

12. Of the three roots of a maxillary molar, which is most likely to help differentiate the maxillary first, second, and third molars from each other?

13. Which cusp is more likely to be smaller on a maxillary second molar than on a maxillary first molar?

a. distobuccal cusp

b. distolingual cusp

14. The roots of a maxillary second molar lie closer together than the roots of which tooth?

a. maxillary first molar

b. maxillary third molar

15. Which two cusp ridges make up the transverse oblique ridge?

16. Identify the tooth in Fig. 33-20.

17. Maxillary molars usually have three root canals, but if four root canals are present, which molar and which root are most likely to contain the fourth canal?

a. first molar—lingual root

b. first molar—two canals in the mesiobuccal root

c. second molar—mesiobuccal root

d. third molars

18. A six-year-old patient is given tetracycline antibiotics. If tetracycline can discolor teeth that are in their formative stages, which molars might have discoloration in their crowns?

a. maxillary and mandibular

b. first and second permanent molars

c. second and third secondary molars

d. only third molars

19. If a maxillary third molar only has three cusps, which three cusps are they most likely to be?

a. mesiobuccal

b. mesiolingual

c. distolingual

d. distobuccal

e. cusp of Carabelli

20. A tooth that is an obvious maxillary molar is found with four roots fused to each other, but is severely dilacerated at the apical third. Which molar is the tooth most likely to be?

a. first

b. second

c. third

d. first or second

MANDIBULAR MOLARS

The permanent mandibular molars are larger than any other mandibular teeth. They function as chewing or grinding tools. There are three on each side—the first, second, and third mandibular molars. They occupy the posterior segment of each mandibular quadrant. Like their maxillary antagonists, they show a progressive decrease in size the more posterior the tooth. Which molars are therefore the smallest?

The crowns of the mandibular molars are shorter cervicoocclusally than those of the teeth anterior to them, but in all other dimensions the molars are larger. The roots are not as long as some of the mandibular roots, but their bifurcation results in excellent anchorage.

The crowns of the mandibular molars are

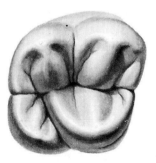

FIG. 33-20

wider mesiodistally than buccolingually. Is this also true of the maxillary molars? If not, how is it different?

Certain traits distinguish mandibular molars from maxillary molars.

1. Mandibular molars as a rule have only two roots, one mesial and one distal. How many do the maxillary molars have?
2. Generally there are four major cusps on mandibular molars; if a fifth cusp is present, it is a minor cusp.
3. The crowns are always broader mesiodistally than buccolingually.
4. Mandibular molars have two buccal cusps that are nearly equal in size. They also have two lingual cusps that are almost equal in size.

First Molars

Evidence of calcification	Birth
Enamel completed	3 years
Eruption	6 years
Root completed	9-10 years

The mandibular first molars (Fig. 33-21) are usually the first permanent teeth to erupt, with eruption occurring around 6 years of age. They are the only mandibular molars that usually have five cusps—two buccal and two lingual, which are major, and one distal, which is minor. The mandibular first molars are normally the largest teeth in the mandibular arch, with a crown usually about 1 mm longer mesiodistally than buccolingually.

Mandibular molars generally have two roots, one mesial and one distal. What other teeth have two roots? Are the roots mesial and distal or buccal and lingual?

Facial (buccal) aspect

From the buccal view (Fig. 33-22; see also Fig. 33-21, A) the one distal and two buccal cusps can be seen. The mesiobuccal cusp is the widest of the three; the distal cusp is the smallest. The mesiobuccal and distobuccal cusps are approximately equal in height and are separated by the mesiobuccal groove. This mesiobuccal groove often ends in a buccal pit. The distal cusp is much more conical in shape and is smaller in height and width than the other two. It is separated from a distobuccal cusp by a distobuccal groove. The cervical line on a mandibular first molar dips apically toward the root bifurcation. Whereas the entire distal profile of the crown is convex, only the mesial profile of the crown is convex at the middle and occlusal thirds; the cervical third is concave. Both the mesial and distal crown profiles converge toward the cervical side so that the cervical third of the crown is narrower than the occlusal third.

The roots of this tooth are well formed. The mesial root is almost perpendicular to the middle third of the root. From this point it curves distally toward its apex, which is located directly below and in line with the mesiobuccal cusp. The distal root shows little curvature and projects distally from the root base. The two roots are widely separated at their apices but share a common root base.

Lingual aspect

Two cusps of almost equal size, mesiolingual and distolingual, make up the lingual profile (Fig. 33-23; see also Fig. 33-21, B). The lingual developmental groove separates these two cusps. The lingual cusps are higher and more pointed than the two buccal cusps.

A portion of the distal cusp can be seen from the mesial aspect. The tooth is wider on the buccal than on the lingual side. From the lingual view notice the convergence from the distal side to the distolingual cusp.

The mesial and distal profiles of the lingual aspect are both convex. The crest of contour, which represents the contact area, is somewhat higher on the mesial than on the distal side; however, both are in the middle third of the tooth.

The bifurcation of the two roots begins with the bifurcation groove on the root trunk located directly in line with the lingual developmental groove.

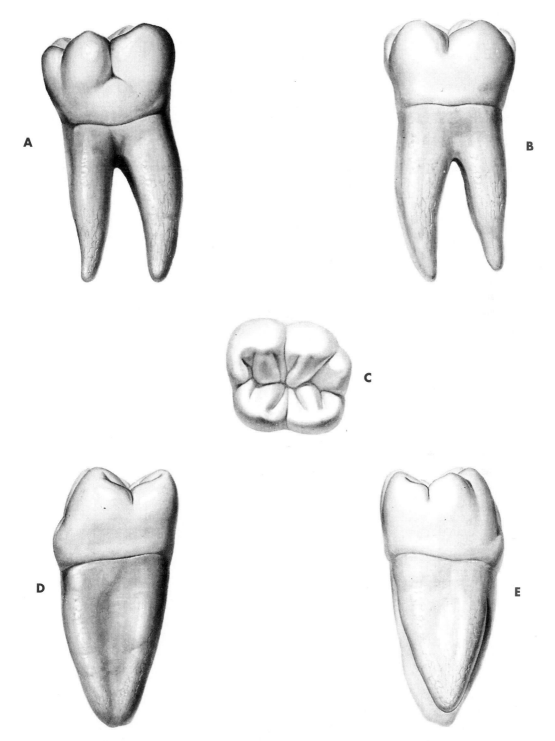

FIG. 33-21. A mandibular right first molar. **A,** Buccal view. **B,** Lingual view.
C, Occlusal view. **D,** Mesial view. **E,** Distal view. (From Zeisz RC, Nuckolls J:
Dental anatomy, St Louis, 1949, Mosby.)

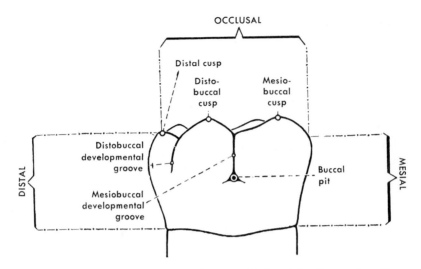

FIG. 33-22.   The buccal surface of a mandibular right first molar. (From Zeisz RC, Nuckolls J: *Dental anatomy,* St Louis, 1949, Mosby.)

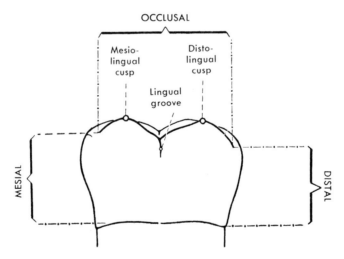

FIG. 33-23.   The lingual surface of a mandibular right first molar. (From Zeisz RC, Nuckolls J: *Dental anatomy,* St Louis, 1949, Mosby.)

The lingual surface is rather flat in comparison with the convex buccal surface. The cervical line is straight mesiodistally.

Mesial aspect

From the mesial aspect (Fig. 33-24; see also Fig. 33-21, *D*) two cusps can be seen, the mesiolingual and the mesiobuccal. The mesiolingual is the higher and more conical of the two.

Only one root, the mesial, can be seen from the mesial view.

The mesial marginal ridge has a prominent crest, which is divided by the mesial marginal groove, located lingual to the center of the crown.

The buccal profile is marked by the buccocervical ridge, a slight bulge in the cervical third of the buccal surface.

The lingual height of contour is located at the center of the middle third of the tooth on the lingual surface.

The cervical line tends to curve occlusally about 1 mm in the center of the mesial surface. It is located higher on the lingual side than on the buccal side by almost 1 mm.

The buccolingual measurements of the crown, root, and cusps are all greater on the mesial surface than on the distal surface. The mesial cusp is also higher than the distal cusp.

Distal aspect

The distolingual cusp is the largest of the three cusps visible from the distal aspect (Fig. 33-25; see also Fig. 33-21, *E*). The distobuccal cusp is next in size, and the distal cusp is the smallest. The distobuccal groove can be seen separating the latter two cusps. The distal marginal ridge, not as wide as the mesial marginal ridge, is bisected by the distal marginal groove. This groove is lingual to the center of the tooth.

The crown of a first molar tapers and converges distally, so that if a specimen of the tooth is held with the distal surface of the crown at a right angle to the line of vision, a greater portion of the occlusal surface is visible than from the mesial aspect.

The distal contact area is located on the distal cusp and is centered over the distal root.

Occlusal aspect

The occlusal view (Fig. 33-26; see also Fig. 33-21, *C*) of a mandibular first molar shows five

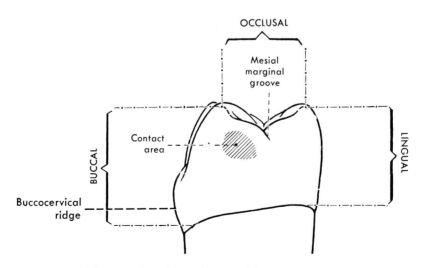

FIG. 33-24.   The mesial surface of a mandibular right first molar. (From Zeisz RC, Nuckolls J: *Dental anatomy,* St Louis, 1949, Mosby.)

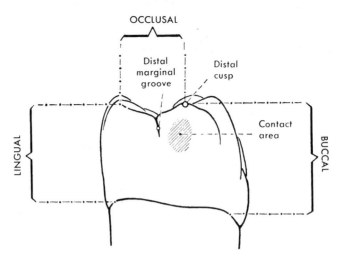

FIG. 33-25. The distal surface of a mandibular right first molar. (From Zeisz RC, Nuckolls J: *Dental anatomy,* St Louis, 1949, Mosby.)

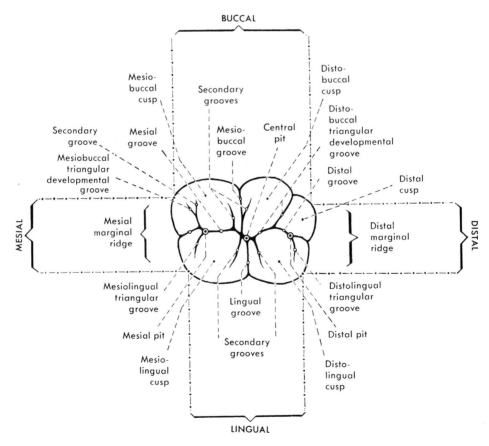

FIG. 33-26. The occlusal surface of a mandibular right first molar. (From Zeisz RC, Nuckolls J: *Dental anatomy,* St Louis, 1949, Mosby.)

cusps, four major and one minor. All five are functional. What is the minor cusp? What differentiates a major cusp from a minor cusp?

The occlusal outline of the tooth is pentagonal and shows a tapering convergence toward the distal and lingual sides. Not only are the mesial cusps wider buccolingually than the distal cusps, but the mesiodistal measurement of the three buccal cusps together is much larger than the same measurement for two lingual cusps combined.

The mesiobuccal cusp is wider than either of the lingual cusps, which are about the same size.

The distobuccal cusp is the smallest of the four major cusps, and the distal is the smallest of all five.

The developmental grooves that separate these cusps are the **central developmental groove,** the **mesiobuccal developmental groove,** the **distobuccal developmental groove,** and the lingual developmental groove. All the developmental grooves converge at the central pit in the center of the central fossa. The central fossa of the occlusal surface is a concave area bordered by the distal slope of the mesiofacial cusp, the mesial and distal slopes of the distofacial cusp, the mesial slope of the distal cusp, the distal slope of the mesiolingual cusps, and the mesial slope of the distolingual cusp. Two other fossae are present, the mesial triangular fossa (just inside the mesiodistal marginal ridge) and the distal triangular fossa (a slight depression just mesial to the central portion of the distal marginal ridge).

The mesiobuccal groove separates the mesiofacial and distofacial cusps and extends onto the buccal surface. The distobuccal groove separates the distofacial and distal cusps. The lingual groove separates the two lingual cusps and continues onto the lingual surface. The two buccal grooves and the lingual groove form a Y-shaped pattern on the occlusal surface of the crown.

Mesial and distal marginal ridge grooves may also be present. Several supplemental grooves radiate from the mesial and distal pits, which are usually found in the mesial and distal triangular fossae, respectively.

Second Molars

Evidence of calcification	2-3 years
Enamel completed	7-8 years
Eruption	11-13 years
Root completed	14-15 years

The mandibular second molars (Fig. 33-27) resemble the mandibular first molars buccally and lingually, except that there usually is not a fifth or distal cusp. The roots of the second molar are shorter, closer together, and more distally inclined than those of the first molar.

All four cusps of the mandibular second molars are nearly equal in size. Occlusally the second molars have a more rectangular shape than the first molars have.

Facial (buccal) aspect (Fig. 33-28; see also Fig. 33-27, *A*)

Facially the first and second molars are similar, except that a second molar crown is not as long mesiodistally and is slightly shorter cervicoocclusally. A second molar has only two buccal cusps separated by a single buccal groove. These two cusps, the mesiobuccal and the distobuccal, are equal in their mesiodistal measurements.

The roots of a second molar may be somewhat shorter and are usually located closer together than the roots of a first molar. They are also more distally inclined in relation to the occlusal plane of the crown.

Lingual aspect (Fig. 33-29; see also Fig. 33-27, *B*)

The crown of a mandibular second molar converges far less lingually than that of a first molar because there is no distal cusp. The two lingual cusps, mesiolingual and distolingual, are nearly the same size and are separated by a lingual groove, which sometimes terminates in a lingual pit. The contact areas are at a lower level mesially and especially distally.

Mesial aspect

From the mesial view of the mandibular second molar (Fig. 33-30; see also Fig. 33-27, *D*), the cervical line shows less curvature than a first molar does, and the mesial root is less broad.

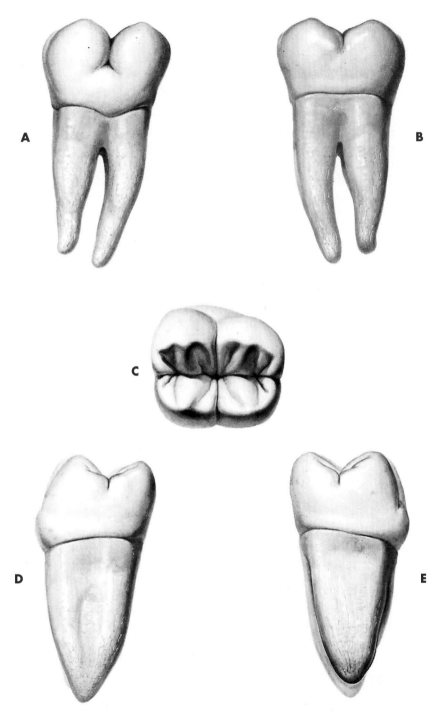

FIG. 33-27.   A mandibular right second molar. **A,** Buccal view. **B,** Lingual view. **C,** Occlusal view. **D,** Mesial view. **E,** Distal view. (From Zeisz RC, Nuckolls J: *Dental anatomy,* St Louis, 1949, Mosby.)

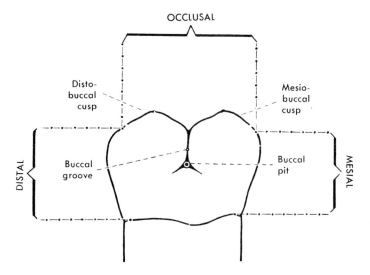

FIG. 33-28.   The buccal surface of a mandibular right second molar. (From Zeisz RC, Nuckolls J: *Dental anatomy,* St Louis, 1949, Mosby.)

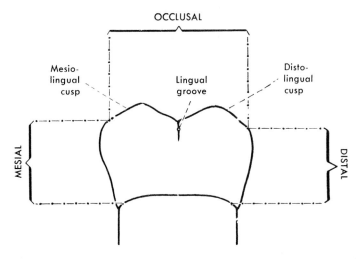

FIG. 33-29.   The lingual surface of a mandibular right second molar. (From Zeisz RC, Nuckolls J: *Dental anatomy,* St Louis, 1949, Mosby.)

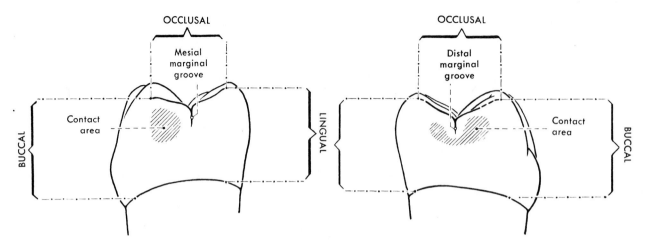

FIG. 33-30.   The mesial surface of a mandibular right second molar. (From Zeisz RC, Nuckolls J: *Dental anatomy,* St Louis, 1949, Mosby.)

FIG. 33-31.   The distal surface of a mandibular right second molar. (From Zeisz RC, Nuckolls J: *Dental anatomy,* St Louis, 1949, Mosby.)

Otherwise the mesial view is the same for both molars.

Distal aspect

On the distal view (Fig. 33-31; see also Fig. 33-27, *E*) the most noticeable difference between the first and second molars is the absence of a distal cusp. The contact area is therefore centered both buccolingually and cervicoocclusally.

Occlusal aspect

The occlusal outline (Fig. 33-32; see also Fig. 33-27, *C*) of a second molar is rectangular. All four cusps are equal in size. The developmental grooves are the buccal groove, the lingual groove, and the central developmental groove, and they traverse the occlusal surface in a cross pattern. There are more secondary grooves than on a first molar. The four triangular grooves include a distofacial, a distolingual, a mesiofacial and a mesiolingual. Three pits may be present—a mesial, a distal, and a central.

Third Molars

Evidence of calcification	8-10 years
Enamel completed	12-16 years
Eruption	17-21 years
Root completed	18-15 years

Like the maxillary third molars, the mandibular third molars are irregular and unpredictable. The crown is usually shorter in all dimensions than second molars, although it is possible to find a third molar larger than even a first molar. This, however, is an exception and not the rule.

The occlusal outline of the crown is more oval than rectangular, though the crown usually resembles that of a mandibular second molar. The two mesial cusps are larger than the two distal cusps. The occlusal surface has a very wrinkled appearance, with an irregular groove pattern and numerous pits (Fig. 33-33).

The roots of the third molars are usually shorter than those of the second molars and are inclined acutely to the distal side. They are also very close together and often fused.

Roots

Mandibular molars have two roots (Figs. 33-34 and 33-35), one mesial and one distal, with a single root trunk (bifurcated root). The mesial root is the longer and stronger of the two. It curves mesially and then turns distally in the

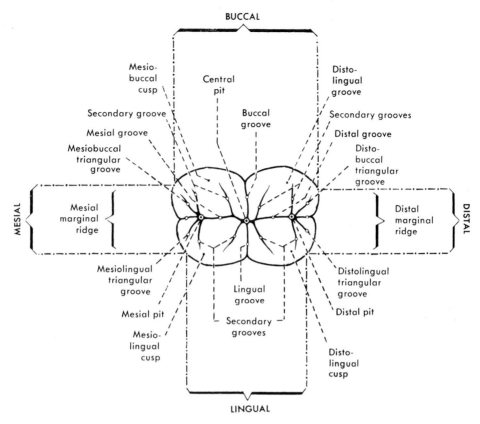

FIG. 33-32. The occlusal surface of a mandibular right second molar. (From Zeisz RC, Nuckolls J: *Dental anatomy*, St Louis, 1949, Mosby.)

Comparison Chart of Mandibular Molars

Aspect	First molar	Second molar	Third molar
Buccal	Crown has widest mesiodistal diameter	Smaller crown than first molar	Smallest crown
	Three buccal cusps—mesiobuccal, distobuccal, and distal	Two buccal cusps—mesiobuccal and distobuccal	Two buccal cusps—mesiobuccal and distobuccal
	Two buccal grooves	One buccal groove	One buccal groove
	Roots widely separated and relatively vertical	Roots closer together and inclined distally	Roots short and fused, with pronounced distal inclination
Mesial	Mesial root broad	Mesial root not as broad	Same as second molar
Occlusal	Pentagonal outline	Rectangular outline	Ovoid outline
	Mesial and distal profiles straight, converging lingually	Mesial and distal profiles curved; no lingual convergence	Mesial and distal profiles highly curved; no lingual convergence
	Main grooves form Y pattern	Main grooves form a cross (+)	Grooves show no set pattern
	Large occlusal surface relative to total crown area seen from occlusal side	Occlusal table same as in first molar	More supplementary and accessory grooves
Roots	Wide apart and longest	Closer together	Usually fused, curved, and shorter

apical portion. The distal root is usually quite straight and may curve mesially or distally at its apical third.

The root trunk is bifurcated very close to the cervical line. The trunk is short and is grooved

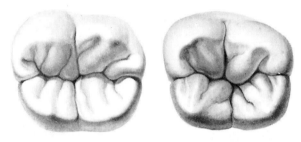

FIG. 33-33. Occlusal view of two mandibular right third molars. (From Zeisz RC, Nuckolls J: *Dental anatomy,* St Louis, 1949, Mosby.)

on the buccal and lingual surfaces toward the bifurcation.

The following are characteristics of mandibular molar roots:

1. The roots become shorter the more posterior the molar is; the mandibular first molar is therefore the longest.
2. The roots are less divided the further posterior the molar is.
3. The roots become more varied in shape, size, and direction the more posterior the tooth is.

Pulp Cavity

The pulp cavity of the mandibular molars (Figs. 33-36 and 33-37) consists of a pulp chamber and three pulp canals—the distal, the mesiobuccal, and the mesiolingual.

The distal root canal is much larger than the other two canals and is the only canal in the dis-

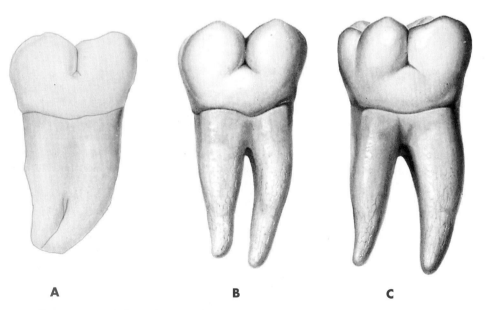

A   **B**   **C**

FIG. 33-34. A buccal view of mandibular right molars. **A,** Third molar. **B,** Second molar. **C,** First molar. Notice how the roots get closer together and become shorter from the first molar to the third molar. Third molar roots are often fused.

tal root. The mesial root houses two root canals, the mesiobuccal and the mesiolingual. Often these two canals join into one single apical foramen; sometimes there is only one canal in the mesial root. On rare occasions there are two canals in the distal root, just as in the mesial root.

There are five pulp horns, one for each cusp. In the four-cusp form there are only four pulp horns. Which pulp horn is missing? (Hint: In the four-cusp form, which cusp is missing?)

The first molar is more likely to have three root canals (distal, mesiobuccal, and mesiolingual) and five pulp horns. Although the second molar may have two canals (the mesial and the distal, one in each root), it is more likely to have three root canals. The second molar has only four pulp horns. Third molars resemble second molars in pulpal anatomy.

Pertinent Data

Mandibular first molars

	Right	Left
Universal Code	30	19
International Code	46	36
Palmer notation	6⌋	⌊6
Number of roots	2	
Number of pulp horns	5	
Number of cusps	5	
Number of developmental lobes	5	

Location of proximal contact areas.
Mesial: Middle third
Distal: Middle third
Height of contour.
Facial: Cervical third, 0.5 mm
Lingual: Middle third, 1 mm
Identifying characteristics. The five cusps make these the largest mandibular teeth. They

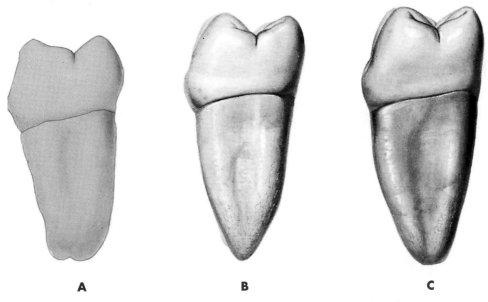

FIG. 33-35. A mesial view of mandibular right molars. **A,** Third molar. **B,** Second molar. **C,** First molar. (From Zeisz RC, Nuckolls J: *Dental anatomy,* St Louis, 1949, Mosby.)

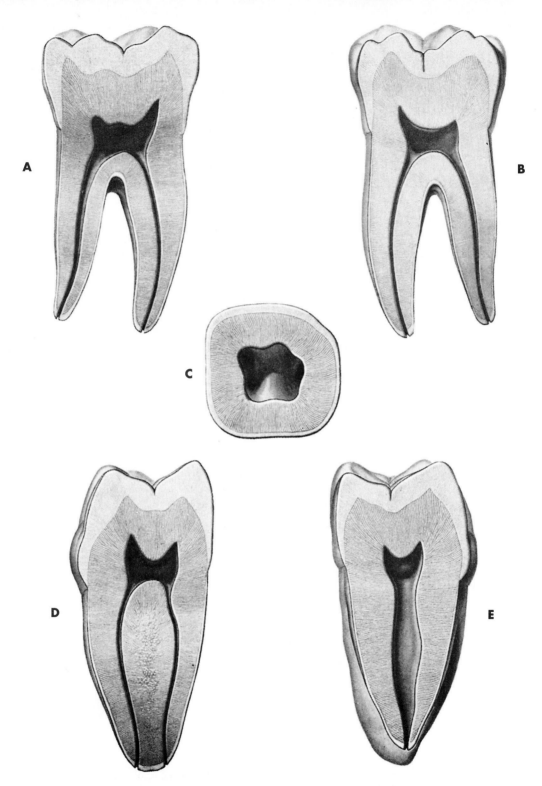

FIG. 33-36.   The pulp cavity of a mandibular right first molar. **A**, Mesiodistal section, buccal view. **B**, Distomesial section, lingual view. **C**, Cross section, occlusal view. **D**, Linguobuccal section, mesial view. **E**, Buccolingual section, distal view.

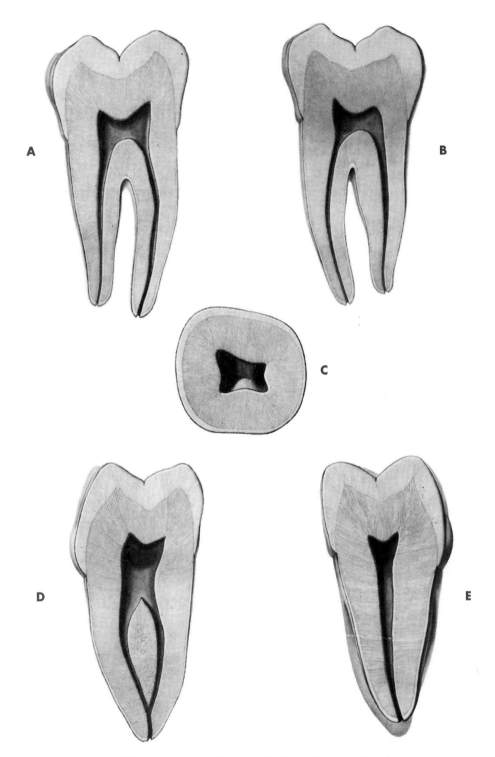

FIG. 33-37. The pulp cavity of a mandibular right second molar. **A,** Distomesial section, buccal view. **B,** Mesiodistal section, lingual view. **C,** Cross section, occlusal view. **D,** Buccolingual section, mesial view. **E,** Linguobuccal section, distal view. (From Zeisz RC, Nuckolls J: *Dental anatomy*, St Louis, 1949, Mosby.)

are wider mesiodistally than buccolingually. The crown converges lingually and slightly distally. The three buccal cusps are separated by two buccal grooves, and the two lingual cusps are separated by one lingual groove. These three grooves converge to form a Y pattern. There are two roots, a mesial and a distal, and three root canals (the mesial root has two root canals).

Mandibular second molars

	Right	Left
Universal Code	31	18
International Code	47	37
Palmer notation	7⌐	⌐7
Number of roots	2	
Number of pulp horns	4	
Number of cusps	4	
Number of developmental lobes	4	

Location of proximal contact areas.
Mesial: Middle third
Distal: Middle third
Height of contour.
Facial: Cervical third, 0.5 mm
Lingual: Middle third, 1 mm
Identifying characteristics. These molars have four cusps of nearly equal size. The crown is smaller in all dimensions and has less lingual convergence. There is only one buccal groove and one lingual groove, which join together on the occlusal surface as they bisect the central developmental groove; the groove pattern is therefore a cross. The two roots are closer together and incline slightly distally. There is one root canal in the distal root. The mesial root can have one or two root canals.

Mandibular third molars

	Right	Left
Universal Code	32	17
International Code	48	38
Palmer notation	8⌐	⌐8
Number of roots	2 (fused into 1)	
Number of pulp horns	4 or 5	
Number of cusps	4 or 5	
Number of developmental lobes	4 or 5	

Location of proximal contact areas.
Mesial: Middle third
Distal: Middle third
Height of contour.
Facial: Cervical third, 0.5 mm
Lingual: Middle third, 1 mm
Identifying characteristics. These are the most variable mandibular teeth in form. They usually resemble the mandibular second molars, with four cusps, a shallower, smaller central fossa, and more secondary and tertiary grooves. A five-cusp form is not unusual. The two roots (mesial and distal) are often fused and inclined distally.

Review Questions

PART B

1. When the first and second molars of the mandibular arch are compared, which of the following is not true?
   a. There is only one groove visible from the facial surface on a second molar.
   b. The crown is larger both mesiodistally and faciolingually on a second molar.
   c. There is less lingual convergence on a second molar.
   d. Both have two roots.
2. When the mandibular first and second molars are compared, in what way are the two different?
   a. The first has more roots and root canals.
   b. The second has more pulp horns.
   c. The second does not have a distal cusp.
   d. The first has a different height of contour.
3. The lingual height of contour on all mandibular molars:
   a. measures 0.5 mm.

b. measures more than 0.5 mm.

c. measures less than 0.5 mm.

d. varies considerably from the first to the third molar.

4. An important factor concerning personal oral hygiene is that the mandibular molars:

a. do not have an oblique ridge, which helps deflect the food onto the gums.

b. are more difficult to clean because of their lingual contours.

5. Which of the following is least true of a mandibular second molar?

a. It has four cusps of nearly equal size.

b. It has three root canals, with two in the mesial root.

c. It has five cusps.

d. It has four developmental lobes.

6. Which of the following is a list of correct names for the cusps of a mandibular first molar?

a. mesiolingual, mesiofacial, distolingual, distofacial, cusp of Carabelli

b. central, mesial, distal, facial, lingual

c. mesiolingual, mesiofacial, distolingual, distofacial, distal

d. distolingual, distofacial, mesiolingual, mesiofacial

7. The roots of a mandibular first molar are:

a. facial and lingual.

b. mesial, distal, and central.

c. facial, lingual, and middle.

d. mesial and distal.

8. When comparing all maxillary and mandibular molars, fused roots would most likely be found on which of the following?

a. first molars

b. second molars

c. third molars

d. all of the above

9. What is a major difference between first and second molars, whether maxillary or mandibular?

a. First molars usually have four cusps, and second molars have three.

b. First molars usually have five cusps, and second molars have four.

c. First molars have more supplemental grooves.

d. Second molars are wider mesiodistally.

10. Which of the following is true concerning maxillary and mandibular molars?

a. Both have oblique ridges.

b. Only maxillary molars have oblique ridges.

c. Neither have oblique ridges.

d. Only mandibular molars have oblique ridges.

11. Two root canals are commonly found in:

a. the lingual root of maxillary first molars.

b. the distal root of mandibular first molars.

c. the mesial root of mandibular first molars.

d. none of the above.

12. Furcation refers to:

a. the absence of a particular characteristic of the root anatomy.

b. the splitting of a root trunk into terminal roots.

c. the division of root canals from the root trunk.

d. none of the above.

13. Name the smallest permanent mandibular molar cusp.

14. A buccal pit is found at the end of the:

a. buccal groove of a mandibular second molar

b. mesiobuccal developmental groove of a mandibular first molar

c. distobuccal developmental groove of a mandibular first molar

d. distobuccal groove of a mandibular second molar

e. a and b

f. a and d

15. Name the occlusal pits of mandibular first molars.

a. mesial

b. distal

c. central

d. all of the above

CHAPTER 34

DECIDUOUS DENTITION

OBJECTIVES

- To identify the various deciduous teeth
- To recognize whether a tooth is primary or secondary
- To know the eruption dates of the primary and secondary teeth
- To understand the essential differences between deciduous and permanent teeth
- To understand the importance and functions of deciduous teeth
- To compare the dental anatomic features of deciduous teeth, not only with the other deciduous teeth but also with their permanent counterparts

THE DECIDUOUS dentition is made up of primary teeth in humans. These teeth are shed and then replaced by permanent successors. This process of shedding the deciduous teeth and replacement by the permanent teeth is called *exfoliation.* Exfoliation begins 2 or 3 years after the deciduous root is completely formed. At this time the root begins to resorb at its apical end, and resorption continues in the direction of the crown until the entire root is resorbed and the tooth finally falls out.

The primary or deciduous dentition consists of 20 teeth, each quadrant containing two incisors, one canine, and two molars (Fig. 34-1).

The first deciduous teeth to erupt, about 8 months after birth, are the mandibular central incisors. The maxillary central incisors usually erupt about a month later. As in the permanent teeth, the primary mandibular teeth usually erupt before the maxillary. Following is an approximate eruption schedule of the deciduous teeth. (Also see Fig. 24-6.)

Central incisors	8-12 months
Lateral incisors	9-13 months
First molars	13-19 months
Canines	16-22 months
Second molars	25-33 months

ESSENTIAL DIFFERENCES BETWEEN DECIDUOUS AND PERMANENT TEETH

1. The deciduous anteriors are smaller than their permanent successors in both their crown and root proportions. Deciduous molars are wider mesiodistally than the permanent premolars, which will take their places.

2. The roots of deciduous anterior teeth are narrower and longer in crown length as well as tooth length and width as compared with the permanent teeth roots.

3. The roots of deciduous posterior teeth are very narrow at their cervical enamel junctions (CEJ) where the crowns join the roots. In addition the root trunks of deciduous molars are very short.

4. The cervical ridge of enamel at the cervical third of the anterior crown labially and lingually is much more prominent in deciduous dentition. These bulky ridges extend out from the very narrow cervical necks of the teeth.

5. The buccocervical ridges on the deciduous molars are much more pronounced, especially on first molars. These cervical prominences give deciduous crowns a bulbous appearance and accentuate the narrow cervical portion of deciduous roots.

6. The buccal and lingual surfaces of deciduous molars taper occlusally above the cervical curvatures much more so than the permanent molar buccal and lingual surfaces. This results in a much narrower **occlusal table** of the occlusal surface buccolingually.

7. The roots of the deciduous molars are longer and more slender than the roots of the permanent teeth. These roots also flare apically to allow room in between for the developing permanent tooth crowns (Fig. 34-2).

8. The deciduous teeth are usually lighter in color than the permanent teeth. They have a whiter color with a bluish cast. Permanent teeth have more yellow, grey, or brown tones.

9. The pulp chambers of deciduous teeth are relatively large in comparison with the crowns that envelop them.

10. The pulp horns of deciduous teeth extend rather high occlusally, placing them much closer to the enamel than the pulp horns in permanent teeth.

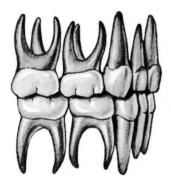

FIG. 34-1. Deciduous teeth. (From Massler M, Schour I: *Atlas of the mouth in health and disease,* ed 2, Chicago, 1975, American Dental Association.)

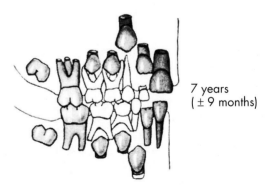

7 years
(± 9 months)

FIG. 34-2. Premolars rest between deciduous molar roots. Gray teeth are permanent; white teeth are primary. (From Massler M, Schour I: *Atlas of the mouth in health and disease,* ed 2, Chicago, 1975, American Dental Association.)

11. The dentin thickness between the pulp chambers and the enamel is much thinner than in permanent teeth.
12. The enamel of deciduous teeth is relatively thin and has a consistent depth (Fig. 34-3).

THE IMPORTANCE OF DECIDUOUS TEETH

The importance of deciduous teeth cannot be stressed enough. These teeth are extremely important for the proper development of the muscles of mastication, the formation of the bones of the jaws, and the eventual location, alignment, and occlusion of the permanent teeth. Indeed, the succedaneous teeth develop as buds from the deciduous tooth buds.

The deciduous teeth maintain a place for the permanent teeth. It is their function to allow for bone growth of the dental arches. As the bone continues to grow, the deciduous teeth develop spaces between them called *primate spaces*.

The spaces between the deciduous canines and first molars and those between the first and second molars are called *leeway spaces*. They allow an extra margin of space for the eruption of the permanent canine, and the first and second premolars. Leeway space is necessary because several offsetting factors are present. First, the mesiodistal measurement of the two permanent premolars combined is less than the sum of the mesiodistal measurements of the deciduous molars. Although this allows extra room for the premolars, the permanent canine requires more room than the deciduous canine. Second, bone growth allows for leeway space, but this is offset by the phenomenon of mesial drift. The first permanent molar tends to move mesially; thus the amount of space reserved for the permanent premolars is shortened. If a deciduous molar is pre-

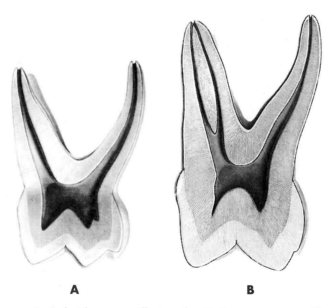

A **B**

FIG. 34-3.   **A,** A deciduous maxillary molar. **B,** A permanent maxillary molar. (From Zeisz RC, Nuckolls J: *Dental anatomy,* St Louis, 1949, Mosby.)

maturely lost or a decayed interproximal space is not restored, a permanent molar will push into this space and block out the premolar. There is little if any extra space (see Fig. 25-3).

In addition, the resorption of the deciduous roots helps guide their erupting permanent replacements into the proper location. The succedaneous teeth follow the resorbing root through the bone until the deciduous tooth exfoliates from a lack of root anchorage. When a deciduous tooth exfoliates, its permanent replacement can often be seen directly underneath it. Sometimes a thin layer of gum may be covering it; usually it is not completely impacted with bone.

Maxillary Central Incisors (Fig. 34-4)

Labial aspect (Fig. 34-5; see also Fig. 34-4, *A*)

A deciduous central incisor's mesiodistal diameter is greater than its cervicoincisal length, whereas a permanent central incisor's cervicoin-

cisal length is greater than its mesiodistal diameter. No mamelons are visible on the deciduous tooth.

Lingual aspect

From the lingual aspect (Fig. 34-6; see also Fig. 34-4, *B*) the crown shows well-developed marginal ridges and a highly developed cingulum.

Mesial and distal aspects

From the proximal aspects (Fig. 34-7; see also Figs. 34-4, *D* and *E*) the crown appears wide in relation to its total length. Because of its short length, the labiolingual measurements make the crown appear thick, even at the incisal third. The mesiocervical curvature is greater than the distal curvature.

Incisal aspect

From the incisal surface (see Fig. 34-4, *C*) the crown appears much wider mesiodistally than labiolingually. The incisal edge appears nearly straight.

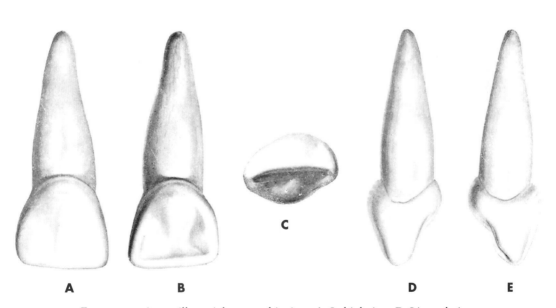

A   **B**   **C**   **D**   **E**

FIG. 34-4.   A maxillary right central incisor. **A**, Labial view. **B**, Lingual view. **C**, Incisal view. **D**, Mesial view. **E**, Distal view. (From Zeisz RC, Nuckolls J: *Dental anatomy*, St Louis, 1949, Mosby.)

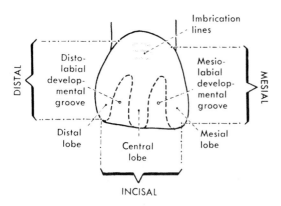

FIG. 34-5. The labial surface of a maxillary right central incisor. (From Zeisz RC, Nuckolls J: *Dental anatomy*, St Louis, 1949, Mosby.)

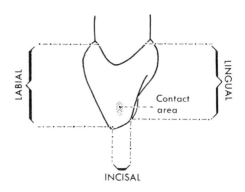

FIG. 34-7. The mesial surface of a maxillary right central incisor. (From Zeisz RC, Nuckolls J: *Dental anatomy*, St Louis, 1949, Mosby.)

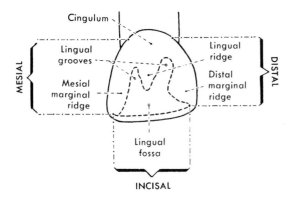

FIG. 34-6. The lingual surface of a maxillary right central incisor. (From Zeisz RC, Nuckolls J: *Dental anatomy*, St Louis, 1949, Mosby.)

Maxillary Lateral Incisors

A lateral incisor's crown is smaller than a central incisor's crown in all dimensions, except that the cervicoincisal length is greater than its mesiodistal width. In all other ways it appears similar to a central incisor. The root appears much longer in proportion to the crown when compared with the central (Fig. 34-8).

Roots of Maxillary Incisors

The root of a deciduous maxillary incisor appears constricted at its cervical third. It is twice as long as the crown and tapers evenly toward a blunt apex. There is a mesial concavity on the root surface, but the distal surface is generally convex. The lateral incisor surface is longer and more tapered than that of the central incisor.

Mandibular Central Incisors (Fig. 34-9)

Labial aspect

Mamelons or grooves may be visible in a labial view of a deciduous mandibular incisor (Fig. 34-10). The crown appears wide in comparison with its permanent successor. The mesial and distal sides of the crown taper evenly from the contact areas. The root may be two to three times the height of the crown. It is very narrow and is also conical in shape.

Lingual aspect

The lingual surface (Fig. 34-11; see also Fig. 34-9, *B*) appears smoothly contoured and tapers toward the cingulum. The marginal ridges are less pronounced than those of the primary maxillary incisors.

Mesial and distal aspects

From the mesial aspect the incisal ridge is centered over the root. The labial and lingual cervi-

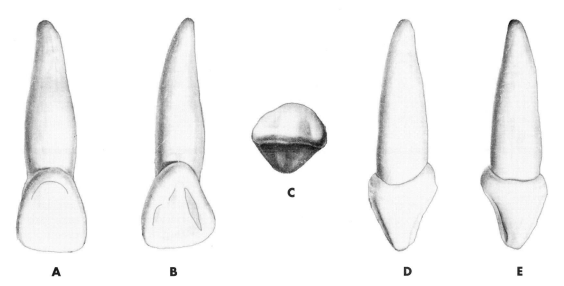

FIG. 34-8.   A maxillary right lateral incisor. **A,** Labial view. **B,** Lingual view. **C,** Incisal view. **D,** Mesial view. **E,** Distal view. (From Zeisz RC, Nuckolls J: *Dental anatomy,* St Louis, 1949, Mosby.)

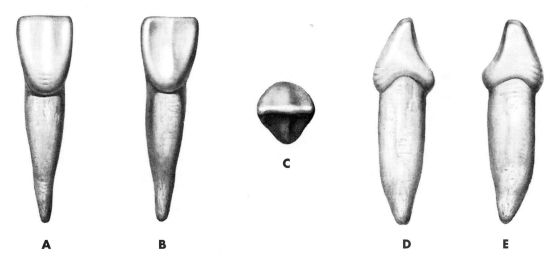

FIG. 34-9.   A mandibular right central incisor. **A,** Labial view. **B,** Lingual view. **C,** Incisal view. **D,** Mesial view. **E,** Distal view. (From Zeisz RC, Nuckolls J: *Dental anatomy,* St Louis, 1949, Mosby.)

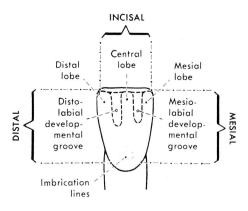

FIG. 34-10.   The labial surface of a mandibular right central incisor. (From Zeisz RC, Nuckolls J: *Dental anatomy,* St Louis, 1949, Mosby.)

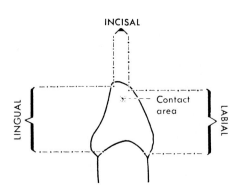

FIG. 34-12.   The distal surface of a mandibular right central incisor. (From Zeisz RC, Nuckolls J: *Dental anatomy,* St Louis, 1949, Mosby.)

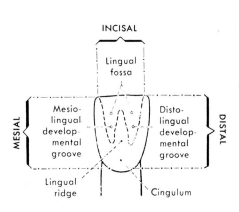

FIG. 34-11.   The lingual surface of a mandibular right central incisor. (From Zeisz RC, Nuckolls J: *Dental anatomy,* St Louis, 1949, Mosby.)

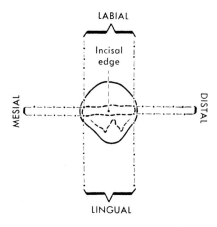

FIG. 34-13.   The incisal edge of a mandibular right central incisor. (From Zeisz RC, Nuckolls J: *Dental anatomy,* St Louis, 1949, Mosby.)

cal contours are quite convex, much more so than those of the permanent mandibular incisors. Cervical curvature is greater on the mesial side than on the distal side (Fig. 34-12; see also Figs. 34-9, *D* and *E*).

Incisal aspect

The incisal view (Fig. 34-13; see also Fig. 34-9, *C*) shows the incisal ridge centered over the crown of the tooth. The labial surface appears flat with a slight convexity, whereas the lingual surface appears concave.

Mandibular Lateral Incisors

The mandibular lateral incisors (Fig. 34-14) are wider and longer than the central incisors, and their cingula are more developed. Labiolin-

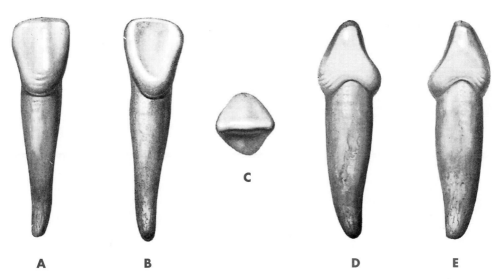

FIG. 34-14.   A mandibular right lateral incisor. **A,** Labial view. **B,** Lingual view. **C,** Incisal view. **D,** Mesial view. **E,** Distal view. (From Zeisz RC, Nuckolls J: *Dental anatomy,* St Louis, 1949, Mosby.)

gually the lateral incisors are also wider. There is a tendency for the incisal ridge to slope distally, and its distal margin is more rounded.

Roots of Mandibular Incisors

The root of the deciduous mandibular lateral incisor is longer, narrower, and more tapered than that of the central. It also is less blunt at the apex. The lateral has a distal longitudinal groove and a mesial depression running lengthwise.

The mandibular central incisor's root is just a little shorter and does not have any grooves or depressions on its root surfaces.

Maxillary Canines (Fig. 34-15)

Labial aspect (Fig. 34-16; see also Fig. 34-15, *A*)

A primary canine is bulkier than the primary incisors in every aspect. The crown is more constricted at the cervix in relation to its mesiodistal width and more convex on its mesial and distal surfaces. The facial lobes are well developed, and a sharp cusp is evident. The root is about

twice as long as the crown and more slender than that of its permanent successor.

Lingual aspect

From the lingual view (Fig. 34-17; see also Fig. 34-15, *B*) the mesial and distal marginal ridges, incisal ridges, and cingulum are all very pronounced. A tubercle may extend from the cusp tip to the lingual ridge. The lingual ridge extends from the cusp tip to the cingulum and divides the lingual surface into mesiolingual and distolingual fossae.

Mesial and distal aspects (Fig. 34-18; see also Figs. 34-15, *D* and *E*)

The outline form is similar to that of a lateral or central incisor, except that a canine is much wider at the cervical third of the crown. Both the crown and the root at the cervical third are wider labiolingually than the incisors.

Incisal aspect

From the incisal view (Fig. 34-19; see also Fig. 34-15, *C*), the crown is rhomboidal—like a square that has been slightly shifted. The labial ridge is relatively pronounced, and the cingulum

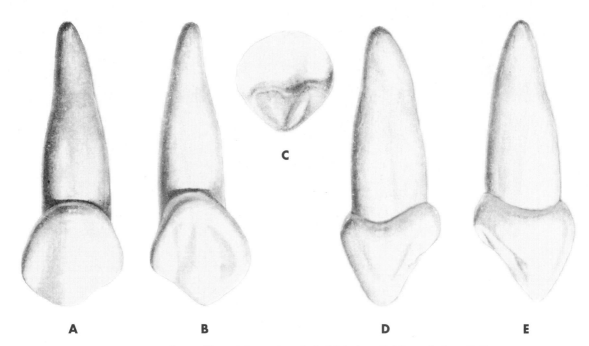

A   **B**   **C**   **D**   **E**

FIG. 34-15.   A maxillary right canine. **A,** Labial view. **B,** Lingual view. **C,** Incisal view. **D,** Mesial view. **E,** Distal view. (From Zeisz RC, Nuckolls J: *Dental anatomy,* St Louis, 1949, Mosby.)

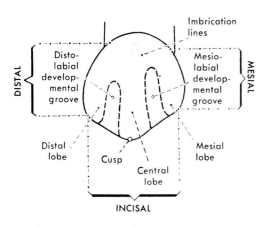

FIG. 34-16.   The labial surface of a maxillary right canine. (From Zeisz RC, Nuckolls J: *Dental anatomy,* St Louis, 1949, Mosby.)

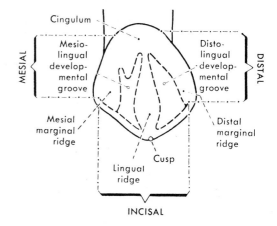

FIG. 34-17.   The lingual surface of a maxillary right canine. (From Zeisz RC, Nuckolls J: *Dental anatomy,* St Louis, 1949, Mosby.)

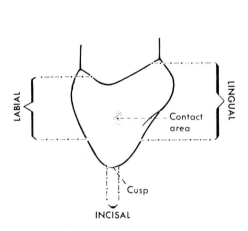

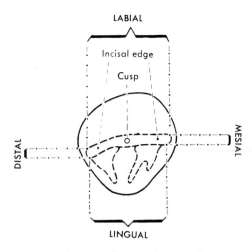

FIG. 34-18.   The mesial surface of a maxillary right canine. (From Zeisz RC, Nuckolls J: *Dental anatomy,* St Louis, 1949, Mosby.)

FIG. 34-19.   The incisal edge of a maxillary right canine. (From Zeisz RC, Nuckolls J: *Dental anatomy,* St Louis, 1949, Mosby.)

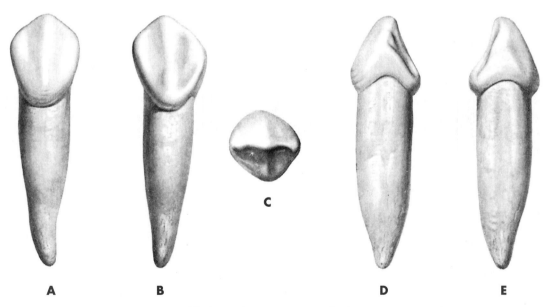

FIG. 34-20.   A mandibular right canine. **A,** Labial view. **B,** Lingual view. **C,** Incisal view. **D,** Mesial view. **E,** Distal view. (From Zeisz RC, Nuckolls J: *Dental anatomy,* St Louis, 1949, Mosby.)

is obvious. The tip of the cusp is slightly distal to the center of the tooth.

Mandibular Canines (Fig. 34-20)

Labial aspect

Compared with a maxillary canine, the labial surface of a mandibular canine (Fig. 34-21; see also Fig. 34-20, *A*) is much flatter, with shallow developmental grooves. The distal cusp ridge is longer than that of a maxillary canine. The root

is long, narrow, and almost twice the length of the crown, though shorter and more tapered than that of a maxillary canine.

Lingual aspect

The most obvious difference between the maxillary and mandibular canines is the presence of a slight concavity called the lingual fossa. Instead of two lingual fossae, there is one. The lingual surface (Fig. 34-22; see also Fig. 34-20, *B*) is less prominent than that of a maxillary canine, and the crown converges lingually so that it is narrower on the lingual side than on the labial.

Mesial and distal aspects (Fig. 34-23; see also Figs. 34-20, *D* and *E*)

The outline form of a mandibular canine resembles an incisor, with the incisal ridge centered over the crown labiolingually. The labiolingual measurements are smaller than those of a maxillary canine.

Incisal aspect

The incisal ridge (Fig. 34-24; see also Fig. 34-20, *C*) is straight and centers over the crown labiolingually. The lingual surface shows a definite tapering toward the cingulum. The labial surface from this aspect presents a flat surface with a slight convexity, whereas the lingual surface presents a flattened surface that is slightly concave.

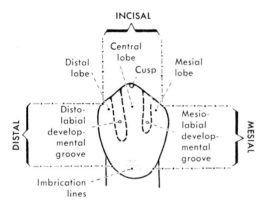

FIG. 34-21.   The labial surface of a mandibular right canine. (From Zeisz RC, Nuckolls J: *Dental anatomy,* St Louis, 1949, Mosby.)

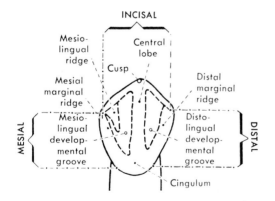

FIG. 34-22.   The lingual surface of a mandibular right canine. (From Zeisz RC, Nuckolls J: *Dental anatomy,* St Louis, 1949, Mosby.)

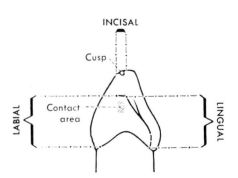

FIG. 34-23.   The mesial surface of a mandibular right canine. (From Zeisz RC, Nuckolls J: *Dental anatomy,* St Louis, 1949, Mosby.)

Roots of Canines

The roots of the deciduous canines are almost twice as long as their crowns, are thicker than the roots of the incisors, and their apices are more blunt. The mandibular root is slightly shorter than the maxillary root and is more tapered. Both have roots that taper lingually as well as apically. They are triangular in cross section.

Maxillary First Molars (Fig. 34-25)

Buccal aspect (Fig. 34-26; see also Fig. 34-25, *A*)

The deciduous maxillary first molar is a blend of premolar and molar. It does not resemble any other tooth, deciduous or permanent. This is the most atypical of all maxillary molars. However, like all other maxillary molars, it is wider buccolingually than mesiodistally.

It has two major cusps, a mesiobuccal and a mesiolingual. There is a distobuccal cusp, but it is only about half as large as the mesiobuccal cusp.

Lingual aspect

The lingual view (Fig. 34-27; see also Fig. 34-25, *B*) shows that the crown of a deciduous maxillary first molar converges toward the lingual surface.

The mesiolingual cusp is the longest and sharpest cusp on this tooth. The distolingual cusp is

small and rounded, if present at all. There is also a type of deciduous maxillary first molar that has only three cusps—one lingual and two buccal.

The lingual root is larger than the other two roots. A tiny tubercle can sometimes be seen on the mesiolingual cusps, but it cannot be called a cusp of Carabelli.

Mesial aspect (Fig. 34-28; see also Fig. 34-25, *D*)

The buccolingual measurement of a deciduous maxillary first molar at the cervical third is greater than the same measurement at the occlusal third. This is true of all molar teeth but is more evident on the deciduous teeth. The mesiolingual cusp is more pronounced and longer in size than the mesiobuccal cusp. The most obvious difference between the deciduous and permanent molars is that the deciduous first molars have an extreme convexity in the cervical third of the buccal surface (buccocervical ridge). This convexity appears to be overdeveloped when compared with that of the permanent teeth. It is a major characteristic of the deciduous maxillary first molars. The cervical line curves slightly toward the occlusal side.

Distal aspect (Fig. 34-29; see also Fig. 34-25, *E*)

The crown appears to be narrower distally than mesially. The distobuccal cusp is more developed than the distolingual cusp, which is not always present. The cervical convexity (buccocervical ridge) on the buccal surface does not continue onto the distal surface.

Occlusal aspect

The occlusal view (Fig. 34-30; see also Fig. 34-25, *C*) shows that the crown converges in a lingual direction so that the occlusal table appears triangular. The crown may have three or four cusps. If four are present, two will be on the buccal side and two on the lingual. If three cusps develop, only one will be lingual.

The occlusal surface is similar to that of the permanent molars except that the occlusal table is smaller in comparison. On the three-cusp form there is only a central and a mesial pit (no distal pit), and an oblique ridge often

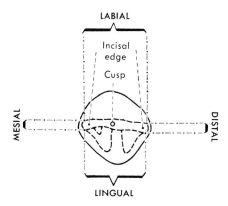

FIG. 34-24. The incisal edge of a mandibular right canine. (From Zeisz RC, Nuckolls J: *Dental anatomy*, St Louis, 1949, Mosby.)

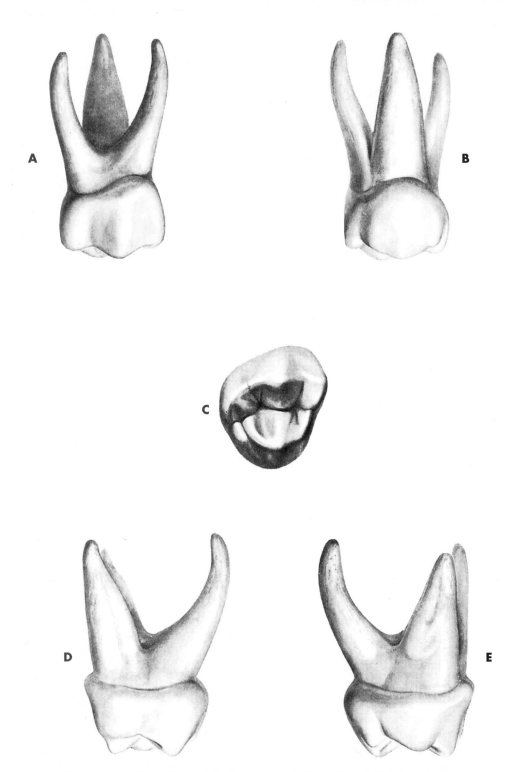

FIG. 34-25.   A maxillary right first molar. **A,** Buccal view. **B,** Lingual view.
C, Occlusal view. **D,** Mesial view. **E,** Distal view. (From Zeisz RC, Nuckolls J:
Dental anatomy, St Louis, 1949, Mosby.)

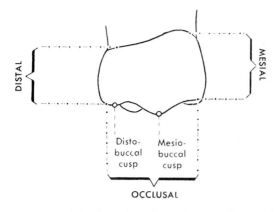

FIG. 34-26.   The buccal surface of a maxillary right first molar. (From Zeisz RC, Nuckolls J: *Dental anatomy,* St Louis, 1949, Mosby.)

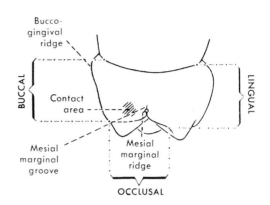

FIG. 34-28.   The mesial surface of a maxillary right first molar. (From Zeisz RC, Nuckolls J: *Dental anatomy,* St Louis, 1949, Mosby.)

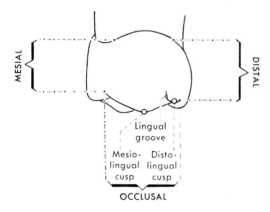

FIG. 34-27.   The lingual surface of a maxillary right first molar. (From Zeisz RC, Nuckolls J: *Dental anatomy,* St Louis, 1949, Mosby.)

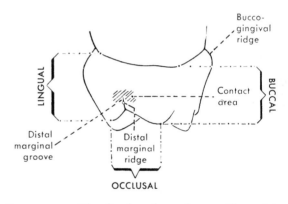

FIG. 34-29.   The distal surface of a maxillary right first molar. (From Zeisz RC, Nuckolls J: *Dental anatomy,* St Louis, 1949, Mosby.)

unites the mesiolingual with the distofacial cusps. The central groove connects the two fossae, the central fossa and the mesial triangular fossa. The buccal developmental groove is well developed and divides the two buccal cusps occlusally. The mesial, mesiofacial triangular, mesial marginal, and mesiolingual triangular grooves originate in the mesial pit. The distal, facial, and mesial developmental grooves radiate from the central pit.

On the four-cusp form, there are three fossae: mesial, central, and distal. A small pit is usually

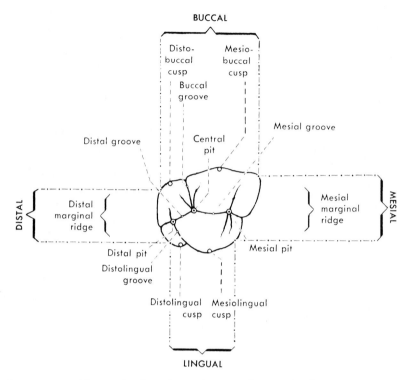

FIG. 34-30. The occlusal surface of a maxillary right first molar. (From Zeisz RC, Nuckolls J: *Dental anatomy*, St Louis, 1949, Mosby.)

present in each fossa. Grooves originating at the distal pit are the distofacial triangular, the distolingual, and the distal marginal grooves. An oblique ridge runs from the distobuccal cusp to the mesiolingual cusp.

Roots of Maxillary First Molars

Maxillary first molars have three roots, two buccal and one lingual. They are long, slender, and very flared. The lingual root is longer, more curved and tips back buccally at the apex. The mesiobuccal root is the next longest; the distobuccal is the shortest and the straightest.

The root trunk becomes trifurcated immediately above the cervical line. The root trunk is proportionately small when compared with the

length of the roots. Each root has a single root canal.

Maxillary Second Molars (Fig. 34-31)

Buccal aspect

A deciduous maxillary second molar resembles a permanent maxillary first molar, although it is much smaller. From the buccal view (Fig. 34-32; see also Fig. 34-31, *A*) two equal-sized buccal cusps with a buccal groove between them are visible. As on a deciduous first molar, the crown is narrow at its cervix, compared with its mesiodistal measurement at the contact area. A deciduous second molar is much larger than a deciduous first molar both in crown and root formation. The two buccal cusps are about equal

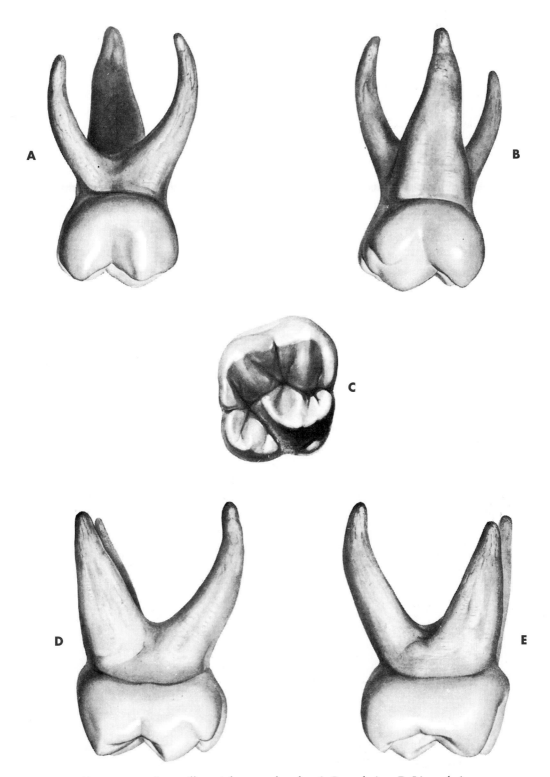

FIG. 34-31.   A maxillary right second molar. **A,** Buccal view. **B,** Lingual view.
C, Occlusal view. **D,** Mesial view. **E,** Distal view. (From Zeisz RC, Nuckolls J:
Dental anatomy, St Louis, 1949, Mosby.)

in size. How is this different from the cusps of a deciduous first molar?

Lingual aspect

From the lingual view (Fig. 34-33; see also Fig. 34-31, *B*) the crown shows three cusps—a mesiolingual, a distolingual, and a tubercle of Carabelli. The mesiolingual cusp is large and well developed. The distolingual cusp is more developed than that of a deciduous first molar but still small in comparison with the two buccal and the mesiolingual cusps. The tubercle of Carabelli is a fifth cusp on this tooth. It is poorly developed and is located on the lingual surface of the mesiolingual cusp. It is separated from the mesiolingual cusp by a developmental groove. A lingual developmental groove separates the mesiolingual and distolingual cusps.

Mesial aspect

From the mesial view (Fig. 34-34; see also Fig. 34-31, *D*) this tooth resembles a permanent molar, only smaller. In comparison with a deciduous first molar, the crown is 0.5 mm longer and about 2 mm wider buccolingually, and the roots are up to 2 mm longer. The lingual root curves much the same way as those of the first molars. The cusp of Carabelli is visible lingual and apical to the mesiolingual cusp, which is large in comparison with the mesiobuccal cusp.

Distal aspect

From the distal view (Fig. 34-35; see also Fig. 34-31, *E*) the crown appears smaller than from a mesial aspect, but not to the same degree as found on a deciduous maxillary first molar. The distobuccal and distolingual cusps are about the same length. A rather straight cervical line is evident both distally and mesially.

Occlusal aspect

From the occlusal view (Fig. 34-36; see also Fig. 34-31, *C*) the deciduous maxillary second molar resembles a permanent first molar. It has four well-developed cusps—mesiobuccal, distobuccal, mesiolingual, distolingual—and a cusp of Carabelli. The developmental grooves, although less defined, are almost identical to those found on a permanentfirst molar. The mesiolingual cusp is the largest, and the distolingual the smallest, except for the fifth cusp.

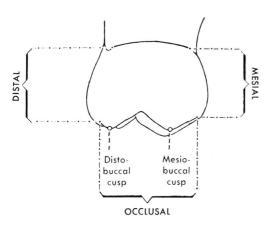

FIG. 34-32. The buccal surface of a maxillary right second molar. (From Zeisz RC, Nuckolls J: *Dental anatomy,* St Louis, 1949, Mosby.)

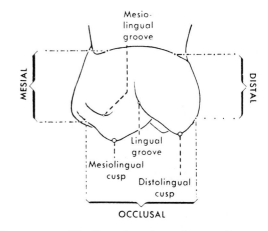

FIG. 34-33. The lingual surface of a maxillary right second molar. (From Zeisz RC, Nuckolls J: *Dental anatomy,* St Louis, 1949, Mosby.)

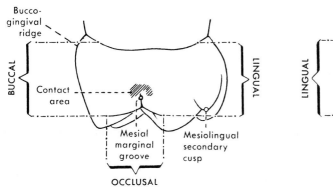

FIG. 34-34. The mesial surface of a maxillary right second molar. (From Zeisz RC, Nuckolls J: *Dental anatomy,* St Louis, 1949, Mosby.)

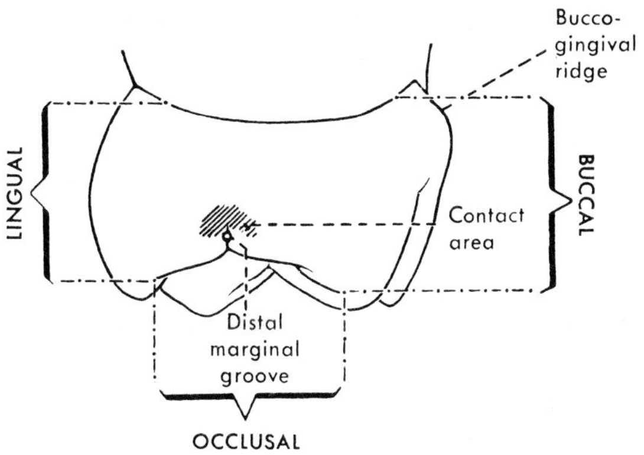

FIG. 34-35. The distal surface of a maxillary right second molar. (From Zeisz RC, Nuckolls J: *Dental anatomy,* St Louis, 1949, Mosby.)

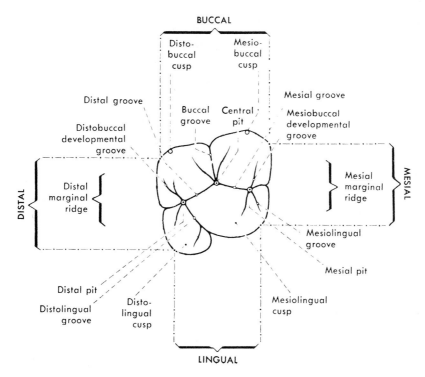

FIG. 34-36. The occlusal surface of a maxillary right second molar. (From Zeisz RC, Nuckolls J: *Dental anatomy,* St Louis, 1949, Mosby.)

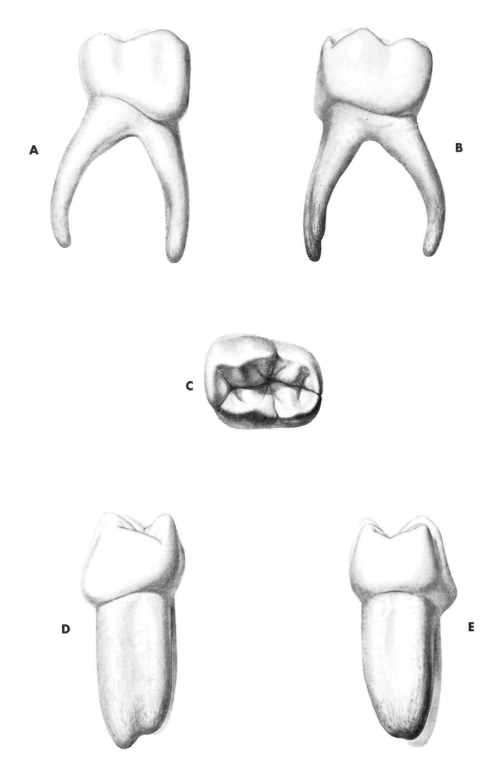

Fig. 34-37. A mandibular right first molar. **A,** Buccal view. **B,** Lingual view. **C,** Occlusal view. **D,** Mesial view. **E,** Distal view. (From Zeisz RC, Nuckolls J: *Dental anatomy,* St Louis, 1949, Mosby.)

Roots of Maxillary Second Molars

There are three roots, two buccal and one lingual. Like the deciduous first molar, the deciduous maxillary second molar's longest root is the lingual, and its shortest is the distobuccal. Unlike the first molar the mesiobuccal root may be as long as the lingual. The root trunk is short, and each of the roots has only one root canal.

Mandibular First Molars (Fig. 34-37)

Buccal aspect (Fig. 34-38; see also Fig. 34-37, *A*)

A primary mandibular first molar does not resemble any of the other teeth, deciduous or permanent. Its mesial outline is rather flat straight up and down, whereas the distal outline is convex, converging sharply toward the cervical line. This makes the distal contact area fairly convex. The distal portion of the crown is shorter than the mesial portion.

Two distinct buccal cusps are present, but the developmental groove between them is not always evident. The mesial cusp is larger than the distal cusp. The crown is wider mesiodistally than buccolingually.

The roots are long, slender, and flared, with the mesial root curving slightly distally in its apical third. The point of bifurcation is very close to the cervical line of the crown, a characteristic of all deciduous molars. Observe the curvature of the cervical line (see Fig. 34-38).

Lingual aspect (Fig. 34-39; see also Fig. 34-37, *B*)

The crown and root converge lingually on the mesial half of the crown; distally they do not converge. The mesiolingual cusp is long and sharp, whereas the distolingual cusp is more rounded and not as long. The mesial marginal ridge is so well developed that it almost appears to be another cusp.

The cervical line is almost straight across, being quite different from the cervical line on the buccal aspect. Buccally the cervical line curves apically on the mesial half of the tooth.

Mesial aspect

The most characteristic feature of this tooth is an extremely bulbous curvature on its buccal surface at the cervical third. This buccocervical convexity can easily be seen from the mesial view (Fig. 34-40; see also Fig. 34-37, *D*) and causes the occlusal table to appear rather narrow from cusp tip to cusp tip.

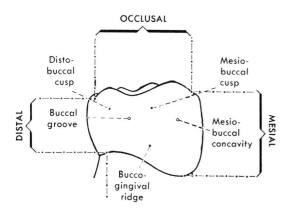

FIG. 34-38. The buccal surface of a mandibular right first molar. (From Zeisz RC, Nuckolls J: *Dental anatomy,* St Louis, 1949, Mosby.)

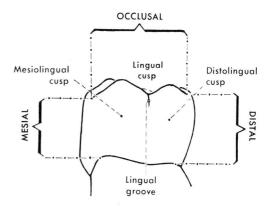

FIG. 34-39. The lingual surface of a mandibular right first molar. (From Zeisz RC, Nuckolls J: *Dental anatomy,* St Louis, 1949, Mosby.)

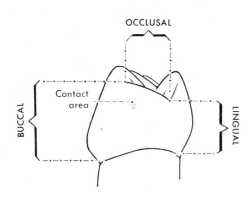

FIG. 34-40.   The mesial surface of a mandibular right first molar. (From Zeisz RC, Nuckolls J: *Dental anatomy*, St Louis, 1949, Mosby.)

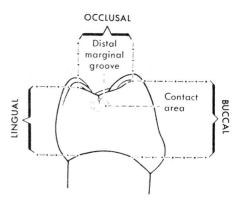

FIG. 34-41.   The distal surface of a mandibular right first molar. (From Zeisz RC, Nuckolls J: *Dental anatomy*, St Louis, 1949, Mosby.)

The mesiobuccal cusp is longer than the mesiolingual cusp because the cervical line curves up from the buccal to the lingual side. The buccal surface is flat from the tip of the mesiobuccal cusp to the crest of the buccocervical curvature. Although this buccocervical curvature is quite pronounced, the remainder of the buccal surface above the curvature is rather flat and tipped at a sharp angle toward the buccal cusp.

Distal aspect

The distal aspect (Fig. 34-41; see also Fig. 34-37, *D*) of the crown does not display such an extreme buccocervical curvature. The height of the cusps, buccal and lingual, appears more uniform, and the cervical line is almost straight across buccolingually. The distobuccal and distolingual cusps are not as developed as the two mesial cusps. Furthermore, the distal marginal ridge is not as well defined as the mesial marginal ridge. The distal root is rounder and shorter than the mesial root, tapers apically, and houses only one root canal.

The distal surface is more convex than the mesial surface; therefore the distal contact area is more rounded and convex than the mesial contact area.

Occlusal aspect

The occlusal outline (Fig. 34-42; see also Fig. 34-37, *C*) of the crown is rhomboidal. From this view the prominence of the mesiobuccal surface is evident. The mesiobuccal cervical ridge is also pronounced and gives the tooth a rhomboidal shape that tapers distally. The mesiolingual cusp appears to be the widest cusp, and the mesial marginal ridge is well developed. A buccal developmental groove may be present. A distinct transverse ridge runs between the mesiofacial and the mesiolingual cusps. This ridge divides the occlusal surface into two fossae: one contains the mesial pit, the other the central and distal pits, and all are joined by a central developmental groove. A lingual groove radiates from the central pit between the two lingual cusps. A facial groove runs from the central pit to the buccal surface between the two buccal cusps. Mesial and distal triangular fossae, as well as mesial and distal marginal and triangular grooves, can be seen in Fig. 34-37, *C*.

Roots of Mandibular First Molars

The deciduous mandibular first molar has two roots, a mesial and a distal. They are flat, broad, and flared widely apart. The mesial root has a longitudinal developmental groove run-

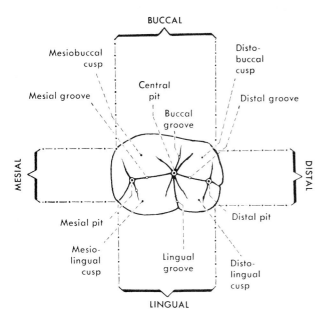

BUCCAL

Mesiobuccal cusp

Mesial groove

Central pit

Buccal groove

Disto-buccal cusp

Distal groove

MESIAL

DISTAL

Mesial pit

Mesio-lingual cusp

Lingual groove

Distal pit

Disto-lingual cusp

LINGUAL

FIG. 34-42.   The occlusal surface of a mandibular right first molar. (From Zeisz RC, Nuckolls J: *Dental anatomy,* St Louis, 1949, Mosby.)

ning its length, and it has two root canals. The distal root is the shorter and thinner of the two; it has only one canal.

Mandibular Second Molars (Fig. 34-43)

Buccal aspect (Fig. 34-44; see also Fig. 34-43, *A*)

A primary mandibular second molar resembles a permanent mandibular first molar except that it is smaller and has the typical deciduous molar constriction at the cervix of the crown.

Mesiobuccal and distobuccal developmental grooves divide the buccal surface occlusally into three cusps. The three buccal cusps are the mesiofacial, the distofacial, and the distal. The term *buccal* can be substituted for *facial*. What would the names of the three cusps then be? These cusps are about equal in length and width; the distobuccal (distofacial) cusp is slightly longer than the other two.

Characteristically the roots of a second molar

are long and slender, flaring mesiodistally at their middle and apical thirds. These roots are often twice as long as or longer than the crown. The point of bifurcation of the roots starts immediately below the cervical line of the crown. How is this different from a permanent first molar's roots?

Lingual aspect

From the lingual view (Fig. 34-45; see also Fig. 34-43, *B*) a short lingual groove can be seen dividing two cusps of about equal dimensions. The two lingual cusps, the mesiolingual and the distolingual, are not as wide as the three buccal cusps. The tooth therefore converges lingually. The cervical line is straight.

Mesial aspect

The mesial view (Fig. 34-46; see also Fig. 34-43, *D*) of the crown resembles that of a permanent mandibular first molar. However, its buccal surface shows a cervical bulge typical of deciduous molars. This crest of contour on the buccal side is notably less than that of a deciduous first molar. Like a deciduous first molar, a flattened buccal surface angles occlusally from this crest of contour, which presents a proportionately smaller occlusal table than on the permanent mandibular molars.

The mesial marginal ridge is rather high, giving the cusp the appearance of being shorter. The lingual cusp is longer than the buccal cusp because the cervical line extends up from the buccal to the lingual side.

The mesial root is broad, flat, blunted at its apex, and houses two canals.

Distal aspect (Fig. 34-47; see also Fig. 34-43, *E*)

The crown is not as wide distally as it is mesially, nor is the distal marginal ridge as high or as long as the mesial marginal ridge. The cervical line has the same upper inclination buccolingually as the mesiocervical line.

Three cusps can be seen from the distal view: the distofacial, the distal, and the distolingual. Because the tooth converges distally, portions of the mesiofacial and mesiolingual cusps are also visible from the distal view.

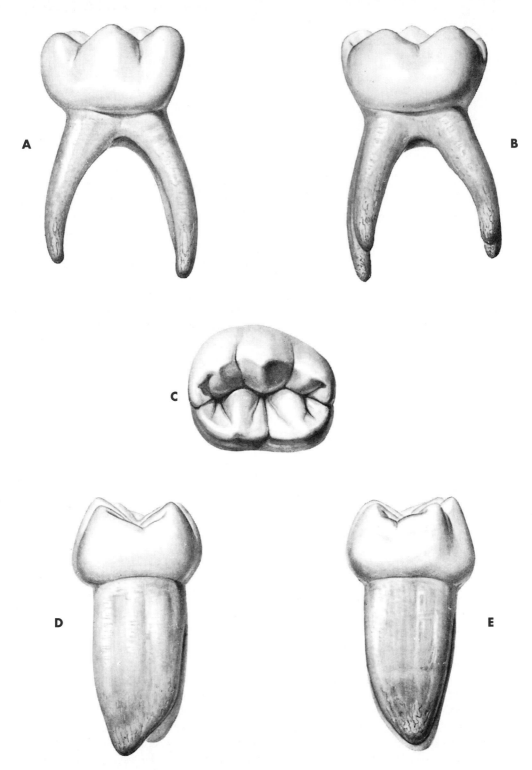

FIG. 34-43. A mandibular right second molar. **A,** Buccal view. **B,** Lingual view. **C,** Occlusal view. **D,** Mesial view. **E,** Distal view. (From Zeisz RC, Nuckolls J: *Dental anatomy,* St Louis, 1949, Mosby.)

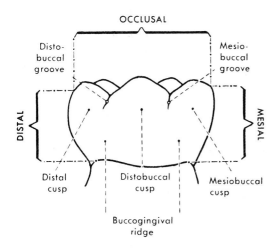

FIG. 34-44.   The buccal surface of a mandibular right second molar. (From Zeisz RC, Nuckolls J: *Dental anatomy*, St Louis, 1949, Mosby.)

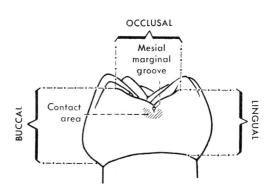

FIG. 34-46.   The mesial surface of a mandibular right second molar. (From Zeisz RC, Nuckolls J: *Dental anatomy*, St Louis, 1949, Mosby.)

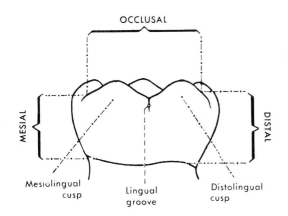

FIG. 34-45.   The lingual surface of a mandibular right second molar. (From Zeisz RC, Nuckolls J: *Dental anatomy*, St Louis, 1949, Mosby.)

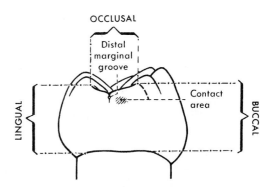

FIG. 34-47.   The distal surface of a mandibular right second molar. (From Zeisz RC, Nuckolls J: *Dental anatomy*, St Louis, 1949, Mosby.)

Although the distal root is more tapered than the mesial root at its apical end, it does resemble the mesial root with its broad and flattened surface. The distal root has one canal. Does this differ from the distal root of a deciduous mandibular first molar?

Occlusal aspect (Fig. 34-48; see also Fig. 34-43, C)

The three buccal cusps are similar in size, as are the two lingual cusps. However, the total mesiodistal width of the three buccal cusps is much more than the total mesiodistal width of the two

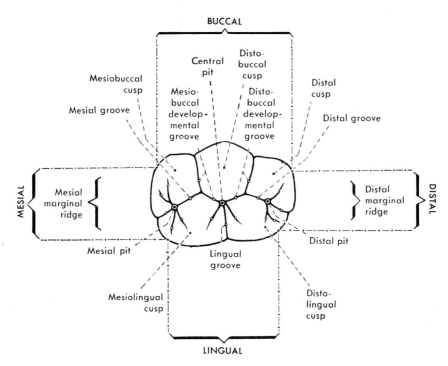

BUCCAL

Central
pit

Disto-
buccal
cusp

Mesiobuccal
cusp

Mesio-
buccal
develop-
mental
groove

Disto-
buccal
develop-
mental
groove

Distal
cusp

Mesial groove

Distal groove

MESIAL

Mesial
marginal
ridge

DISTAL

Distal
marginal
ridge

Mesial pit

Lingual
groove

Distal pit

Mesiolingual
cusp

Disto-
lingual
cusp

LINGUAL

Fig. 34-48.   The occlusal surface of a mandibular right second molar. (From Zeisz RC, Nuckolls J: *Dental anatomy,* St Louis, 1949, Mosby.)

lingual cusps. This allows the tooth to converge lingually.

The mesiofacial, distofacial, and lingual grooves radiate from the central pit in a Y shape. A central developmental groove joins the mesial triangular fossa and pit. Scattered over the occlusal surface are supplemental grooves located on the triangular ridges and fossae. The mesial marginal ridge is more pronounced than the distal marginal ridge.

The crown converges both distally and lingually. This convergence is similar to that seen in a permanent first molar, but the distal cusp in a permanent molar is much smaller than the two other buccal cusps. On a deciduous molar the three buccal cusps are almost equal in size and development. All three buccal cusps of the de-

ciduous molars are small in comparison with those of the permanent molars. This gives the deciduous tooth crown a narrower buccolingual dimension in comparison with its mesiodistal dimensions.

Roots of Mandibular Second Molars

The roots of the deciduous mandibular second molar are twice as long as the crown. They are long, slender, and flared. The root trunk, like all deciduous molars, is short, bifurcating immediately below the cervix of the tooth.

The two roots are the mesial and the distal. The mesial root has two root canals and may have a longitudinal groove dividing it buccolingually. The distal root has only one root canal, and no grooves divide the root surface itself.

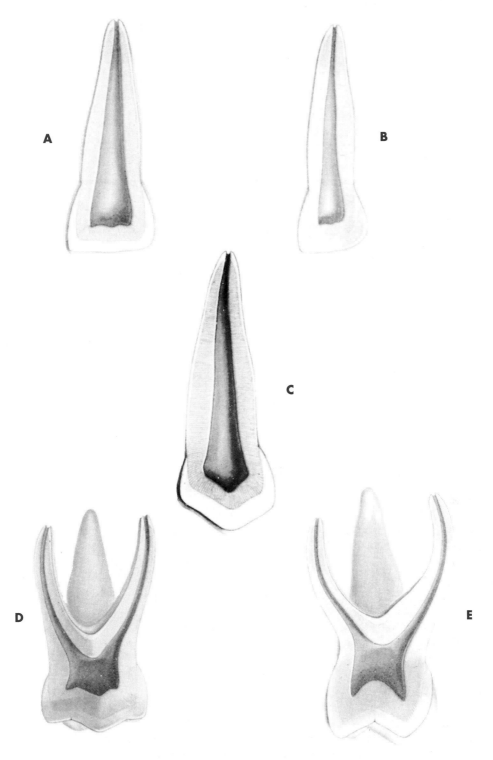

FIG. 34-49. Maxillary right deciduous teeth, facial views. **A,** Central incisor. **B,** Lateral incisor. **C,** Canine. **D,** First molar. **E,** Second molar. (From Zeisz RC, Nuckolls J: *Dental anatomy,* St Louis, 1949, Mosby.)

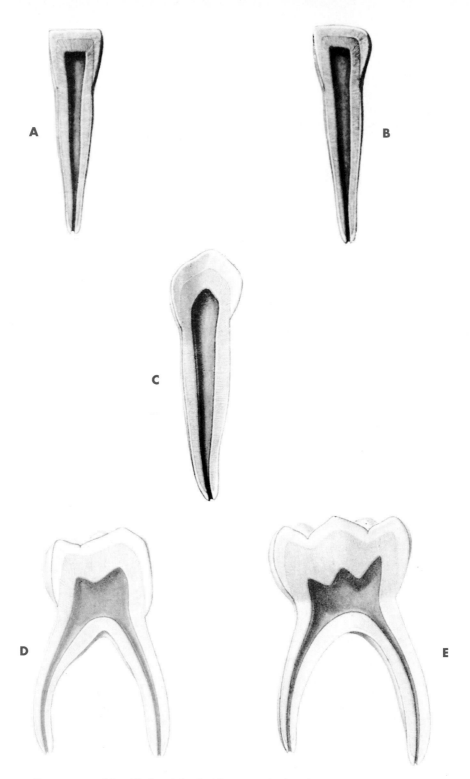

FIG. 34-50. Mandibular right deciduous teeth, facial views. **A,** Central incisor. **B,** Lateral incisor. **C,** Canine. **D,** First molar. **E,** Second molar. (From Zeisz RC, Nuckolls J: *Dental anatomy,* St Louis, 1949, Mosby.)

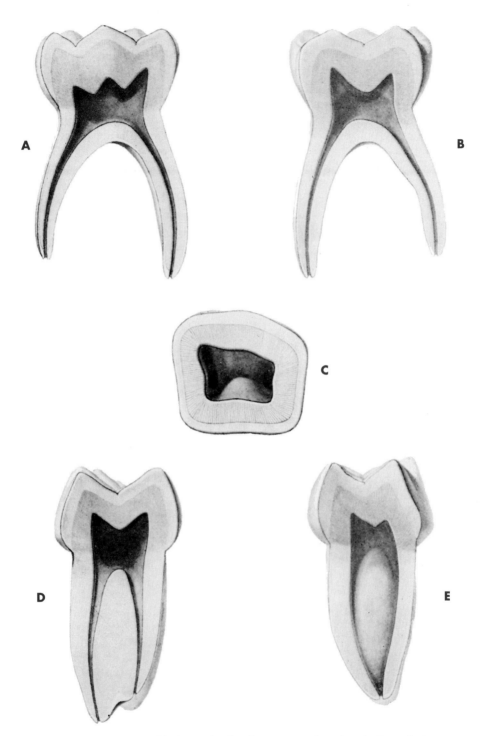

FIG. 34-51. A mandibular right deciduous second molar. A, Buccal view. B, Lingual view. C, Occlusal view. D, Mesial view. E, Distal view. (From Zeisz RC, Nuckolls J: *Dental anatomy,* St Louis, 1949, Mosby.)

Pulp Cavities of Deciduous Teeth

The pulp cavities of deciduous teeth mirror the outer form of the teeth except that the pulp horns are longer and more pointed (Figs. 34-49 and 34-50). Compared with the pulp chambers of the permanent teeth, the pulp chambers of deciduous teeth are large in proportion to the tooth size and the pulp horns are more extreme. The mandibular deciduous molars are like miniature permanent teeth with larger-sized pulp chambers, root canals, and pulp horns (Fig. 34-51).

Review Questions

1. Give two terms that are synonymous with the commonly used term *baby teeth*.
2. What is meant by the term *exfoliation*, and how does exfoliation occur?
3. How many deciduous teeth are there? How many are molars? Incisors? Premolars?
4. What are the eruption dates of the following?
   a. deciduous maxillary incisors
   b. deciduous mandibular incisors
   c. deciduous canines
   d. deciduous first molars
5. Which teeth usually erupt first, maxillary or mandibular?
6. Name 12 essential differences between deciduous and permanent teeth.
7. What cervical bulge of enamel is more pronounced on the deciduous teeth than on the permanent teeth?
8. Which deciduous tooth is least like any in the permanent dentition?
   a. primary maxillary second molar
   b. primary mandibular first molar
   c. primary mandibular second molar

9. Give one special characteristic that is unique to each type of deciduous molar.
10. Rewrite the 12 essential differences between deciduous and permanent teeth in summary form.
11. Caries in deciduous teeth can lead to nerve involvement more easily than in permanent teeth. Which of the reasons for this are true?
    a. There is less thickness of the dentin between the enamel and the pulp chamber in deciduous teeth.
    b. The pulp horns extend rather high occlusally in deciduous teeth.
    c. The pulp chambers of deciduous teeth are relatively large compared to their crowns.
    d. a, b, and c
12. The cervical ridges of deciduous teeth are _____ compared with permanent teeth.
    a. more prominent
    b. less bulky
    c. thinner
13. Roots of deciduous teeth are wider than permanent teeth. T or F?
14. Roots of deciduous teeth are longer in comparison to the crowns than permanent teeth. T or F?
15. Roots of deciduous teeth are bulkier and thicker at their cervical junction. T or F?
16. Deciduous molars flare their roots more than permanent molars. T or F?
17. The smallest tooth in the human dentition is a deciduous mandibular central incisor. T or F?
18. Deciduous molars do not have a cusp of Carabelli. T or F?

UNIT IV

TEST

1. A small elevation of enamel that may be found on the surface of a tooth is a
   a. cusp.
   b. tubercle.
   c. sulcus.
   d. fossa.
2. Of the permanent premolars, the one most likely to have two root canals is the
   a. maxillary first premolar.
   b. maxillary second premolar.
   c. mandibular first premolar.
   d. mandibular second premolar.
3. Which of the following is *least* typical for the maxillary second premolar?
   a. The lingual cusp is slightly shorter than the facial cusp.
   b. The facial cusp is slightly larger than the lingual cusp.
   c. The two cusps are approximately the same length.
   d. The facial cusp is shorter and more blunt compared with the lingual cusp.
4. When the two cusps of the maxillary first premolars are compared,
   a. the facial cusp is longer but not wider.
   b. the lingual cusp is both shorter and narrower.
   c. the facial cusp is shorter but wider.
   d. the lingual cusp is both longer and wider.

5. Which of the following is *not* true of maxillary first premolars?
   a. commonly bifurcated root
   b. single root trunk
   c. facial cusp tip displaced to the distal from midline
   d. the roots are the mesial and distal
6. The last of these teeth to erupt are
   a. the mandibular first premolars.
   b. the maxillary canines.
   c. the maxillary first premolars.
   d. the mandibular canines.
7. Of the following, the least likely to bifurcate is the
   a. maxillary second premolar.
   b. mandibular canine.
   c. mandibular first premolar.
   d. mandibular second premolar.
8. The least likely to have two root canals is
   a. the mesiobuccal root of a maxillary molar.
   b. the mesial root of the mandibular molar.
   c. an upper premolar.
   d. a mandibular canine.
9. Which of the following are the first permanent teeth to erupt?
   a. maxillary first molars
   b. mandibular first molars
   c. mandibular centrals
   d. maxillary centrals
10. Which of the following have the least cervical contact areas?
   a. central incisors
   b. third molars
   c. canines
   d. premolars
11. Which of the following are class traits of all molars?
   a. Molars have the largest occlusal surfaces of any teeth in the dentition.
   b. Molars have three to five major cusps.
   c. Molars have two functional cusps and two afunctional cusps.
   d. Molars have two or three roots.
   e. a, b, d

12. The distobuccal and mesiolingual cusps on the occlusal table of a maxillary molar are usually connected by a ridge. This ridge is termed
    a. the transverse ridge.
    b. the triangular ridge.
    c. the Carabellian ridge.
    d. the oblique ridge.
    e. a and d.
13. The maxillary incisors in a class II, division II, malocclusion are
    a. retruded.
    b. protruded.
    c. edge to edge.
    d. end to end.
14. Maxillary laterals exhibit
    a. the same number of lobes as first molars.
    b. the same number of lobes as first premolars.
    c. two labial and two lingual lobes.
    d. three lobes only.

A 9-year-old boy presents himself with a large gingival abscess at the gingival crest of his deciduous maxillary first right molar. The tooth is loose and painful upon percussion.

15. We could expect this 9-year-old patient to exhibit
    a. no permanent teeth at all other than first molars.
    b. a mixed dentition.
    c. evidence of facial trauma.
    d. evidence of severe periodontal disease.
16. We would consider the following types of treatment appropriate for an abcessed deciduous 2nd molar
    a. root resection
    b. periodontal surgery
    c. removal of the affected tooth
    d. splinting the deciduous molars together
17. If this molar was removed, which of the following is *not* true?
    a. A space maintainer is probably not needed.
    b. The permanent replacement could be expected soon.

c. His eruption pattern is earlier than that of most children his age.
    d. Not much evidence of the deciduous root would be present.
18. From the occlusal view, which tooth is wider on the lingual than on the buccal?
    a. maxillary central incisor
    b. mandibular first molar
    c. maxillary first molar
    d. mandibular first premolar
    e. mandibular second premolar
19. The cusp of Carabelli of the permanent maxillary first molar may be
    a. absent.
    b. located lingual to the distolingual cusp.
    c. the third largest cusp.
    d. all of the above.
20. The longest and shortest cusps of the maxillary first molar are the
    a. mesiofacial and distofacial.
    b. mesiolingual and distofacial.
    c. mesiolingual and distolingual.
    d. distofacial and distolingual.
21. In class I occlusion, the mandibular lateral incisor
    a. opposes the maxillary lateral incisor and canine.
    b. opposes only the maxillary lateral incisor.
    c. opposes maxillary central and lateral incisors.
    d. is free of contact with opposing teeth.
22. As compared with the permanent mandibular central incisor, the root of the mandibular lateral incisor is
    a. larger in all dimensions.
    b. longer but not wider.
    c. wider but not longer.
    d. the same size.
23. Morphologically, the mandibular lateral incisor is almost identical to the mandibular central incisor, with which difference?
    a. The mandibular lateral incisor is usually slightly larger.
    b. The mandibular lateral incisor has an

elongation of the distoincisal angle distolingually.

c. When the mandibular lateral incisor is
viewed incisally, the crown appears to be
slightly rotated on its base.

d. All of the above are true.

24. In comparison with the permanent maxillary
canine, the permanent mandibular canine
has a mesiodistal crown width that is
a. somewhat wider.
b. somewhat narrower.
c. identical.
d. a great deal wider.

25. In comparison with the mandibular canine,
the maxillary canine
a. has a relatively longer crown.
b. is less likely to be bifurcated.
c. has a less pronounced cingulum.
d. has less prominent lingual features.

26. Which of the following anterior teeth
exhibits the most deviation in tooth morphology?
a. mandibular central incisor
b. maxillary canine
c. maxillary lateral incisor
d. mandibular lateral incisor

27. The smallest permanent tooth in the mouth
is the
a. maxillary central incisor.
b. mandibular central incisor.
c. maxillary lateral incisor.
d. mandibular lateral incisor.

28. Which of the following anterior teeth is
most likely to have two root canals?
a. mandibular lateral incisor
b. maxillary canine
c. maxillary central incisor
d. mandibular canine

29. Mesiodistal measurements of the crowns of
anterior teeth as seen from an incisal view
indicate that the crowns are
a. wider at the mesial than the distal.
b. wider at the distal than the mesial.
c. wider at the lingual than the facial.
d. wider at the facial than the lingual.

30. Which of the following is the largest, longest,
and strongest root of the maxillary molar?
a. facial
b. lingual
c. mesiofacial
d. distofacial

31. Which of the following cusps is frequently
missing from the maxillary third molar?
a. mesiofacial
b. distofacial
c. distolingual
d. mesiolingual

32. The oblique ridge of maxillary molars
crosses the occlusal surface obliquely from
a. mesiofacial to mesiolingual.
b. mesiolingual to distofacial.
c. distofacial to distolingual.
d. mesiofacial to distolingual.

33. Where is the lingual height of contour located on the mandibular molars?
a. middle third
b. occlusal third
c. cervical third
d. at the junction of occlusal and middle third

34. The mandibular molars are aligned in
the alveolar bone in such a way that their
crowns are
a. tilted to the distal and facial side.
b. tilted to the lingual but upright otherwise.
c. upright in all directions.
d. tilted to the mesial and lingual side.

35. The permanent mandibular first molar usually has
a. two root canals in the mesial root, one in
the distal.
b. one root canal in the lingual root, one in
the facial.
c. two root canals in both the mesial and
distal roots.
d. one root canal in each root.

36. The four most frequently found congenitally
missing teeth are
a. maxillary first premolar, maxillary lateral, mandibular lateral, and third molar.
b. maxillary third molar and lateral, and

mandibular canine and third molar.
c. maxillary third molar, mandibular third molar, maxillary lateral, and mandibular second bicuspid.
d. maxillary third molar and first bicuspid, and mandibular third molar and canine.

37. The greatest convexity of the facial surface of anterior teeth is
a. different from that of the posterior teeth.
b. the cervical third.
c. the middle third.
d. the junction of middle and incisal thirds.

38. Which of the following is *not* a set trait of the deciduous dentition?
a. Most primary teeth are smaller than the analogous permanent teeth.
b. The crowns of primary teeth seem long relative to their total length when compared with the permanent teeth.
c. In the anterior primary teeth, the labial and lingual surfaces bulge conspicuously in the cervical third.
d. Primary crowns are milk white in color.
e. The enamel is thinner in primary teeth and the pulp chamber is larger.

39. What is the most distinguishing feature of the maxillary first deciduous molar?
a. cusp relationship
b. buccal cervical ridge
c. mesial profile
d. occlusal outline

40. A child 14 months of age should normally have which deciduous teeth present in the mouth (all four quadrants)?
a. centrals, laterals, canines, first molars, second molars
b. centrals, laterals, canines, first molars
c. centrals, laterals, first molars, second molars
d. centrals, laterals, canines
e. centrals, laterals, first molars

41. Which of the following deciduous teeth do not resemble any other deciduous teeth or permanent teeth?

a. deciduous mandibular first molar
b. deciduous mandibular second molar
c. deciduous maxillary first molar
d. deciduous maxillary second molar
e. a and c

42. Which has three roots?
a. mandibular molars
b. maxillary premolars
c. deciduous maxillary molars
d. maxillary molars
e. a, c, and d
f. c and d

43. The cusp of Carabelli of the permanent maxillary first molar is sometimes
a. located on the distolingual cusp.
b. missing entirely.
c. located on the lingual surface.
d. located on the mesiolingual cusp.
e. a, c, and d.
f. b, c, and d.

44. The smallest tooth in the human dentition is the
a. deciduous mandibular central.
b. deciduous mandibular lateral.
c. permanent mandibular central.
d. permanent lower lateral.

45. The permanent mandibular incisors differ from the permanent maxillary incisors in the following way.
a. Maxillary incisors are smaller.
b. Mandibular lateral is larger than the central.
c. Maxillary have fewer pits and less developed marginal ridges.
d. Mandibular have more developed cingula.

46. What is the excess space called that is available for the permanent canine and premolars?
a. freeway space
b. primate space
c. interdental space
d. leeway space
e. horizontal overjet

Suggested Readings

Andrews LF: The six keys to normal occlusion, Amer J Orthod 62(3):296, 1972.

Angle EH: Treatment of malocclusion of the teeth and fractures of the maxillae: Angle's system, ed 6, Philadelphia, 1900, SS White Dental Manufacturing Co.

Ash MM: Wheeler's atlas of tooth form, ed 5, Philadelphia, 1984, WB Saunders Co.

Ash MM: Wheeler's dental anatomy, physiology, and occlusion, ed 6, Philadelphia, 1984, WB Saunders Co.

Ayer WA: Thumb-finger sucking and bruxing habits in children. In Bryant P, Gale E, Rugh J, (editors): Oral motor behavior: impact on oral conditions and dental treatment, NIH Publications No. 79-1845, Washington, DC, 1979, US Government Printing Office.

Begg PR: Stone age man's dentition, Amer J Orthod 40:298, April 1954.

Begg PR: Stone age man's dentition, Amer J Orthod 40:373, May 1954.

Begg PR: Stone age man's dentition, Amer J Orthod 40:462, June 1954.

Begg PR: Stone age man's dentition, Amer J Orthod 40:517, July 1954.

Begg PR, Kesling PC: Begg orthodontic theory and technique, Philadelphia, 1977, WB Saunders.

Berry DC, Singh BP: Effect of electromyographic biofeedback therapy on occlusion contacts, J Prosthet Dent 51:397, 1984.

Dawson PE: Evaluation, diagnosis, and treatment of occlusal problems, ed 2, St Louis, 1989, Mosby.

DuBrul EL: Sicher's oral anatomy, ed 8, St Louis, 1988, Ishiyaku EuroAmerica, Inc.

Farman AG, Escobar V: Duplication of oral and maxillofacial structures, Quintessence International, 17(11):731, 1986.

Fuller JL, Denehy GE: Concise dental anatomy and morphology, ed 2, Chicago, Iowa Year Book Med Pub.

Grahnen H, Granath LE: Numerical variations in primary dentition and their correlation with permanent dentition, Odontol Rev 12:348, 1961.

Kessler HP, Kraut RA: Dentigerous cyst associated with an impacted mesiodens, Gen Dent 48:47, 1989.

King NM, Wei SH: Developmental defects of enamel: a study of 12 year olds in Hong Kong, JADA 112:835, 1986.

Kraus BS, Jordan E, Abrams L: Dental anatomy and occlusion, St. Louis, 1992, Mosby.

Mangold WG et al: New community residents' preferences for dental service information, JADA 112:840, 1986.

Massler M, Schour I: Atlas of the mouth in health and disease, ed 2, Chicago, 1975, American Dental Association.

Mohl ND: A textbook of occlusion, Lombard, Ill, 1988, Quintessence.

Mourino AP, Camm JH: Multiple anomalies of a newborn: report of a case, JADA 114:335, 1987.

Proffit WR, Fields HW, Nixon WL: Occlusal forces in normal and long-face adults, J Dent Res 62:566, 1983.

Ramfjord S, Ash MM: Significance of occlusion in the etiology and treatment of early, moderate, and advanced periodontitis, J Periodontal 52:511, 1981.

Ramfjord S, Ash MM: Occlusion, ed 3, Philadelphia, 1983, WB Saunders Co.

Renner RP: An introduction to dental anatomy and esthetics, Lombard, Ill., 1985, Quintessence.

Woelfel JB: Dental anatomy: its relevance to dentistry, ed 4, Philadelphia, 1990, Lea & Febiger.

Answers to Review Questions

CHAPTER 1

1. Tori and exostoses are bony outgrowths of the mandible and maxilla. They can become traumatized by many things and may become painful. Many times they need to be removed before denture construction to allow for proper fit of the denture.
2. The vestibule is the space between the lips or cheeks and the teeth.
3. The frenum attachments contain no muscle, only connective tissue.
4. The alveolar mucosa is redder because the epithelium, or mucous membrane is thin and the red color from the underlying blood vessels shows through. The gingiva is thicker and the redness does not show through as much, hence the pink color.
5. The palate is divided into a hard palate and a soft palate. The anterior transverse ridges of tissue are the rugae.
6. The posterior nasal spine is the pointed area at the middle part of the posterior end of the hard palate. It serves as a partial attachment for the anterior end of the soft palate.
7. The mylohyoid muscle supports the floor of the mouth.
8. The sublingual caruncle is a reddened elevation of tissue at the base of the lingual frenum that is the opening of the duct of the submandibular gland and one of the major ducts of the sublingual gland.
9. The palatoglossal and palatopharyngeal muscles make up the anterior and posterior pillars, and the palatine tonsil lies between them.
10. The fauces is the space between the left and right tonsillar pillars.
11. The oral cavity consists of the vestibule and the oral cavity proper, which lies between the teeth and back to the tonsils. Its upper and lower boundaries are the palate and the floor of the mouth.
12. Knowledge of normal anatomy is important so that one can recognize the abnormal.
13. Some generalized disease states that may be recognized by signs in the oral cavity are leukemia, vitamin deficiencies, measles, AIDS, and many others.
14. Fordyce's granules are sebaceous glands that develop with no relationship to hair follicles. They are small yellowish spots found on the lips, cheeks and retromolar triangle. They are not a problem and seem to have no real clinical significance.

CHAPTER 2

1. The main cell organelles and their function are the:
   a. Nucleus—control center of cell. Contains DNA and RNA to control function.
   b. Mitochondria—provide energy for cell metabolism.
   c. Endoplasmic reticulum—produces cell product.
   d. Golgi apparatus—packages cell product with a membrane.
   e. Lysosomes—enzyme-filled droplets that scavenge up the dead or unneeded substances within the cell.
   f. Cytoskeleton—microfilaments and microtubules of protein that maintain shape of cells and aid in movements of cilia.
2. Pinocytosis is the process of taking liquids into a cell. The cell membrane is pushed inward until a portion of it is then pinched off, surrounding the liquid to keep it separate from the cytoplasm of the cell.

496

3. Organelles are functioning parts of the cell, while inclusions are passively stored structures, generally not produced by the cell.

4. The cell membrane functions to keep the cytoplasm and organelles within the cell while allowing for molecules or substances to pass in and out of the cell.

5. Epithelium is a covering or lining membrane of the body.

6. Stratified squamous epithelium is the most common epithelium of the body.

7. Epithelial cells arise in the bottom or basal layer, and as that layer multiplies, the cells are pushed up through the various layers until they are shed from the outer layer.

8. Desmosomes are points of modification on the cell membrane at which cells are held together.

9. Glands arise from downgrowths of epithelium into the connective tissue beneath the epithelium.

10. Glands are classified by their presence or absence of ducts, the mechanism by which they secrete their product, the arrangement of their components, and the type of product they produce.

11. The embryonic germ layers are ectoderm, mesoderm, and entoderm. Epithelium comes from all three layers.

12. The outer cell mass of the blastocyst forms the placenta and sacs surrounding the embryo/fetus. The inner cell mass is the group of cells that actually forms the embryo/fetus.

13. The components of general irregular connective tissue are cells such as fibroblasts, macrophages, mesenchymal cells, plasma cells, etc.; ground substance; fibers such as collagen, elastic, and reticular; and intercellular fluid that is a filtrate of blood plasma. Within many connective tissues there may also be nerves, blood vessels, and lymphatics.

14. Cartilage and bone differ in several ways. One is that bone grows only by adding to or taking away from the surface, while cartilage grows by surface addition as well as interstitial growth. They also differ in that bone is calcified and vascular and most cartilage is not.

15. Bone is made hard by the presence of hydroxyapatite crystals.

16. A Haversian system is a vascular system within bone that makes it a vital tissue.

17. In endochondral development you have two epiphyses (end pieces) and a diaphysis (shaft, or middle piece). Between those are blocks of cartilage known as epiphyseal plates that allow for the lengthening of bone.

18. Blood cells are generally divided into red blood cells and white blood cells. The presence or absence of granules in the cells further categorizes the white blood cells.

19. Neutrophils are phagocytes and function in inflammatory responses; eosinophils function in combating allergic reactions and in inflammation; basophils produce histamine to combat allergic reactions; lymphocytes combat infection and function in the immune response; plasma cells come from lymphocytes and also function in immune response; monocytes are macrophages and probably form osteoclasts, which destroy bone and other calcified substances; platelets are not blood cells but remains of the stem cell megakaryocyte and play an important role in blood clotting.

20. Hemoglobin is found in red blood cells and has the ability to carry oxygen to other cells and to carry carbon dioxide away from cells.

21. Three types of muscle tissue are skeletal, which is throughout the body and produces willful movements of the structures to which it is attached; cardiac, which is the muscle of the heart; and smooth, which is found in the digestive tract, lungs, many blood vessels, and other organs of the body.

22. Myofiber—the cell that makes up striated muscle. The cell is as long as the muscle. Myofibril—the subunit of the myofiber, which when grouped together forms the muscle cell. Myofilament—the subunit of actin and myosin, which slide over each other and cause the muscle to contract.

23. The sarcomere is the smallest functional unit of muscle cells. Sarcomeres contain the actin and myosin filaments and by their arrangement cause the striations seen in muscle.

24. Skeletal muscle contracts by a chemical reaction that pulls the actin filaments along the myosin filaments and causes shortening of the sarcomere.

25. The parts of a neuron are the axon, cell body, and dendrite.

26. *Afferent* means "toward" and refers to sensory messages going to the brain. *Efferent* means "away from" and refers to motor messages traveling from the brain to cause muscle contraction or glandular secretion.

27. A myelin sheath is the covering of some nerves and partially controls the speed of the depolarization and the ability for a nerve to repair itself.

28. The myelin sheath helps provide a tube along which the nerve can regrow until it reaches its original location.

29. Nerve impulses travel from dendrite to cell body to axon.

CHAPTER 3

1. The three embryonic periods and their times are:
Period of the ovum—fertilization through week 2.
Period of the embryo—weeks 3 through 8.
Period of the fetus—weeks 9 through 36 or birth.

2. The lips form between the third and sixth embryonic weeks.

3. The buccopharyngeal membrane is the primitive wall between the stomodeum and the foregut. The stomodeum side of the wall forms from ectoderm, while the foregut side of the wall forms from entoderm. It ruptures at about 4 to 4½ weeks.

4. The upper lip is formed by the maxillary processes and the medial nasal processes.

5. The primary palate, from the medial nasal processes and the palatal shelves from the maxillary processes, forms the hard and soft palate. The palate forms from about weeks 6½ to 11.

6. Epithelial rests are remnants of the epithelial covering of the palatal shelves that break down in fusion of the palate. In later life they may form cysts.

7. A cyst is an epithelial-lined, fluid-filled sac, which may grow and push aside teeth if they are nearby.

8. Unilateral cleft lip is lack of migration and then breakdown of the tissue between one maxillary process and one medial nasal process. Bilateral cleft lip happens on both sides. Unilateral cleft palate occurs when one palatal shelf fuses with the nasal septum but not with the other palatal process. Bilateral cleft palate occurs when the palatal shelves and nasal septum do not fuse with each other.

9. Cleft lips form at about 3½ to 6 weeks, and cleft palates from 6½ to 11 weeks.

10. The muscles of mastication, mylohyoid, anterior digastric, tensor tympani, and tensor veli palatini form from the first pharyngeal arch. The malleus and incus bones of the middle ear also form from that arch.

11. The muscles of facial expression arise from the second pharyngeal arch. They are innervated by the VII (facial) nerve, and we know that the VII nerve is the nerve of the second arch.

12. The muscles of the pharynx, larynx, and most of the soft palate form from the fourth and sixth arches.

13. Rathke's pouch is an upward embryologic growth from the roof of the primitive oral cavity. It forms the anterior and intermediate lobe of the pituitary gland at the base of the brain.

14. A lingual thyroid is a red, raised mound of tissue growing up out of the dorsum of the tongue right behind the circumvallate papillae. It develops because the thyroglossal duct fails to form, and the thyroid gland therefore grows where it originated and not down in the neck where it migrated.

15. The upper lip develops as a result of migration of connective tissue, which fills in the groove between the two structures. Palates form from a breakdown of the epithelium of the palatal shelves and a fusion of the underlying connective tissue of both shelves.

CHAPTER 4

1. The dental lamina is the first sign of tooth development, and it is first seen during the sixth embryonic week.
2. Oral epithelium is an example of stratified squamous epithelium.
3. The enamel organ comes from ectoderm.
4. The three stages of the enamel organ are:
   • Bud stage—when localized thickening begins in dental lamina and a bloblike cluster of cells bulges into the connective tissue deep to the dental lamina
   • Cap stage—when the deep part of the bud begins to develop a depression on the surface, and we begin to see a dental papilla condensing beneath it; three layers present
   • Bell stage—begins to take on the shape of the future tooth on the deep surface of the organ; four layers present
5. Ectodermal dysplasia is a developmental problem affecting structures that arise from ectoderm. The significance of the origin of the enamel organ is that any developmental problem that affects ectodermally derived structures will affect enamel. Other structures affected are hair, nails, sweat glands, sebaceous glands, and salivary glands.

6. The four layers of the bell stage and their function are:
   • Outer enamel epithelium—protects and later aids in nourishment
   • Inner enamel epithelium—forms ameloblasts, which form enamel
   • Stellate reticulum—protection and nourishment
   • Stratum intermedium—nourishment of ameloblasts from inner enamel epithelium; also produces protein for possible use by ameloblasts and receives secretions from ameloblasts

7. Following are the definitions and roles of:
   • Successional lamina—a budding off of the dental lamina; develops the enamel organs of the 20 succedaneous permanent teeth
   • Vestibular lamina—the thickening of oral tissue facial to the dental lamina; splits and forms the vestibular or mucobuccal mucolabial fold.
   • Dental papilla—mesodermal condensation of cells next to the inner enamel epithelium; eventually forms the dentin and pulp of the tooth
   • Dental sac—surrounds part of the dental papilla and part of the outer enamel epithelium; forms cementum, the periodontal ligament, and part of the alveolar bone.

CHAPTER 5

1. IEE cells elongate and increase their cellular organelles.
2. Preameloblasts continue an increase in their organelles, and the nucleus shifts from the middle of the cell toward the stratum intermedium to be closer to the new pathway of nutrients. Then they are considered ameloblasts.

3. It is the early dentinal tissue, the dental papilla, that controls the form the enamel organ will take. The dental papilla initiates the change in the IEE cell that causes it to become a preameloblast. From that time forward, the changes in dentin influence enamel, and the control seems to switch back and forth. If it goes wrong at any one point, all growth in that area of enamel and dentin may be affected.

4. If enamel crystals do not grow to full size, the enamel will be less dense or hypocalcified.

5. The crystals in the wide upper end of the keyhole are aligned parallel to the long axis, while the crystals in the narrow bottom part of the keyhole begin to angle away from the long axis until the lowest ones are almost 60 degrees off the long axis of the rod.

6. Nasmyth's membrane is the protective cuticular layer formed by the reduced enamel epithelium and deposited on the surface of the completed enamel.

7. Enamel lamellae are spaces or cracks between enamel rods formed either by trauma or developmental problems.

8. The three distinct areas of primary dentin are:
   a. Dentinal tubules
   b. Peritubular dentin
   c. Intertubular dentin

9. Secondary dentin has tubules and is about the same in density as the primary dentin. Reparative dentin has few if any tubules and is more dense than secondary dentin.

10. Dead tracts are empty dentinal tubules caused by relatively sudden death of the odontoblasts, and sclerotic or transparent dentin is a filling in of the dentinal tubule as the odontoblastic process retracts or degenerates.

11. As the pulp grows older, its chamber becomes smaller and it becomes more fibrous, whereas the younger pulp is more cellular. The decrease in cells also tends to decrease the reparative potential of the pulp.

12. Pulp stones are calcified areas within or adjacent to the pulp. They may be formed from odontoblasts or more frequently from degenerating cells of the pulp that calcify.

13. Pulp stones have very little affect on the health of the pulp, although they may cause some problems in endodontics.

CHAPTER 6

1. The epithelial root sheath develops from the inner and outer enamel epithelia of the enamel organ.

2. After dentin starts to develop, the epithelial root sheath begins to break up.

3. Epithelial rests are remnants of the epithelial root sheath and may form periodontal cysts in later life.

4. Cells of the dental sac form:
   a. Cementum
   b. Periodontal ligament
   c. Cribriform plate, or alveolar bone proper

5. The two types of cementum are acellular and cellular cementum. Acellular cementum is found in the cervical one third of enamel and at the dentinocemental junction on the other two thirds of the root. Cellular cementum is found in the middle third and increasing in the apical third.

6. Sharpey's fibers are the embedded portion of the periodontal ligament in both alveolar bone proper and cementum.

7. Alveolar bone has compact bone buccally and lingually, cribriform plate plus bundle bone lining the socket, and spongy or cancellous bone between the two.

8. The lamina dura is the radiographic representation of the cribriform plate area. It is a white radiopaque line around the outside of the radiolucent periodontal ligament

space. If it is thickened in one or more teeth, it is an indication of occlusal trauma on that part of the dentition.

9. Gingival fibers support and hold gingiva against the tooth. Transseptal fibers hold the teeth in interproximal contact. The alveolar crest and horizontal fibers of the alveolodental fibers support the tooth horizontally. The oblique fibers of the alveolodental fibers support the tooth against occlusal forces. The apical group of alveolodental fibers resist removing the tooth from the socket. The other groups can also play a role in this. In multirooted teeth, the interradicular fibers perform the function of all of the previously mentioned alveolodental fibers.

10. Mesial drift is the physiologic tendency for teeth to move mesially. With missing teeth and interproximal wear, this can occur more rapidly.

11. Bone resorption is caused by pressure on the bone from the tooth. This pressure reduces the blood flow in the area, and osteoclasts are formed to accomplish this. Apposition is caused by the periodontal fibers that are stretched in tooth movement, placing tension on the bone, which tension causes bone production.

Chapter 7

1. Active eruption is the total life span of the tooth, from the time of crown development until the tooth is lost or the individual dies.

2. The three stages of tooth eruption and their span are:
   a. Preeruptive stage—from the beginning of calcification of the crown until root formation starts
   b. Eruptive stage—from the beginning of root formation until the tooth erupts and comes into contact with the opposing tooth

   c. Posteruptive stage—from the time teeth come into contact with opposing teeth until they are lost or the individual dies.

3. Supraeruption is the eruption of the tooth above the occlusal plane because of loss of the opposing tooth or malalignment of the opposing tooth that allows for this supraeruption.

4. Theories of tooth eruption, and which one is the most likely cause are:
   a. Root elongation
   b. Alveolar bone formation and changes
   c. Periodontal ligament
   d. Vascular pressures in dental tissues
   Active eruption is multifactorial and it is likely that they all have important roles.

5. It is probably caused by digestive enzymes secreted by the reduced enamel epithelium.

6. The positions of permanent teeth to primary teeth in eruption are:
   a. Anterior permanent teeth develop apically and lingually to primary teeth.
   b. Permanent premolars develop between the roots of the primary molars.

7. Ankylosis is the fusion of alveolar bone with cementum in the region of the cervical line. It may cause retained primary teeth. It is treated by breaking the fusion and extracting the tooth.

8. Three causes of retained primary teeth are:
   a. Ankylosis
   b. No permanent successor
   c. Permanent tooth not erupting in normal position

Chapter 8

1. The divisions of the oral mucosa are specialized mucosa, masticatory mucosa, and lining mucosa. Specialized mucosa is found on the dorsum of the tongue. Masticatory mucosa is found in the gingiva and hard palate. Lining mucosa is all other areas.

2. Three variations of stratified squamous

epithelium are nonkeratinized, parakeratinized, and keratinized.

3. Stratum basalis is basically unchanged in all three types of stratified squamous epithelium. Stratum spinosum thickens as you go from nonkeratinized to keratinized. Stratum granulosum is not seen in nonkeratinized and becomes more obvious with keratinization. Stratum corneum has fairly normal cell nuclei in nonkeratinized, shriveled nuclei and decreased numbers of nuclei in parakeratinized, and no nuclei in keratinized. In thick keratinized skin there is also an additional layer, the stratum lucidum, between the granulosum and the corneum.

4. The mobility of the mucosa is determined by the length of the connective tissue ridges and pegs projecting up into the epithelium and by the kind of tissue to which the mucosa is connected to the connective tissue layer. If there is no submucosa the mucosa will be more tightly attached.

5. Changes in color of mucosa are affected by thickness of epithelium and excessive blood flow in the mucosa because of inflammation.

6. In the submucosa we might find nerves, blood vessels, minor salivary glands, fat cells, collagen fibers, and/or elastic fibers.

7. The average depth of the gingival sulcus is about 2 mm (many will be so specific as to quote 1.8 mm).

8. The interdental papilla protects the interproximal areas beneath the contact point and prevents food from packing in between them and causing periodontal disease.

9. The col is the protected area of gingival epithelium immediately apical to the interproximal contact point or area of the teeth. It may be damaged when there is interproximal decay that destroys the contact point or when a tooth is improperly restored without a contact point or area.

10. Normal gingival appearance is described as pink and stippled.

11. The relationship of the attachment epithelium to the tooth in the four stages of passive eruption are:
Stage I—attachment epithelium entirely on enamel
Stage II—attachment epithelium mostly on enamel with part on cementum
Stage III—attachment epithelium extends from the CEJ onto cementum
Stage IV—attachment epithelium is entirely on cementum apical to CEJ

CHAPTER 9

1. The tongue is derived from all three germ layers: ectoderm, mesoderm, and entoderm.

2. Extrinsic muscles originate outside the tongue and end inside, whereas intrinsic muscles begin and end in the tongue.

3. The intrinsic muscles shorten, flatten, and narrow the tongue. The palatoglossus and styloglossus pull the tongue up and back, the hyoglossus pulls the lateral edges down, and the genioglossus either extends the tongue or pulls the tip back.

4. The papillae are:
   a. Circumvallate or vallate—a V-shaped row of large, rounded papillae that separates the anterior two thirds of the tongue from the posterior one third; taste
   b. Fungiform—small, rounded elevations that frequently appear as red spots on the anterior two thirds of the tongue; taste on anterior two thirds of tongue
   c. Filiform—elongated processes that have no taste buds and are simply for general sensation; anterior two thirds of the tongue
   d. Foliate—vertical folds on the lateral border of the tongue two thirds of the way back; taste

5. Most of the cells are supporting cells, while only a few are taste cells.

6. The tongue can become reddened and smooth in conditions such as vitamin defi-

ciencies, and the filiform papillae can get elongated and stained in some inflammatory processes or changes in microorganisms in the oral cavity.

CHAPTER 10

1. Acini are the secretory endpieces in glands. The three types are serous, mucous, and seromucous.
   a. Serous acini have granular apices, and intercellular walls are not easily seen. The nucleus is round and located at the basal end of the cell.
   b. Mucous acini have frothy cytoplasm, and one can see the intercellular walls. Nuclei are flattened against the basal end of the cell.
   c. Seromucous acini have mucous acini with a cap of serous cells on their end. Nuclei of these two cells have the same orientation.
2. A myoepithelial cell is a squid-shaped connective tissue cell that has contractile properties. Myoepithelial cells are spread over the ends of the acini and, with their contractions, help the acini to secrete.
3. Define:
   a. Intercalated ducts—ducts that carry acini secretion into striated intralobular ducts
   b. Striated duct—intralobular secretory ducts that have infoldings of the basal cell membrane and trap mitochondria between the folds, giving a striated appearance to the duct.
   c. Secretory duct—a duct that modifies the secretion of the duct and conserves inorganic ions and water
   d. Excretory duct—a duct that transports the secretions without modifying them
   e. Intralobular duct—duct within the lobule
   f. Interlobular duct—duct between lobules that carries secretions to duct end

4. Serous demilunes are serous cells that sit as a cap on mucous acini.
5. Salivary glands secretion is controlled by the parasympathetic portion of the autonomic nervous system.
6. Amylase is the enzyme found in saliva. It begins the breakdown of long-chain starches into smaller carbohydrate components.
7. Saliva functions to prepare the bolus of food, buffer pH, and play a role in immune functions.

CHAPTER 11

1. There are 22 bones in the skull, excluding the six ossicles of the middle ear.
2. The bones of the skull are subdivided into the eight bones that surround the brain, known as the neurocranium, and the 14 bones that form the face, known as the viscerocranium.
3. Define:
   a. Suture—the joining together of two or more bones
   b. Foramen—a short opening in a bone
   c. Canal—a long, tubelike opening in a bone
   d. Fossa—a shallow depression
   e. Alveolar process—that portion of the mandible and maxilla that forms the sockets for the teeth
4. The hard palate is formed by the palatal processes of the maxillae and the horizontal portion of the palatine bones.
5. a. Coronal suture—frontoparietal suture
   b. Sagittal suture—interparietal suture
   c. Lambdoid suture—parietooccipital suture
6. The largest of the paranasal sinuses is in the body of the maxilla.
7. The area behind the maxillary third molars is the maxillary tuberosity.
8. The mandible is divided into a body, alveolar process, and ramus.

9. Major landmarks of
   a. Maxilla—body and sinus, alveolar process with canine eminence, zygomatic process, frontal process, palatal process with incisive foramen
   b. Mandible—body with mental protuberance, mental foramen, with mylohyoid lines and genial tubercles on the medial side; alveolar process; ramus with the neck of the condyle, condyle, mandibular notch, coronoid process, mandibular foramen, and lingula on medial side

10. Growth of maxilla and mandible:
    a. Maxilla—There is growth in the height and width of the alveolar process as well as the palatal process, but the growth in arch length occurs at the maxillary tuberosity.
    b. Mandible—There is also growth in height and width of body and alveolar process, while the main increase in arch length comes about from the resorption of the anterior ramus of the mandible and apposition on the posterior surface of the ramus.

11. The parts of the sphenoid bone are:
    a. Body
    b. Lesser wing of sphenoid
    c. Greater wing of sphenoid
    d. Pterygoid process
       1. medial pterygoid plate and hamulus
       2. lateral pterygoid plate
       3. pterygoid fossa
    The sphenoid sinus is found in the body of the sphenoid bone.

12. The rim of the orbit is made up equally of parts of the:
    a. Maxilla
    b. Frontal
    c. Zygomatic

13. The lesser wing of the sphenoid divides the anterior from the middle cranial fossa. The petrous temporal bone divides the middle from the posterior cranial fossa.

CHAPTER 12

1. The lower part of the nasal septum is formed from the vomer bone, whereas the upper portion is formed from the perpendicular plate of the ethmoid bone. The anterior end of the nasal septum is formed from the nasal septal cartilage.

2. The lateral wall is formed on the upper portion from the ethmoid bone and the lower portion from the maxilla. Close to the point of union of those two bones is the inferior nasal concha.

3. A meatus is the space underneath the projections of the nasal conchae.

4. Respiratory epithelium functions to trap contaminants entering the nasal cavity and move them out of the nasal cavity.

5. Opening into the:
   a. Inferior meatus—the nasolacrimal duct
   b. Middle meatus—in the hiatus semilunaris, from anterior to posterior, the openings for the frontal sinuses, anterior ethmoid air cells, and maxillary sinus; onto the ethmoid bulla, the opening of the middle ethmoid air cells.
   c. Superior meatus—posterior ethmoid air cells
   d. Sphenoethmoidal recess—sphenoid sinuses

6. Olfactory epithelium is found in the roof of the nasal cavity. It extends down over the superior surface of the superior nasal concha and about 10 mm down the nasal septum.

7. Maxillary sinuses may cause infections because the opening is high in the medial wall and may have small openings, both of which can cause drainage problems. The sinus may dip in between the bent roots of maxillary posterior teeth and make them difficult to extract.

8. A sinus infection may seem to come from teeth because the same nerve that supplies a tooth also supplies a part of the mucosa of

the maxillary sinus. Daily messages go to the brain from the teeth, and then during a sinus infection a message is sent from an infected mucosa of the sinus. The brain is so used to getting messages from the tooth that it interprets the sinus pain as being tooth-originated pain.

Chapter 13

1. In general, the origin is the more fixed part of a muscle, and the insertion is the more movable part. In some muscles these could be reversed.
2. The action of the muscle is to create an action or a function by shortening or tensing.
3. Terms in relation to mandibular movements are:
   a. Elevation—raising the mandible and closing the jaw
   b. Protrusion—moving the mandible forward
   c. Retrusion—moving the mandible posteriorly
   d. Depression—lowering the mandible or opening the mouth
   e. Lateral excursion—forward movement of one condyle; mandible moves laterally
4. The muscles used in creating the above movements are:
   a. Elevation—masseter, temporal, medial pterygoid
   b. Protrusion—both lateral pterygoids together
   c. Retrusion—posterior fibers of temporal and digastric, when infrahyoid muscles are relaxed
   d. Depression—suprahyoids and infrahyoids working together; also the inferior head of the lateral pterygoids
   e. Lateral excursion—lateral pterygoid on one side acting alone
5. The difference in innervation indicates that the anterior belly arose from the first pha-

ryngeal arch, which is innervated by the trigeminal nerve, while the posterior belly arose from the second pharyngeal arch, which is innervated by the facial nerve.
6. The larynx movement is accomplished by contraction of the suprahyoid muscles and the thyrohyoid muscle. There is also help from the pharyngeal constrictors.
7. The internal jugular vein and lymph nodes are found beneath the sternomastoid muscle.
8. Referred pain is pain that originates in one area but is felt in another area. The sternomastoid and trapezius muscles have muscle spasms that are felt in the area of the TMJ.
9. The geniohyoid, sternohyoid, sternothyroid, thyrohyoid, and omohyoid muscles are innervated by cervical nerves.

Chapter 14

1. A synovial cavity is a sac that contains minor amounts of a lubricating fluid. It is interposed between two bones or between muscles and joints and allows the two surfaces to glide over each other without irritation.
2. The TMJ capsule is a collagenous capsule that surrounds the entire joint. It is strengthened on its lateral side by a thickening known as the *temporomandibular ligament*. This ligament prevents the condyle from being displaced too far inferiorly and posteriorly.
3. The two movements of the TMJ are rotating and gliding movements. The rotating movement takes place between the condyle and the disc, while the gliding movement takes place between the disc and the temporal bone. The first few millimeters of jaw opening are purely rotational, whereas the continued opening is rotational and gliding.
4. The posterior superior elastic lamina helps pull the disc posteriorly to its normal posi-

tion from the open position. The lower collagenous lamina prevents the disc from being pulled too far anteriorly and damaging the elastic lamina and causing anterior displacement. The lower head of the lateral pterygoid and some of the upper head pull the condyles forward and cause the jaw to protrude and depress or move into lateral excursion and depress if only contracting on one side. The upper head fibers that are attached to the disc relax their tension in the closing movement and allow for smooth posterior movement in closure.

5. TMJ pain can be caused by referred pain from adjacent muscles that may be in spasm. It may also be caused by arthritis, torn portions of the disc, bruxism, and malocclusion, as well as other possible conditions.

6. TMJ sounds are caused by sudden anterior or posterior movements of the disc as well as separation of the synovial cavities and possible arthritic surfaces rubbing over one another.

7. Disc derangement is the condition when the disc is either trapped or torn so that it does not function properly.

Chapter 15

1. The muscles of facial expression are located in the areas of the neck, scalp, ears, eyes, nose, and mouth.

2. These muscles are innervated by the VII (facial) nerve.

3. The buccinator plays a role in mastication by taking the food that is moved off the occlusal surface into the vestibule and pushing it back up onto the occlusal surfaces to continue to be masticated.

4. The muscles around the oral cavity are:
   a. Levator labii superioris—from the lower rim of the orbit down into the medial part of the upper lip; raises the upper lip as in sneer

   b. Zygomaticus minor—from the cheek at the lateral corner of the eye down and medial into the medial part of the upper lip; pulls the upper lip up and laterally as in smile

   c. Zygomaticus major—from the prominence of the cheek down and forward into the corner of the lip; pulls the corner of the mouth up and laterally as in a broad smile

   d. Levator anguli oris—from just below the infraorbital foramen, down and lateral into the corner of the lip; pulls the upper lip up and medially in a cherubic sort of smile

   e. Depressor labii inferioris—from beneath the depressor anguli oris, up and medial to insert into the midline of the lower lip; pulls the lower lip down as in a pout

   f. Depressor anguli oris—from the inferior border of the mandible below the canines; ascends and converges to insert into the lower corner of the lip; pulls the corner of the mouth down as in a pout or grimace

   g. Buccinator—from the pterygomandibular raphe running forward in the cheek into the corner of the mouth; pulls the corner of the mouth laterally as in flat smile

Chapter 16

1. The palatoglossal and palatopharyngeal muscles narrow the fauces. The palatoglossal originates from the posterolateral hard palate and the anterolateral soft palate. The palatoglossal runs down and forward to insert into the posterolateral tongue, pulling the tongue up and posteriorly, while the palatopharyngeal runs down and inserts into the pharyngeal wall and thyroid cartilage, elevating the pharynx.

2. The palatopharyngeal and salpingopharyngeal muscles elevate the pharynx and are innervated by nerve XI in X. The stylopharyngeal muscle elevates and dilates the pharynx and is innervated by IX.

3. All pharyngeal constrictors insert into the median raphe and are innervated by nerve XI in X. Their origins are:
   a. Superior constrictor—medial pterygoid plate and hamulus, medial mandibular alveolar process, and pterygomandibular raphe
   b. Middle constrictor—from the posterior part of the hyoid bone and stylohyoid ligament
   c. Inferior constrictor—posterior part of the thyroid cartilage of the larynx

4. Nasal speech sounds occur because of an inability to adequately seal off the oral pharynx from the nasal pharynx with the soft palate.

5. The levator veli palatini muscle closes off the oral from the nasal pharynx in speech. It is innervated by the nerve XI in X

6. Sequence of food digestion:
   a. Masticate, mix with saliva, and form bolus
   b. Elevate tongue and move food toward posterior tongue
   c. Elevate soft palate to close off oral from nasal pharynx
   d. Elevate and dilate pharynx
   e. Narrow fauces and seal off oral pharynx from oral cavity
   f. Start pharyngeal constriction from superior to inferior
   g. Move food into esophagus and down about halfway
   h. Allow peristaltic contractions to move food from there

7. Food sometimes seems to get caught halfway down the esophagus because that is where voluntary skeletal muscle ends and involuntary smooth muscle begins. It then waits for peristalsis to move it.

CHAPTER 17

1. Blood enters the right atrium→right ventricle→pulmonary artery→lungs→pulmonary veins→left atrium→left ventricle→aorta→common iliac arteries→external iliac arteries→femoral arteries→leg→femoral veins→external iliac veins→common iliac veins→inferior vena cava→right atrium of heart.

2. Blood leaves the heart and enters the aorta. On the right side, the common carotid artery and the right subclavian artery come off of the brachiocephalic artery. On the left, the common carotid artery arises directly from the aortic arch. Just below the larynx, the common carotid splits into external and internal carotid arteries. The external supplies the teeth and oral cavity.

3. The common carotid artery divides into external and internal carotids.

4. Teeth and the oral cavity are supplied by the lingual and maxillary arteries.

5. Blood supply to the muscles of mastication comes off of the maxillary artery in the infratemporal fossa.

6. Blood supply to all areas of oral cavity:
   a. Lingual—to the tongue and mucosal floor of the mouth
   b. Inferior alveolar and mental—to the lower teeth and lower lip mucosa and gingiva
   c. Posterior superior alveolar—To the maxillary molars and probably the premolars, as well as the maxillary sinus
   d. Anterior superior alveolar—to the maxillary anterior teeth
   e. Infraorbital—to the mucosa and gingiva of the upper lip
   f. Greater and lesser palatine arteries—to the hard and soft palates, respectively
   g. Buccal artery—To the mucosa of the cheek and most buccal gingiva

7. The major vein that drains most of the head and neck is the internal jugular vein.

8. The pterygoid plexus of veins lies just posterior to the maxillary tuberosity; it may be injured in a posterior superior alveolar injection if care is not taken. If injury occurs, a hematoma would result, causing some discomfort to the patient.

9. Blood in the internal jugular system joins with the subclavian vein to form the brachiocephalic vein, which flows into the superior vena cava and into the right atrium. Blood in the external jugular vein goes to the subclavian vein and into the brachiocephalic vein, the superior vena cava and on to the heart.

10. If the anterior retromandibular vein is missing, the external jugular vein will be larger than usual. If the posterior retromandibular vein is missing the internal jugular will be larger than normal and the external jugular will be smaller than normal.

CHAPTER 18

1. The major salivary glands and their ducts are:
   a. Parotid—opens into the buccal vestibule opposite the maxillary second molar
   b. Submandibular—Opens onto the sublingual caruncle
   c. Sublingual—opens onto the sublingual caruncle and sublingual fold in the floor of the mouth
   All of these glands produce saliva to help prepare the bolus of food and begin breakdown of starches with their production of amylase.

2. The minor salivary glands and their ducts are:
   a. Labial—mucosa of the lip; many openings
   b. Buccal—cheeks; many openings
   c. Palatine—soft palate and posterolateral hard palate; many openings
   d. Glossopalatine—palatoglossal fold; many ducts

e. Anterior lingual glands—underside of the anterior tongue; many ducts
   f. Glands of von Ebner—under the vallate papillae on the tongue; many ducts
   g. Posterior lingual glands—mixed with lingual tonsils on the posterior one third of the tongue; many ducts
   Their function is to secrete minor amounts of saliva to keep mucosal surfaces moist.

3. Saliva mixes with food to produce a bolus of food for ease in swallowing. It also lubricates the mucosa and makes speech and swallowing easier. It buffers the pH and contains other substances which can control the carious process.

CHAPTER 19

1. The subdivisions of the nervous system are:
   Central nervous system (brain and spinal cord)
   Peripheral nervous system (spinal nerves, cranial nerves, and autonomic motor system)

2. The dorsal root and dorsal root ganglion, the ventral root, and the dorsal and ventral primary rami are the parts of a spinal nerve. The two things seen in cross section of the spinal cord are the centrally placed gray matter and the peripherally placed white matter.

3. Stimulation of sympathetic nervous system results in increased heart and respiratory rate, shutdown of blood supply to the viscera, dilation of the pupil of the eye, dryness of the mouth, and clammy skin.

4. Stimulation of the parasympathetic nervous system results in decreased heart and respiratory rate, a significant increase to the blood supply of the viscera, and stimulation of most glands of the body.

5. The cranial nerves and their functions are:
   I—smell
   II—vision

III—eye movements, pupil constriction, and lens accommodation
IV—eye movements
V—sensory supply to the anterior head and the oral cavity and motor supply to the muscles of mastication and other muscles
VI—eye movements
VII—muscles of facial expression, taste to the tongue, and parasympathetic innervation to the salivary glands
VIII—hearing and equilibrium
IX—taste and general sensation to the posterior one third of the tongue, sensory innervation to the pharynx, motor innervation to the stylopharyngeal muscle, and parasympathetic innervation to the salivary gland
X—taste and sensation to the root of the tongue and epiglottis, motor innervation to the pharynx, larynx, and soft palate, motor innervation to the cardiac muscle and smooth muscle of the respiratory and GI systems, and glandular supply to most glands below the neck
XI—motor innervation to the pharynx, larynx, soft palate, trapezius, and sternocleidomastoid
XII—motor supply to the intrinsic and extrinsic tongue muscles, except the palatoglossus

6. Nerves III, VII, IX, and X, as well as sacral 2-4, carry parasympathetic fibers.
7. Nerve supply to the teeth:
Mandibular teeth—inferior alveolar nerve
Maxillary anteriors—anterior superior alveolar
Maxillary premolars and mesiobuccal root of the maxillary first molar—middle superior alveolar
Maxillary molars, except for the mesiobuccal root of the first molar—posterior superior alveolar
8. Nerve supply to the oral mucosa:
Inferior alveolar nerve (mental branch)—gingiva, mucosa of lower lip

Buccal nerve—mucosa of cheek and most buccal gingiva
Lingual nerve—mandibular lingual gingiva, mucosa of the floor of the mouth, and the epithelial anterior two thirds of tongue
Posterior superior alveolar nerve—posterior maxillary buccal gingiva
Nasopalatine nerve—lingual gingiva of the maxillary central and lateral incisors
Greater palatine nerve—hard palate and the maxillary lingual gingiva
Lesser palatine nerve—soft palate
IX nerve—posterior one third of the tongue
Infraorbital nerve—maxillary labial mucosa and gingiva

9. Nerve supply to major salivary glands:
Submandibular and sublingual glands—VII nerve→chorda tympani→runs in lingual nerve→submandibular ganglion→to glands
Parotid gland—IX nerve→lesser petrosal nerve→otic ganglion→auriculotemporal nerve→parotid gland
10. Taste to the anterior two thirds of the tongue is from nerve VII via the chorda tympani→lingual nerve
11. The submandibular and sublingual salivary glands and the lacrimal gland of the eye would have their functions affected if the seventh cranial nerve was damaged.
12. If the parotid gland had to be removed, the seventh (facial) nerve might be affected, and there could be loss of function of the muscles of facial expression.

CHAPTER 20

1. Lymph nodes aid in combating infection through the production of lymphocytes.
2. The major groups of nodes in the head and neck are:
   a. Submental
   b. Submandibular

c. Upper deep cervical
d. Lower deep cervical
e. Retropharyngeal
f. Parotid or preauricular
g. Occipital

3. The structures that drain primarily into groups are:
   a. Submental—the mandibular incisors, the tip of the tongue, the lower lip, and the chin
   b. Submandibular—the rest of mandibular and maxillary teeth except, generally, the third molars; the face, the maxillary sinus, most of the tongue, the anterior nasal cavity, and the submental nodes
   c. Upper deep cervical—the third molars, the posterior nasal cavity, the root of the tongue, the retropharyngeal nodes, the parotid nodes, and the submandibular nodes
   d. Lower deep cervical—the upper deep cervical nodes and the occipital nodes
   e. Retropharyngeal—the posterior throat wall and possibly some of the posterior nasal cavity
   f. Parotid or preauricular—the parotid gland and the anterior area of the ear
   g. Occipital—behind the ear and the occipital region

4. Fascial spaces are potential spaces between muscle layers that interconnect with one another and through which infections can spread.

5. Fascial space infections may eventually end in the posterior mediastinum and may be fatal.

6. Submental space infections come from lingual abscesses of mandibular molars.

7. Swellings below the eye generally come from a periapical infection of the maxillary canine, which breaks out of the bone.

8. The upper deep cervical nodes are the first group noticed in a throat infection.

CHAPTER 21

1. The cervical line separates the enamel from the cementum of the tooth.

2. If a tooth is not completely erupted, that part of the anatomic crown that is still under the gum is considered the clinical root. The clinical root is any part of the tooth as yet unerupted under the gum, no matter what part of the tooth it is.

3. Trifurcated is three rooted, and bifurcated is two rooted.

4. Upper

5. Dentin

6. Enamel

7. Pulp

8. Pulp, dentin, and cellular cementum

9. Cementum

10. Pulp

11. The pulp cavity is divided into the pulp chamber and the pulp canal.

12. The pulp horn is part of the pulp chamber.

13. The pulp tissue comprises blood vessels (arteries and veins), lymph vessels, connective tissues, nerve tissue, and odontoblasts.

14. Two

15. The alveolar process is that part of the maxillary bone that forms the bony sockets that hold the roots of the teeth. One of these bony sockets is called an alveolus.

16. Clinical

17. Enamel, 96%; dentin, 70%; cementum 45% to 55%

18. The more inorganic material there is in the tooth tissue, the harder the tooth tissue.

19. The incisors cut, the canines hold and tear, the premolars help hold and help grind, and the molars crush or grind the food. The more cusps a tooth has, the more it functions as a grinding tool rather than a holding tool. The incisors do not have cusps but sharp edges, which function to cut rather than hold or crush food.

20. The canines are the longest teeth in the mouth because they have the longest roots and the longest crowns. The maxillary canines are usually longer than the mandibular canines.
21. The term *premolar* is more accurate than the term *bicuspid* because some premolars have three cusps instead of two, as implied by the prefix bi- in the term bicuspid.
22. The many broad cusps of molars function as one set of gears interlocking with another set of gears to crush or pulverize.
23. There are 8 premolars and 12 molars.
24. Five: occlusal, buccal, mesial, distal, and lingual.
25. The mesial is closest to the midline, and the distal is farther from the midline.
26. Anterior teeth have an incisal edge.
27. A line angle is a place on the tooth where two surfaces meet. The anterior line angles are: distolabial, mesiolabial, distolingual, mesiolingual, linguoincisal, and labioincisal; the posterior line angles are: distobuccal, mesiobuccal, distolingual, mesiolingual, distoocclusal, mesioocclusal, buccoocclusal, and linguoocclusal.
28. A point angle is a place on the tooth where three surfaces meet.
29. Four
30. Lingual fossa
31. Tubercle
32. Pit
33. A tubercle is a small elevation of enamel on the crown of a tooth. A cusp is a much larger mound on the crown that makes up a major division of its occlusal or incisal surface.
34. Items a, b, c, f, and h are concave; d, e, and g are convex.
35. A developmental groove separates the primary parts of a crown or root. The deepest part of a developmental groove ends in a pit.
36. Distal, occlusal, and lingual

37. Four lobes (three facial, and one lingual)
38. The triangular ridge of the buccal cusp is the lingual ridge of the buccal cusp; the triangular ridge of the lingual cusp is the buccal ridge of the lingual cusp.
39. c
40. d
41. a
42. Three

CHAPTER 22

1. The interproximal spaces are normally filled with gingival tissue called papillary gingiva or interdental papilla. If this is missing, the space is filled with a void called a cervical or gingival embrasure.
2. The embrasures are facial, lingual, incisal, occlusal, and gingival. They allow for food to be deflected away from the teeth and not forced into the contact area between the teeth. The gingival embrasure, also called the cervical embrasure, is not present if the interproximal space is occupied by gingiva.
3. Anterior teeth have a greater curvature of the cementoenamel junction (CEJ), and the mesial curvature of a tooth is greater than the distal.
4. Cervical line and CEJ
5. A coarse, fibrous diet composed of fruits, whole grains, uncooked vegetables, and nuts offers mechanical stimulation of the gingival tissues. This massage and friction not only help clean the teeth and gums from bacteria but also help stimulate the gingival tissues. A soft diet such as mashed potatoes, pudding, ice cream, and scrambled eggs does not offer enough frictional massage. People who deny themselves fibrous foods end up with puffy, bleeding, edematous gums, resulting in periodontal disease.
6. An overhanging restoration causes food

and debris to be trapped between the restoration and the gum tissue. This results in a buildup of bacteria that can either attack the gum tissue or the tooth, depending on the type of bacteria. Either caries, periodontal disease, or both are the result.

7. An open contact between two teeth allows food to pack between the teeth, which can cause gingival tissues to be chronically inflamed and eventually result in bone destruction and periodontal disease. If, however, the space is the size of a diastema, which is relatively large, it is possible that food impaction may not occur. The food would have enough space to slide through the diastema without impacting.

8. A contact point refers to where the occlusal cusp of one tooth hits the occlusal portion of a tooth in the opposing arch (e.g., an upper tooth hitting a lower tooth or vice versa). A contact area is on the mesial or distal surface of a tooth where one tooth touches the tooth immediately next to it within the same arch. The mesial contact area of the lower first premolar touches the distal contact area of the lower canine.

9. The interproximal space distal to the upper first molar is the most likely to create food impaction because the contact area between the distal surface of the upper first molar and the mesial surface of the upper second molar is displaced the most, resulting in a long vertical cervical interproximal space. This space would be much harder to clean than either of the other two. A large edentulous area does not usually allow food impaction anyway.

10. a. a
    b. a
    c. a
    d. b

11. b. They are interchangeable terms and mean the same thing.

12. e

CHAPTER 23

1. The primary dentition has 20 teeth, and the secondary dentition has 32 teeth.
2. The maxillary and mandibular arches each comprise 10 deciduous or 16 permanent teeth.
3. There are four quadrants: upper right, upper left, lower right, and lower left.
4. No, only a permanent tooth can be a succedaneous tooth because by definition a succedaneous tooth is a permanent tooth that succeeds or replaces a deciduous tooth.
5. All the maxillary and mandibular permanent molars. All other permanent teeth are succedaneous.
6. Yes
7. Mixed
8. Three—primary, secondary, and mixed.
9. a. 3—Permanent maxillary right first molar
       5—Permanent maxillary right first premolar
       19—Permanent mandibular left first molar
       28—Permanent mandibular right first premolar
       32—Permanent mandibular right third molar
       A—Primary maxillary right second molar
       E—Primary maxillary right central
       J—Primary maxillary left second molar
       M—Primary mandibular left canine
       S—Primary mandibular right first molar
10. a. F
    b. S
    c. C
    d. 4
    e. 25
11. a. Permanent maxillary left third molar
    b. Primary maxillary right second molar
    c. Permanent maxillary left central
    d. Permanent maxillary right first molar

12. a. 16
    b. A
    c. 9
    d. 3
13. Palmer—6⌐
    Universal—30
    FDI—46
14. a. Universal—Permanent maxillary right central
    b. Palmer—Permanent maxillary right third molar
    c. Universal—Primary maxillary right central
    d. Palmer—Permanent maxillary right central
    e. FDI—Permanent maxillary right central, or Universal—Permanent maxillary left canine
    f. FDI—Permanent maxillary right third molar, or Universal—Permanent mandibular left second molar

CHAPTER 24

1. F
2. c
3. The joining of two lobes of a tooth
4. Developmental lobes
5. Lingual lobe
6. Lobe of Carabelli
7. The deciduous first molars usually erupt before the canines.
8. a
9. Mandibular first molars usually erupt before the maxillary first molars. The central incisors sometimes erupt before the molars but more often do not.
10. F
11. b
12. If a deciduous molar is lost, especially a second molar, the permanent first molar will move mesially into the space once occupied by the deciduous tooth. Thus less

space is left for the eruption of the permanent second premolar. The second premolar then could erupt out of alignment or be blocked out entirely.
13. Mesial drift is associated with all permanent molars. It is a phenomenon whereby the molars have a tendency to move in a mesial direction toward the midline.
14. c
15. Mamelons
16. 5
17. Mixed dentition with the deciduous mandibular second molars and/or maxillary canines still present; or permanent dentition with all the deciduous teeth replaced by their succedaneous replacements and first molars and possibly second molars present
18. The period of primary dentition ends when the first permanent tooth erupts; this usually is a first permanent molar or a central incisor.
19. Deciduous mandibular canines and first and second molars; deciduous maxillary canines and first and second molars
20. When the last deciduous tooth is lost and only permanent teeth remain
21. F
22. T
23. T
24. T
25. a. From birth to 16 years to be completely safe
    b. From the third or fourth month of fetal life to birth (Tetracycline is such a drug and its package insert states such a warning precaution.)

CHAPTER 25

1. The horizontal alignment of teeth is affected by the balance of forces from the tongue pushing the teeth out and the lips and cheeks holding the teeth in. It can also

be affected if one or more teeth are missing genetically; by the pattern and sequence of eruption; by the presence or absence of diastemas, primate spaces, or leeway spaces; or by the fact that one or more teeth may be missing because of impaction, delayed eruption or improper positioning in eruption. It is not uncommon for the space held for a permanent tooth to be decreased because of decay or because of the premature loss of a deciduous tooth. Horizontal alignment changes constantly on account of changing the balance of forces within the mouth: the premature loss of permanent teeth, bone support, and opposing dentition or adjacent tooth structure as occurs with decay or trauma.

2. The tongue, cheek, and lip muscles affect the alignment of the teeth.

3. The curve of Wilson can be seen from the buccal of one side to the buccal of another. The curve of Spee rises in an anterior to posterior direction.

4. a. Open bite—space left between the teeth when the jaws close

   b. Over bite—extension of the incisal ridges of the maxillary anterior teeth below the incisal edges of the lower anterior teeth

   c. Overjet—condition in which the incisal ridges or facial cusps or the maxillary teeth extend facially from the incisal ridges or cusps of the mandibular teeth

   d. Centric occlusion—maximum intercuspation of the teeth when the jaws are closed

   e. Working side—the side to which the mandible is moved

   f. Balancing side—the side where the buccal cusps of mandibular teeth are located directly under the lingual cusps of the maxillary teeth when the jaw is moved toward the opposite side

5. Class II

6. Class I

7. The mandibular molars are situated more mesially than their maxillary counterparts.

8. a

9. All influence occlusion.

10. Elements of ideal occlusion:

    a. The maxillary and mandibular bones are in proper relationship so that the teeth occlude in a class I relationship.

    b. The condyles of the mandible are in their most favorable location within the glenoid fossae.

    c. Muscles of the face and jaws are in harmony with the bones in the class I relationship.

    d. Occlusion of the teeth is most stable when they interlock.

    e. Molars and canines are in a class I occlusal relationship.

    f. The curve of Spee is fairly flat.

    g. The teeth have good, tight proximal contacts with no spaces between teeth.

    h. There are no rotated, tipped, extruded, or missing teeth.

    i. The upper and lower arches are symmetrical and well formed.

    j. The teeth have a slight mesial tip in that their occluding surfaces are more mesial than their gingival surfaces.

    k. The incisors flair labially, and the rest of the teeth flair lingually.

    l. The maxillary first molar is stolarized by touching the mandibular second molar, which causes it to have a more mesial tip.

11. Some differentiating features of primitive occlusions were:

    a. Primitive people had flat occlusions because of severe attrition.

    b. They had little or no overbite for the same reason, and the incisors were severely abraded.

    c. There was a slight loss of vertical dimension caused by occlusal wear.

    d. There was a smaller overall mesial-to-distal arch length caused by interproximal wear.

e. There were fewer impacted teeth because there was more room for third molar eruption.

f. There was a tendency toward mandibular advancement and an edge-to-edge bite of the anterior teeth.

12. The eruption of the primary teeth.

13. The eruption of the primary molars.

14. The relationship of the cusps of the molars and/or premolars of one jaw with those of the opposing jaw when the teeth occlude.

15. Flush terminal plane.

CHAPTER 26

1. An anomaly is something that deviates noticeably from that which is ordinary.

2. Some extrinsic factors are physical or chemical trauma, biologic agents such as viruses, bacteria, or nutritional deficiencies. Some intrinsic factors are heredity, metabolic dysfunction, and genetic mutations.

3. Factors originating from heredity are determined by the individual's genetic makeup, which is inherited from the individual's parents. These inherited characteristics may or may not show up at birth. Sometimes they show up years later. Congenital factors occur at birth. They may or may not be the result of heredity.

4. Hyperdontia means having more teeth than usual, as opposed to anodontia, which means having no teeth.

5. An odontoma is a collection of calcified dental tissues such as a mixture of enamel, dentin, cementum, and/or pulp. This accumulation may or may not resemble a tooth. Its composition varies in the amount of the above tissues.

6. Gemination occurs when a single tooth germ tries to divide itself into two teeth by splitting one tooth germ. Fusion occurs when two separate tooth germs unite to form one tooth.

7. Congenital syphilis is the cause of Hutchinson's incisors and mulberry molars. It is caused by the mother's being infected with syphilis before the baby is born.

8. Amelogenesis imperfecta is a hereditary developmental anomaly that affects the calcification of enamel. The enamel is discolored, very thin, and easily fractured. Dentinogenesis imperfecta is also a hereditary developmental anomaly, but it affects the dentin rather than the enamel. The dentin becomes unusually translucent and discolored and continues to fill the pulp chamber until it completely obliterates the pulp chamber and root canals.

9. Tetracycline staining is a yellowish, brownish, or grayish dental stain that occurs because the pregnant mother or young child takes the antibiotic tetracycline during the developmental stage of tooth formation.

10. Mottled enamel is a form of enamel fluorosis that discolors the teeth. The teeth have white spots, opaque areas, and in severe cases, brownish blotches or striations that badly discolor the teeth. It is caused by too much fluoride in the tooth structure during tooth formation.

11. Familial tendency occurs when a trait (anomaly, good or bad characteristics, possibly hereditary tendency) occurs more frequently in one family generation after generation than that trait occurs in the general population.

12. Third molars

13. Upper (90% of supernumerary teeth occur in the maxilla.)

14. f

CHAPTER 27

1. b, c, and d

2. a

3. c and d

4. a, b, and c

5. a. Rete peg formation is the irregular binding of the epithelium to the bone by collagen fibers. These collagen fibers connect the epithelium and the underlining connective tissue, which results in a dimpled effect to the attached gingiva because of the spacing of the attaching fibers.
    b. Stratified squamous epithelium is the most common multiple-layered epithelium. It is composed of the following layers of epithelia: stratum corneum, stratum granulosum, stratum spinosum, and stratum basale.
6. d
7. See Fig. 27-2.
8. T
9. F
10. F
11. T
12. T

CHAPTER 28

1. i
2. All will happen.
3. If the nerve of a tooth becomes inflamed it can cause sensitivity to hot and/or cold, and pain upon biting. The resulting edema within the root canal can cause pressure upon the vein that drains the tooth. This can result in an obstruction of arterial blood and eventual death of the nerve because of oxygen deprivation.
4. The following are the pathologic situations that could be present in Fig. 28-6:
    a. A periodontal involvement on the mesial and distal surfaces of the maxillary first molar
    b. Extrusion, tipping, and resulting occlusal interferences of the maxillary first molar
    c. Recession of the gingiva as a result of the extrusion of the maxillary first molar

    d. Occlusal trauma from premature occlusal contacts as a result of the maxillary first molar tipping and extruding, the maxillary second molar moving forward, and the mandibular second molar tipping and or moving forward
    e. Lateral interferences, balancing and working interferences, and protrusive interferences for the same reasons as above
    f. Fracture and breakage of the molars because of premature occlusal contacts
    g. Temporomandibular joint dysfunction, muscle spasms, and headaches from trying to avoid the occlusal interferences
    h. Periodontal and pulpal abscesses
5. d
6. e
7. e
8. d

CHAPTER 29

1. Maxillary incisors
2. Central incisors
3. Mandibular centrals and mandibular laterals—the centrals are almost identical and the laterals are very similar to the centrals (the laterals are wider mesiodistally).
4. Mesial
5. Maxillary
6. Distal
7. Mandibular
8. Mandibular lateral
9. Maxillary
10. Inside
11. Mesial
12. Maxillary first premolars
13. Mandibular second premolar
14. Maxillary first premolar
15. First
16. Distal
17. Mesiolingual
18. Second

19. First
20. Mandibular first molar
21. a
22. b
23. b

Chapter 30

1. a
2. d
3. c
4. d
5. c
6. c
7. a
8. c
9. b
10. b
11. b
12. d
13. d
14. d
15. d
16. a
17. d
18. d
19. b
20. b

Chapter 31

1. d
2. c
3. b
4. d
5. b
6. d
7. canine eminence
8. T
9. F
10. F

Chapter 32

1. b
2. b
3. d
4. a
5. a
6. a
7. a
8. b
9. a
10. c
11. b
12. c
13. c
14. b
15. a
16. d
17. T
18. F
19. F
20. T

Chapter 33 — Part A

1. Mesiolingual cusp
2. Distobuccal and mesiolingual cusps
3. Fifth cusp (also called the cusp of Carabelli)
4. Distolingual cusp
5. Mesiolingual cusp
6. Mesiolingual, mesiobuccal, and distobuccal cusps
7. yes
8. no
9. no
10. c
11. c
12. Mesiobuccal root, because it can have two root canals
13. b
14. a
15. The lingual cusp ridge of the distobuccal

cusp and the distolingual cusp ridge of the mesiolingual cusp

16. This tooth would most likely be a maxillary right first molar; but from this very limited single view it is difficult to see the fifth cusp. It therefore, could also be a maxillary right second molar. The only thing we can tell for sure is that it is a maxillary right molar.
17. b
18. c
19. a, b, d
20. c. These three things are more common in third molars: fused roots, dilacerated roots, and more than or less than the usual three roots.

CHAPTER 33 — PART B

1. b
2. c
3. b
4. b
5. c
6. c
7. d
8. c
9. b
10. b
11. c
12. b
13. Distal—usually found on the first molars
14. e
15. d

CHAPTER 34

1. Deciduous teeth and primary teeth
2. *Exfoliation* means the shedding of baby teeth. It occurs during the process of the permanent teeth's eruption when pressure is placed on the roots of the deciduous teeth. This triggers a response within the body to resorb the roots of the baby teeth.
3. There are 20 deciduous teeth: 8 molars, 8 incisors, 4 canines, and no premolars.
4. a. 8-12 months
   b. 6-8 months
   c. 16-22 months
   d. 13-19 months
5. Mandibular
6. See p. 463
7. Facial or buccocervical ridge
8. b
9. The deciduous maxillary first molar does not resemble a permanent molar or premolar. It has only two major cusps, a buccal and a lingual, but its major characteristic is its extremely developed buccocervical ridge. The deciduous maxillary second molar is a smaller version of the permanent maxillary first molar but with a buccocervical ridge. The deciduous mandibular first molar does not resemble a permanent molar or premolar. The crown tapers distally. Its major characteristic is its extreme buccocervical ridge. The deciduous mandibular second molar has five cusps, and all three buccal cusps are about equal in size. It resembles the permanent first molar except that it is smaller and it constricts at the cervix of the crown.
10. Summarize in your own words answer number six above.
11. d
12. a
13. False
14. True
15. False
16. True
17. True
18. False

Unit Test Answers

UNITS I AND II

1. b
2. c
3. c
4. d
5. c
6. d
7. c
8. b
9. d
10. f
11. b
12. b
13. b
14. c
15. a
16. e—None of the above. It is transitional.
17. b
18. b
19. e
20. b
21. b
22. c
23. b
24. d
25. d
26. b
27. b
28. b
29. c
30. c
31. a
32. b
33. c
34. e
35. e
36. d
37. d
38. d
39. e
40. c
41. c
42. a
43. c
44. d
45. b
46. a
47. a
48. c
49. b
50. a
51. d
52. e—None of the above. They develop posterior teeth.
53. c
54. c
55. c
56. c
57. a
58. d
59. e—None of the above. It is the hyoglossus.
60. b
61. d
62. c
63. d
64. d
65. c

UNIT III

1. e—None of the above. There are 22 bones.
2. f
3. f
4. e—None of the above. It is in body of mandible.

5. d
6. f
7. c
8. b
9. c
10. d
11. b
12. d
13. d
14. a
15. e
16. f
17. d
18. d
19. a
20. c
21. b
22. c
23. d
24. c
25. d
26. d
27. b
28. c
29. c
30. a
31. a
32. b
33. c
34. e—None of the above. The buccinator does it.
35. b
36. c
37. d
38. e
39. e
40. d
41. a
42. d
43. b
44. c
45. e
46. f—None of the above. The internal carotid artery has no branches in the neck.
47. d

48. b
49. f
50. b
51. a
52. d
53. b
54. d
55. e
56. c
57. d
58. d
59. d
60. e—None of the above. It is the anterior superior alveolar.
61. d
62. e
63. b
64. e
65. e
66. b
67. b
68. d
69. d
70. d

UNIT IV

1. b
2. a
3. d
4. b
5. d
6. b
7. d
8. d
9. b
10. a
11. e
12. e
13. a
14. b
15. b
16. c

17. c
18. c
19. a
20. c
21. c
22. a
23. d
24. b
25. b
26. c
27. b
28. d
29. d
30. b
31. c
32. b

33. a
34. d
35. a
36. c
37. b
38. b
39. b
40. e
41. e
42. f
43. f
44. a
45. b
46. d

Appendix

Wheeler RC: *A textbook of dental anatomy and physiology,* ed 4, Philadelphia, 1965, WB Saunders Co.

Average Permanent Teeth Dimensions as Recorded by Dr. Russell C. Wheeler

	Length of crown	Length of root	Mesio-distal diameter of crown*	Mesio-distal diameter at cervix	Labio- or bucco-lingual diameter	Labio- or bucco-lingual diameter at cervix	Curvature of cervical line (mesial)	Curvature of cervical line (distal)
Maxillary teeth								
Central incisor	10.5	13.0	8.5	7.0	7.0	6.0	3.5	2.5
Lateral incisor	9.0	13.0	6.5	5.0	6.0	5.0	3.0	2.0
Canine	10.0	17.0	7.5	5.5	8.0	7.0	2.5	1.5
First premolar	8.5	14.0	7.0	5.0	9.0	8.0	1.0	0.0
Second premolar	8.5	14.0	7.0	5.0	9.0	8.0	1.0	0.0
First molar	7.5	b l 12 13	10.0	8.0	11.0	10.0	1.0	0.0
Second molar	7.0	b l 11 12	9.0	7.0	11.0	10.0	1.0	0.0
Third molar	6.5	11.0	8.5	6.5	10.0	9.5	1.0	0.0
Mandibular teeth								
Central incisor	9.0†	12.5	5.0	3.5	6.0	5.3	3.0	2.0
Lateral incisor	9.5†	14.0	5.5	4.0	6.5	5.8	3.0	2.0
Canine	11.0	16.0	7.0	5.5	7.5	7.0	2.5	1.0
First premolar	8.5	14.0	7.0	5.0	7.5	6.5	1.0	0.0
Second premolar	8.0	14.5	7.0	5.0	8.0	7.0	1.0	0.0
First molar	7.5	14.0	11.0	9.0	10.5	9.0	1.0	0.0
Second molar	7.0	13.0	10.5	8.0	10.0	9.0	1.0	0.0
Third molar	7.0	11.0	10.0	7.5	9.5	9.0	1.0	0.0

*The sum of the mesiodistal diameters, both right and left, which gives the arch length, is maxillary 128 mm, mandibular 126 mm.

†Lingual measurement is approximately 0.5 mm longer.

Nerve Supply of Oral Cavity

Nerve	Mucosa	Teeth	Sinus
Maxillary division (V₂)			
Posterior superior alveolar	Buccal; maxillary gingiva	Maxillary molars	Maxillary sinus
Middle superior alveolar	—	Maxillary premolars and mesiobuccal root of first molar	Maxillary sinus
Anterior superior alveolar	Labial gingiva of maxilla	Maxillary anteriors	—
Infraorbital (superior labial)	Labial gingiva of maxilla	—	—
Nasopalatine	Lingual gingiva of maxillary incisors	—	—
Descending palatine			
Greater palatine	All hard palate except lingual gingiva of maxillary incisors	—	—
Lesser palatine	Soft palate	—	—
Mandibular division (V₃)			
Inferior alveolar	—	All mandibular teeth	—
Mental	Facial gingivae from mandibular premolar to central incisor, mucosa and skin of lower lip	—	—
Lingual	All mandibular lingual gingivae, floor of mouth, and anterior two thirds of tongue	—	—
Buccal	Cheek and mandibular buccal gingivae from first premolar on back	—	—
Facial nerve (VII)			
Chorda tympani	Taste in anterior two thirds of tongue	—	—
Glossopharyngeal nerve (IX)	Taste and sensation to posterior third of tongue	—	—

Glossary

A

A band Dark microscopic band in the middle of a muscle sarcomere. The A band contains the myosin and parts of the actin myofilaments.

abducens Sixth cranial nerve (VI); related to eye movement.

abrasion Mechanical wearing away of teeth by abnormal stresses. Can result from abnormal tooth brushing habits or other abnormal stresses on the teeth.

abutment A tooth or prosthetic "stump" that serves to support one end of a fixed or a removable bridge.

accessional Permanent teeth that do not replace deciduous teeth but rather become an accession (an addition) to the deciduous or succedaneous teeth or to both types.

accessory nerve Eleventh cranial nerve (XI); supplies motor control to the trapezius and sternomastoid muscles in the neck as well as to the muscles of the pharynx, larynx, and soft palate.

accessory root canals Extra openings into the pulp; usually located on the sides of the roots or in the bifurcations.

accidental grooves Tertiary grooves that occur on third molars; smaller than primary or secondary grooves and occuring with no uniformity.

acellular cementum Cementum in which no cells are trapped.

acetylcholine A neuron-produced substance that aids in the transmission of impulses from one neuron to another and from many neurons to muscles in contraction.

acini Bulbous or tubular secretion-producing endpieces of a gland; pronounced a-sin-I.

acquired Pertaining to something obtained by oneself rather than inherited.

acquired occlusion See *centric occlusion.*

acquired centric occlusion See *centric occlusion.*

acromegaly Disease resulting from an excess of growth hormone, which causes some bones in the body to continue growing after normal growth has completed.

actin One of the myofilaments in muscle; it is thinner than myosin and located in the I band and part of the A band. It is also found as a component of microfilaments in cell cytoskeleton.

action Function of a muscle; the work accomplished when a muscle contracts or shortens.

adduct To move toward the midline, as in muscle movement of extremities.

adipocyte A fat cell found as a component of connective tissue. These cells increase or decrease in number as fat is accumulated or depleted.

adrenalin A substance produced primarily by the adrenal gland that increases activity of the heart and lungs.

afferent A type of nerve fiber carrying sensory messages to the brain.

afunctional Not performing a purpose or action.

agranulocytes White blood cells without granules in their cytoplasm; lymphocytes and monocytes.

ala   Latin for *wing;* referring to the sides of the nostrils; plural *alae.*

alignment   How the teeth are arranged in a row mesially, distally, facially, and lingually.

allergenic   Capable of producing an allergic reaction.

allergic reaction   Body's reaction to an allergen, as in hives.

alpha-tubulin   One of two major protein components of microtubules; help make up the cytoskeleton.

alveolar bone   Bone that forms the sockets for the teeth.

alveolar bone proper   See *cribriform plate.*

alveolar crest   Highest part of the alveolar bone closest to the cervical line of the tooth.

alveolar crest group   Alveolodental fibers running from the cementum to the alveolar crest of bone.

alveolar eminences   Bulges on the facial surface of alveolar bone that outline the position of the roots.

alveolar mucosa   Mucosa between the mucobuccal fold and gingiva.

alveolar process   Part of the bone in the maxillae and mandible that forms the sockets for the teeth. See *alveolar bone.*

alveolodental fibers   Periodontal fibers that run between the tooth and alveolar bone.

alveolus (alveoli)   Cavity or socket in the alveolar process in which the root of the tooth is held.

ameloblast   Enamel-forming cell that arises from oral ectoderm.

amelogenesis imperfecta   A hereditary form of enamel hypocalcification.

amylase   Digestive enzyme that breaks starch into simpler compounds.

anatomic crown   The part of the tooth covered by enamel.

anemia   Deficiency of red blood cells or hemoglobin to carry oxygen.

angle of the mandible   Point at the lower border of the mandible body where it turns up onto the ramus.

Angle's classification   System of dental classifications based primarily on the relationship of the permanent first molars to each other and to a lesser degree on the relationship of the permanent canines to each other.

ankyloglossia   See *tongue-tie.*

ankylosis   Fusion of the cementum of a tooth with alveolar bone.

anodontia   No teeth at all are present in the jaw.

anomaly   Any noticeable difference or deviation from that which is ordinary or normal.

antagonists   Having an opposing action to something else.

anterior   Situated in front of; a term commonly used to denote the incisor and canine teeth or the area toward the front of the mouth.

anterior auricular muscle   Muscle of facial expression that extends from in front of the ear into the skin of the ear.

anterior coupling   The touching of the anterior teeth during centric occlusion.

anterior cranial fossa   The anterior part of the cranial cavity that houses the frontal lobes of the brain.

anterior ethmoidal nerve   The branch of the nasociliary nerve of V_1 that passes through the anterior ethmoidal foramen into the anterior ethmoid air cells and sends a branch to the external nose.

anterior ethmoid sinus   Frontmost group of ethmoid air cells.

anterior nasal spine   Small projection of the maxillae at the bottom of the nasal aperture.

anterior pillar   Fold of tissue extending down in front of the tonsil.

anterior superior alveolar artery   Branch of the infraorbital artery to the maxillary incisors, canines, and premolars.

anterior superior alveolar nerve   Branch of the infraorbital nerve that serves the maxillary incisors and canines.

antibodies   Defensive proteins, called immunoglobulins, produced by cells such as lymphocytes and plasma cells.

antihistamine   Drug that controls the body's histamine reaction, which causes congestion of tissues.

aorta   Large vessel carrying oxygenated blood from the heart to the remainder of the body.

A-P film   Anterior-posterior film that is taken with a radiograph source in front and film behind.

apatite crystals   Small crystals of mineral deposits.

apex (apices)   Endpoint or farthest tip, as of the tooth root.

apical end of a cell   Narrow end of a pyramidal cell forming the lumen of a duct.

apical foramen   Aperture or opening at or near the apex of a tooth root through which the blood and nerve supply of the pulp enters the tooth.

apical group   Alveolodental fibers that attach from the base of the alveolus to the apex of the tooth.

apposition   Addition, as to the surface of bone or any hard substance. One of the processes that takes place in bone growth and remodeling.

appositional growth   The process of adding to the surface of bone or any hard substance. See *apposition*.

arch, dental   See *dental arch*.

arthritis   Inflammation of body joints.

articular disc   Fibrous disc between the condyle and the mandibular fossa.

articular eminence   Slope of temporal bone in front of the mandibular fossa.

atrophic   Pertaining to the wasting away of a tissue, organ, or part from disease, defective nutrition, or lack of use.

atrophy   Wasting away of a tissue, organ, or part from disease, defective nutrition, or lack of use.

attached gingiva   Tightly adherent gingiva that extends from free gingiva to alveolar mucosa.

attachment apparatus   See *attachment unit*.

attachment epithelium   The cells that attach the gingiva to the tooth. These originally are cells of the reduced enamel epithelium.

attachment unit   Subdivision of the periodontium: cementum, periodontal ligament, and alveolar bone.

attrition   Process of normal wear on the crown.

auditory tube   See *pharyngotympanic tube*.

auriculotemporal nerve   Branch of the third division of the trigeminal nerve that supplies the skin over the ear and the parotid gland.

autonomic nervous system   Automatic nervous system of the body that is not willfully controlled. It controls the functions of the glands and smooth and cardiac muscle.

axon   Process of the neuron that carries the message from the cell body to the next neuron.

B

balancing side   Term used in denture construction to denote the side of the denture that must be balanced to prevent the denture from tipping. In natural dentition it occurs when the buccal cusps of the mandibular teeth are located directly under the lingual cusps of the maxillary teeth. These cusps actually touch.

basal end of cell   Broad outer end of a pyramidal cell forming a duct; end of any tall cell resting on a basement membrane.

basal layer   Bottom layer in multiple-layered epithelium; layer that undergoes cell division.

basement membrane   Ultrastructural layer of connective tissue on which epithelial cells rest; they rest on the side of the cell farthest from the free cell surface.

basophils   White granulocyte blood cells that play a role in phagocytosis and possible allergic reactions.

bell stage   Third stage of enamel organ formation in which the crown form is established.

beta-tubulin   One of two major protein components of microtubules, which help make up the cytoskeleton.

biconcave discs   Discs that have a depression in the middle on both sides.

bicuspid   See *premolars*.

bifurcation   Division into two parts or branches, as any two roots of a tooth.

bisecting angle technique   Technique of taking radiographs that slightly compromises accuracy of the image.

blade-vent implants   Wedge-shaped implants that are driven into a premade trough in the bone; bone grows into the holes in the blade of the implant.

blastocyst   Hollow ball of cells that results from division of a fertilized ovum. It becomes the outer and inner cell mass of an embryo.

B-lymphocyte   A cell of connective tissue that, when antigenically stimulated, becomes plasma cell producing antibodies.

body of the mandible   Horizontal portion of the mandible, excluding the alveolar process.

bolus of food   A ball of food that has been chewed and mixed with saliva and is ready to be swallowed.

bone   Hard connective tissue that forms the framework of the body. The hardness is attributable to the hydroxyapatite crystal.

brachiocephalic artery   Branch of the aorta that carries blood to the right arm and right side of the head.

brachiocephalic veins   Paired veins that drain the right and left arms and sides of the head. These two veins unite to form the superior vena cava.

branchial arches   See *pharyngeal arches*.

bruxism   Abnormal grinding of the teeth.

bucca   Latin word for *cheek*.

buccal   Pertaining to the cheek; toward the cheek or next to the cheek. Also called *facial*.

buccal branch   Branch of the maxillary artery that goes to the cheek and buccal gingiva.

buccal contour   Posterior teeth; see *facial contours*.

buccal developmental groove   Groove that separates the buccal cusps on a buccal surface.

buccal embrasure   See *embrasure*.

buccal glands   Small minor salivary glands in the cheek.

buccal nerve   Branch of the third division of the trigeminal nerve that supplies the skin and mucosa of the cheek and buccal gingiva.

buccinator   Muscle of facial expression that extends from the back buccal portion of the maxillae, mandible, and pterygomandibular raphe forward in the cheek to the corner of the mouth.

buccopharyngeal membrane   Membrane that separates the stomodeum from the foregut.

bud stage   First stage of development of the enamel organ. It develops from the dental lamina.

bundle bone   Extra thickness of bone added to the cribriform plate.

C

calcification   Process by which organic tissue becomes hardened by a deposit of calcium salts within its substance. The term, in a liberal sense, connotes the deposition of any mineral salts that contribute to the hardening and maturation of hard tissue.

canal   Long tubular opening through a bone.

cancellous bone   See *spongy bone.*

canine eminence   Extra bulk of bone on the labial aspect of the maxillae; it overlies the roots of the canine teeth.

canine fossa   Depression in the maxillae below the infraorbital foramen.

canine rise   During lateral excursion, the only teeth to touch are the maxillary and mandibular canines on the side toward which the jaw is moving.

canines   Third teeth from the midline, at the corner of the mouth; used for grasping; also called *cuspids.*

cap stage   Second stage of enamel organ development.

capsule   Fibrous sheet of tissue surrounding a joint.

cardiac muscle   Striped, involuntarily controlled muscle of the heart.

carotene   A yellow pigment that is found in varying amounts in the skin.

carotid canal   Canal in the base of the skull for the passage of the internal carotid artery.

carotid sheath   A fibrous sheath that surrounds the carotid arteries, internal jugular vein, and vagus nerve.

cartilage   Type of firm connective tissue that gives form to different parts of the body, such as the ears, trachea, and larynx.

CAT scan   Computer Assisted Tomography. A scan of all or part of the body that allows the information to be digitally stored and reconstructed to give virtually any view.

cell   Basic functioning component of the body; capable of reproducing itself in most instances. Tissues are made up of groups of cells.

cell body   Central part of a neuron containing the nucleus.

cell membrane   Wall surrounding the cell.

cellular cementum   Cementum in which cells are trapped.

cellular inclusions   Storage products in a cell not actually used to maintain the cell under normal circumstances.

cementoblasts   Cells that form cementum.

cementocytes   Cementoblasts that have become entrapped in cementum.

cementoenamel junction (CEJ)   Junction of enamel of the crown and cementum of the root. This junction forms the cervical line around the tooth.

cementoma   Cementum tumor at root tip that destroys surrounding bone.

cementum   Layer of bonelike tissue covering the root of the tooth.

central developmental groove   Developmental groove that crosses the occlusal surface of a tooth from the mesial to the distal side; divides the tooth into buccal and lingual parts.

central developmental pit   Pit that occurs in the central fossa.

central fossa   Fossa that occurs in the center of the central groove.

central groove   See *central developmental groove.*

central nervous system   Brain and spinal cord.

central occlusion   A system of classifying the occlusion based on the relationship of the mandibular teeth to the maxillary teeth.

centric occlusion   Relationship of the occlusal surfaces of one arch to those of the other when the jaws are closed and the teeth are in maximum intercuspation.

centric relation   Arch-to-arch relationship of the maxillae to the mandible when the condyles are in their most upward position, the mandible is in its most posterior position, and the jaw is most braced by its musculature.

cephalometric film   Film of skull taken from a side view so that cephalometric tracings can be done for orthodontic evaluation.

cervical   That portion of a tooth near the junction of the crown and root. Pertaining to the neck region (e.g., nerves of the neck).

cervical crest   Gingival tissue located near the cervical line of the tooth.

cervical embrasure   Embrasure or spillway located cervical to the contact area of the teeth.

cervical line   Line formed by the junction of the enamel and cementum on a tooth.

cervical loop   The deepest part of the inner and outer enamel epithelium seen in the bell stage; there is no interposing stellate reticulum or stratum intermedium; aids in root formation.

cervical third   That portion of the crown or root of a tooth at or near the cervical line.

cervicoenamel ridge   Any prominent ridge of enamel immediately near the cervical line on the crown of a tooth.

cervix   Constricted structure; the narrow region at the junction of the crown and root of the tooth.

choana   Region at the posterior end of the nasal septum where it opens into the nasal pharynx; means "funnel."

chondroblasts   Cells that form cartilage.

chondrocytes   Cartilage-forming cells that have surrounded themselves with their secretory product.

chorda tympani   Branch of the facial nerve (VII) that joins with the lingual nerve to carry taste sensations from the anterior two thirds of the tongue and secretomotor fibers to the submandibular and sublingual glands.

cilia   Movable, hairlike structures on the apical end of a columnar cell that helps to move substances over the surface of the cells.

cingulum   Lingual lobe of anterior teeth.

circumferential lamellae   Growth layers in bone around the outermost portion of the bone.

circumvallate papillae   Large V-shaped row of papillae lying on the posterior dorsum of the tongue.

class I occlusal relationship   Normal relationship between maxillary and mandibular molars.

class II occlusal relationship   Condition when a mandibular molar is posterior to its normal position.

class III occlusal relationship   Condition when a mandibular molar is anterior to its normal position.

cleft lip   Gap in the upper lip occurring during development.

cleft palate   Lack of joining together of the hard or soft palates.

clinical crown That part of the tooth protruding out of the gingiva.

clinical root That part of the tooth embedded in the gingiva and socket.

coalescence Joining of two lobes of a tooth.

coccygeal Relating to the tailbone area; a single pair of nerves in the tailbone region.

col Area of an interdental papilla that lies cervical to the interproximal contact of the tooth.

collagen Nonelastic, primary fiber of connective tissue.

common carotid artery Main blood vessel on either side of the neck that supplies most of the head.

compound tubuloalveolar gland Glandular arrangement that has a branching duct system with secreting cells at the ends of the ducts arranged like tubes with a bulbous endpiece.

compressor naris Muscle in flared part of nostrils that closes them.

concavity Depression in a surface.

concha See *superior nasal concha.*

concrescence Two adjacent teeth that fuse by their cementum.

condylar neck Constricted part of the ramus of the mandible, just below the condyle.

congenital Occurring at or before birth; may or may not be hereditary.

congenitally missing Condition of having never been developed.

conical tooth A supernumerary tooth that is cone shaped.

connective tissue One of the four basic tissues made up of cells, fibers, ground substance (glue), and sometimes crystal. Bone, cartilage, and blood are special types of connective tissue.

contact area Area of contact of one tooth with another in the same arch.

contact point Specific point at which a tooth from one arch occludes with another tooth from the opposing arch.

contour Shape of a tooth.

convenience occlusion See *centric occlusion.*

convexity Bulge in a surface.

copula Pharyngeal-arch structure that forms the posterior third of the tongue.

coronal suture Suture between the frontal bone and the two parietal bones; also called the *frontoparietal suture.*

coronoid notch Notch in the upper surface of the mandibular ramus, just anterior to the condyle.

coronoid process Bony projection at the upper anterior ramus of the mandible; point of attachment for the temporal muscle.

corrugator Muscle from the bridge of the nose to the lateral part of the eyebrow.

cortical plate Dense bone on the buccal and lingual surfaces of the alveolar bone.

cortisone An antiinflammatory drug.

cranial nerves Twelve pairs of nerves originating from the brain.

craniofacial deformities Abnormal development of the head and face region.

craniosacral outflow Another name for the parasympathetic nervous system.

cribriform plate Bone that forms the actual wall of the tooth socket.

cribriform plate of ethmoid Small perforations of ethmoid bone beside the crista galli that provide passages for olfactory nerves from the nasal to the cranial cavity.

cristae   The inner leaflike projections of a mitochondrion; enzymes attached to them enhance cellular activity.

crista galli   Small bony projection of ethmoid bone in the anterior cranial fossa; helps attach the dura mater covering of the brain.

crossbite   Condition in which the cusps of a tooth in one arch exceed the cusps of a tooth in the opposing arch, buccally or lingually.

cross section   Cutting through a tooth perpendicular to the long axis.

crown   That part of the tooth covered with enamel.

crypt   Term used to describe the early tooth socket.

curve of Spee   Anatomic line beginning at the tip of the canines and following the buccal cusps of premolars and molars when viewed from the buccal aspect of the first molars.

curve of Wilson   Curve that follows the cusp tips, as seen from a frontal view.

cusp   Major pointed or rounded eminence on or near the occlusal surface of a tooth.

cusp of Carabelli   Fifth lobe of a maxillary first molar.

cyst   Epithelium-lined sac of fluid that may grow to varying sizes.

cytoplasm   Fluid substance of cells.

D

dead tracts   Empty dentinal tubules resulting from death of odontoblasts and their processes in that area.

debrided   Having already accomplished the removal (debridement) of nerve tissue and other debris from the pulp cavity to leave a surgically cleaned area.

deciduous   That which will be shed; specifically, the first dentition of human or animal.

deep petrosal nerve   Sympathetic nerve from the carotid plexus that supplies blood vessels to glands in the palate, nose and lacrimal gland.

deglutition   Action of swallowing.

dendrite   Single process or multiple processes of a neuron that pick up impulses from other neurons and carry them to the cell body of its neuron.

dens in dente   An invagination of the outer surface of the tooth crown turning inward on itself.

dental arch   All the teeth in either the maxillary or mandibular jaw that form an arch.

dental classification   A system of classifying the relationship of the upper teeth to the lower teeth.

dental follicle   See *dental sac.*

dental lamina   Embryonic downgrowth of oral epithelium that is the forerunner of the tooth germ.

dental papilla   Mesodermal structure partially surrounded by the inner enamel epithelial cells. The dental papilla forms the dentin and pulp.

dental sac   Several layers of flat mesodermal cells partially surrounding the dental papilla and enamel organ; forms the cementum, periodontal ligament, and some alveolar bone.

dentin (formerly dentine)   Hard calcified tissue forming the inside body of a tooth, underlying the cementum and enamel and surrounding the pulpal tissue.

dentinal tubule   Space in the dentin occupied by odontoblastic process.

dentinocemental junction   Location in the root where the dentin joins the cementum.

dentinoenamel junction   Line marking the junction of the dentin and the enamel.

dentinogenesis imperfecta   Hereditary imperfect dentin formation.

dentition   General character and arrangement of the teeth, taken as a whole, as in carnivorous, herbivorous, and omnivorous dentitions. Primary dentition refers to the deciduous teeth, secondary dentition to the permanent teeth. Mixed dentition refers to a combination of permanent and deciduous teeth in the same dentition.

depression   Lowering of the mandible or opening of the mouth.

depressor anguli oris   Muscle of facial expression that extends from the lower border of the mandible at the canine area up to the corner of the lower lip.

depressor labii inferioris   Muscle that goes from the chin area up into the middle part of the lower lip.

descending palatine artery   Branch of the maxillary artery that supplies the hard and soft palates.

descending palatine nerve   Branch of the second division of the trigeminal nerve to the hard and soft palates.

desmosome   Ultrastructural part of a cell next to the cell wall that helps hold cells together.

developmental depression   Noticeable concavity on the formed crown or root of a tooth; occurs at the junction of two lobes, as on the mesial surface of maxillary first premolars, or at the furcation of roots.

developmental grooves   Fine depressed lines in the enamel of a tooth that mark the union of the lobes of the crown.

developmental lines   See *developmental grooves.*

developmental lobes   Major growth centers of a tooth.

developmental pit   Small hole formed by the junction of two or more developmental lines.

diaphysis   The central shaft of a developing long bone.

diastema   Any spacing between teeth in the same arch.

digastric fossae   Two small depressions on the inferior surface of the mandible at the midline.

digastric muscle   Suprahyoid muscle extending from the mastoid process area to the midline of the mandible; retracts and lowers the mandible.

dilacerated   Said of developing tooth roots that become bent and crooked because of developmental problems.

dilacerated tooth   Tooth with sharply bent roots.

dilaceration   A sharp bend in the root or crown of the tooth.

dilator naris   Muscle that goes over the tip of the nose and opens the nostrils.

diploë   Thin layer of cancellous bone between the outer and inner plates of skull bones.

disc derangement   When there is damage and displacement to the articular disc of the temporomandibular joint.

distal   Distant; farthest from the median line of the face or from the origin of a structure.

distal contact area   See *contact area.*

distal marginal groove   Groove that crosses the distal marginal ridge.

distal oblique groove   Groove that separates the distolingual cusp from the remainder of the occlusal surface of an upper molar.

distal pit   Pit found in the distal fossa.

distal proximal surface   Proximal surface on the posterior side of a tooth.

distal step   The mandibular molars are more posterior than the maxillary molars.

distal third   Viewed from the facial or lingual surface, the third of a surface farthest from the midline.

distobuccal developmental groove   Developmental groove that extends on the buccal surface of a lower first or third molar between the distobuccal and distal cusps.

distoclusion   See *class II occlusal relationship*.

distolingual cusp   Most distal of the lingual cusps.

distolingual groove, distolingual developmental groove   See *distal oblique groove*.

distomolars   Fourth molars

DNA   Deoxyribonucleic acid; the substance in a cell nucleus that builds the genetic information to enable the cell to build a duplicate of itself or control products produced by the cell.

dorsal primary ramus   Dorsal branch of the mixed spinal nerve that goes to the midline of the back.

dorsal root   Sensory root of a spinal nerve entering the spinal cord.

dorsal root ganglion   Cell bodies of sensory nerves to the spinal cord. A ganglion is located in the dorsal root of a spinal nerve.

dorsum of the tongue   Top surface of the tongue.

dwarfed roots   Tooth with very short roots in comparison with the crown.

E

ectoderm   Outer embryonic germ layer that forms skin, salivary glands, hair, sweat glands, sebaceous glands, nerves, and so on.

ectodermal dysplasia   A pathologic condition in which all structures developing from embryonic ectoderm have their growth interrupted. This involves skin, hair, sebaceous glands, sweat glands, salivary glands, and enamel of teeth.

edema   Swelling of tissue.

edge, incisal   See *incisal edge*.

edentulous   An area without the presence of teeth.

efferent   Refers to a nerve fiber carrying motor messages from the brain.

elastic cartilage   Type of cartilage that has a large number of elastic fibers in it; for example, the ear.

elastic fiber   Fiber of connective tissue that has elastic properties. Many of these are found in the walls of large arteries.

elastin   Major component of elastic fibers of connective tissue.

elevation   Raising the mandible, or closing the mouth.

embrasure   Open space between the proximal surfaces of two teeth where they diverge buccally, labially, or lingually and occlusally from the contact area.

enamel   Hard calcified tissue that covers the dentin of the crown portion of a tooth.

enamel cuticle   Nasmyth's membrane; a thin membrane that covers the crown of a tooth at eruption.

enamel dysplasia   Abnormality of enamel growth.

enamel fluorosis   A form of enamel hypocalcification where enamel is discolored because of an excess of fluoride in the tooth structure.

enamel hypocalcification   Enamel that is not as dense as regular enamel.

enamel hypoplasia   Enamel that is thin or pitted.

enamel lamellae   Imperfections or cracks in enamel formed by trauma or imperfect enamel formation.

enamel organ   Ectodermal epithelial structure that leads to the formation of tooth enamel.

enamel pearls   Small rounded elevations of enamel, usually developing in the bifurcations or trifurcations of teeth; considered abnormal structures.

enamel rod   Individual pillars of enamel formed by ameloblasts.

enamel spindle   Odontoblastic process trapped in enamel at the dentinoenamel junction.

enamel tuft   Area of hypocalcified enamel at the dentinoenamel junction.

endochondral bone formation   Bone that forms by replacing a hyaline cartilage model.

endocrine   Gland or type of secretion that is carried away from the producing cells by blood vessels; the secretion is used in other parts of the body to control certain functions; has no duct system.

endoplasmic reticulum   Tubular system in a cell related to the cell's production of secretions such as protein.

endosteal   Inside bone; in the center marrow area.

endosteal lamellae   Layers of bone lining the walls of the marrow cavity of the bone.

endosteum   See *endosteal.*

entoderm   Inner germ layer of an embryo that forms the epithelial lining of organs such as the digestive tract, liver, lungs, and pancreas.

enzyme   A protein that aids in increasing the speed of reaction in many types of cells and systems of the body.

eosinophils   White granulocyte cells that have some phagocytosing properties and allergic properties.

epicranius   Muscle of facial expression in the scalp region extending from front to back.

epiglottis   Cartilage that helps cover the laryngeal opening.

epinephrine   Substance produced either synthetically or by the body and that causes many reactions; in dentistry it is used to constrict blood flow in tissues; see also *adrenalin.*

epiphyseal plate   Block of cartilage between the diaphysis and epiphysis in long bones; allows for longitudinal growth.

epiphysis   The end components of growing bone found in long bones.

epithelial   Pertaining to epithelium.

epithelial attachment   The substance produced by the reduced enamel epithelium that helps secure the attachment epithelium at the base of the gingival sulcus to the tooth.

epithelial diaphragm   Deep part of the epithelial root sheath that is turned horizontally.

epithelial rests   Cells from the epithelial root sheath that remain in the periodontal space and cells that remain at areas of embryonic fusion.

epithelial rests of Malassez   See *epithelial rests.*

epithelial root sheath   Downgrowth of the inner and outer enamel epithelium that outlines the shape and number of the roots.

epithelium   Layer or layers of cells that cover the surface of the body or line the tubes or cavities inside the body; one of the four basic tissues.

equilibrium   Sense of balance.

eruption   Movement of the tooth as it emerges through surrounding tissue so that the clinical crown gradually appears longer.

eruptive stage   Period of eruption from the completion of crown formation until the teeth come into occlusion.

ethmoid air cells   Small, interconnecting bony compartments in the lateral nasal wall that form the ethmoid sinuses.

ethmoid bone   Bone that forms a very small part of the anterior neurocranium, part of the medial wall of the orbit, and a large part of the nasal cavity.

ethmoid bulla   Oblong bulge in the middle meatus above the hiatus semilunaris, onto which opens the middle ethmoid air cells.

ethmoid sinus   Group of small air cavities in the bone of the lateral wall of the nasal cavity.

excretory duct   Duct that is surrounded by connective tissue between the lobules of a gland or is outside the gland and carrying the salivary fluid to the surface without changing it.

exfoliation   Shedding or loss of a primary tooth.

exocrine   Gland or type of secretion that is carried away from the producing cells by a duct system.

exostoses   Small extra growths of bone on a bone surface; usually seen on the buccal cortical plate.

external auditory meatus   Opening of the ear on the side of the skull.

external carotid artery   Branch of the common carotid artery that supplies most of the head except the inside of the skull.

external jugular vein   Vein that drains the superficial structures of the neck and flows eventually into the subclavian vein in the neck.

external nasal nerve   Branch of the anterior ethmoidal nerve of V_1 that supplies the upper bridge of the nose.

external oblique line   The bony ridge running downward from the anterior border of the ramus of the mandible and out onto the lateral alveolar process and body.

extracellular fluid   Fluid between cells; consists primarily of blood plasma.

extrinsic   Originating outside a structure.

extrinsic factors   External factors.

F

facial   Term used to designate the outer surfaces of the teeth collectively (buccal or labial).

facial artery   Branch of the external carotid artery that supplies the superficial face area.

facial contours   Curvature of the facial surface of a tooth.

facial embrasure   See *embrasure.*

facial nerve   Seventh cranial nerve (VII), which serves the muscles of facial expression as well as most taste and gland control.

facial surface   See *facial.*

facial third   From a proximal view, the third of the surface closest to the facial side.

familial tendency   When an anomaly occurs more frequently than usual in one family.

fascia   Connective tissue covering muscles and separating muscle layers.

fascial spaces   Potential spaces between layers of muscles or layers of connective tissue.

fat cell   See *adipocyte.*

fauces   Space between the left and right palatine tonsils.

FDI system   The Federation Dentaire Internationale (International Dental Federation) system for tooth identification.

fibroblast   Basic cell of connective tissue that produces the collagen fiber.

fibrocartilage   Type of cartilage containing large quantities of collagen fibers.

fifth-cusp developmental groove   Groove that separates the cusp of Carabelli from the lingual surface on an upper molar.

fight-or-flight mechanism   Another term for the re-actions of the sympathetic nervous system.

filiform papillae   Small pointed projections that heavily cover most of the dorsum of the anterior two thirds of the tongue.

fissure   Deep cleft; developmental line fault usually found in the occlusal or buccal surface of a tooth; commonly the result of the imperfect fusion of the enamel of the adjoining dental lobes.

flange   Projecting edge; the edge of a denture.

flexion   A bend or a twist in the root, not involving the crown.

fluorosis   Discolored enamel resulting from exces-sive fluoride intake while the crown is developing.

flush terminal plane   The mandibular and maxillary second molars are even, with neither being anterior or posterior.

foliate papillae   Poorly developed papillae that appear as small vertical folds in the posterior part of the sides of the tongue.

foramen   Short circular opening through a bone (plural often foramina).

foramen cecum   Depression in the tongue two thirds of the way back that marks the beginning point of development of the thyroid gland; means "blind aperture."

foramen lacerum   A jagged opening in the base of the skull that is part of the anterior floor of the carotid canal. In life this foramen is filled with a piece of cartilage and nothing of any importance passes through it.

foramen magnum   Large foramen in the base of the occipital bone.

foramen ovale   Oval-shaped foramen in the sphe-noid bone at the base of the skull.

foramen rotundum   Foramen in the front part of the middle cranial fossa that opens into the pterygo-palatine fossa behind and below the eye.

foramen spinosum   Small opening in base of the skull just posterior to the foramen ovale; it transmits the middle meningeal artery to the covering of the brain.

Fordyce granules   Misplaced sebaceous glands in the lips, cheek, or retromolar pad area.

foregut   Front end of the gastrointestinal tube in the early developing embryo.

fossa   Round, wide, relatively shallow depression in the surface of a tooth as seen commonly in the lin-gual surfaces of the maxillary incisors or between the cusps of molars; also a shallow depression in bone.

fovea palatinae   Small depressions in mucosa on either side of the posterior nasal spine, indicating the junction of the hard and soft palates.

free gingiva   Gingiva that forms the gingival sulcus.

frenulum   Little frenum or fold of tissue.

frontal bone   Bone that forms the forehead.

frontal nerve   One of the three main branches of the ophthalmic division of the trigeminal nerve.

frontal prominence   Bulge in the forehead region that forms the upper facial area in the embryo.

frontal sinus   Air sinus in the frontal bone above the eye that opens into the hiatus semilunaris in the middle meatus.

frontooccipitalis   See *occipitofrontalis*.

frontoparietal suture   See *coronal suture*.

functional eruptive stage   See *posteruptive stage*.

fungiform papillae   Small circular papillae scattered throughout the anterior two thirds of the dorsum of the tongue.

fusion   Two teeth that fuse at their dentin while they are developing. Also, a term used for the process of formation of the hard and soft palates.

G

ganglion   An accumulation of nerve cell bodies outside of the brain or spinal cord.

gemination   A tooth that partially or fully divides into two teeth while developing.

genial tubercles   Small projections for muscle attachment on the lingual surface of the mandible at the midline.

genioglossus   Extrinsic tongue muscle running from the center of the mandible up into the tongue.

geniohyoid muscle   Suprahyoid muscle that extends from the genial tubercles to the hyoid bone.

germinative layer   See *basal layer.*

gingiva   Part of the gum tissue that immediately surrounds the teeth and alveolar bone.

gingival crest   Most occlusal or incisal extent of gingiva.

gingival crevice   Subgingival space that, under normal conditions, lies between the gingival crest and the epithelial attachment.

gingival embrasure   See *cervical embrasure.*

gingival fibers   Periodontal fibers in the gingiva.

gingival papillae   That portion of the gingiva found between the teeth in the interproximal spaces gingival to the contact area; also called *interdental papillae.*

gingival sulcus   Space between the free gingiva and the tooth surface.

gingival tissue   See *gingiva.*

gingival unit   Subdivision of the periodontium.

gingivitis   Inflammation involving the gingival tissues only.

glands of von Ebner   Small, minor, serous salivary glands (lingual glands) that open into the crypts of the vallate papillae.

globulomaxillary cyst   Cyst that forms between the maxillary lateral incisor and canine.

glossitis   Inflammation of the tongue wherein the tongue is red and smooth.

glossopharyngeal glands   Small minor salivary glands in the tonsillar pillars.

glossopharyngeal nerve   Ninth cranial nerve (IX), serving a muscle of the pharynx, taste, general sensation, and salivary glands.

glycogen   Form of starch that by enzymes makes glucose (body sugar) or is made from glucose, depending on bodily needs; stored as a cellular inclusion and readily available as instant energy.

glycoproteins   One of the two main classes of proteins found in the ground substance of connective tissue.

goblet cells   Single-celled glands that secrete mucus; found in the epithelium of respiratory and digestive tracts from the stomach through the gastrointestinal tract.

Golgi apparatus   Flat saclike layers in a cell that "package" the cell products for transportation outside the cell.

granular layer of Tomes   Interglobular dentin in the root.

granulocytes   White blood cells that have small or large granules in their cytoplasm; neutrophils, basophils, and eosinophils.

gray matter   Central portion of the spinal cord containing cell bodies of motor and sensory neurons.

greater auricular nerve   Branch of the cervical plexus from C2-C3 that innervates the skin over the angle of the jaw.

greater palatine artery   Branch of the descending palatine artery to the hard palate.

greater palatine foramen   Foramen on either side of the hard palate between the maxillae and palatine bones.

greater palatine nerve   Branch of the descending palatine nerve that serves the hard palate.

greater petrosal nerve   A parasympathetic branch of the VII (facial) cranial nerve that supplies all glands from the hard palate, nasal cavity, and the lacrimal gland.

greater wing of the sphenoid   Part of the sphenoid bone projecting onto the side of the skull behind the zygomatic bone as well as the posterior part of orbit.

ground substance   Gluelike substance that serves as the background for connective tissue, including cartilage and bone; composed of a substance known as a mucopolysaccharide.

group function   During lateral excursion, several teeth, not just a solitary canine, touch simultaneously. Usually the maxillary canine and the first and second premolars touch at the same time.

gubernacular canal   A small canal in the alveolar bone of a mixed dentition individual, located just lingual to its primary tooth. This canal was occupied by the successional lamina of the permanent tooth.

H

habitual occlusion   See *centric occlusion*.

hamular process   See *pterygoid hamulus*.

hard tissue   Calcified or mineralized tooth tissues or bone.

hairy tongue   A condition wherein the filiform papillae on the tongue have elongated, giving the tongue a hairy appearance.

hare lip   A midline cleft of the upper lip that resembles the upper lip of a rabbit. Very rare.

haversian lamellae   Concentric layers of bone around blood vessels in bone.

Haversian system   System of blood vessels located within the bones to provide them with nourishment.

hematoma   Escape of blood from an injured blood vessel into tissue spaces.

hemoglobin   Component in red blood cells that carries oxygen.

hereditary   Inherited through the genes of parents.

Hertwig's epithelial root sheath   See *epithelial root sheath*.

hiatus of the maxillary sinus   The opening from the middle meatus of the nasal cavity into the maxillary sinus.

hiatus semilunaris   Curving depression beneath the middle nasal concha in the middle meatus. It has openings in it for the frontal, anterior ethmoid, and maxillary sinuses.

hindgut   The lower third of the embryonic gut tube that forms the lower part of the large intestine from the descending colon to the anus.

histamine   Substance produced by some cells that causes swelling or edema of the tissues.

holocrine   Method of secretion wherein the cell dies and releases its products.

horizontal group   Group of alveolodental fibers.

hormones   Chemical substances produced by the body that have certain effects on other organs or glands of the body.

Hutchinson's incisors   Notched central incisors that develop as a result of congenital syphilis.

hyaline cartilage   Type of cartilage that is very firm; sometimes replaced by bone. The larynx and trachea are examples of hyaline cartilage.

hydroxyapatite (sometimes spelled hydroxylapatite) The crystal that is found in hard substances of the body such as bone, cementum, dentin, and enamel.

hyoglossus   Extrinsic tongue muscle running from the hyoid bone up into the lateral border of the tongue.

hyoid   Horseshoe-shaped bone in the neck between the mandible and larynx.

hyoid arch   Second pharyngeal arch, which forms some of the structures in the neck.

hyoid muscles   Muscles that attach to the free-floating hyoid bone in the neck.

hypercementosis   Increased thickness of cementum, usually seen at the apex of the root.

hyperdontia   More than the usual number of teeth.

hyperemia   Congestion of blood seen in pulp.

hypocalcified enamel   Condition in which there is either an insufficient number of enamel crystals or insufficient growth of the crystals.

hypoglosssal nerve   Twelfth cranial nerve (XII); supplies motor control to the tongue muscles.

hypophyseal fossa   Saddle-shaped depression on the body of the sphenoid bone located in the middle cranial fossa containing the pituitary gland.

hypoplastic enamel   Thin enamel; may be hypocalcified as well.

I

I band   Light microscopic band at either end of the sarcomere. The I band contains only actin myofilaments.

imbrication lines   Horizontal lines best seen on the labial surfaces of anterior teeth. These are surface manifestations of the striae of Retzius.

immunity   Body's resistance to certain organisms or diseases.

impacted   Describing teeth not completely erupted that are fully or partially covered by bone or soft tissue.

incisal edge   Edge formed at the labioincisal line angle of an anterior tooth after an incisal ridge has worn down.

incisal embrasure   See *embrasure.*

incisal ridge   Rounded ridge form of the incisal portion of an anterior tooth.

incisal third   From a proximal, lingual, or labial view of an anterior tooth, the third of the surface closest to the incisal edge.

incisive foramen   Foramen at the midline of the anterior palate region.

incisive papilla   Small, rounded, oblong mound of tissue directly behind or lingual to the maxillary central incisors and lying over the incisive foramen.

incisors   Four center teeth in either arch; essential for cutting.

inferior alveolar branch or artery   Branch of the maxillary artery that supplies the lower teeth.

inferior alveolar nerve   Branch of the third division of the trigeminal nerve to the lower teeth.

inferior border of mandible   Lower edge of the lower jaw.

inferior meatus   Area sheltered by the inferior nasal conchae.

inferior nasal conchae   Small bones that project from the lower lateral walls of the nasal cavity.

inferior orbital fissure   Groove like opening in the inferior lateral part of the orbit.

inferior pharyngeal constrictor muscle   Lowest of three muscles that form the throat wall and help move food down into the esophagus.

inner cell mass Inner thickened layer of a blastocyst that becomes an embryo.

inflammatory reaction Body's mechanism to combat harmful organisms by bringing more plasma and blood cells to an injured area.

infrahyoid muscles Muscles below the hyoid bone that attach to it.

infraorbital artery Termination of the maxillary artery that passes out of the floor of the orbit through the infraorbital foramen; supplies the skin of the lower eyelid, upper lip, and side of the nose.

infraorbital foramen Foramen just below the lower rim of the orbit in the maxillary bone.

infraorbital nerve Termination of the second division of the trigeminal nerve that supplies the skin of the lower eyelid, nose, and upper lip.

infratemporal fossa Area on the side of the skull immediately below the temporal fossa; pterygoid muscles and the maxillary artery are located there.

infratrochlear nerve A branch of the ophthalmic division of the trigeminal nerve that supplies the skin in the lower medial corner of the eye.

inherited Passed on from parents or grandparents.

inner cell mass The clump of cells on the inside of an embryonic blastocyst that forms the three germinal layers.

inner enamel epithelium (IEE) Group of epithelial cells in the enamel organ that eventually form the enamel of the crown.

inorganic matrix Hydroxyapatite crystals in the early matrix.

inorganic matter Mineral deposits such as calcium or phosphorus.

insertion End of a muscle attached to a more movable structure.

intercalated ducts Short, small ducts that carry saliva from acini to striated ducts.

intercuspal position (ICP) See *centric occlusion.*

intercuspation Relationship of the cusps of the premolars and molars of one jaw to those of the opposing jaw during any of the occlusal relationships.

interdental Located between the teeth.

interdental papilla Projection of gingiva between the teeth.

interdental space See *interproximal space.*

interglobular dentin Areas of hypocalcified dentin between normal areas of dentin; found in both crown and root dentin.

interlobular ducts Ducts between lobules of glands.

intermaxillary suture Suture between the maxillae. It is seen below the nasal cavity and in the front portion of the hard palate.

internal acoustic meatus Opening in the lateral part of the posterior cranial fossa for the facial and stato-acoustic cranial nerves.

internal carotid artery Branch of the common carotid artery that supplies the brain and inside of the skull.

internal jugular vein Main vein that drains the brain and deep structures of the head and neck; flows into the brachiocephalic vein.

interparietal suture See *sagittal suture.*

interproximal Between the proximal surfaces of adjoining teeth in the same arch.

interproximal space Triangular space between adjoining teeth; the proximal surfaces of the teeth form the sides of the triangle; the alveolar bone, the base, and the contact area of the teeth form the apex.

interstitial growth   Growth from within, as seen in cartilage formation when chondrocytes divide and enlarge.

interstitial lamellae   Parts of old bone layers found between newly formed layers of bone.

intertubular dentin   All dentin that is not tubular or peritubular.

intralobular ducts   Ducts surrounded by acini in a gland. Some of them help change the saliva before it leaves the gland.

intramembranous bone formation   Bone formed directly from mesenchymal cells that become osteoblasts.

intrinsic   Lying entirely inside a structure.

intrinsic factors   Internal factors.

involuntary muscle   Not voluntary; unable to be willfully controlled.

J

jugular foramen   See *jugular fossa.*

jugular fossa   Depression in the base of the skull with an opening for the passage of the internal jugular vein and the IX, X, and XI cranial nerves from the skull.

junctional epithelium   Epithelium that functions to hold mucosa in the base of the gingival sulcus to the tooth.

K

keratin   Substance that makes up the surface cells of skin, hair, and nails.

keratinized cells   Dead cells of the stratum corneum.

keratinized stratified squamous epithelium   Multilayered epithelium, like skin; upper layers are dead cells; makeup is similar to the composition of hair.

keratohyalin granules   Granules in the stratum granulosum that help produce the dead layer of cells on the skin surface.

L

labia   Latin word for lips; singular labium.

labial   Of or pertaining to the lips; toward the lips.

labial frenum   Fold of tissue that attaches the lip to the labial mucosa at the midline of the lips.

labial glands   Small minor salivary glands in the lips.

lacrimal bone   Small bone at the inner front of the orbit, forming part of the canal from the eye to the nose.

lacrimal groove   Groove in the lacrimal bone for the lacrimal duct.

lacrimal nerve   Branch of the ophthalmic division of the trigeminal nerve that provides sensation for the lacrimal gland and for skin lateral to and above the eye.

lambdoid suture   Inverted V-shaped suture between the occipital and parietal bones; also known as the parietooccipital suture.

lamina dura   Radiographic term denoting the cribriform plate and bundle bone.

laryngeal pharynx   That part of the common pathway of the respiratory and digestive systems from the base of the tongue to the opening of the larynx.

larynx   Voice box; trachea begins just below it.

lateral excursion   Movement of the jaws sideways.

lateral head film   See *cephalometric film.*

lateral lingual swellings   Paired structures arising from the internal pharyngeal arches and forming the anterior two thirds of the tongue.

lateral nasal process   Embryologic structure that forms the side of the nose and the area beneath the medial corner of the eye.

lateral pharyngeal   Area or fascial space beside the throat wall.

lateral pharyngeal space   See *lateral pharyngeal*.

lateral pterygoid muscle   Muscle that extends from the pterygoid plate to the condyle and protrudes the mandible.

lateral pterygoid plate   Thin wall of bone projecting back from the pterygoid process on the lateral side.

leeway space   The difference between the sum of the mesiodistal measurements of the deciduous canines and the deciduous molars compared with the mesiodistal measurements of the permanent canines and premolars in any one quadrant.

lesser palatine artery   Branch of the descending palatine artery that goes to the soft palate.

lesser palatine foramen   Foramen at the posterior end of the hard palate that transmits the lesser palatine nerve and artery to the soft palate.

lesser palatine nerve   Branch of the descending palatine nerve that supplies the soft palate.

lesser petrosal nerve   Branch of the glossopharyngeal nerve (IX) that carries secretomotor function to the parotid gland via the auriculotemporal nerve.

lesser wing of sphenoid   Projection of the sphenoid bone that forms the posterior border of the anterior cranial fossa.

leukemia   Cancer of white blood cells that chokes out red blood cell production.

levator anguli oris   Muscle that goes from beneath the eye to the corner of the upper lip.

levator labii superioris   Muscle that extends from below the eye to the middle part of the upper lip.

levator palpebri superioris   Muscle inside the eye that is supplied by the oculomotor nerve that elevates the upper eyelid.

levator veli palatini   Muscle of the soft palate that helps pull it back against the throat wall.

ligament   Regularly arranged group of collagen fibers that attach bone to bone.

line angle   Angle formed by two surfaces, for example, mesial and lingual; the junction is called the mesiolingual line angle.

lingual   Pertaining to or affecting the tongue; next to or toward the tongue.

lingual artery   Branch of the external carotid artery that supplies the tongue and floor of the mouth.

lingual contours   Curvature of the lingual surface of a tooth.

lingual crest of curvature   Most convex or widest portion of the lingual surface of a tooth.

lingual developmental groove   Groove on the lingual surface that separates two lingual cusps; see *lingual groove*.

lingual embrasure   See *embrasure*.

lingual frenum   Fold of tissue that attaches the undersurface of the tongue to the floor of the mouth.

lingual glands   Minor salivary glands of the tongue.

lingual groove   Developmental groove that occurs on the lingual side of the tooth.

lingual nerve   Branch of the third division of the trigeminal nerve that supplies general sensation to the tongue and floor of the mouth.

lingual surface   See *lingual*.

lingual third   From a proximal view, the third of a surface closest to the lingual side.

lingual thyroid   A thyroid gland that does not descend to the neck in development. It is found on the surface of the tongue posterior to the circumvallate papillae.

lingual tonsils   Tonsil tissue on the dorsum of the posterior part of the tongue.

lingula   Small projection of bone just in front of the mandibular foramen.

lining mucosa   Mucosa of the soft palate, lips, cheeks, vestibule, and floor of the mouth.

lipid   Fatty substance found in cells as an inclusion; used as a reserve source of energy.

lobe   Part of a tooth formed by any one of the major developing centers that begin the calcification of the tooth.

lobe of Carabelli   See *cusp of Carabelli.*

long buccal nerve   Lower branch of the buccal nerve that supplies the mandibular buccal gingiva.

lower deep cervical   Group of lymph nodes in the lower lateral neck beneath the sternomastoid muscle.

Ludwig's angina   Infection in the fascial spaces beneath the chin.

lumbar   Relating to the lower back, for example, vertebrae or nerves of the lower back.

lumen   Inside of a tube or duct; inside diameter of the opening.

lymph nodes   Small bean-shaped structures connected to one another by very small tubules. They combat infections in the body.

lymphadenopathy   Enlarged lymph glands or nodes; may be seen or felt when one has a sore throat, infected ears, and so on.

lymphatic vessels   Small tubes throughout the body that carry fluid from between the cells back into the vascular system.

lymphocytes   Kind of agranulocyte; active in the inflammatory process.

lymphoid tissue   Tissues made up of lymphocytes, which fight infections.

lysosomes   Small membrane-bound structures in a cell that act as a "garbage can" for the nonusable or harmful substances that find their way inside the cell.

M

macrodontia   Teeth that are too large for the jaw.

macrophage   Cell of connective tissue that destroys other cells, usually from outside the body.

malocclusion   Abnormal occlusion of the teeth.

mamelon   One of the three rounded protuberances of the incisal surface of a newly erupted incisor tooth.

mandible   Lower jaw.

mandibular   Pertaining to the lower jaw.

mandibular arch   First pharyngeal arch that forms the area of the mandible and maxillae; the lower dental arch.

mandibular condyle   Rounded top of the mandible that articulates with the mandibular fossa.

mandibular division   Third part of the trigeminal nerve (V); frequently represented as V_3.

mandibular foramen   Opening on the medial surface of the ramus of the mandible for the entrance of nerves and blood vessels to the lower teeth.

mandibular fossa   Depression on the inferior surface of the skull in the temporal bone that articulates with the condyle of the mandible.

mandibular notch   See *coronoid notch.*

mandibular process   That portion of the mandibular pharyngeal arch that goes to form the mandible.

mandibular tori   Bony growths on the lingual cortical plate of bone opposite the mandibular canines; also called *torus mandibularis.*

marginal developmental groove   See *marginal groove.*

marginal gingiva   See *free gingiva.*

marginal groove   Groove that crosses a marginal ridge.

marginal ridge   Ridge or elevation of enamel forming the margin of the surface of a tooth; specifically, at the mesial and distal margins of the occlusal surfaces of premolars and molars and at the mesial and distal margins of the lingual surfaces of incisors and canines.

marrow cavity   Hollow center of bone responsible for blood cell production and, later in life, for fat storage.

masseter muscle   Muscle on the lateral surface of the mandible that elevates it.

masseteric branch   Branch of the maxillary artery to the masseter muscle.

mast cells   Cells in connective tissue that release histamines.

mastication   Act of chewing or grinding.

masticatory mucosa   Mucosa of the hard palate and gingiva.

mastoid process   Large projection of temporal bone behind the ear.

matrix   Framework for a material; the framework for hard-tissue formation.

maturation stage   The stage of hard tissue development where the crystals that have been deposited grow in size.

maxillae   Paired main bones of the upper jaw.

maxillary   Pertaining to the upper arch.

maxillary arch   Upper dental arch.

maxillary artery   Major branch of the external carotid artery that supplies the teeth, gingiva, cheeks, palate, and several other areas.

maxillary division   Second part of the trigeminal nerve (V); usually represented as V_2.

maxillary process   Upper portion of the mandibular pharyngeal arch that forms the maxillae.

maxillary sinus   Largest of the paired paranasal sinuses; located in the maxillae.

maxillary tuberosity   Bulging posterior surface of the maxillae posterior to the third molar region.

meatus   Space beneath the shelter of each of the nasal conchae.

medial nasal processes   Embryologic structures that form the bridge of the nose, the middle part of the upper lip, part of the nasal septum, and part of the anterior hard palate.

medial pterygoid muscle   Muscle that runs between the mandible and pterygoid process and elevates the mandible.

medial pterygoid plate   Thin wall of bone projecting back from the pterygoid process on the medial side.

median line   Vertical (central) line that divides the body into right and left; the median line of the face.

median palatine cyst   Cyst that forms along lines of fusion of palatal shelves of maxillae.

median palatine suture   Suture that goes down the middle of the hard palate. The anterior part of the suture may also be called part of the intermaxillary suture.

median raphe   A midline joining of the left and right pharyngeal constrictor muscles in the posterior throat wall; runs from the base of the skull above to the esophagus below.

megakaryocyte   Large cell in marrow that is the forerunner of white blood cells.

melanin   Brown pigment in the skin. An increase in the amount of pigment is seen after sunburn and is produced by the melanocytes.

melanocytes   Pigment-producing cells located below the basal layer of epithelium. The pigment granules are incorporated into the basal cells and move up through the layers to the surface.

mental artery   Branch of the inferior alveolar artery that supplies the lower lip and gingiva adjacent to the lip.

mental branch   See *mental artery.*

mental foramen   Foramen on the lateral side of the mandible, below the premolars.

mental nerve   Branch of the inferior alveolar nerve that supplies the skin and mucosa of the lower lip and labial gingiva.

mental protuberance   Point of the chin on the anterior inferior surface of the midline of the mandible.

mental spines   See *genial tubercles.*

mentalis   Muscle that extends from the bone on the chin into the skin of the chin.

merocrine   Method of secretion wherein the droplets pass out of the cell by fusing with the cell membrane, eliminating the possibility of damage to the cell.

mesenchymal cell   Primitive cell of the mesodermal embryonic layer. This cell has the ability to form a number of different tissues. Some of these cells are available throughout life.

mesial   Toward or situated in the middle, for example, toward the midline of the dental arch.

mesial contact area   See *contact area.*

mesial developmental depression   Indented area on the mesial surface of a tooth.

mesial drift   Phenomenon of permanent molars continuing to move mesially after eruption.

mesial marginal developmental groove   See *mesial marginal groove.*

mesial marginal groove   Developmental groove that crosses the mesial marginal ridge.

mesial pit   Pit found in the mesial fossa.

mesial proximal surface   Proximal surface closest to the midline.

mesial step   The mandibular molars are more anterior than the maxillary molars.

mesial third   From a facial or a lingual view, third of the surface closest to the midline.

mesiobuccal developmental groove   Developmental groove that runs on the buccal surface of a lower first or third molar between the mesiobuccal and distobuccal cusps.

mesioclusion   See *class III occlusal relationship.*

mesiodens   Supernumerary teeth arising in the midline of the maxilla.

mesiolingual cusp   Most mesial of the lingual cusps.

mesiolingual developmental groove   Lingual developmental groove that separates the mesiolingual and distolingual cusps.

mesiolingual groove   See *mesiolingual developmental groove.*

mesoderm   Middle germ layer of the embryo that forms connective tissue, muscle, bone, cartilage, blood, and so on.

metabolism   Building up or breaking down of food accompanied by the production or use of energy.

microdontia   Teeth that are too small for the jaw.

microfilament   The ultrastructural solid filament that is part of the cytoskeleton. Composed of actin.

microtubule   The hollow ultrastructural filament of cytoskeleton; usually associated with motility of cilia or flagella.

microvilli   Ultrastructural elongations of the surface of epithelial cells that absorb; for example, the gut, which increases the surface area of the cell so that it can absorb more.

middle cranial fossa   The middle concavity in the floor of the skull that houses the temporal lobes and base of brain.

middle ethmoid sinus   Middlemost group of ethmoid air cells.

middle meatus   Area sheltered by the middle nasal concha.

middle meningeal artery   Branch of the first part of the maxillary artery that is the main blood supply to the meninges of the brain.

middle nasal concha   Small projection of thin bone from the middle of the lateral nasal wall.

middle pharyngeal constrictor muscle   The middle of three muscles that form the throat wall and help move food down into the esophagus.

middle superior alveolar nerve   Branch of the infraorbital nerve that supplies the maxillary premolars and usually the mesiobuccal root of the maxillary first molar.

middle third   See *mesial third.*

midgut   That part of the early digestive tract that will develop from the mid duodenum to the left colic flexure of the large intestine.

midline   Imaginary line that divides the body into right and left halves.

midsagittal plane   Divides the body vertically into right and left halves.

migration (movement)   The flow of connective tissue in the upper lip that aids in the formation of the lip.

mineralization stage   The stage in which hydroxyapatite crystals are laid down in developing hard tissue.

mitochondria   Small organelles in a cell that produce energy and control the metabolism of the cell; singular, mitochondrion.

mitotic division   Process of cell division that leads to the development of two cells from one.

mixed dentition   State of having primary and permanent teeth in the dental arches at the same time.

molars   Large posterior teeth used for grinding.

monocytes   White agranulocytes that have phagocytic properties.

mortality rate   Death rate; the number of deaths in a certain population for a certain reason; usually measured in a percentage, or may be the number of deaths per 1000, 10,000, 100,000, and so on.

mottled enamel   Enamel that has been discolored by excess fluorides in naturally fluoridated water or by excessive fluoride intake.

MRI scan   A computer-generated body scan using magnetic fields instead of ionizing radiation.

mucocele   A traumatized minor salivary gland, usually in the lip, that causes a blister like lesion; generally will rupture and heal.

mucogingival junction   Point at which the alveolar mucosa becomes gingiva.

mucosa   Moist epithelial linings of the oral cavity and the respiratory and digestive systems.

mucous   Pertaining to mucus, the thick viscous secretion of a gland.

mucous acini   Salivary unit that produces viscous saliva.

mulberry molars   Molars with multiple cusps; caused by congenital syphilis.

multiple root   Root with more than one branch.

muscle   One of the four basic tissues; has the property of contraction or shortening of the fibers, which accomplishes work. There are three types of muscle: skeletal, cardiac, and smooth.

muscle of uvula   The small muscular projection that extends down from the posterior of the soft palate.

myelin sheath   Covering around axons or dendrites of some nerves.

myelinated   Covered with myelin; a nerve that has a myelin sheath.

mylohyoid line   Diagonal line on the medial surface of the mandible for attachment of the mylohyoid muscle.

mylohyoid muscle   Suprahyoid muscle that forms the floor of the mouth.

mylohyoid nerve   Branch of the inferior alveolar nerve to the mylohyoid muscle and anterior belly of the digastric muscle.

myoepithelial cell   An epithelial-like cell that is found around glands and can contract like a muscle to help squeeze the secretions out of the ducts of the glands.

myofiber   Single muscle fiber or muscle cell.

myofibril   Component of muscle fiber; when grouped together, myofibrils make up a myofiber.

myofilaments   Smallest thick and thin filaments in a myofibril that are responsible for contraction.

myosin   One of the myofilaments located in the A band; thicker than actin.

N

nasal aperture   Opening of the nasal cavity in the skull.

nasal bone   Bones that form the bridge of the nose.

nasal pharynx   That part of the nasal region from the posterior end of the nasal septum down to the level of the soft palate.

nasal pits   Depressions in the developing facial area that deepen into the nasal passages.

nasal septum   Wall between the left and right sides of the nasal cavity; made up of the ethmoid and vomer bones.

nasalis   Nasal muscle of facial expression; divided into dilator naris and compressor naris.

Nasmyth's membrane   See *primary enamel cuticle.*

nasociliary nerve   Branch of the first division of the trigeminal nerve that supplies the ethmoid air sinuses, the skin in the lower medial corner of the eye, and the bridge of the nose.

nasopalatine nerve   Continuation of the sphenopalatine nerve that supplies the lingual gingiva of the maxillary incisors.

nervous tissue   One of the four basic tissues. Groups of cells (neurons) carry messages to and from the brain and perform many other tasks.

neurocranium   Part of the skull that surrounds the brain.

neuron   Nerve cell.

neutroclusion   See *class I occlusal relationship.*

neutrophils   Granulocytes whose granules do not stain brightly. This is one of the major cell groups involved in the inflammatory process.

nodular   Characterized by nodes or knotlike swellings.

nonkeratinized   Lack of any keratinization.

nonsuccedaneous   Permanent teeth that do not succeed or replace deciduous teeth.

nonworking side   Opposite side from which the mandible is moved.

nucleolus   Circular, dense area within the nucleus that contains most of the RNA within the nucleus.

nucleus   Control center of the cell. DNA and RNA are found here to control cell division and production.

O

oblique groove   See *distolingual groove.*

oblique group   Group of alveolodental fibers.

oblique ridge   Ridge running obliquely across the occlusal surface of the upper molars. It is formed by the union of the triangular ridge of the distobuccal cusp with the distal portion of the triangular ridge of the mesiolingual cusp.

occipital bone   Bone of the base and back of the skull. The foramen magnum is found in the basal portion.

occipital condyles   Thick, smooth surfaces on the basal part of the occipital bone just lateral to the foramen magnum. They articulate with the cervical vertebrae.

occipitofrontalis   See *epicranius.*

occluding   Contacting, opposing teeth.

occlusal   Articulating or biting surface.

occlusal embrasure   See *embrasure.*

occlusal plane   Side view of the occlusal surfaces.

occlusal relationship   Way in which the maxillary and mandibular teeth touch one another.

occlusal stress   Pressures on the occlusal surfaces of teeth.

occlusal surface   See *occlusal.*

occlusal table   As seen from an occlusal view, the area bordered by the cusp tips and marginal ridges.

occlusal third   From a proximal, lingual, or buccal view of a posterior tooth, the third of a surface closest to the occlusal surface.

occlusal trauma   Injury brought about by one tooth prematurely hitting another during closure of the jaws.

occlusion   Relationship of the mandibular and maxillary teeth when closed or during excursive movements of the mandible; when the teeth of the mandibular arch come into contact with the teeth of the maxillary arch in any functional relationship.

oculomotor nerve   Third cranial nerve (III); aids in the movement of the eye.

odontoblast   Dentin-forming cell that originates from the dental papilla.

odontoblastic process   Cellular extension of the odontoblast, which is located along the full width of the dentin.

odontoma   A tumor made up of enamel, dentin, cementum, and pulp.

olfactory epithelium   Modified respiratory epithelium found in the superior nasal cavity containing nerves that allow the sensation of smell.

olfactory nerve   First cranial nerve (I); transmits sensations of smell.

omohyoid muscle   Infrahyoid muscle that extends from the shoulder blade to the hyoid bone.

opaque   Not easily able to transmit light.

open bite   Space left between the teeth when the jaws close.

open contact   Space between adjacent teeth in the same arch; an interproximal opening instead of a contact area where the teeth touch.

ophthalmic division   First part of the trigeminal nerve (V); usually represented as V_1.

optic foramen   Opening into the posterior orbit that contains the optic nerve.

optic nerve   Second cranial nerve (II); conducts visual stimuli.

oral cavity proper   That area of the oral cavity bounded anteriorly and laterally by the teeth and posteriorly by the palatine tonsil.

oral epithelium   Lining membrane of the oral cavity; stratified squamous epithelium.

oral pharynx   The area behind the oral cavity that runs from the palatine tonsils to the back wall of the throat.

orbicularis oculi   Muscle that goes around the eye and eyelid.

orbicularis oris   Muscle that encircles the mouth; has many muscles running into it and blending with it.

orbit   Bony opening for the eye in the skull.

organelles   Means "little organs"; the functioning components in cells; they aid in the vital functions of the cells.

organic matrix   Noncalcified framework in which crystals grow.

origin   End of a muscle that is attached to the less movable structure.

osseointegrated implant   An implant with openings or grooves that allow for bone to grow into and anchor the implant.

ossicles   Small bones of the middle ear.

osteoblasts   Cells that form bone.

osteoclast   Multinucleated cell that is responsible for destroying bone as well as cementum and dentin.

osteocyte   Osteoblast that has surrounded itself with bone and become relatively inactive.

ostium of the maxillary sinus   Opening of the maxillary sinus into the nasal cavity beneath the middle nasal concha.

otic ganglion   Parasympathetic ganglion from the ninth cranial nerve (IX) that is attached to the medial side of the mandibular division of the trigeminal nerve and helps provide parasympathetic innervation to the parotid gland.

outer cell mass   That outer layer of a blastocyst that becomes part of the membranes surrounding an embryo and fetus and helps form the placenta.

outer enamel epithelium (OEE)   Outer epithelial layer of the enamel organ; serves as a protection for the developing enamel.

overbite   Relationship of the teeth in which the incisal ridges of the maxillary anterior teeth extend below the incisal edges of the mandibular anterior teeth when the teeth are placed in a centric occlusal relationship.

overhanging restoration   Excess of filling material extending past the confines of the tooth preparation; an overextension of filling material.

overjet   Relationship of teeth in which the incisal ridges or buccal cusp ridges of the maxillary anterior teeth extend facially to the incisal ridges or buccal cusp ridges of the mandibular teeth when the teeth are in a centric occlusal relationship.

P

P-A films   Radiographs taken with the ionizing source in the posterior position and the film in the anterior position.

palatal   Pertaining to the palate or roof of the mouth.

palatal process of the maxillae   Part of the maxillae that forms the anterior part of the hard palate.

palatal process of palatine bone   Horizontal part of palatine bone that forms the posterior part of the hard palate.

palatal root   Lingual root on any maxillary multi-rooted tooth.

palatal shelves   Projections of the maxillary processes that form the hard and soft palates.

palatine bone   Bone that forms the posterior part of the hard palate and the lateral nasal cavity.

palatine glands   Minor salivary glands in the hard and soft palates.

palatine tonsils   Normally just called *tonsils;* found at the side of the throat opposite the back of the tongue.

palatoglossal arch   See *anterior pillar.*

palatoglossal fold   See *anterior pillar.*

palatoglossus muscle   Muscle that extends from the soft palate down into the sides of the tongue. The mucosa over this muscle forms the anterior pillar of the throat.

palatomaxillary suture   See *transverse palatine suture.*

palatopharyngeal arch   See *posterior pillar.*

palatopharyngeal fold   See *posterior pillar.*

palatopharyngeal muscle   Muscle that extends from the soft palate down into the lateral pharyngeal wall. The mucosa over this muscle forms the posterior pillar of the throat.

Palmer notation system   System of coding the teeth, using brackets, numbers, and letters.

palpebral   Referring to the eyelids.

pancreas   Organ in the abdominal cavity behind the stomach that produces many of the enzymes necessary for the digestion of food.

papillary gingiva   Gingiva that forms the interdental papillae.

parakeratinized layer   Stratum corneum where some cells are dead and some are still alive.

parakeratinized stratified squamous epithelium   Multilayered epithelium in which top layers of cells are not completely dead.

paralleling technique   Method of taking radiographs that supposedly gives the most accurate representation of proper tooth dimensions; requires the use of special film holders.

paramolar   Small supernumerary tooth located buccally or lingually to a molar.

paranasal sinuses   Four pairs of cavities in the bones around the nasal cavity.

parapharyngeal   See *lateral pharyngeal.*

parasympathetic nervous system   Part of the autonomic (automatic) nervous system that originates from some of the cranial nerves and some of the sacral nerves. It controls a number of functions, including stimulation of the salivary glands.

parathyroid gland   Small gland embedded in the thyroid gland that helps control calcium metabolism in the body.

parietal bone   Pair of bones that forms the upper lateral part of the skull.

parietooccipital suture   See *lambdoid suture.*

parotid gland   Large salivary gland on the side of the face in front of the ear.

passive eruption   Condition in which the tooth does not move but the gingival attachment moves farther apically.

peg-shaped lateral   Poorly formed maxillary lateral incisor with a cone-shaped crown.

periapical   Around the tip of a tooth root.

pericardium   Sac that surrounds the heart and allows it to contract without irritation of heart muscle.

perichondrium   The fibrous and cellular covering of cartilage; provides new cells for appositional growth.

periodontal   Surrounding a tooth.

periodontal membrane or ligament   Collagen fibers attached to the teeth roots and alveolar bone and serving as an attachment of the tooth to the bone.

periodontium   Supporting tissues surrounding the teeth.

periosteum   Fibrous and cellular layer that covers bones and contains cells that become osteoblasts.

peripheral nervous system   Made up of the nerves originating from the spinal cord and brain (spinal and cranial nerves).

periphery   Circumferential boundary; outer border.

peristaltic contractions   The rhythmic waves of contraction of the smooth muscle of the gut wall that moves the food through the digestive tract.

peritubular dentin   Dentin immediately surrounding the tubule; slightly more calcified than the rest of the dentin.

petrous temporal bone   The hard portion of the temporal bone that houses the middle and inner ear and separates the middle from the posterior cranial fossa.

phagocytes   Cells that destroy various microorganisms.

pharyngeal   Relating to the pharynx or throat.

pharyngeal arches   Development tissue in the upper throat areas from which develop a number of structures in that region.

pharyngeal grooves or clefts   The exterior grooves in the neck region of a developing embryo between the pharyngeal arches.

pharyngeal plexus of nerves   Fibers of the glossopharyngeal (IX), vagus (X), and accessory (XI)

cranial nerves that supply the pharyngeal or throat wall with both motor and sensory.

pharyngeal pouches   The internal grooves in the embryonic neck region between the pharyngeal arches.

pharyngotympanic tube   Bony and cartilaginous tube that leads from the middle ear into the posterior-lateral nasal pharynx.

pharynx   Throat area, from the nasal cavity to the larynx.

pheresis   Process of removing platelets from a blood donor and then pumping the collected blood, minus the platelets, back into the donor.

philtrum   Small depression at the midline of the upper lip.

pillars   Folds of tissue appearing in front of and behind the palatine tonsils.

pinocytosis   The procedure wherein cells take in fluids without losing cytoplasm.

piriform aperture   See *nasal aperture.*

pit   Small pointed depression in dental enamel, usually at the junction of two or more developmental grooves; a small hole anywhere on the crown.

pituitary gland   Master controlling endocrine gland located in the middle cranial fossa.

plasma   Fluid part of the blood without the cells.

plasma cell   One of the cells that helps produce antibodies.

platysma   Broad muscle in the neck going from the mandible down into the upper chest region.

point angles   Meeting of three surfaces at a point to form a corner; angles formed by the junction of three surfaces, for example, the mesiolingual occlusal point angle.

posterior   Situated toward the back, as premolars and molars.

posterior auricular muscle   Muscle extending from behind the ear into the back of the ear.

posterior cranial fossa   The posterior depression in the cranial cavity, behind the petrous temporal bone. It houses the cerebellum and part of the brainstem.

posterior ethmoidal nerve   Branch of the nasociliary nerve of V_1 that passes through the posterior ethmoidal foramen and supplies the posterior ethmoid air cells.

posterior ethmoid sinus   Posterior most group of ethmoid air cells.

posterior mediastinum   Space in the chest behind the heart and between the lungs.

posterior nasal aperture   See *choana*.

posterior nasal spine   Pointed bony projection at the posterior end of the hard palate.

posterior pillar   Folds of tissue behind the tonsil that contain the palatopharyngeus muscle.

posterior superior alveolar artery   Branch of the maxillary artery that enters the maxillary tuberosity and supplies the maxillary molars.

posterior superior alveolar nerve   Part of the second division of the trigeminal nerve that enters the maxillary tuberosity and supplies the maxillary molars, generally excluding the mesiobuccal root of the first molar.

posterior teeth   Teeth of either jaw to the rear of the incisors and canines.

posteruptive stage   Period of eruption from the time the teeth occlude until they are lost and characterized by occlusal wear of teeth and compensating eruption.

potential spaces   Areas between two layers of tissue that are normally closed but may be spread apart, as in a tissue space infection.

preameloblast   Cell in the intermediate stage between an inner enamel epithelial cell and an ameloblast.

preeruptive stage   Period when the crown of the tooth is developing.

prefunctional eruptive stage   See *eruptive stage*.

premature contact area   The area where an upper and a lower tooth touch and hit each other before the rest of the teeth occlude together.

premaxilla   Bony area of the upper jaw that includes the alveolar ridge for the incisors and the area immediately behind it.

premolars   Permanent teeth that replace the primary molars.

preventive considerations   Ideas relating to the prevention of dental disease rather than the treatment of the disease after it occurs.

primary anatomy   Refers to the basic arrangement and number of developmental and triangular grooves on a tooth.

primary attachment epithelium   Remains of reduced enamel epithelium that provides for the initial attachment of mucosa at the base of the gingival sulcus.

primary dentin   Dentin formed from the beginning of calcification until tooth eruption.

primary dentition   First set of teeth; baby teeth; milk teeth; deciduous teeth.

primary enamel cuticle   Keratin-like covering on the surface of the enamel; the final product of the ameloblast.

primary nodes   First group of lymph nodes to be involved in the spread of infection.

primary palate   The early developing part of the hard palate that comes from the medial nasal process and forms a V-shaped wedge of tissue that runs from the incisive foramen forward and laterally between the lateral incisors and canines of the maxilla.

primary teeth   See *deciduous.*

primate spaces   The diastema present mesial to the maxillary canine and distal to the mandibular canine. A characteristic usually present in primates such as apes, monkeys, and humans.

procerus   Muscle going from the bridge of the nose to the medial part of the eyebrow.

prosthetic appliance   Any constructed appliance that replaces a missing part.

protein   One of the basic components of many foodstuffs and much of the body. Proteins are made up of small units known as amino acids strung together in long chains.

proteoglycans   One of two classes of carbohydrates and proteins that are found in the ground substance of connective tissue.

protrude   See *protrusion.*

protrusion   Condition of being thrust forward, referring to the teeth being too far labial; the forward movement of the mandible.

proximal   Nearest, next, immediately adjacent to; distal or mesial.

proximal contact areas   Proximal area on a tooth that touches an adjacent tooth on the mesial or distal side.

proximal surface   See *proximal.*

pseudostratified columnar epithelium   Single layer of cells appearing as many layers because the cells have various heights; found primarily in the respiratory tract.

pterygoid branches   Branches of the maxillary artery that supply the medial and lateral pterygoid muscles.

pterygoid fossa   Depression between the medial and lateral pterygoid plates.

pterygoid hamulus   Small curving process projecting down from the medial pterygoid plate of the sphenoid bone.

pterygoid plexus of veins   Meshwork of veins behind the maxillary tuberosity that flows into the maxillary veins.

pterygoid processes   Large downward projections of the sphenoid bone behind the maxillae.

pterygomandibular raphe   Band of connective tissue of the tendon that connects the posterior end of the buccinator muscle with the anterior end of the superior constrictor of the pharynx.

pterygomaxillary fissure   Elongated opening between the maxillary tuberosity and the pterygoid process of the sphenoid bone. The third part of the maxillary artery enters the pterygopalatine fossa through this opening.

pterygopalatine artery   Branch of the maxillary artery for the nasal cavity that joins the greater palatine artery in the anterior hard palate.

pterygopalatine fossa   Space behind and below the orbit; location of the maxillary nerve and the last part of the maxillary artery.

pterygopalatine ganglion   Parasympathetic ganglion associated with the seventh cranial nerve (VII), but attached to the maxillary part of the fifth cranial nerve (V). It supplies the glands of the palate, nasal cavity, and lacrimal gland.

pterygopalatine nerves   Two small branches of the second division of the trigeminal nerve that attaches the pterygopalatine ganglion to the main part of the maxillary division of V.

pulmonary artery   Blood vessel that carries blood from the heart to the lungs to pick up oxygen.

pulmonary veins   Blood vessels that carry blood back to the heart from the lungs.

pulp canal   Canal in the root of a tooth that leads from the apex to the pulp chamber. Under normal conditions it contains dental pulp tissue.

pulp cavity   Entire cavity within the tooth, including the pulp canal and pulp chamber.

pulp chamber   Cavity or chamber in the center of the crown of a tooth that normally contains the major portion of the dental pulp. The pulp canals lead into the pulp chambers.

pulp, dental   Highly vascular and innervated connective tissue contained within the pulp cavity of the tooth. The dental pulp is composed of arteries, veins, nerves, connective tissues and cells, lymph tissue, and odontoblasts.

pulp horn (horn of pulp)   Extension of pulp tissue into a thin point of the pulp chamber in the tooth crown.

pulp stones   Small dentinlike calcifications in pulp.

Purkinje's fibers   Specialized heart muscle fibers that carry nerve impulses.

pyramidal cells   Cuboidal cells in smaller ducts that are pushed into a pyramid shape because of the smaller diameter of the inside (lumen) versus the outside.

Q

quadrants   One fourth of the dentition. The four quadrants are divided into right and left, maxillary and mandibular.

R

radiopacities   Whitish region on a radiograph.

ramus of the mandible   Vertical portion of the mandible.

raphe   Term generally used to refer to the fusion of paired muscles at the middle; it is actually a collagenous union.

Rathke's pouch   Outpouching in the embryonic oral cavity that becomes part of the pituitary gland.

recession   Migration of the gingival crest in an apical direction, away from the crown of the tooth.

red blood cells   Most numerous of the blood cells; responsible for carrying oxygen to the rest of the body; erythrocytes.

reduced enamel epithelium   Fusion of the ameloblast layer with the outer enamel epithelium.

referred pain   Pain that seems to originate in one area but actually originates in another area.

reflex arc   Sensory message that goes to the spinal cord and meets with a motor nerve to cause an action. The reflex action occurs without the message's first reaching the brain to voluntarily cause the action.

reparative dentin   Localized formation of dentin in response to local trauma such as occlusal trauma or caries.

resorption   Physiologic removal of tissues or body products, as of the roots of deciduous teeth or of some alveolar process after the loss of the permanent teeth.

respiratory epithelium   Pseudostratified columnar ciliated epithelium that is found in the nose and most of the rest of the respiratory tract.

rete peg formation   Development of interdigitation between the epithelium and the underlying connective tissue.

reticular fiber   Smaller collagen-like fiber that forms the framework for a number of organs.

retrodiscal pad   Vascular and nerve tissue behind the disc of the temporomandibular joint.

retromandibular vein   Vein lying behind the mandible. It drains the side of the head and sends blood to both the external and internal jugular veins.

retromolar pad   Pad of tissue behind the mandibular third molars found in retromolar triangle.

retromolar triangle   Triangular area of bone just behind the mandibular third molars.

retropharyngeal   Group of lymph nodes behind the posterior throat wall; refers to the area behind the pharynx.

retropharyngeal nodes   See *retropharyngeal.*

retropharyngeal space   Space behind the pharynx and in front of the cervical vertebrae.

retrusion   Act or process of retraction or moving back, as when the mandible is placed in a posterior relationship to the maxillae.

ribosomes   Small granules of RNA found free in the cytoplasm of cells or attached to endoplasmic reticulum.

ridge   Long narrow elevation or crest, as on the surface of a tooth or bone.

risorius   Small muscle that lies on the surface of and parallel to the buccinator muscle.

RNA   Ribonucleic acid; the substance in the cell nucleus and cytoplasm that carries the DNA "message" to build other cells or cell products.

rod sheath   Material surrounding the enamel rod. It is slightly more organic than the enamel rod.

root   That portion of a tooth embedded in the alveolar process and covered with cementum.

root canal   See *pulp canal.*

root planing   Process of smoothing the cementum of the root of a tooth.

root trunk   That portion of a multirooted tooth found between the cervical line and the points of bifurcation or trifurcation of roots.

rudimentary lobe   Small underdeveloped lobe of a tooth; less than a minor lobe.

rugae   Small ridges of tissue extending laterally across the anterior of the hard palate.

S

sacral   Relating to the hip region; for example, sacral nerves and vertebrae.

sagittal suture   Suture that extends along the middle of the top of the skull between the parietal bones.

salpingopharyngeal muscle   Muscle that runs from the end of the auditory tube in the nasal pharynx down into the lateral wall of the pharynx and helps elevate it in the swallowing process.

sarcomere   Smallest functional unit of a striated muscle fiber, composed of an A band with half of an I band at either end and running from Z line to Z line.

sclerotic dentin   Condition in which the tubules have been filled in with dentin because of damage to the odontoblast.

sebaceous glands   Small oil-producing glands that are usually connected to hairs to lubricate them.

secondary anatomy   Extra grooves and pits in addition to the main primary anatomy on a tooth.

secondary attachment epithelium   Epithelium of free gingiva that produces mucosal attachment at the base of the gingival sulcus.

secondary dentin   Dentin formed throughout the pulp chamber and pulp canal from the time of eruption.

secondary dentition   Permanent dentition.

secondary enamel cuticle   Mucopolysaccharide cementing substance secreted by the reduced enamel epithelium that functions in cementing the base of the gingival sulcus to the tooth.

secondary groove   See *supplemental groove.*

secondary nodes   Second group of lymph nodes involved in the spread of infection.

seromucous   Pertaining to a mixture of serum- and mucus-secreting cells in the same gland.

seromucous acini   Glandular acini that have both mucous and serous cells.

serotonin   Compound that can affect blood flow in different parts of the body.

serous   Pertaining to a thin watery type of glandular secretion; serum.

serous acini   Glandular cells that produce watery secretion.

serous demilunes   Cluster of serous salivary cells that sits like a cap or half-moon on a mucous acinus. This acinus therefore secretes both mucus and serum.

Sharpey's fibers   Part of the periodontal ligament; embedded in cementum or alveolar bone.

short palate   Palate of insufficient length to meet the back wall of the throat.

sickle cell anemia   Disease in which the red blood cells are defective and cannot properly carry oxygen.

simple columnar epithelium   Single layer of tall cells found lining the digestive tract and other ducts of the body.

simple cuboidal epithelium   Single layer of square or cubelike cells that line many of the ducts of the body.

simple squamous epithelium   Single layer of flat cells that are found lining blood vessels, chest and abdominal cavities, and many other areas.

single root   Root with one main branch.

skeletal classification   A system of classifying bones based on the position of the maxilla in relation to that of the mandible. This classification does not pertain to the teeth.

skeletal muscle   Striped, voluntarily controlled muscle that allows for body movement.

sleep apnea   A condition in which an individual ceases breathing for 20 or more seconds many times per hour.

slough   Loss of dead cells from the surface of tissue.

smooth muscle   Unstriped, involuntarily controlled muscle found in the digestive tract and other organs; helps move food along the digestive tract.

soft tissue   Noncalcified tissues, such as epithelium, nerves, arteries, veins, and connective tissue.

spasm   Constant contraction of muscle.

specialized mucosa   Mucosa found on the top or dorsum of the tongue that includes the papillae and taste buds.

sphenoethmoidal recess   Most posterosuperior area of the nasal cavity.

sphenoid bone   Large bone that helps form the base of the skull in front of the occipital bone and part of the side of the skull.

sphenoid sinus   One of the paired paranasal sinuses located in the body of the sphenoid bone.

sphenomandibular ligament   Ligament running from the spine of the sphenoid to the lingula of the mandible.

sphenooccipital synchondrosis   Area of endochondral bone growth between the sphenoid and occipital bones that allows for growth of the cranial base and helps determine future occlusion.

sphenopalatine artery   See *pterygopalatine artery.*

sphenopalatine nerve   Branch of the second division of the trigeminal nerve that goes to the mucosa of the nasal cavity and anterior hard palate.

sphere of Monson   Imaginary sphere that theoretically could rest on the mandibular arch.

spillway   See *embrasure.*

spinal accessory nerve   Another name for the eleventh cranial nerve (XI). See *accessory nerve.*

spinal nerve   The joining together of the dorsal and ventral roots to form a mixed spinal nerve.

spinal nerves   Thirty-one pairs of nerves that exit from the spinal cord at each vertebral level.

spongy bone   Less dense bone in the middle of a bone, frequently referred to as the marrow area. In alveolar bone, the layer between the cribriform plate and the cortical plate.

squamosal suture   Suture between the temporal and parietal bones.

stapedius muscle   Small muscle in the middle ear supplied by the seventh cranial nerve (VII) that is attached to the stapes bone and protects the inner ear from loud sounds.

statoacoustic nerve   Eighth cranial nerve (VIII); related to hearing and balance.

stellate reticulum   Ectodermally and epithelially derived middle layer of the enamel organ. It serves as a cushion for the developing enamel.

sternocleidomastoid muscle   Muscle extending from the mastoid process down and forward in the lateral neck to the sternum and clavicle.

sternohyoid muscle   Infrahyoid muscle from the sternum to the hyoid bone.

sternomastoid muscle   See *sternocleidomastoid muscle.*

sternothyroid muscle   Muscle that goes from the sternum to the thyroid cartilage of the larynx.

stolarized molar   The permanent maxillary first molar is tipped mesially so that the distal marginal ridge of the upper first molar touches the mesial marginal ridge of the lower second molar.

stomodeum   Depression in the facial region of the embryo that is the beginning of the oral cavity.

stratified columnar epithelium   Epithelium that is rather rare but, when seen in large ducts, consists of two, or more, rows of columnar cells.

stratified cuboidal epithelium   See *stratified columnar epithelium.*

stratified squamous epithelium   Most common of the multiple-layered epithelia; found as skin and mucosa.

stratum basale   Bottom layer of stratified squamous epithelium; see also *basal layer.*

stratum corneum   Top layer of stratified squamous epithelium.

stratum germinativum   See *basal layer.*

stratum granulosum   Layer above the stratum spinosum in stratified squamous epithelium. Granules in this layer indicate the beginning of cell death.

stratum intermedium   Fourth developing layer of the enamel organ; responsible for aiding ameloblast nourishment.

stratum lucidum   Clear layer of epithelial cells found between stratum granulosum and stratum corneum in thick skin such as palms of hands and soles of feet.

stratum spinosum   Layer immediately above the basal layer in stratified squamous epithelium. The cells produced in the basal layer move up into the spinous layer.

striae of Retzius   Incremental growth lines seen in sections of enamel.

striated ducts   Salivary intralobular and interlobular ducts that look as if they have stripes at the base of the cells because of infolding of basal cell membrane and mitochondria trapped in between the infoldings.

styloglossus muscle   Extrinsic tongue muscle running from the styloid process into the tongue.

stylohyoid muscle   Suprahyoid muscle going from the styloid process to the hyoid bone.

styloid process   Small pointed projection of bone that points down and forward from the base of the skull just behind the mandible.

stylomastoid foramen   Small foramen between the mastoid and styloid process. The facial nerve exits from the skull here.

stylopharyngeal muscle   Muscle that runs from the styloid process down into the lateral wall of the pharynx; helps elevate and dilate the pharynx in the swallowing process.

subclavian vein   Vein that drains blood from the arm. It joins with the internal jugular vein to form the brachiocephalic vein.

sublingual caruncle   Small elevation of soft tissue at the base of the lingual frenum that is the opening for the submandibular duct.

sublingual fold   Fold of tissue extending backward on either side of the floor of the mouth; duct of the submandibular gland lies below it.

sublingual fossa   Depression for the sublingual gland on the medial surface of the mandible above the mylohyoid line in the canine region.

sublingual gland   Major salivary gland that lies in the floor of the mouth adjacent to the mandibular canines.

subluxation   Dislocation of the mandible.

submandibular   Referring to the region below the mandible; a group of lymph nodes around the submandibular gland.

submandibular fossa   Depression for the submandibular gland on the medial surface of the mandible below the mylohyoid line in the molar region.

Submandibular ganglion   Parasympathetic ganglion of the seventh nerve (VII) suspended from the lingual nerve. Postganglionic nerves go to the submandibular and sublingual glands.

submandibular gland   Large major salivary gland that lies beneath the mandible near the angle of the mandible.

submandibular nodes   See *submandibular*.

submaxillary gland   See *submandibular gland*.

submental   Area below the chin; a group of lymph nodes beneath the chin.

submental nodes   See *submental*.

submucosa   Supporting layer of loose connective tissue under a mucous membrane; may contain fat or minor salivary glands.

subperiosteal implants   A prosthetic appliance resembling a denture framework that is implanted beneath the mucosa and periosteum of an edentulous area and has projections protruding up through the mucosa for attachment of a denture or bridge.

succedaneous   Permanent teeth that succeed or take the place of the deciduous teeth after the latter have been shed—that is, the incisors, canines, and premolars.

successional lamina   Lingual growth off of the dental lamina that forms permanent incisors, canines and premolars.

sulcus   Long V-shaped depression or valley in the surface of a tooth between the ridges and the cusps. A sulcus has a developmental groove at the apex of its V. Sulcus also refers to the trough around the teeth formed by the gingiva.

superior auricular muscle   Muscle extending from above the ear down into the upper part of the ear.

superior constrictor muscle   Uppermost of the three pharyngeal constrictor muscles.

superior lateral nasal nerves   Branch of the spheno-palatine nerve that supplies the superior and lateral parts of the nasal cavity.

superior nasal concha   Small projection of ethmoid bone from the upper lateral nasal wall.

superior nuchal line   Horizontal line on the external surface of the occipital bone for the attachment of neck muscles.

superior orbital fissure   Groove in the upper lateral part of the orbit between the greater and lesser wings of the sphenoid.

superior pharyngeal constrictor muscle   The upper of three muscles that forms the throat wall and helps move food down into the esophagus. Part of the muscle joins anteriorly with the buccinator muscle of the cheek.

superior vena cava   Vein that drains blood from the head and arms into the heart.

supernumeraries   Extra teeth in the jaw.

supplemental canal   See *accessory root canals.*

supplemental groove   Shallow linear groove in the enamel of a tooth. It differs from a developmental groove in that it does not mark the junction of lobes; it is a secondary or smaller groove.

supplemental tooth   Supernumerary tooth that re-sembles a regular tooth.

supraeruption   Eruption of a tooth beyond the oc-clusal plane.

suprahyoid muscles   Muscles above the hyoid bone that attach to it.

supraorbital foramen   Supraorbital notch when it has a small projection of bone extending across it.

supraorbital nerve   Branch of the ophthalmic divi-sion of V; innervates the skin of the forehead.

supraorbital notch   Small notch in the upper rim of the orbit.

supraperiosteal   Tissue lying on the surface of bone.

supratrochlear nerve   Branch of the frontal nerve that innervates the skin in the upper medial corner of the eye.

surfaces   Four sides and the top of a tooth.

suture   Line where two bones join together.

sympathetic system   Part of the autonomic (auto-matic) nervous system that originates from the tho-racic and lumbar levels of the spinal cord.

synovial cavity   Epithelium-lined space that secretes tiny amounts of fluid, synovia, and is found in joints that are free moving.

synovial fluid   Thin, watery fluid secreted in joints that lubricates articulating surfaces.

T

taste buds   Small structures primarily found in vallate, fungiform, and foliate papillae that detect taste.

temporal bone   Bone that forms part of the side of the skull, including the ear area.

temporal branches   Branches of the maxillary artery that serve the temporal muscle.

temporal fossa   Large flattened area on the side of the skull that is the origin of the temporal muscle.

temporal muscle   Muscle on the side of the head attached to the mandible; elevates and pulls the mandible back.

temporalis muscle   See *temporal muscle.*

temporomandibular joint   Jaw joint between the temporal bone and mandible.

temporomandibular ligament   Thickened part of the temporomandibular joint (TMJ) capsule on the lateral side.

tendon   Regularly arranged group of collagen fibers that connects skeletal muscle to bone.

tensor tympani muscle   Small muscle in the middle ear attached to the malleus bone and supplied by the mandibular division of V. Dampens loud sounds and protects the inner ear.

tensor veli palatini   Muscle that runs from the auditory tube region down, forward, and around the lateral side of the hamular process and then turns medially into the anterior part of the soft palate. As its name indicates, when it contracts, it tenses the soft palate in swallowing and speech.

tertiary anatomy   Very shallow and numerous grooves, pits, and lines often seen in third molars giving it a wrinkled appearance.

tertiary grooves   See *accidental grooves*.

tertiary nodes   Third group of lymph nodes involved in the spread of infection.

tetracycline staining   Discolored teeth that result when an expectant mother or a young child takes the antibiotic tetracycline while tooth crowns are still developing.

therapeutic considerations   Treating diseased teeth.

thoracolumbar outflow   Another name for the sympathetic nervous system.

thorax (thoracic)   Chest region; pertaining to nerves of the chest.

thymus   Gland in the chest above the heart that is responsible for early establishment of immune cells to protect the body.

thyrohyoid muscle   Muscle going from the thyroid cartilage of the larynx to the hyoid bone.

thyroid gland   Gland in the neck that controls much of the body's metabolic rate.

T-lymphocyte   Type of lymphocyte that multiples in the thymus and fights virus-infected cells, tumors, and tissue and organ grafts.

Tomes' process   See *odontoblastic process*.

tongue-tie, tongue-tied   Condition in which the lingual frenum is short and attached to the tip of the tongue, making normal speech difficult.

tonsillar pillars   The vertical folds of tissue that lie in front of and behind the palatine tonsils in the lateral throat wall.

tooth germ   Soft tissue that develops into a tooth.

tooth migration   Movement of the tooth through the bone and gum tissue.

torus palatinus   Large bony growth in the hard palate.

trabeculae   Interlacing meshwork that makes up the cancellous bony framework.

transitional epithelium   Multiple rows of epithelial cells that seem to change in thickness when stretched or relaxed; found in the ureters, urinary bladder, and part of the urethra.

transparent dentin   See *sclerotic dentin*.

transseptal fibers   Periodontal fibers that extend from the cementum of one tooth to the cementum of the adjacent tooth.

transverse groove of oblique ridge   See *oblique groove*.

transverse palatine suture   Suture that runs across the posterior part of the hard palate between the maxillae and the palatine bones.

transverse ridge   Ridge formed by the union of two triangular ridges, traversing the surface of a posterior tooth from the buccal to the lingual side.

trapezius   Muscle at the back of the neck that goes down and out to the lateral part of the clavicle and scapula.

trauma   Wound; bodily injury or damage.

triangular fossa   Depression formed by the triangular groove between the triangular ridge and the marginal ridge.

triangular ridge   Any ridge on the occlusal surface of a posterior tooth that extends from the point of a cusp to the central groove of the occlusal surface.

trifurcation   Division of three tooth roots at their point of junction with the root trunk.

trigeminal nerve   Fifth cranial nerve (V); supplies motor control to the muscles of mastication and sensation to the teeth, oral cavity, and face.

trochlear nerve   Fourth cranial nerve (IV); aids in movements of the eye.

tubercle   Overcalcification of enamel resulting in a small cusplike elevation on some portion of a tooth crown.

tubercle tooth   Very small rudimentary supernumerary tooth.

tuberculum impar   Structure from the first pharyngeal arch that forms the midline of the tongue about one half to two thirds of the way back.

Turner's teeth   Hypocalcification of a single tooth.

type I collagen   The type of collagen fiber found most frequently in irregular and regular connective tissue.

U

ultraviolet radiation   One of the wavelengths in the electromagnetic spectrum; found in sunlight and produced by sunlamps.

united oral epithelium   Joining of the reduced enamel epithelium with the oral epithelium.

Universal system, Universal Code   System of coding teeth using the numbers 1 to 32 for permanent teeth and the letters A to T for the deciduous teeth.

upper deep cervical   Group of lymph nodes in the upper lateral neck beneath the sternomastoid muscle.

uvula   Small hanging fold of tissue in back of the soft palate.

V

V_1 First or ophthalmic division of the trigeminal nerve.

V_2 Second or maxillary division of the trigeminal nerve.

V_3 Third or mandibular division of the trigeminal nerve.

vagus nerve   Tenth cranial nerve (X); controls the muscles of the larynx and pharynx, muscles and glands of the digestive tract, and muscle of the heart.

vallate papillae   See *circumvallate papillae.*

vascular   Relating to blood supply.

vasoconstrictor   Substance that constricts blood vessels.

ventral primary ramus   The major branch of a spinal nerve, which we recognize as a nerve.

ventral root   Motor root of spinal nerve

vermilion zone   Red part of the lip where the lip mucosa meets the skin.

vestibule   Space between the lips or cheeks and the teeth.

visceral   Referring to the organs of the body and the structures supplied by involuntary muscle, such as the heart and digestive tract.

viscerocranium   Facial part of the skull.

Volkmann's canals   Blood vessel canal in bone that runs into bone from the outside.

voluntary muscle   Muscle able to be willfully controlled by the person or organism.

vomer   Bone that forms the lower part of the nasal septum.

W

white blood cells   Least numerous of the blood cells; responsible for the inflammatory process and other protective functions of the body; leukocytes.

white matter   The whitish appearing peripheral part of the spinal cord made up of myelinated axons of motor and sensory nerves.

working side   Side to which the mandible is moved.

Z

Z line   Junction between two sarcomeres in skeletal and cardiac muscle.

zygomatic arch   Arch of bone on the side of the face or skull formed by the zygomatic bone and temporal bone.

zygomatic bone   Bone that forms the cheek area.

zygomatic nerve   Branch of the maxillary division of V that innervates the skin of the cheek bone and temple and also carries parasympathetic fibers from VII to the lacrimal gland.

zygomaticoalveolar crest   Heavy ridge of maxilla and zygomatic bone that forms a heavy supporting ridge running up from the alveolar process of the maxillary premolar-molar region.

zygomaticus major   Muscle that extends from the cheek to the corner of the upper lip.

zygomaticus minor   Muscle that extends from the cheek toward the middle part of the upper lip.

Index

565

NOTES

NOTES

NOTES

NOTES

NOTES

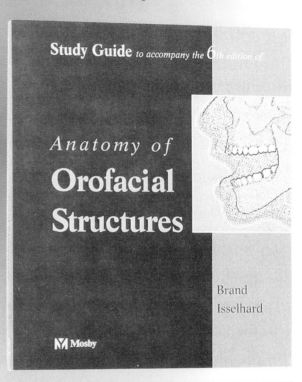

FLASH CARDS

Permanent Maxillary

Right Central Incisor

	RIGHT
Universal Code	8
International Code	11
Palmer notation	1⌋
Number of roots	1
Number of pulp horns	3
Number of developmental lobes	4

Location of proximal contact areas
MESIAL: Incisal third
DISTAL: Junction of incisal and middle thirds

Height of contour
FACIAL: Cervical third, 0.5 mm
LINGUAL: Cervical third, 0.5 mm

Identifying characteristics: These incisors are the largest and most prominent incisors. The distoincisal is more rounded than the mesioincisal angle. The lingual surface has a prominent cingulum, broad lingual fossa, and distinct marginal ridges. The pulp cavity is one large single chamber and root canal.

Permanent Maxillary

Right Lateral Incisor

	RIGHT
Universal Code	7
International Code	12
Palmer notation	2⌋
Number of roots	1
Number of pulp horns	1 to 3
Number of developmental lobes	4

Location of proximal contact areas
MESIAL: Junction of incisal and middle thirds
DISTAL: Middle third

Height of contour
FACIAL: Cervical third, 0.5 mm
LINGUAL: Cervical third, 0.5 mm

Identifying characteristics: The lingual anatomical features are similar to those of the central incisors but are more highly developed and have more prominent marginal ridges and deeper lingual fossae. Lateral incisors are more likely to have a lingual pit. The cingulum may be smaller, almost absent. The labial surface resembles that of a central incisor except that the labial surface is more convex. The crown-root ratio is less than in a central incisor because the crown is usually smaller, whereas the root is almost as long. In all other ways the lateral incisors appear as smaller, more rounded versions of the central incisors.

Permanent Maxillary

Right Canine

	RIGHT
Universal Code	6
International Code	13
Palmer notation	3⌋
Number of roots	1
Number of pulp horns	1
Number of cusps	1
Number of developmental lobes	4

Location of proximal contact areas
MESIAL: Junction of incisal and middle thirds
DISTAL: Middle third

Height of contour
FACIAL: Cervical third, 0.5 mm
LINGUAL: Cervical third, 0.5 mm

Identifying characteristics: The maxillary canines are the longest teeth in the mouth. They have a single cusp with mesial and distal ridges forming an incisal edge. A prominent facial ridge is off-center toward the mesial. Cingulum is prominent. The prominent mesiofacial lobe forms this facial ridge of the cusp. The centrofacial lobe forms the lingual ridge of the cusp. This lingual ridge divides the mesial and distal fossae. The distofacial ridge is longer and more rounded than the mesiofacial.

Permanent Maxillary

Right First Premolar

	RIGHT
Universal Code	5
International Code	14
Palmer notation	4⌋
Number of roots	2
Number of pulp horns	2
Number of cusps	2
Number of developmental lobes	4

Location of proximal contact areas
MESIAL AND DISTAL: Just cervical to the junction of occlusal and middle thirds

Height of contour
FACIAL: Cervical third, 0.5 mm
LINGUAL: Middle third, 0.5 mm

Identifying characteristics: These premolars have bifurcated roots. A longitudinal groove is present on the root. The mesial surface shows a developmental fossa. The mesial marginal groove crosses the mesial marginal ridge and extends onto the mesial surface. The facial cusp is wider and longer than the lingual cusp. The mesial ridge of the facial cusp may have a slight concavity.

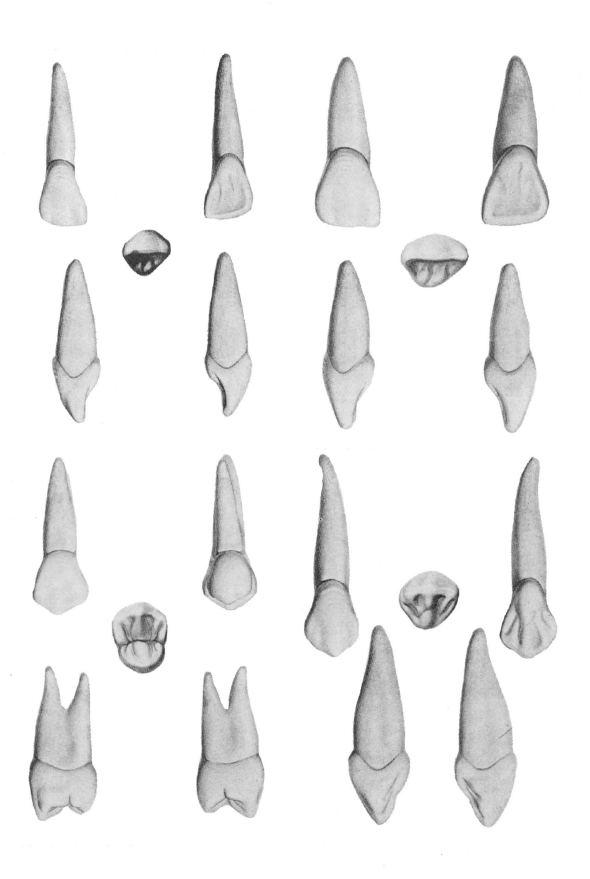

Permanent Maxillary

Right Second Premolar

	RIGHT
Universal Code	4
International Code	15
Palmer notation	5⌋
Number of roots	1
Number of pulp horns	2
Number of cusps	2
Number of developmental lobes	4

Location of proximal contact areas
MESIAL AND DISTAL: Just cervical to the junction of occlusal and middle thirds

Height of contour
FACIAL: Cervical third, 0.5 mm
LINGUAL: Middle third, 0.5 mm

Identifying characteristics: These premolars usually have a single root. About 40% have two root canals. The buccal and lingual cusps are nearly equal in length. The buccal cusp is shorter than that of a first premolar. The entire crown, especially the occlusal outline, is less angular and more rounded. The occlusal surface has more supplemental grooves. The occlusal developmental grooves are shorter, shallower, and more irregular.

Permanent Maxillary

Right First Molar

	RIGHT
Universal Code	3
International Code	16
Palmer notation	6⌋
Number of roots	3
Number of pulp horns	4
Number of cusps	4
	5 (including cusp of Carabelli)
Number of developmental lobes	5

Location of proximal contact areas
MESIAL: Middle third
DISTAL: Middle third

Height of contour
FACIAL: Cervical third, 0.5 mm
LINGUAL: Middle third, 0.5 mm

Identifying characteristics: A cusp of Carabelli may be present. The occlusal outline is square or rhomboidal rather than triangular. The distolingual cusp is well developed. There is a prominent oblique ridge and distal facial and lingual grooves. The crown is nearly as wide mesiodistally as buccolingually. The three roots are widely separated.

Permanent Maxillary

Right Second Molar

	RIGHT
Universal Code	2
International Code	17
Palmer notation	7⌋
Number of roots	3
Number of pulp horns	4
Number of cusps	4
Number of developmental lobes	4

Location of proximal contact areas
MESIAL: Middle third
DISTAL: Middle third

Height of contour
FACIAL: Cervical third, 0.5 mm
LINGUAL: Middle third, 0.5 mm

Identifying characteristics: These teeth are similar to maxillary first molars except that the fifth cusp is usually absent and the distolingual cusp is less well developed. The oblique ridge is less prominent. The crown is shorter occlusocervically and narrower mesiodistally. It is just as wide buccolingually. The occlusal outline of the crown is rhomboidal to heart shaped. The three roots are less separated.

Permanent Maxillary

Right Third Molar

	RIGHT
Universal Code	1
International Code	18
Palmer notation	8⌋
Number of roots	1 to 4
Number of pulp horns	1 to 4
Number of cusps	3 to 5
Number of developmental lobes	4

Location of proximal contact areas
MESIAL: Middle third
DISTAL: None

Height of contour
FACIAL: Cervical third, 0.5 mm
LINGUAL: Middle third, 0.5 mm

Identifying characteristics: These teeth vary more in form than any others. They usually do not have a distolingual cusp. The occlusal outline is heart shaped, with three cusps. The roots, usually three, have a tendency to be very close together or to fuse with an extreme distal inclination.

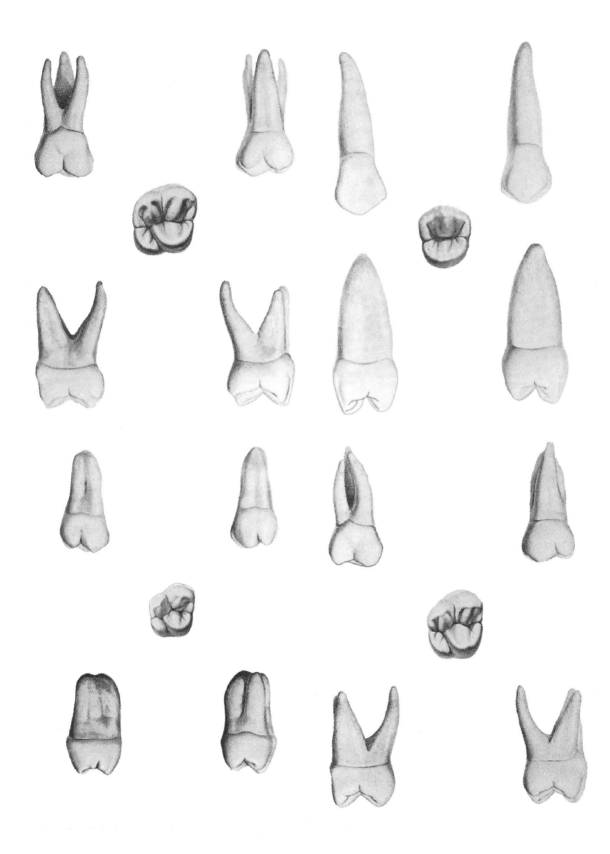

Permanent Mandibular

Right Central Incisor

	RIGHT	
Universal Code	25	
International Code	41	
Palmer notation	1⌋	
Number of roots		1
Number of pulp horns		3
Number of developmental lobes		4

Location of proximal contact areas
MESIAL: Incisal third
DISTAL: Incisal third

Height of contour
FACIAL: Cervical third, less than 0.5 mm
LINGUAL: Cervical third, less than 0.5 mm

Identifying characteristics: The distoincisal and mesioincisal angles are nearly identical. The lingual surface is shallow, with no prominent features. The crown is wider faciolingually than mesiodistally. The root is oval shaped in cross section. The incisal edge shows wear on the facioincisal edge. From a proximal view the incisal edge appears to be tilted toward the lingual side.

Permanent Mandibular

Right Lateral Incisor

	RIGHT	
Universal Code	26	
International Code	42	
Palmer notation	2⌋	
Number of roots		1
Number of pulp horns		3
Number of developmental lobes		4

Location of proximal contact areas
MESIAL: Incisal third
DISTAL: Incisal third

Height of contour
FACIAL: Cervical third, less than 0.5 mm
LINGUAL: Cervical third, less than 0.5 mm

Identifying characteristics: The crown is similar to that of the mandibular central incisors. The distal lobe is more highly developed than the mesial. The distal incisal ridge angles toward the lingual as if rotating on the root axis. The crown and the root are slightly larger than those of the central incisors.

Permanent Mandibular

Right Canine

	RIGHT	
Universal Code	27	
International Code	43	
Palmer notation	3⌋	
Number of roots		1 or 2
Number of pulp horns		1
Number of cusps		1
Number of developmental lobes		4

Location of proximal contact areas
MESIAL: Incisal third
DISTAL: Just cervical to the junction of incisal and middle thirds

Height of contour
FACIAL: Cervical third, less than 0.5 mm
LINGUAL: Cervical third, less than 0.5 mm

Identifying characteristics: The crown is similar to the crown of the maxillary canines but narrower and smoother. It has less prominent lingual features. From a proximal view, the cusp tip is inclined to the lingual. From an incisal view, the distal end of the incisal edge is rotated to the lingual. They have the longest roots in the mandibular arch, with longitudinal grooves on the root.

Permanent Mandibular

Right First Premolar

	RIGHT	
Universal Code	28	
International Code	44	
Palmer notation	4⌋	
Number of roots		1
Number of pulp horns		1 or 2
Number of cusps		2
Number of developmental lobes		4

Location of proximal contact areas
MESIAL AND DISTAL: Just cervical to junction of occlusal and middle thirds

Height of contour
FACIAL: Cervical third, 0.5 mm
LINGUAL: Middle third, 1 mm

Identifying characteristics: These premolars have two cusps, one large buccal and one small lingual. The buccal cusps are centered directly over the root. The lingual cusps are centered lingual to the root and are afunctional and nonoccluding. The occlusal surface slopes sharply lingual in a cervical direction. The mesiobuccal cusp ridge is shorter than the distobuccal cusp ridge. It has a mesiolingual developmental groove and one root.

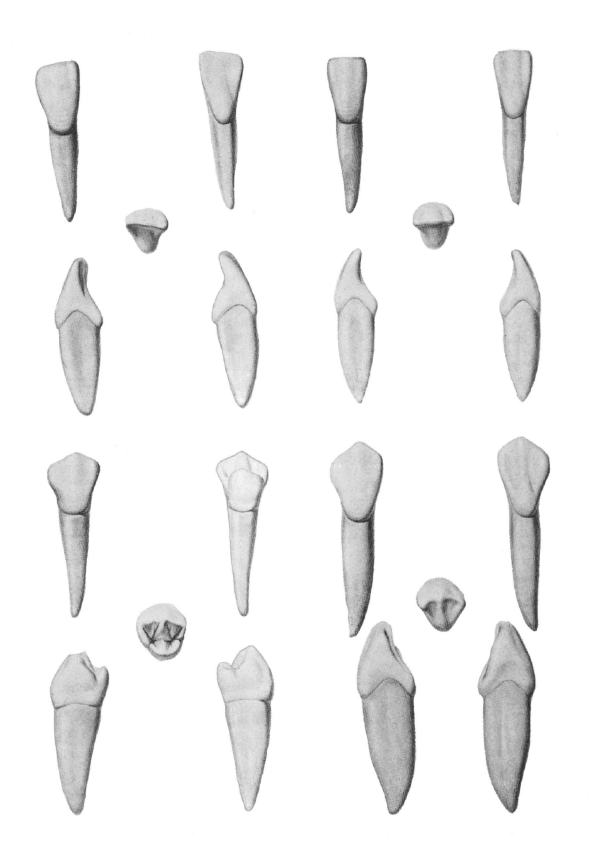

Permanent Mandibular

Right Second Premolar

	RIGHT	
Universal Code	29	
International Code	45	
Palmer notation	5⌐	
Number of roots		1
Number of pulp horns		2 or 3
Number of cusps		2 or 3
Number of development lobes		4

Location of proximal contact areas

MESIAL AND DISTAL: Just cervical to junction of occlusal and middle thirds

Height of contour

FACIAL: Cervical third, 0.5 mm
LINGUAL: Middle third, 1 mm

Identifying characteristics: These premolars have two or three cusps. The buccal cusp is very large. If two lingual cusps are present, the mesiolingual is the larger. Although the lingual cusps are larger than on a first premolar, they are afunctional and do not occlude with the maxillary teeth. A second premolar has more secondary anatomical features and more variation than any other tooth except a third molar. The two-cusp form has a U- or H-groove pattern. A mesiolingual groove is rare and is poorly developed if present. The three-cusp form has a lingual developmental groove between the two lingual cusps. The single root is longer and larger than that of a first premolar.

Permanent Mandibular

Right First Molar

	RIGHT	
Universal Code	30	
International Code	46	
Palmer notation	6⌐	
Number of roots		2
Number of pulp horns		5
Number of cusps		5
Number of developmental lobes		5

Location of proximal contact areas

MESIAL: Middle third
DISTAL: Middle third

Height of contour

FACIAL: Cervical third, 0.5 mm
LINGUAL: Middle third, 1 mm

Identifying characteristics: The five cusps make these the largest mandibular teeth. They are wider mesiodistally than buccolingually. The crown converges lingually and slightly distally. The three buccal cusps are separated by two buccal grooves. The two lingual cusps are separated by one lingual groove. These three grooves converge to form a Y pattern. There are two roots, a mesial and a distal, and three root canals (the mesial root has two root canals).

Permanent Mandibular

Right Second Molar

	RIGHT	
Universal Code	31	
International Code	47	
Palmer notation	7⌐	
Number of roots		2
Number of pulp horns		4
Number of cusps		4
Number of developmental lobes		4

Location of proximal contact areas

MESIAL: Middle third
DISTAL: Middle third

Height of contour

FACIAL: Cervical third, 0.5 mm
LINGUAL: Middle third, 1 mm

Identifying characteristics: These molars have four cusps of nearly equal size. The crown is smaller in all dimensions and has less lingual convergence. There is only one buccal groove and one lingual groove, which join together on the occlusal surface as they bisect the central developmental groove. The groove pattern is therefore a cross (+). The two roots are closer together and incline slightly distally. There is one root canal in the distal root. The mesial root can have one or two root canals.

Permanent Mandibular

Right Third Molar

	RIGHT	
Universal Code	32	
International Code	48	
Palmer notation	8⌐	
Number of roots		2 (fused into 1)
Number of pulp horns		4 or 5
Number of cusps		4 or 5
Number of developmental lobes		4 or 5

Location of proximal contact areas

MESIAL: Middle third
DISTAL: Middle third

Height of contour

FACIAL: Cervical third, 0.5 mm
LINGUAL: Middle third, 1 mm

Identifying characteristics: These are the most variable mandibular teeth in form. They usually resemble the mandibular second molars, with four cusps and a shallower, smaller central fossa, with more secondary and tertiary grooves. A five-cusp form is not unusual. The two roots (mesial and distal) and often fused and inclined toward the distal side.

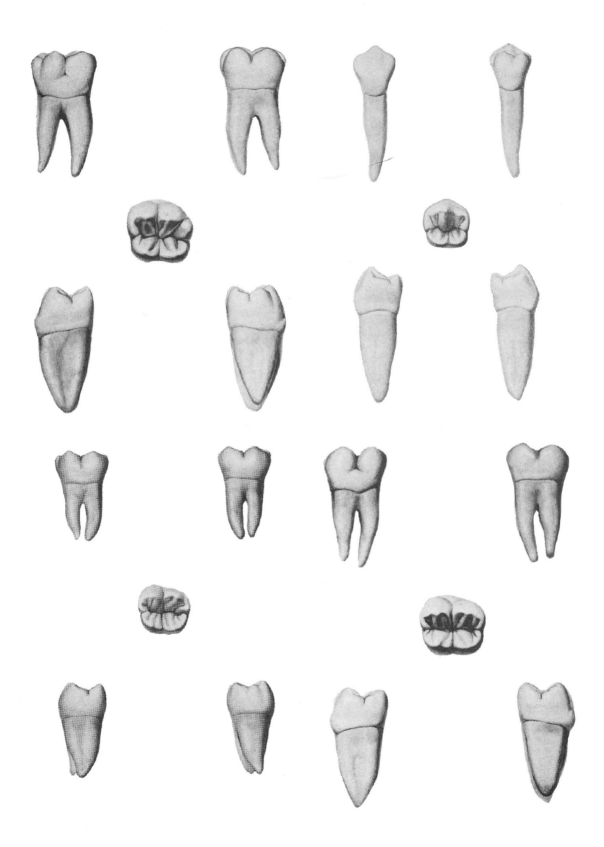

Deciduous Maxillary

Right Central Incisor

	RIGHT
Universal Code	E
International Code	51
Palmer notation	A⌋
Number of roots	1
Number of pulp horns	3
Number of developmental lobes	4

Location of proximal contact areas
MESIAL: Incisal third toward incisal angle
DISTAL: Incisal third toward middle third

Height of contour
FACIAL: Cervical third (more accentuated than permanent teeth)
LINGUAL: Cervical third (more accentuated than permanent teeth)

Identifying characteristics: Crown is wider mesiodistally than longer cervicoincisally. It is more rounded and more bulbous than the permanent central. It is also smaller and constricts more at the cementoenamel junction. Lingual features are more distinct. The facial and lingual height of contours are more convex than the permanent incisors. The pulp horn is larger in relation to the permanent teeth.

Deciduous Maxillary

Right Lateral Incisor

	RIGHT
Universal Code	D
International Code	52
Palmer notation	B⌋
Number of roots	1
Number of pulp horns	3
Number of developmental lobes	4

Location of proximal contact areas
MESIAL: Incisal third toward incisal angle
DISTAL: Incisal third toward middle third

Height of contour
FACIAL: Cervical third (more accentuated than permanent teeth)
LINGUAL: Cervical third (more accentuated than permanent teeth)

Identifying characteristics: The crown is longer cervicoincisally than wider mesiodistally. The crown is smaller and narrower mesiodistally. It is more slender than the primary centrals. The lateral is less squatier and resembles the permanent incisors more closely than the primary maxillary centrals. In proportion to the primary maxillary central the root is much longer. The lingual features are less distinctive, and the cervical constriction is greater.

Deciduous Maxillary

Right Canine

	RIGHT
Universal Code	C
International Code	53
Palmer notation	C⌋
Number of roots	1
Number of pulp horns	3
Number of cusp	1
Number of developmental lobes	4

Location of proximal contact areas
MESIAL: Incisal part of middle third
DISTAL: Incisal part of middle third

Height of contour
FACIAL: Cervical third (more accentuated than the incisors)
LINGUAL: Cervical third (more accentuated than the incisors)

Identifying characteristics: The cusp tip is in the center of the crown from the proximal view. The mesial slope is indented incisally and the distal slope is more rounded (obtuse). The crown is much wider labiolingually than the incisors. The root of the primary canine is proportionally longer than the root of the secondary maxillary canine. The root of the primary canine is long, slender, and tapering and is more than twice the crown length.

Deciduous Maxillary

Right First Molar

	RIGHT
Universal Code	B
International Code	54
Palmer notation	D⌋
Number of roots	3
Number of pulp horns	3
Number of cusps	3
Number of developmental lobes	4

Location of proximal contact areas
MESIAL: Junction of middle and occlusal third
DISTAL: Middle third

Height of contour
FACIAL: Extremely prominent mesiobuccal cervical bulge
LINGUAL: Cervical convexity

Identifying characteristics: Resembles a premolar and a molar. This is a three-cusped molar. The mesiolingual cusp is the largest and sharpest. The most characteristic thing about this tooth is the well-pronounced convexity on the mesiobuccal outline in the cervical third. Three roots—two buccal and one lingual roots.

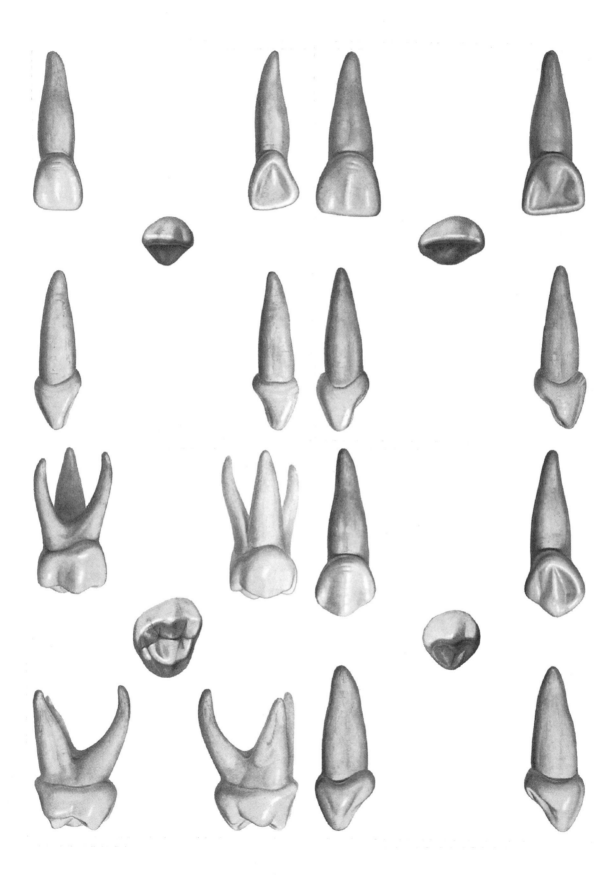

Deciduous Maxillary

Right Second Molar

	RIGHT
Universal Code	A
International Code	55
Palmer notation	E⌋
Number of roots	3
Number of pulp horns	5 or 4
Number of cusps	5 or 4
Number of developmental lobes	5

Location of proximal contact areas
MESIAL: Junction of occlusal and middle third
DISTAL: Middle third

Height of contour
FACIAL: Junction of occlusal and middle third
LINGUAL: Junction of occlusal and middle third

Identifying characteristics: Resembles permanent maxillary first molar, even has prominent oblique ridge. Three roots—two buccal and one lingual. Roots are long, slender, and flared widely apart. The faciolingual measurement of the crown is greater than the mesiodistal.

Deciduous Mandibular

Right Central Incisor

	RIGHT
Universal Code	P
International Code	81
Palmer notation	A⌋
Number of roots	1
Number of pulp horns	3
Number of developmental lobes	4

Location of proximal contact areas
MESIAL: Incisal angle
DISTAL: Incisal angle

Height of contour
FACIAL: Cervical of crown
LINGUAL: Cervical of crown

The prominences of the facial and lingual at the cervical are as pronounced as any other deciduous teeth and more so than the permanent mandibular incisors.

Identifying characteristics: The incisal ridge is straight from an incisal view. From a facial view the crown is flat. The distal and mesial are almost identical. The crown is wide in proportion to its length in comparison with its permanent successor. The root is long and tapered. It is almost twice as long as the crown.

Deciduous Mandibular

Right Lateral Incisor

	RIGHT
Universal Code	Q
International Code	82
Palmer notation	B⌋
Number of roots	1
Number of pulp horns	3
Number of developmental lobes	4

Location of proximal contact areas
MESIAL: Near incisal angle
DISTAL: Slightly lower than mesial

Height of contour
FACIAL: Cervical third
LINGUAL: Cervical third

As all anterior deciduous teeth, they exhibit pronounced cervical prominences.

Identifying characteristics: The incisal ridge runs slightly toward the distal. The lateral is longer and larger than the mandibular primary central incisor and the root is also longer. The lateral has a more rounded (obtuse) distoincisal angle.

Deciduous Mandibular

Right Canine

	RIGHT
Universal Code	R
International Code	83
Palmer notation	C⌋
Number of roots	1
Number of pulp horns	3
Number of cusps	1
Number of developmental lobes	4

Location of proximal contact areas
MESIAL: Junction of middle third and incisal third
DISTAL: Junction of middle third and incisal third

Height of contour
FACIAL: Distinct cervical bulge
LINGUAL: Distinct cervical bulge

Identifying characteristics: Similar to primary maxillary canine, except it is slightly shorter and much narrower labiolingually. The mandibular canine also has a shorter root.

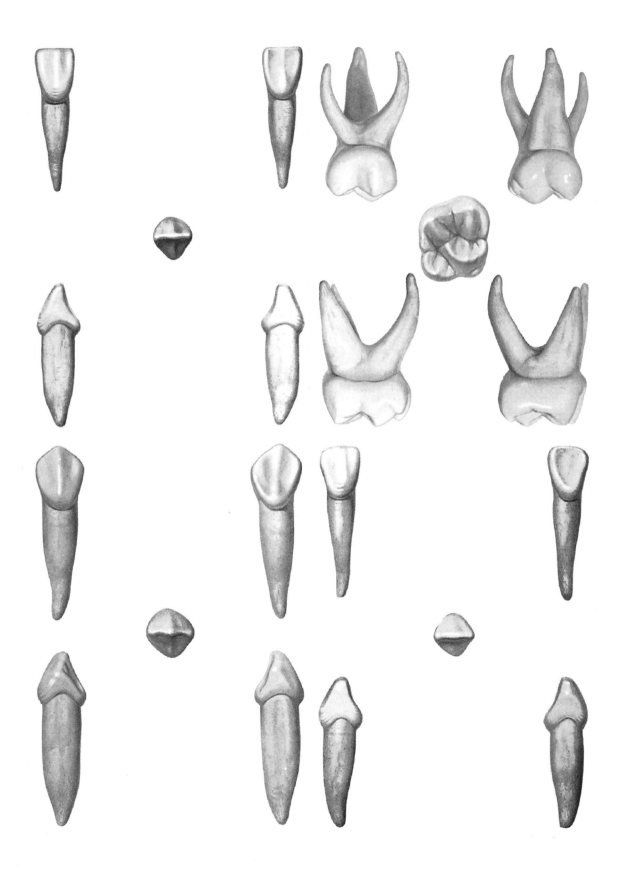

Deciduous Mandibular
Right First Molar

	RIGHT
Universal Code	S
International Code	84
Palmer notation	D⌋
Number of roots	2
Number of pulp horns	4
Number of cusps	4
Number of developmental lobes	4

Location of proximal contact areas
MESIAL: Middle third
DISTAL: Middle third

Height of contour
FACIAL: An extremely bulbous curvature on the mesiobuccal cervical third
LINGUAL: Middle third

Identifying characteristics: This tooth does not resemble any of the other teeth, deciduous or permanent. This tooth varies so much it appears strange and primitive. The mesial root is much larger than the distal, and the mesial half of the crown is much larger than the distal. The most characteristic thing about this tooth is the extreme convexity on the mesiobuccal at the cervical third. There are two roots, a mesial and a distal.

Deciduous Mandibular
Right Second Molar

	RIGHT
Universal Code	T
International Code	85
Palmer notation	E⌋
Number of roots	2
Number of pulp horns	5
Number of cusps	5
Number of developmental lobes	5

Location of proximal contact areas
MESIAL: Junction of occlusal and middle third
DISTAL: Middle third

Height of contour
FACIAL: Buccal cervical ridge
LINGUAL: Middle third

Identifying characteristics: Resembles the permanent mandibular first molar. There are three buccal cusps and two lingual cusps; two roots, a mesial and a distal. The roots are longer than the deciduous first molars and flared far apart.

Additional Notes

Additional Notes

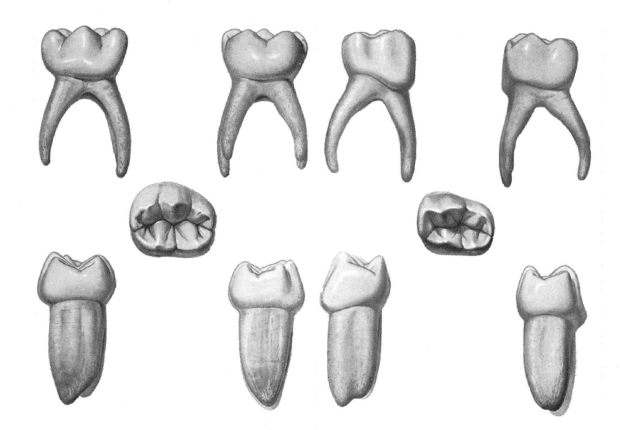

Permanent Maxillary

Left Central Incisor

	LEFT
Universal Code	9
International Code	21
Palmer notation	⌐1
Number of roots	1
Number of pulp horns	3
Number of developmental lobes	4

Location of proximal contact areas
MESIAL: Incisal third
DISTAL: Junction of incisal and middle thirds

Height of contour
FACIAL: Cervical third, 0.5 mm
LINGUAL: Cervical third, 0.5 mm

Identifying characteristics: These incisors are the largest and most prominent incisors. The distoincisal is more rounded than the mesioincisal angle. The lingual surface has a prominent cingulum, broad lingual fossa, and distinct marginal ridges. The pulp cavity is one large single chamber and root canal.

Permanent Maxillary

Left Lateral Incisor

	LEFT
Universal Code	10
International Code	22
Palmer notation	⌐2
Number of roots	1
Number of pulp horns	1 to 3
Number of developmental lobes	4

Location of proximal contact areas
MESIAL: Junction of incisal and middle thirds
DISTAL: Middle third

Height of contour
FACIAL: Cervical third, 0.5 mm
LINGUAL: Cervical third, 0.5 mm

Identifying characteristics: The lingual anatomical features are similar to those of the central incisors but are more highly developed and have more prominent marginal ridges and deeper lingual fossae. Lateral incisors are more likely to have a lingual pit. The cingulum may be smaller, almost absent. The labial surface resembles that of a central incisor except that the labial surface is more convex. The crown-root ratio is less than in a central incisor because the crown is usually smaller, whereas the root is almost as long. In all other ways the lateral incisors appear as smaller, more rounded versions of the central incisors.

Permanent Maxillary

Left Canine

	LEFT
Universal Code	11
International Code	23
Palmer notation	⌐3
Number of roots	1
Number of pulp horns	1
Number of cusps	1
Number of developmental lobes	4

Location of proximal contact areas
MESIAL: Junction of incisal and middle thirds
DISTAL: Middle third

Height of contour
FACIAL: Cervical third, 0.5 mm
LINGUAL: Cervical third, 0.5 mm

Identifying characteristics: The maxillary canines are the longest teeth in the mouth. They have a single cusp with mesial and distal ridges forming an incisal edge. A prominent facial ridge is off-center toward the mesial. Cingulum is prominent. The prominent mesiofacial lobe forms this facial ridge of the cusp. The centrofacial lobe forms the lingual ridge of the cusp. This lingual ridge divides the mesial and distal fossae. The distofacial ridge is longer and more rounded than the mesiofacial.

Permanent Maxillary

Left First Premolar

	LEFT
Universal Code	12
International Code	24
Palmer notation	⌐4
Number of roots	2
Number of pulp horns	2
Number of cusps	2
Number of developmental lobes	4

Location of proximal contact areas
MESIAL AND DISTAL: Just cervical to the junction of occlusal and middle thirds

Height of contour
FACIAL: Cervical third, 0.5 mm
LINGUAL: Middle third, 0.5 mm

Identifying characteristics: These premolars have bifurcated roots. A longitudinal groove is present on the root. The mesial surface shows a developmental fossa. The mesial marginal groove crosses the mesial marginal ridge and extends onto the mesial surface. The facial cusp is wider and longer than the lingual cusp. The mesial ridge of the facial cusp may have a slight concavity.

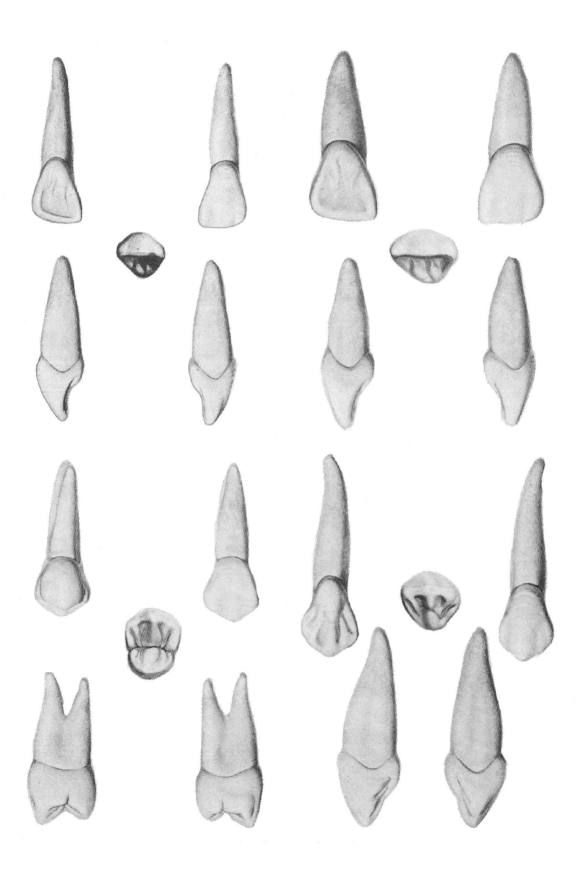

Permanent Maxillary

Left Second Premolar

	LEFT
Universal Code	13
International Code	25
Palmer notation	⌐5
Number of roots	1
Number of pulp horns	2
Number of cusps	2
Number of developmental lobes	4

Location of proximal contact areas
MESIAL AND DISTAL: Just cervical to the junction of occlusal and middle thirds

Height of contour
FACIAL: Cervical third, 0.5 mm
LINGUAL: Middle third, 0.5 mm

Identifying characteristics: These premolars usually have a single root. About 40% have two root canals. The buccal and lingual cusps are nearly equal in length. The buccal cusp is shorter than that of a first premolar. The entire crown, especially the occlusal outline, is less angular and more rounded. The occlusal surface has more supplemental grooves. The occlusal developmental grooves are shorter, shallower, and more irregular.

Permanent Maxillary

Left First Molar

	LEFT
Universal Code	14
International Code	26
Palmer notation	⌐6
Number of roots	3
Number of pulp horns	4
Number of cusps	4
	5 (including cusp of Carabelli)
Number of developmental lobes	5

Location of proximal contact areas
MESIAL: Middle third
DISTAL: Middle third

Height of contour
FACIAL: Cervical third, 0.5 mm
LINGUAL: Middle third, 0.5 mm

Identifying characteristics: A cusp of Carabelli may be present. The occlusal outline is square or rhomboidal rather than triangular. The distolingual cusp is well developed. There is a prominent oblique ridge and distal facial and lingual grooves. The crown is nearly as wide mesiodistally as buccolingually. The three roots are widely separated.

Permanent Maxillary

Left Second Molar

	LEFT
Universal Code	15
International Code	27
Palmer notation	⌐7
Number of roots	3
Number of pulp horns	4
Number of cusps	4
Number of developmental lobes	4

Location of proximal contact areas
MESIAL: Middle third
DISTAL: Middle third

Height of contour
FACIAL: Cervical third, 0.5 mm
LINGUAL: Middle third, 0.5 mm

Identifying characteristics: These teeth are similar to maxillary first molars except that the fifth cusp is usually absent and the distolingual cusp is less well developed. The oblique ridge is less prominent. The crown is shorter occlusocervically and narrower mesiodistally. It is just as wide buccolingually. The occlusal outline of the crown is rhomboidal to heart shaped. The three roots are less separated.

Permanent Maxillary

Left Third Molar

	LEFT
Universal Code	16
International Code	28
Palmer notation	⌐8
Number of roots	1 to 4
Number of pulp horns	1 to 4
Number of cusps	3 to 5
Number of developmental lobes	4

Location of proximal contact areas
MESIAL: Middle third
DISTAL: None

Height of contour
FACIAL: Cervical third, 0.5 mm
LINGUAL: Middle third, 0.5 mm

Identifying characteristics: These teeth vary more in form than any others. They usually do not have a distolingual cusp. The occlusal outline is heart shaped, with three cusps. The roots, usually three, have a tendency to be very close together or to fuse with an extreme distal inclination.

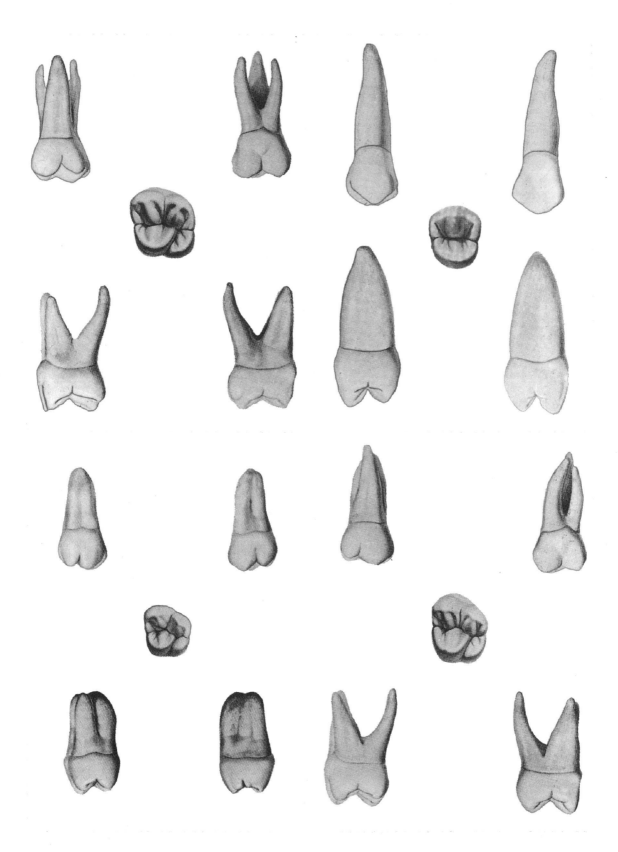

Permanent Mandibular

Left Central Incisor

	LEFT
Universal Code	24
International Code	31
Palmer notation	⌐1
Number of roots	1
Number of pulp horns	3
Number of developmental lobes	4

Location of proximal contact areas
MESIAL: Incisal third
DISTAL: Incisal third

Height of contour
FACIAL: Cervical third, less than 0.5 mm
LINGUAL: Cervical third, less than 0.5 mm

Identifying characteristics: The distoincisal and mesioincisal angles are nearly identical. The lingual surface is shallow, with no prominent features. The crown is wider faciolingually than mesiodistally. The root is oval shaped in cross section. The incisal edge shows wear on the facioincisal edge. From a proximal view the incisal edge appears to be tilted toward the lingual side.

Permanent Mandibular

Left Lateral Incisor

	LEFT
Universal Code	23
International Code	32
Palmer notation	⌐2
Number of roots	1
Number of pulp horns	3
Number of developmental lobes	4

Location of proximal contact areas
MESIAL: Incisal third
DISTAL: Incisal third

Height of contour
FACIAL: Cervical third, less than 0.5 mm
LINGUAL: Cervical third, less than 0.5 mm

Identifying characteristics: The crown is similar to that of the mandibular central incisors. The distal lobe is more highly developed than the mesial. The distal incisal ridge angles toward the lingual as if rotating on the root axis. The crown and the root are slightly larger than those of the central incisors.

Permanent Mandibular

Left Canine

	LEFT
Universal Code	22
International Code	33
Palmer notation	⌐3
Number of roots	1 or 2
Number of pulp horns	1
Number of cusps	1
Number of developmental lobes	4

Location of proximal contact areas
MESIAL: Incisal third
DISTAL: Just cervical to the junction of incisal and middle thirds

Height of contour
FACIAL: Cervical third, less than 0.5 mm
LINGUAL: Cervical third, less than 0.5 mm

Identifying characteristics: The crown is similar to the crown of the maxillary canines but narrower and smoother. It has less prominent lingual features. From a proximal view, the cusp tip is inclined to the lingual. From an incisal view, the distal end of the incisal edge is rotated to the lingual. They have the longest roots in the mandibular arch, with longitudinal grooves on the root.

Permanent Mandibular

Left First Premolar

	LEFT
Universal Code	21
International Code	34
Palmer notation	⌐4
Number of roots	1
Number of pulp horns	1 or 2
Number of cusps	2
Number of developmental lobes	4

Location of proximal contact areas
MESIAL AND DISTAL: Just cervical to junction of occlusal and middle thirds

Height of contour
FACIAL: Cervical third, 0.5 mm
LINGUAL: Middle third, 1 mm

Identifying characteristics: These premolars have two cusps, one large buccal and one small lingual. The buccal cusps are centered directly over the root. The lingual cusps are centered lingual to the root and are afunctional and nonoccluding. The occlusal surface slopes sharply lingual in a cervical direction. The mesiobuccal cusp ridge is shorter than the distobuccal cusp ridge. It has a mesiolingual developmental groove and one root.

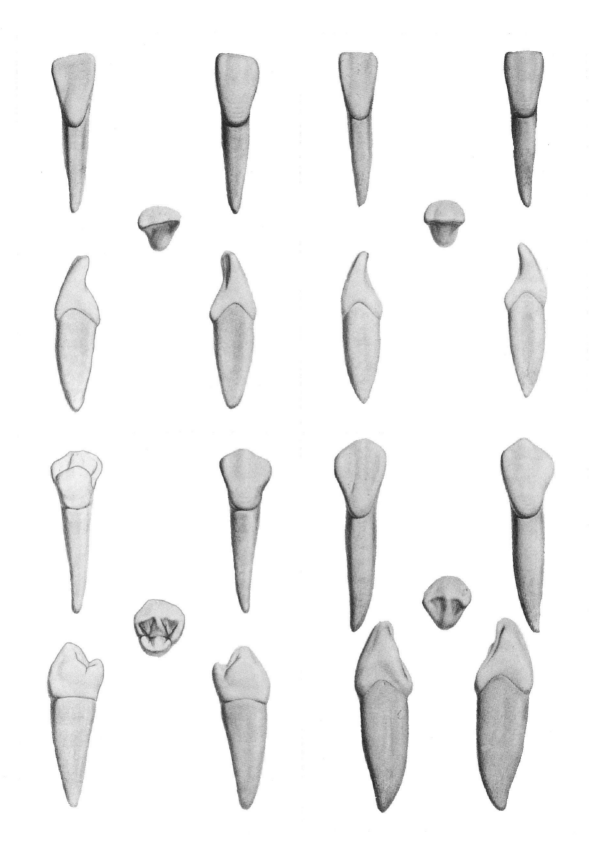

Permanent Mandibular

Left Second Premolar

	LEFT
Universal Code	20
International Code	35
Palmer notation	⌐5
Number of roots	1
Number of pulp horns	2 or 3
Number of cusps	2 or 3
Number of development lobes	4

Location of proximal contact areas
MESIAL AND DISTAL: Just cervical to junction of occlusal and middle thirds

Height of contour
FACIAL: Cervical third, 0.5 mm
LINGUAL: Middle third, 1 mm

Identifying characteristics: These premolars have two or three cusps. The buccal cusp is very large. If two lingual cusps are present, the mesiolingual is the larger. Although the lingual cusps are larger than on a first premolar, they are afunctional and do not occlude with the maxillary teeth. A second premolar has more secondary anatomical features and more variation than any other tooth except a third molar. The two-cusp form has a U- or H-groove pattern. A mesiolingual groove is rare and is poorly developed if present. The three-cusp form has a lingual developmental groove between the two lingual cusps. The single root is longer and larger than that of a first premolar.

Permanent Mandibular

Left First Molar

	LEFT
Universal Code	19
International Code	36
Palmer notation	⌐6
Number of roots	2
Number of pulp horns	5
Number of cusps	5
Number of developmental lobes	5

Location of proximal contact areas
MESIAL: Middle third
DISTAL: Middle third

Height of contour
FACIAL: Cervical third, 0.5 mm
LINGUAL: Middle third, 1 mm

Identifying characteristics: The five cusps make these the largest mandibular teeth. They are wider mesiodistally than buccolingually. The crown converges lingually and slightly distally. The three buccal cusps are separated by two buccal grooves. The two lingual cusps are separated by one lingual groove. These three grooves converge to form a Y pattern. There are two roots, a mesial and a distal, and three root canals (the mesial root has two root canals).

Permanent Mandibular

Left Second Molar

	LEFT
Universal Code	18
International Code	37
Palmer notation	⌐7
Number of roots	2
Number of pulp horns	4
Number of cusps	4
Number of developmental lobes	4

Location of proximal contact areas
MESIAL: Middle third
DISTAL: Middle third

Height of contour
FACIAL: Cervical third, 0.5 mm
LINGUAL: Middle third, 1 mm

Identifying characteristics: These molars have four cusps of nearly equal size. The crown is smaller in all dimensions and has less lingual convergence. There is only one buccal groove and one lingual groove, which join together on the occlusal surface as they bisect the central developmental groove. The groove pattern is therefore a cross (+). The two roots are closer together and incline slightly distally. There is one root canal in the distal root. The mesial root can have one or two root canals.

Permanent Mandibular

Left Third Molar

	LEFT
Universal Code	17
International Code	38
Palmer notation	⌐8
Number of roots	2 (fused into 1)
Number of pulp horns	4 or 5
Number of cusps	4 or 5
Number of developmental lobes	4 or 5

Location of proximal contact areas
MESIAL: Middle third
DISTAL: Middle third

Height of contour
FACIAL: Cervical third, 0.5 mm
LINGUAL: Middle third, 1 mm

Identifying characteristics: These are the most variable mandibular teeth in form. They usually resemble the mandibular second molars, with four cusps and a shallower, smaller central fossa, with more secondary and tertiary grooves. A five-cusp form is not unusual. The two roots (mesial and distal) and often fused and inclined toward the distal side.

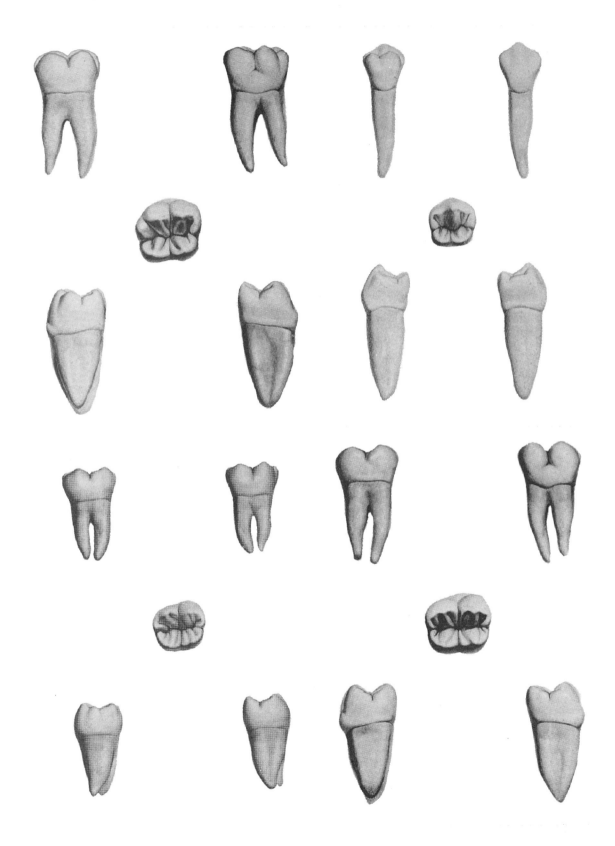

Deciduous Maxillary

Left Central Incisor

	LEFT
Universal Code	F
International Code	61
Palmer notation	⌊A
Number of roots	1
Number of pulp horns	3
Number of developmental lobes	4

Location of proximal contact areas
MESIAL: Incisal third toward incisal angle
DISTAL: Incisal third toward middle third

Height of contour
FACIAL: Cervical third (more accentuated than permanent teeth)
LINGUAL: Cervical third (more accentuated than permanent teeth)

Identifying characteristics: Crown is wider mesiodistally than longer cervicoincisally. It is more rounded and more bulbous than the permanent central. It is also smaller and constricts more at the cementoenamel junction. Lingual features are more distinct. The facial and lingual height of contours are more convex than the permanent incisors. The pulp horn is larger in relation to the permanent teeth.

Deciduous Maxillary

Left Lateral Incisor

	LEFT
Universal Code	G
International Code	62
Palmer notation	⌊B
Number of roots	1
Number of pulp horns	3
Number of developmental lobes	4

Location of proximal contact areas
MESIAL: Incisal third toward incisal angle
DISTAL: Incisal third toward middle third

Height of contour
FACIAL: Cervical third (more accentuated than permanent teeth)
LINGUAL: Cervical third (more accentuated than permanent teeth)

Identifying characteristics: The crown is longer cervicoincisally than wider mesiodistally. The crown is smaller and narrower mesiodistally. It is more slender than the primary centrals. The lateral is less squatier and resembles the permanent incisors more closely than the primary maxillary centrals. In proportion to the primary maxillary central the root is much longer. The lingual features are less distinctive, and the cervical constriction is greater.

Deciduous Maxillary

Left Canine

	LEFT
Universal Code	H
International Code	63
Palmer notation	⌊C
Number of roots	1
Number of pulp horns	3
Number of cusp	1
Number of developmental lobes	4

Location of proximal contact areas
MESIAL: Incisal part of middle third
DISTAL: Incisal part of middle third

Height of contour
FACIAL: Cervical third (more accentuated than the incisors)
LINGUAL: Cervical third (more accentuated than the incisors)

Identifying characteristics: The cusp tip is in the center of the crown from the proximal view. The mesial slope is indented incisally and the distal slope is more rounded (obtuse). The crown is much wider labiolingually than the incisors. The root of the primary canine is proportionally longer than the root of the secondary maxillary canine. The root of the primary canine is long, slender, and tapering and is more than twice the crown length.

Deciduous Maxillary

Left First Molar

	LEFT
Universal Code	I
International Code	64
Palmer notation	⌊D
Number of roots	3
Number of pulp horns	3
Number of cusps	3
Number of developmental lobes	4

Location of proximal contact areas
MESIAL: Junction of middle and occlusal third
DISTAL: Middle third

Height of contour
FACIAL: Extremely prominent mesiobuccal cervical bulge
LINGUAL: Cervical convexity

Identifying characteristics: Resembles a premolar and a molar. This is a three-cusped molar. The mesiolingual cusp is the largest and sharpest. The most characteristic thing about this tooth is the well-pronounced convexity on the mesiobuccal outline in the cervical third. Three roots—two buccal and one lingual roots.

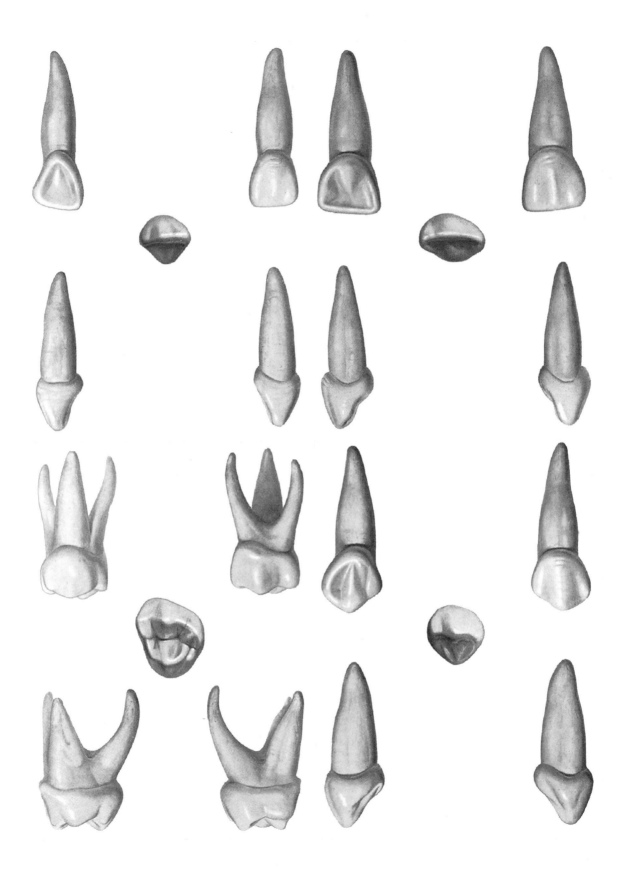

Deciduous Maxillary

Left Second Molar

		LEFT
Universal Code		J
International Code		65
Palmer notation		⌐E
Number of roots	3	
Number of pulp horns	5 or 4	
Number of cusps	5 or 4	
Number of developmental lobes	5	

Location of proximal contact areas
MESIAL: Junction of occlusal and middle third
DISTAL: Middle third

Height of contour
FACIAL: Junction of occlusal and middle third
LINGUAL: Junction of occlusal and middle third

Identifying characteristics: Resembles permanent maxillary first molar, even has prominent oblique ridge. Three roots—two buccal and one lingual. Roots are long, slender, and flared widely apart. The faciolingual measurement of the crown is greater than the mesiodistal.

Deciduous Mandibular

Left Central Incisor

		LEFT
Universal Code		O
International Code		71
Palmer notation		⌐A
Number of roots	1	
Number of pulp horns	3	
Number of developmental lobes	4	

Location of proximal contact areas
MESIAL: Incisal angle
DISTAL: Incisal angle

Height of contour
FACIAL: Cervical of crown
LINGUAL: Cervical of crown

The prominences of the facial and lingual at the cervical are as pronounced as any other deciduous teeth and more so than the permanent mandibular incisors.

Identifying characteristics: The incisal ridge is straight from an incisal view. From a facial view the crown is flat. The distal and mesial are almost identical. The crown is wide in proportion to its length in comparison with its permanent successor. The root is long and tapered. It is almost twice as long as the crown.

Deciduous Mandibular

Left Lateral Incisor

		LEFT
Universal Code		N
International Code		72
Palmer notation		⌐B
Number of roots	1	
Number of pulp horns	3	
Number of developmental lobes	4	

Location of proximal contact areas
MESIAL: Near incisal angle
DISTAL: Slightly lower than mesial

Height of contour
FACIAL: Cervical third
LINGUAL: Cervical third

As all anterior deciduous teeth, they exhibit pronounced cervical prominences.

Identifying characteristics: The incisal ridge runs slightly toward the distal. The lateral is longer and larger than the mandibular primary central incisor and the root is also longer. The lateral has a more rounded (obtuse) distoincisal angle.

Deciduous Mandibular

Left Canine

		LEFT
Universal Code		M
International Code		73
Palmer notation		⌐C
Number of roots	1	
Number of pulp horns	3	
Number of cusps	1	
Number of developmental lobes	4	

Location of proximal contact areas
MESIAL: Junction of middle third and incisal third
DISTAL: Junction of middle third and incisal third

Height of contour
FACIAL: Distinct cervical bulge
LINGUAL: Distinct cervical bulge

Identifying characteristics: Similar to primary maxillary canine, except it is slightly shorter and much narrower labiolingually. The mandibular canine also has a shorter root.

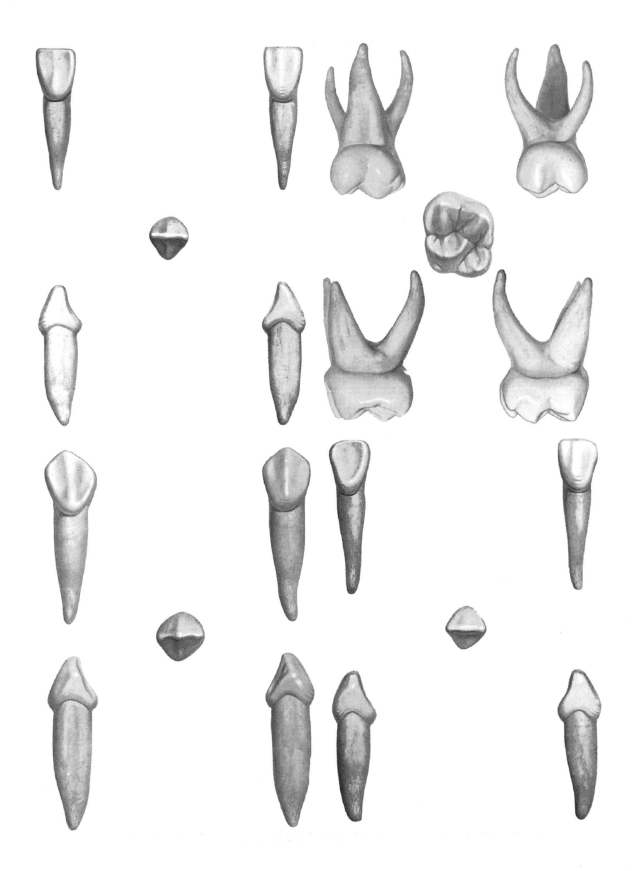

Deciduous Mandibular

Left First Molar

		LEFT
Universal Code		L
International Code		74
Palmer notation		⌐D
Number of roots	2	
Number of pulp horns	4	
Number of cusps	4	
Number of developmental lobes	4	

Location of proximal contact areas
MESIAL: Middle third
DISTAL: Middle third

Height of contour
FACIAL: An extremely bulbous curvature on the mesiobuccal cervical third
LINGUAL: Middle third

Identifying characteristics: This tooth does not resemble any of the other teeth, deciduous or permanent. This tooth varies so much it appears strange and primitive. The mesial root is much larger than the distal, and the mesial half of the crown is much larger than the distal. The most characteristic thing about this tooth is the extreme convexity on the mesiobuccal at the cervical third. There are two roots, a mesial and a distal.

Additional Notes

Deciduous Mandibular

Left Second Molar

		LEFT
Universal Code		K
International Code		75
Palmer notation		⌐E
Number of roots	2	
Number of pulp horns	5	
Number of cusps	5	
Number of developmental lobes	5	

Location of proximal contact areas
MESIAL: Junction of occlusal and middle third
DISTAL: Middle third

Height of contour
FACIAL: Buccal cervical ridge
LINGUAL: Middle third

Identifying characteristics: Resembles the permanent mandibular first molar. There are three buccal cusps and two lingual cusps; two roots, a mesial and a distal. The roots are longer than the deciduous first molars and flared far apart.

Additional Notes

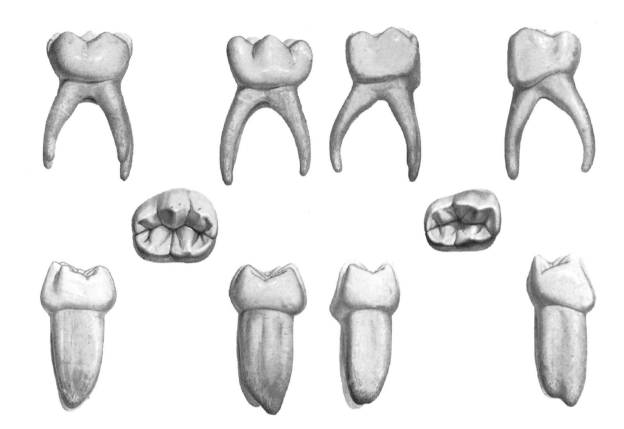